# WORKING TOGETHER
# WHEN FACING CHRONIC PAIN

A book designed for patients and written
by their health professionals

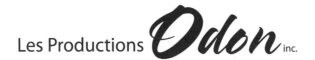

Les Productions *Odon* inc.

Laval, Quebec, Canada
www.productionsodon.com
lesproductionsodon@videotron.ca

**Bibliothèque et Archives nationales du Québec and Library and Archives Canada cataloguing in publication**

Main entry under title:

Working together when facing chronic pain: a book designed for patients and written by their health professionals

Translation of: Faire équipe face à la douleur chronique.
Includes bibliographical references.

ISBN  978-0-9810478-1-2

1. Chronic pain.  2. Chronic pain - Treatment.  3. Patient participation.  I. O'Donnell-Jasmin, Louise, 1957-   . II. Boulanger, Aline, 1959- .

RB127.F3413 2010        616'.0472        C2009-904865-5

Published by Les Productions Odon inc.
Cover design: Katrine Jasmin, Créations DG
Cover art copyright: iStock photo
Linguistic revision: Shannon Bannock, Qu'Appelle Communications, quappelle@accesscomm.ca (foreward, chapters 2, 8, 12, 19, 20, 26, 27, 31, 41, 42, 45, 46, 48, 51, 52, testimonials by Gary Blank, Terry Bremner, Morris K., Louise O'Donnell-Jasmin, Helen Small, Janice Sumpton, Helen Tupper)
Translation: Sheryl Curtis, Les Communications WriteTouch (chapters 1, 3, 4, 5, 6, 7, 9, 10, 13, 14, 15, 16, 17, 18, 22, 24, 25, 28, 29, 30, 32, 33, 34, 35, 36, 37, 38, 39, 44, 47, 49, 50, 53, 54, 55, 56, 57, 58; testimonials by Line Brochu, André Léonelli, Lucie Moisan, Louise O'Donnell-Jasmin, Mélanie R.); Louise O'Donnell-Jasmin (chapter 23)
Production: Katrine Jasmin, Créations DG; Louis-Philippe Verrier, karibü
Proofreading: Les Productions Odon inc

© Les Productions Odon inc.

**To buy or distribute this book:**
Visit our web site at: www.productionsodon.com
Email: lesproductionsodon@videotron.ca

Legal Deposit- 3rd Trimester 2010
Bibliothèque nationale du Québec
Bibliothèque nationale du Canada

Printed in Canada

Please note that the editor has opted for Canadian spelling in this book.

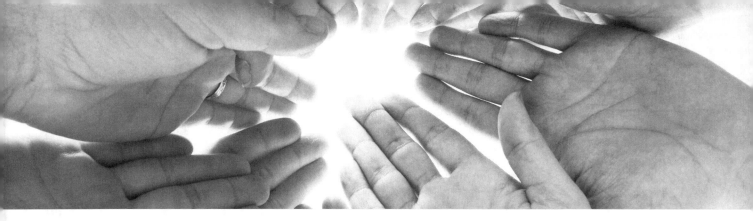

# TABLE OF CONTENTS

## SECTION 5 — PROFESSIONAL ASSOCIATIONS FOR PAIN SPECIALISTS — 365

# FOREWARD

**Lorimer Moseley** NHMRC Senior Research Fellow
Prince of Wales Medical Research Institute & the Université of New South Wales, Sydney, Australia

## WELCOME TO "**THAT** BOOK".

With very few exceptions, everybody hurts. And everybody knows that when they are hurting, they are keen to not hurt anymore. In fact, everybody knows that the more they are hurting, the keener they are to not hurt any longer. This fundamental capacity of pain to make us behave in a certain way is exactly what makes pain our most sophisticated, effective and complex protective device. Pain is, in this sense, our greatest ally. However, pain can persist after the tissues of the body have healed. Pain can become chronic. It can "have a mind of its own." It can take over your life and lead you into a downward spiral of disability, depression and agony. How does this happen? How can pain exist in the absence of injury? How, for that matter, can injury occur without pain? These questions are of fundamental importance to the 20% of Westerners who are currently disabled to some extent by a chronic pain problem.

The past four decades of research into pain have taught us much about these questions. Perhaps the most fundamental insight we have gained is the fact that activity in the nerves that carry danger messages from the tissues to the brain — the so-called "nociceptors" — is not pain, nor is it sufficient for pain or, in fact, even necessary for pain. In fact, pain depends on the brain's evaluation of everything that might be relevant for evaluating danger to body tissue. This means that pain is a measure of the brain's perception of threat to tissues, not the actual threat. Importantly, this process of perceiving threat occurs unconsciously. The pain is the conscious bit — the end product or output of the brain. It is no longer defensible to consider chronic pain as a sign of chronic injury. Instead, we must embrace the true complexity of the human body and consider all of the possible contributions to the brain's evaluation of danger to body tissue. This is not an easy task. To presume pain is simply a message from the body is deliciously simplistic, but it is, alas, fundamentally wrong.

We know that *understanding* the true complexity of pain reduces its impact. Think of how remarkable this really is — if you understand that pain is the result of a complex biological process in the brain, your pain then reduces and affects your life less. There are also very well established methods to help you manage your own pain yourself and the pain of others. That is where books such as this one are critical.

By gathering experts from across pain-relevant fields — more than 50 of them no less — and convincing them to write something for this book, editor Louise O'Donnell-Jasmin has been able to put together a remarkable resource. This resource will be helpful for people in pain and their carers, loved ones and clinicians. I imagine that there is no wider coverage of the management of pain anywhere else — I certainly haven't seen one. I suggest that this book be given pride of place in your library because it stands to be "**that book**" to which one turns when feeling stuck in the journey of returning from pain-related disability to normal life. I heartily commend Louise for what is a most impressive achievement — to get contributions from so many people who are already squeezing the last milliseconds out of their busy clinical or scientific schedules to "add their bit" is a testament to the critical importance of this book and the wonderful tenacity of its editor.

# ACKNOWLEDGEMENTS

First and foremost, I would like to thank Dr. Aline Boulanger[1] who believed in this book from the very start, drew up the first table of contents and referred me to many authors. Throughout the difficulties I experienced as a result of my painful condition, she always encouraged me. I would also like to thank Dr. Jacques Charest[2] for his assistance with my search for authors and for his support.

I would like to honour all those who were involved in my care team, from near or far, those who believed in my pain and those who loved me, even when I was difficult to love.

I owe my return to "normal" life to the Alan Edwards Centre for Research on Pain team at the Montreal General Hospital, and particularly to Dr. Yoram Shir, Louise Lamb[3], to Gaston Brosseau, psychologist[4], and to their faith in me, as well to an extraordinary physiotherapist, Diane Racette[5], who helped me build up my courage and my desire to find myself once again. They have all, of course, helped heal my soul, hurt by long years of pain, sadness and isolation...

I would like to honour the impressive number of authors who devoted their valuable time to writing this book, using plain language to enable each and every one of us to understand all aspects of chronic pain, and sharing their knowledge, their expertise, their commitment and their passion for clinical work. I would also like to honour all those who gave their testimonials in this work. I admire their courage.

This work was made possible by a large number of people. I would like to highlight the excellent work done by Line Brochu[6] who provided support for the French-language version, for her many re-readings and her focus on the "person suffering from chronic pain"; she is a remarkable woman with surprising and invincible determination. I thank my daughters from the bottom of my heart: Katrine Jasmin[7] for the visual design for the cover and the content of the work and for her contribution to the layout, as well as Annie Jasmin Pht and Martine Jasmin who helped re-read the books.

I would never have made my way to this page without the tireless support of my husband, without his faith in me, without his constant support. Every moment of my life is a testimonial to his love for me.

I would also like to thank the many people at Pfizer Canada who supported this project and whose greatly appreciated, non-profit financial contribution provided for the English translation and the first printing of the French and English versions of this book.

**Louise O'Donnell-Jasmin**

1.  Dr. Aline Boulanger MD, FRCPC, MPH, anesthesiologist, Manager – Pain Clinic, Centre hospitalier de l'Université de Montréal (CHUM), Manager – Pain Clinic, Hôpital du Sacré-Cœur, Montreal, Quebec, Canada
2.  Dr. Jacques Charest PhD, psychologist, Rouyn-Noranda, Quebec, Canada
3.  Dr. Yoram Shir MD, Professor - Anaesthesia, Director - Alan Edwards Pain Management Unit, McGill University Health Centre (MUHC), Montreal , Quebec, Canada
    Louise Lamb, RN, Alan Edwards Centre for Research on Pain, McGill University Health Centre (MUHC – Montreal General Hospital)
4.  Gaston Brosseau, psychologist, Saint-Lambert, Quebec, Canada
5.  Diane Racette Pht, FCAMPT, MOPPQ, MACP, Physioactif, Laval, Quebec, Canada
6.  When these words were written, Line Brochu was the secretary on the Board of Directors of the Association québécoise de douleur chronique, Quebec, Canada
7.  Katrine Jasmin, BA, Créations DG, Montreal, Quebec, Canada http://www.creationsdg.com/

# UNDERSTANDING CHRONIC PAIN

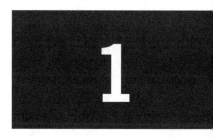

# INTRODUCTION

Louise O'Donnell-Jasmin, BEd, Laval, Quebec, Canada

## «LEARN FROM YESTERDAY, LIVE FOR TODAY, NEVER GIVE UP.»

**Louis Garneau,**
Louis Garneau, President, Louis Garneau Sports Inc., Quebec Canada

## 1. BECOMING AN EXPERT PATIENT

Starting from the principle that the patient is at the heart of the care team, how can we equip the patient so that he/she can become an active member of the team, an expert patient? In social, psychological, physiological, spiritual and emotional terms, the patient can work towards regaining control of his/her condition and life. Patients can choose to self-manage their pain and work with their care team, their loved ones and other patients to become expert patients.

*Working together when facing chronic pain* **is a work that is intended to support the efforts of all those suffering from chronic pain and their loved ones to self-manage chronic pain. Education about this pain is one of the solutions to which this book opens doors. This work is also intended for all health professionals who want to learn more about the issues and aspects specific to chronic pain, and benefit from the experience of their colleagues and the testimonials of patients.**

In addition to the overall goal of informing and educating, this book is also intended to help these people become familiar with:

- The steps in the self-management of pain: regaining physical and psychological control as an individual and as a member of a family, a couple, a community and a workplace;
- The role of the patient and the health care professionals involved in his/her current environment in the treatment of chronic pain;
- The advantages, benefits, positive impacts and responsibilities of the patient playing an active role within the care team.

## 2. PRESENTATION OF THE WORK

*Working together when facing chronic pain* is above all intended to give people suffering from any form of chronic pain food for thought and information about a large number of tools and treatments, as well as about the physiological, psychological and social aspects of pain. The loved ones of an individual suffering from chronic pain may also benefit significantly from this book since it will enable them to encourage him/her to persevere in the search for short-, medium- and long-term solutions, in order to return to a more active, even a normal life.

Each chapter in the first three sections will be of great interest to people of all ages who want to understand chronic pain. **Section 1, Understanding chronic pain**, contains chapters on the biomedical aspects of various painful conditions. **Section 2, Psychological and**

**social aspects of chronic pain**, covers the numerous aspects that affect the lives of those suffering from chronic pain and their loved ones, themes which are all too often neglected in the treatment of pain. **Section 3, Treatment options and pain management**, covers a wide range of treatments available, both medical, complementary and alternative.

The chapters contained in **Sections 1** to **3** were written by health care professionals who have been treating chronic pain for several years. When reading them, you will benefit from the experience, the knowledge, the skill and the wisdom of these authors. These authors were joined, at the end of **Section 3**, by two amazing women, both suffering from chronic pain, who founded pain associations in North America: Helen Small (PARC: Promoting Awareness of RSD in Canada) and Penney

Cowan (American Chronic Pain Association - ACPA); their informed testimonials and the solutions they propose will serve as sources of inspiration and motivation for each and every reader.

Regardless of your painful condition or that of your loved one, each chapter contains pertinent, validated information. Regardless of the importance of the physical activity, the support provided by the care team, or the participatory role played by the individual suffering from pain, each chapter provides information that might change your life, your attitude to pain, your awareness of your role, and the importance to be placed on each aspect of pain.

**Sections 4** and **5** present the various pain associations for people suffering from pain or for health professionals. Each association has its own specific mission and objectives; above all, they have volunteers and members who live with chronic pain on a daily basis and work relentlessly to help their loved ones, their colleagues and their patients. Becoming a member of such associations is essential in terms of representativity to decision-makers. Chronic pain is a scourge of epidemiological proportions that must be known and acknowledged: pain is often more than a symptom, rather a disease in itself.

**Section 6** presents excellent models of adaptation or rehabilitation programmes available in Quebec. Similar models are offered in a great many countries. Millions of people suffer from chronic pain and such programmes provide unparalleled treatment and care teams who can help them and teach them to become expert patients and good managers of their own health. The Quebec examples are inspiring and encouraging for all care teams throughout the world. If you do not have access to such programmes, you will enjoy major tips for forming your own care team.

Testimonials and case studies are provided in a large number of chapters and at the ends of several of them. Chronic pain is first and foremost a condition that affects the lives of those suffering from the pain, their loved ones, their friends and their work colleagues. Often, people suffering from chronic pain do not express what they experience out of fear of bothering their loved ones. Yet, it is through communicating together that we will all learn to understand and accept what each individual affected by pain feels. Also, these testimonials serve, to a certain extent as the "oasis of dialogue" for this book.

## 3. AGAINST ALL ODDS...

For a long time I was merely a shadow of myself, heavily medicated, living in fear of the next pain crisis, locked in a world I no longer recognized, and where I no longer recognized myself. Pain was my jailer... The jailer didn't expect a thing when I decided to regain control of my life.

When this project was designed, I was barely taking the first few steps away from a difficult withdrawal from a long series of drugs prescribed to relieve my chronic pain. I was being treated by a new pain specialist who had understood, from our very first appointment, the dangerous level of intoxication that was mine. He saved me. After noting my pitiful physical and psychological condition, the first thing he did for me was prepare a cup of tea... Six months later, walking once again, in a significantly better condition, eyes filled with emotion and boundless gratitude, I made this promise to him: I would help other people who were suffering from chronic pain as I had been.

This book is a fulfilment of that promise. I had been very active in the chronic pain world in Quebec, then in Canada, as a volunteer within chronic pain associations (*Association québécoise de la douleur chronique*, Canadian Pain Coalition), spokesperson and lecturer. I spoke with and wrote to all of the suffering people who reached out for help.

This book is the best way I found to answer all the appeals for help that were not made or received, that remained unspoken, to answer all the people suffering from chronic pain who no longer have the strength, the faith or the motivation to ask for help. This book is the answer that I would so liked to have found when I called out to for help, as I started my journey through the desert of pain.

When this project was designed, I was suffering from debilitating neuropathic pain following a dental procedure. As you hold this book in your hands, the pain is now behind me. It no longer takes up all the space, **against all odds**. Many factors have contributed to the improvement in my condition and helped me start living again. You can't win such an intense battle on your own... One thing I know for certain is that in many chapters in this book, I found solutions that the members of my care team and, often my loved ones, had suggested to me, as well as those which I found on my own through trial and error.

With this book, I invite you to discover the formidable strength of the human spirit in the fight against chronic pain. The marvellous collaboration of all these people has served to make this book the most important work published on chronic pain to date, conceived by an individual suffering from chronic pain for an audience made up of people suffering from chronic pain and their loved ones, and written by health professionals working in a variety of sectors, as well as by people living with pain on a daily basis.

Whoever you are, if you hold this book in your hands, you are part of the solution to chronic pain by acknowledging its existence, by wanting to understand, by wanting to help, by wanting to retake control of your life. I thank you for being there.

**This book was written for you!**

# PAIN
# ASSESSMENT

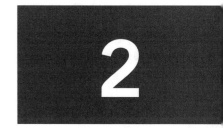

**Mark Ware** MBBS, MRCP (UK), MSc
Assistant professor, Departments of Anesthesia and Family Medicine, McGill University,
Director of clinical research, Alan Edwards Pain Management Unit, McGill University Health Centre (MUHC),
Montreal, Quebec, Canada

## ABSTRACT

The assessment of the patient with chronic pain or a pain syndrome is fundamental to beginning the process of planning pain management options. The physician's approach to a patient with chronic pain follows the same lines as the approach to a patient with any other medical issue. There are two main components to the clinical assessment: the medical history of the patient and the physical examination. In this chapter, we will describe the typical components of these two components to better understand what a patient can expect when seeing a physician for a chronic pain disorder, and to be prepared for the kinds of questions and evaluations that will typically be encountered.

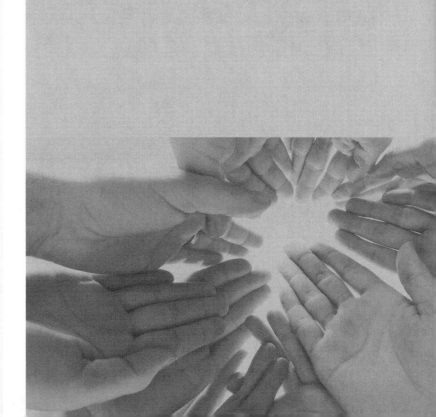

# 1. INTRODUCTION

The purpose of the pain assessment is to determine the diagnosis (or a list of possible other diagnoses, called the differential diagnosis), to evaluate the impact of the pain syndrome on the patient's quality of life, identify his or her goals and expectations, and start to prepare a treatment plan. Chronic pain treatment often includes a range of approaches including pharmacology, physical therapy, psychotherapy and other behavioural approaches, as **sections 2** and **3** of this book so clearly illustrate. However, it always begins with a good preliminary assessment of the patient's condition. Here are the different components of this evaluation.

# 2. THE MEDICAL HISTORY

The medical history is, in a sense, the narrative "story" of the patient's pain in terms of the past and present. When taken by a physician, it is an organized way of capturing as much information as possible regarding the patient and their pain in an efficient and productive manner. Taking the medical history is not only a way to understand what kind of pain the patient has, but also what kind of patient has the pain. This means that the medical history includes questions about the patient's background, family, environment, work, diet, activities, mood and sleep. This section outlines the kind of questions that a patient may expect to be asked. We have prepared this section as though you, the reader, were a patient arriving for the first appointment with your pain doctor.

### TALKING ABOUT PAIN

The first part of a pain evaluation, starting with your medical history, will usually begin with a few questions about your age, work status and immediate situation. This information gives the physician a quick idea about the person with whom they are speaking. Once communication has been established, the physician will usually ask an open-ended question allowing you to talk about your pain such as "Tell me about your pain and why you have come to see me today." This provides you with the opportunity to tell your story. It is worth planning how you will tell your story prepared in advance so that you may use the time efficiently to try to explain to the physician as much about the pain as possible. It is important to have time to bring up your concerns and questions, but also to realize that the physician may be short on time and unable to spend as much time as they would like in hearing all the details about your pain syndrome and how it has come to evolve.

The following guidelines suggest how you may be able to frame your story in a way that conveys the maximum amount of information to the physician in as efficient a way as possible. If the story is not presented in this way, the physician may interrupt or ask specific questions similar to those listed in **Table 1** in order to obtain the information required.

Some specific questions that will be asked concerning the pain are shown in **Table 1**.

TABLE 1: Pain-related questions and examples

| PAIN-RELATED QUESTIONS AND EXAMPLES | |
| --- | --- |
| QUESTIONS | EXAMPLES |
| Onset of pain | Date, gradual or sudden |
| Cause of pain | Surgery accident, infection, etc. |
| Quality of pain | Continuous, fluctuating, episodic, quality of pain: nagging, learning, pressing, heavy |
| Aggravating and alleviating factors | Things that make the pain better or worse |
| Severity of pain | Some physicians ask their patients to rate their pain on a scale from 0 to 10 where zero is no pain at all and 10 is the worst pain ever experienced |
| Location of pain | The pain may be located in one area, and may spread, or radiate to another area |
| Progression of pain | Is the pain returning, getting worse, or staying the same? |

## OTHER PAIN-RELATED ASPECTS OF THE MEDICAL HISTORY

In addition to asking questions about your pain, the physician will then proceed to ask you questions about other aspects of your life, which may include questions about your home environment, for example:

- Do you live alone or with your family?
- Do you have a supportive family that understands your pain and can help you in every day tasks?
- Do you have an environment in which your pain is not well understood and you feel alone and isolated?

Questions may follow concerning your mood, for example:

- Do you feel depressed, angry, anxious or afraid?

It is normal for patients with chronic pain to experience disturbances in mood, and understanding these are important in making an appropriate treatment strategy.

Pain may have a significant impact on sleep, and the physician may ask about your sleep hygiene, for example:

- How much sleep do you typically get every night? Is it of good quality?
- Do you have difficulty falling asleep, or wake up during the night, because of pain or other reasons?
- Do you feel rested in the morning, or drowsy during the day?

The physician will usually perform a review of body systems by asking you a series of focused questions about things that may be related to your pain or its treatment. This may include, among other things, questions about bladder function (e.g. incontinence), bowel function (e.g. constipation), sexual function (e.g. ability to have erections or orgasms), other neurological issues (e.g. headaches or sensory abnormalities) and rheumatologic issues (e.g. joint pain).

## 3. THE PHYSICAL EXAMINATION

After the medical history has been taken, a formal physical examination usually follows. This section tells you what you might expect from this type of examination and the kind of information useful to the physician.

### THE CLINICAL EXAMINATION

The clinical examination begins the first time the physician sees the patient in the waiting room or entering their office. The physician will initially be looking for signs of disability, including the use of aids such as a walking cane, wheelchair or other device. The physician will observe how easily or with what level of difficulty the patient moves and the level of discomfort that registers on the patient's face and in their body movements. It is important that the overall attitude and behaviour of the patient be consistent with the reported levels of pain and disability that are reported, since pain is a subjective experience, and there are no tests that can accurately measure the level of pain. The physician needs to rely on the patient's report of their pain. Therefore, all additional clues as to the location, severity and impact of the pain are extremely important for the physician to observe.

This physical examination usually involves the patient exposing the affected area of the body, sometimes undressing completely and putting on a hospital gown to make the region affected more accessible. The first thing to ask the patient usually is to show the area where the pain is located more specifically. The physician should always ask whether the area affected (or any other areas) is sensitive to touch in order to avoid inconveniencing an extremely sensitive patient during a simple physical examination in which light touch may be painful.

Once the physician has examined the area where the pain is located, a brief general physical examination usually follows, reviewing the head, eyes, lungs and heart. These form part of the routine physical examination and are a quick look at the overall physical health of the patient. The physician will also be looking for more general aspects of health including obesity or general loss of muscle mass.

A physician will often begin a more detailed physical examination by looking at the hands of the patient, as they are a window into the level of activity the patient undertakes. One needs only to think of the difference between the hands of a farm worker and those of an office assistant to appreciate how the appearance of the hands may reflect the kind of activity that the patient undertakes on a daily basis. The hands, wrists and arms may be examined for the presence of swelling, scars and loss of muscle, and to check hair and nail growth, blood flow, sensation and movement. As we are used to touching others with our hands, they a good place to begin the physical examination. This is a less invasive introduction to the examination and useful for beginning the process of a more detailed and sometimes more intimate examination.

The remainder of the examination may be broken down into several general areas.

### THE NEUROLOGICAL EXAMINATION

The neurological examination may consist of an examination of the cranial nerves, which provide our sensory functions such as sight, smell, taste and hearing as well as more central functions of the eyes and the head and neck region.

### THE EXAMINATION OF THE PERIPHERAL NERVOUS SYSTEM

The examination of the peripheral nervous system is one of the most important parts of the pain assessment because it examines the function of the nerves that run from the skin into the spinal cord. The central nervous system is also examined to determine the function of the spinal cord, which relays information up to the brain.

## THE SENSORY EXAMINATION

**The sensory examination** involves a detailed look at the patient's ability to detect sensations such as light touch, pressure, different temperatures, vibration and pain. **Table 2** shows the sensations that are tested and the type of equipment that may be used. Not every physician will perform a detailed examination of this kind, but it is very useful to map out the area of the body affected by pain and any associated sensory abnormalities that are associated with this region. It is usually important for the physician to examine a normal area of the body in order to generate conclusions about the abnormal area where the pain is felt.

Table 2: Examples of equipment used to test sensation

| EXAMPLES OF EQUIPMENT USED TO TEST SENSATION | |
| --- | --- |
| SENSATION TESTED | EQUIPMENT USED |
| Light touch | Cotton wool, soft brush, fingertips |
| Vibration | Tuning fork |
| Pressure | Fingertips, pressure algometer |
| Temperature | Cold object (e.g. side of tuning fork, test tubes with warm/cold water) |
| Pinprick | Toothpick, pin, specialized pin device |

The **sensory examination** detects changes in the way the nerves relay information from the skin toward the brain.

### THE MOTOR EXAMINATION

The **motor examination** will examine the function of the nerves as they relay information from the brain and spinal cord out toward the muscles and joints. Therefore, an examination of muscle movement both active (the movements that the patient can undertake by themselves) and passive (the movements that the physician is able to put the limbs through while the patient is fully relaxed) is very important. This will usually be concluded by a test of reflexes in which the physician taps a part of the tendon of the muscle and observes the response of the muscle, usually by a twitch or contraction. The sensory examination will also usually include an examination of the joints, including the small joints of the hands and the larger joints of the body such as the shoulders, knees and hips.

### THE EXAMINATION OF THE SPINE

The **examination of the spine** from the neck down to the lumbar region (including the buttocks) is a very complex examination and includes both neurological and musculoskeletal components. A typical spine examination includes inspection of the spine for alignment at rest as well as during typical movements such as bending forward, backward and to either side. The physician may feel the muscles along the spine for tenderness and ask the patient to undergo movements while specifically feeling for areas of tenderness. There are several specific examination techniques used under specific conditions to examine for stability of particular joints. These will not be discussed in detail here, but may involve things like straight leg raising, twisting the spine while the patient is lying flat, placing a hand underneath the small of the back while the patient moves the legs, and other such tests.

The remainder of the clinical examination is usually focused on specific aspects of the patient's physical presentation relating to the particular pain syndrome that has been discussed and explored in the medical history.

# 4. INVESTIGATIONS

A primary care physician who is seeing a patient with chronic pain for the first time will usually request a series of investigations that may not be requested by a specialized pain physician treating the same patient. Often, they have already been extensively evaluated prior to the pain clinic visit, sometimes by several physicians. This may explain why not every physician will request additional examinations and investigations.

The purpose of requesting an examination or investigation is to further explore the possible cause of the pain and at times to iden-tify the possible location of treatment approaches. **Table 3** lists the sort of investigations that might be considered by a physician when evaluating a patient with chronic pain. An important question that physicians ask themselves when ordering a test is "How will the result of this test change the way in which I manage this patient's case?" It may be important for patients to ask themselves this question as well. Some tests take a long time to be conducted and should not limit the availability of treatments during this time.

TABLE 3: Examples of investigations used to evaluate chronic pain patients

| EXAMPLES OF INVESTIGATIONS USED TO EVALUATE CHRONIC PAIN PATIENTS | |
| --- | --- |
| TEST | PURPOSE |
| Standard X-rays | Evaluation of structure, bones and joints |
| Myelogram | Form of X-ray where a dye is injected into the spinal cord to see if there is any obstruction of spinal fluid |
| Computed tomography (CT) scan* | More detailed view of tissues such as intervertebral discs, ligaments and tendons, brain and spinal cord |
| Magnetic Resonance Imaging (MRI) | Very detailed view of tissues including brain and spinal cord, discs, joints etc. |
| Nerve conduction studies (NCS) | Tests of how quickly large peripheral nerves are working |
| Electromyography (EMG) | Tests how well nerves carry messages to muscles |
| Quantitative sensory testing (QST) | Detailed tests of how well very small peripheral nerves work at detecting sensations |

\* This test may involve injection of a special dye to see more specific structures.

An additional part of the patient evaluation includes the completion of specialized questionnaires that may be used by the physician to probe further into other aspects of the patient's well being, including psychological status and approaches to pain and functionality. These standardized questionnaires may form part of an initial evaluation package sent to the patient, may be given to the patient in the waiting room for completion or may be requested by the physician in response to specific pain syndromes. Some of these questionnaires are useful as screening tools in determining the kind of pain with which the patient is presenting. Please ask your physician about these questionnaires if you have any issues or problems in completing them, because they may be very important not only for the initial medical evaluation but also in terms of monitoring the response to the treatment plan that is implemented.

# 5. CONCLUDING THE ASSESSMENT

At the end of the process of the medical history, physical examination and ordering of tests and specific investigations, the patient and physician will discuss a treatment plan that will include a range of therapies as further discussed in this book. It is hoped that this chapter will have prepared you for what to expect when seeing a physician for a chronic pain problem, and empower you to go into the evaluation knowing the kind of questions that may be asked and the tests that may be performed, as well as the kind of questions that you may wish to ask the physician when you see them.

# TURNING OVER OLD STONES

Terry Bremner, Stillwater Lake, Nova Scotia, Canada
National Support Group Coordinator, Chronic Pain Association of Canada (CPAC),
President, Action Atlantic, Pain support group leader, Chronic Pain Association of Canada (CPAC)

(See other testimonial, page 374.)

I want to ignore my pain because I don't feel it belongs in my body, or in my life. At all times, I ignore it. Pain is hard to talk about because I have spent so much time pushing it away. There is anger; it isn't easy turning over old stones.

I could have been a better dad, a better adviser, if I hadn't been sick. When the pain level is high, I become very quiet. I'm unable to do this and unable to do that. What's the use of discussing it? I ignore it. I can't wrestle on the floor with my kids or go out in the yard and play rough or play hockey. I see the other fathers or mothers out there doing it. I'd love to be able to do it, too.

When the pain is severe, I remind myself that, somewhere along the way, I've been in greater pain and I made it through. I lie down and try to forget about it.

I don't have a lot of patience. If my children argue or don't do what they are told, I can lose my temper easily. I have to be aware that not everything has to go the way I want it to. I've learned to bite my tongue, take a couple of deep breaths and get through it. It's a real struggle.

I'm still able to go out and do some things. They are not things I liked doing before, or that I wanted to do before, but at least I'm still able to participate in society.

A long time ago, I learned to "make a plan and work a plan." Now if a plan goes into my agenda, I stick to it. I follow through.

I sometimes don't think easily, turning over old stones. I think back and walk the long pain path with all its hurdles. I reflect on the good stops that I have made along the way. To know where I was and where I am today, I know I have come a long way. There are things that I can no longer do, but there are also things that I can do now, and never thought to be able to do in the future. **Never say never!**

## Support group meeting

My psychologist suggested I attend a support group meeting for people in pain. I was so closed down when I first went to a meeting. I'd put in my time, and leave at the coffee break. "*I don't want to be here. Look at this group! Maybe there is a different crowd to hang out with. But why leave when most of the people here know what are our hurdles and struggles?*"

How can I benefit from support group meetings if I don't put any effort into them? I made a commitment to help organize their group's yearly pain conference. While I was organizing the conference, I realized that I was able to use a lot of my effort to encourage others to help. Once a number of group members got involved, the small tasks spread out amongst everyone. It was great sharing ideas and stories with others who struggle with the same issues on a daily basis. What was gained by being a support group member could never have been so by any other means: to have others to offer resources for treatments, experience, struggles and encouragement to live life with better coping strategies. When I was able to make decisions and work with others, my confidence came back. People tell me I eventually opened up like a flower.

I found that no matter the size or age, we can all feel pain and its symptoms. The more strategies we give each other when we need a break from the daily, constant pain, the better our lives with our families will be. Working together with others whose limitations may be greater than mine encourages me to be thankful for all that I have, and be able to share my strengths with all those who suffer, too. This is my very own feel-good medication.

I've accepted that my condition is like luggage. We are not talking the greatest luggage either. There are scrapes, tears in spots, a wobbly wheel and a well-used handle that has grips just my size.

## Learn from the past and build on it

When I look back, I don't know where I would be if it wasn't for my wife. She is a major part of helping me hang in there. So are my children. There are so many weeks and months that I just can't account for.

Now, I'm a dad — for a living. That's what I do. It's a full-time job for me. I'm a stay-at-home dad.

One of my boys said to me one day "Why don't you go out to work like the other dads do? You're home all the time." That hurt. How can I explain the situation to a 10-year-old?

I started to volunteer by helping other pain patients, and now it's my career. My children look at my support group work now as my profession. I'd like to be out selling insurance like I used to, but life has changed. Now, people in the support group look up to me. That's been the healing process. **I have taken what I have learned in my past, and built on it.**

# NEUROPATHIC
## PAIN

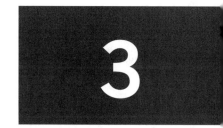

**3**

**René Truchon** MD, FRCPC, anaesthesiologist, Manager, Centre de traitement de la douleur,
Centre hospitalier universitaire de Québec (CHUQ) - Centre hospitalier universitaire de Laval (CHUL),
Quebec, Quebec, Canada

## ABSTRACT

Of the three principal types of pain, neuropathic pain is the one for which enormous progress has been made recently with respect to understanding the mechanisms in question and developing new pharmacological agents for treating this pain.

We stipulate that this pain becomes self-maintaining as a result of a disorder of the nervous system involved in the conduction of pain, causing the pain to be perpetuated by the nerves, the spine and the centres of the brain.

During the evaluation, the physician will look for symptoms and signs that are specific to this type of pain (burning sensation when resting, allodynia, etc.). Moreover, we have specific questionnaires that can serve to guide the diagnosis in the case of more complex pain.

Finally, a specific algorithm for the treatment of neuropathic pain can be used to guide the therapy in keeping with various categories of medication, which are classified according to levels in keeping with studies into their specific effectiveness.

\* The rights to reproduce the pain algorithm on page 17 of this chapter were obtained from the publisher. This algorithm was first published in the "*Cahiers MedActuel dpc*", in the May 7 and May 14 2008 editions of *L'actualité médicale* (Quebec, Canada).

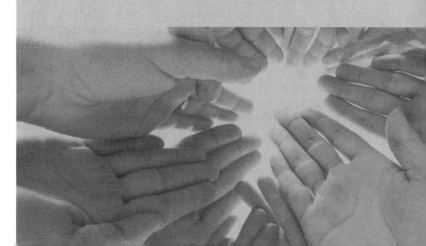

# 1. GENERAL

Chronic pain affects approximately one-fifth of the adult Canadian population, ranking it ahead of diabetes and asthma. Recent Canadian surveys have revealed that 5.7% of the paediatric population (those under the age of 18) also suffer chronic pain. Moreover, neuropathic pain affects 2% to 3% of the Canadian population which represents almost one million Canadians.

# 2. NEUROPATHIC PAIN

Physiopathology can be used broadly to classify pain into three categories: nociceptive pain, idiopathic pain (psychological) and neuropathic pain. The mechanisms involved in pain are complex and involve a multitude of receptors and bodily chemical substances. When the pain process becomes chronic, this often involves intrication (overlapping, mingling) of various types of pain. Pure neuropathic pain, as a result, is clinically rarer. In this chapter, we will discuss only the neuropathic component of chronic pain.

# 3. DEFINITION OF NEUROPATHIC PAIN

Neuropathic pain is caused by a problem with the functioning of the nervous system at all levels (brain, spinal cord and peripheral nerves). Etymologically, the term "neuropathic" has two Greek roots: neuro (from the Greek word "neuron") meaning nerve, and pathic (from the Greek word "pathos") meaning suffering.

It is important to understand that neuropathic pain that has become chronic is independent of the initial damage that had caused the pain, and that the neuropathic pain is **self-maintained** by the patient's nervous system.

Therefore, it is understood that the evolution of this painful syndrome is the result of a disruption in the functioning of the nervous system without necessarily being the consequence of a direct pathology, or an anatomical pathology of the patient's nervous system.

# 4. PATHOPHYSIOLOGY

Unlike nociceptive pain which is experienced when you burn yourself or cut yourself, and which is caused by the trauma of a tissue, neuropathic pain is the consequence of the malfunctioning of the nervous system at various sites throughout the human body. It is maintained by the nervous system itself, whereas the initial painful trauma or injury is healed. The notable changes in the nervous system (brain, spinal cord, nerves) involved in the occurrence of this chronic pain include:
- Spontaneous discharges of painful impulses from the peripheral nerves of the spinal cord, which causes the patient to experience electrical micro-discharges;
- The increase, at the nerves and the spinal cord, of the transmission and amplification of normal nerve impulses (for example, the sense of touch), since these signals are perceived as a burning sensation of the skin rather than a brushing of the skin (allodynia);
- The appearance of spontaneous impulses from the pain coordination center (thalamus, located in the brain may present phenomena similar to those observed in the nerves and spinal cord); these spontaneous discharges of nerve impulses can be painful on their own or through the exaggeration of the pain messages from other regions of the body. Moreover, it is known that, in the case of the spinal cord, the nervous mechanisms that, in a healthy subject, block part of the conduction of pain to the brain, have become very weak or inexistent in the patient

affected, which facilitates the conduction and transmission of pain to the brain and the pain coordination center. Numerous "protective" hormones secreted in the organism, such as endorphin, serotonin, noradrenaline and various neurotransmitters, become much less effective for diminishing or blocking neuropathic pain.

Thus, in order to relieve neuropathic pain, the physician will use different classes of medications that will act on the various sites of the nervous system:
- **On the cutaneous** (or mucous) level by blocking the spontaneous triggering of pain and the conduction of painful impulses: this is how local anaesthetics act, such as when a lidocaine cream is applied directly on the skin of the affected region;
- **On a medullar** (spinal cord) and cerebral level, by blocking the transmission of pain with anti-epileptic medications (pregabalin, neurontin) or anti-depressants (amitriptyline, venlafaxine, duloxetine) that modify the action of the serotonin and the noradrenaline that our body produces on both a peripheral and a central level with medications in which the analgesic action is the principal effect: opiates (morphine, hydromorphone, methadone), tramadol, acetaminophen. We will discuss the algorithm of neuropathic pain treatment later, on **page 17.**

## 5. SYMPTOMS

Chronic pain with a neuropathic component is accompanied by physical signs and numerous symptoms. The most frequent symptoms are indicated in **Table 1**. The specific characteristic of neuropathic pain is the perception of a burning sensation of the skin, or continuous and spontaneous stinging that is often associated with the sensation of tingling or electrical discharges in a specific region of the body.

Other symptoms are **allodynia**, a painful perception of a stimulus that is not normally painful such as the sensation of pain when one's skin is merely touched, **hyperalgesia** (pain that is stronger than normal, such as a when a pinch of the skin is perceived as skin being torn off) or **hyperpathy** (strong pain sensation that persists long after the source of the pain has stopped). The physician will systematically look for pain located in a more distant region that is still relative to the sick zone (for example, pain in the right hand after the right shoulder has been injured).

If there has been a direct injury to the nerve tissue (nerve, spinal column or brain), the healing process attempts to heal the injury in the weeks or months after it occurred. Thus, a nerve that has been cut or crushed tries to regenerate by forming a bud or a ball of small nerve fibres, which is called a neuroma. Neuromas can automatically trigger electrical activity in the damaged nerve, which the patient experiences as an electrical discharge or a muscular contraction (muscle cramp). Moreover, neuromas cause exaggerated responses to touch. The patient describes a great deal of sensitivity to touch and spontaneous tingling sensations in the region where the neuroma is located. Occasionally, the sympathetic component of the nerve may be affected by the nerve damage, resulting in neuropathic pain. This is called complex regional pain syndrome (CRPS).

The components are found in combination with signs and symptoms that are said to be autonomic (autonomic nervous system) and which are characterized by a strong sensation of heat or cold in a painful or injured part of the body. A complete limb may be affected and tend to swell with oedema, present anomalies affecting perspiration (tendency to sweat, dampness, a palm of a hand that is always damp, for example) or hair growth that may increase or can totally disappear (for example, a hand becomes hairier). Very frequently, there are also sudden variations in colour in the painful region (for example, the affected hand becomes deep red or totally white and livid).

Clinically, when the sympathetic component is significant, a limb or an injured region is observed to be cold or hot, hairless, very hairy, swollen, damp, along with joint stiffness. These symptoms and signs occur in addition to the sensations of neuropathic pain.

Without specific treatment, such as a sympathetic block combined with intensive physiotherapy, when a limb is affected by complex regional pain syndrome, it may become totally disabled, with severe atrophy of the muscles, complete ankylosis of the joints, swelling of the fingers, and continual pain. The affected hand may also become a " chicken's ergot" if it is not treated intensively. Pain treatment centres will be responsible for the urgent evaluation and treatment of this condition. (See **chapter 4.**)

TABLE 1: Characteristics of neuropathic pain

| CHARACTERISTICS OF NEUROPATHIC PAIN |
| --- |
| Sensation of a cutaneous burn |
| Spontaneous and continuous stinging |
| Spontaneous or provoked tingling or electrical discharges |
| Allodynia: Pain caused by a stimulus that is not painful |
| Hyperalgesia: Intense pain perceived when the triggering stimulus was only slightly painful |
| Hyperpathy: Long-term, intense pain after the provocation of repetitive pain |

## 6. CAUSE OF NEUROPATHIC PAIN

Depending on the central nervous system site affected, namely the central nervous system in the brain and the spinal column or the peripheral nervous system (the nerves of the limbs or the trunk of the body), neuropathic pain can be identified as central or peripheral. The causes of central neuropathic pain most frequently encountered include: vascular damage to the brain or the spine (following a cerebrovascular accident (CVA) or stroke, trauma to the spine, multiple sclerosis, Parkinson's disease, tumours and infections. The causes of these types of neuropathic pain are listed in **Table 2** (next page).

TABLE 2: Common types of neuropathic pain

| COMMON TYPES OF NEUROPATHIC PAIN | |
| --- | --- |
| CENTRAL | PERIPHERAL |
| Hemicorpus pain following a CVA | Neuralgia of the trigeminal nerve |
| AIDS-related myelopathy | Complex regional pain syndrome |
| Trauma to the spinal cord | Nerve compression in a limb |
| Multiple sclerosis | Nerve damage caused by HIV |
| Phantom limb | Diabetic neuropathies |
| Parkinson's disease | Post-shingles neuralgia |
| Spinal cord injury | Post-thoracotomy and post-thoroscopy neuralgia |
| | Radicular disk herniation |
| | Neuropathy caused by chemotherapy for cancer |
| | Nerve amputation (as part of a limb amputation) |
| | Post-mastectomy pain |

# 7. MULTI-DIMENSIONAL EVALUATION

During the first evaluation of a patient experiencing neuropathic pain, the physician makes an in-depth examination of the events that caused the problem. In addition to an overall and specialized evaluation of the problem, the physician can use specific multi-dimensional tools for evaluating neuropathic pain when searching for the clinical signs of neuropathic pain.

The most commonly used questionnaires for evaluating chronic pain include: EVA, McGill, BECK, MPI, BPI, MMPI-2, SIP, etc. These questionnaires evaluate the functional, psychological and social damage to the individual suffering from chronic pain.

## NEUROPATHIC EVALUATION

**We have specialized questionnaires that enable us to evaluate and quantify the impacts of neuropathic pain.** The principal dedicated questionnaires include: the Neuropathic Pain Scale, the DN4 and Pain Detect. These questionnaires have been validated scientifically and they serve, moreover, to track the progress of the treatments used, both physical and psychosocial.

# 8. TREATMENTS OF NEUROPATHIC PAIN

Three major references can be consulted concerning the treatments of neuropathic pain:
· Canadian consensus statement and guidelines, Canadian Pain Society.
· Journal of Pain Research Management 12:13-21, 2007;
· Quebec consensus statement and guidelines, Société québécoise de la douleur (SQD).

**The treatment of neuropathic pain has three objectives:**
1. To minimize the pain or make it tolerable;
2. Improve the functioning of the body and the individual;
3. To improve quality of life.

These objectives must be attained with a minimum of side effects caused by the treatments and medications used. All therapeutic means **should fit into** the patient's treatment schedules and plans, while relying on his/her active involvement in the therapy.

## NON-PHARMACOLOGICAL TREATMENTS

The non-pharmacological treatments are included in this category:
- Physical treatment, such as physiotherapy, occupational therapy and kinesiology;
- Rehabilitation and psycho-social treatments, such as psychiatric and psychological evaluations and treatments, using individual and group therapies;
- The evaluation of the patient's social and professional circumstances along with the current and future impacts in terms of the evaluation of the neuropathic pain syndrome.

## PHARMACOLOGICAL TREATMENT

The pharmacological treatment of neuropathic pain is handled in keeping with a treatment algorithm developed by experts who met in 2007 in Canada and, following that, in Quebec. These algorithms were based on the evaluation of treatment protocols, randomized and controlled studies and a systematic review of the therapeutic effectiveness of various pharmacological agents.

Treatment starts with the use of a single agent (in Class 1). Following this, a second pharmacological agent may be brought in to be combined with the first or to replace it. When certain symptoms are present, specific treatments, such as the use of a topical anaesthetic (lidocaine) or a ketamine-based cream may be proposed, as is done in the case of post-shingles pain.

Once a diagnosis of neuropathic pain has been established, the first objective is to relieve the pain in keeping with the Quebec treatment algorithm (**Table III, page 18**).

Depending on the circumstances, anti-depressive medication that provides pain relief may be prescribed, for example. The most commonly used anti-depressants include: nortriptyline, amitriptyline, desipramine and venlafaxine. It is also possible to add a medication that prevents painful impulses from being conducted to the spinal cord. Other medications can also be used at the start of the treatment, such as anti-epileptic medications that block pain through their action on an alpha 2 delta nerve receptor in the spinal cord. When the neuropathic pain is located in a precise region of the periphery of the body (a limb, for example), the physician can prescribe medications that are applied directly to the skin (topical) that will block the transmission of the pain by the nerves to the skin and the limb affected. For patients with severe, debilitating pain, a medication that inhibits pain directly (an analgesic), namely a derivative of morphine or tramadol, can be administered concomitantly (in association).

The purpose of adjusting the medication is to relieve the pain with an EVA evaluation of less than 4/10 or pain that is tolerable for the patient.

Thus, pharmacological treatment that effectively inhibits pain will frequently involve a combination of several medications from the four classes of the treatment algorithm. These medications will be adjusted to obtain the fewest side effects possible with effective pain relief.

## 9. SPECIALIZED TREATMENTS AT A PAIN TREATMENT CENTER

In Quebec, pain treatment centres are located in the large urban centres; they are often referred to as pain centres or anti-pain centres or clinics. The advantage of these centres lies in the multidisciplinarity and interdisciplinarity of the treatment team, which helps the patient who is suffering from neuropathic pain. In addition to the multidisciplinary team, these excellent centres also use super-specialized invasive technologies. These services are offered to all the patients in the centre who are treated adequately by the Class I and Class 2 medications in the treatment algorithm while receiving physical and psychological therapies for their condition.

The super-specialized treatments offered in the pain treatment centres are developed in greater detail in **Section 3**. With respect to neuropathic pain syndrome, the most specific treatments will include blocks of the sympathetic nervous system, nerve blocks, chemical or thermal neurolysis, cortisone injections into the skin or near a nerve root, and the destruction of small sensitive fibres or neuromas by means of radiofrequency techniques. The centre may also propose neuromo-dulation, a term that includes the invasive treatments that are intended to alter the perception of pain through the stimulation or inhibition of the nerve paths that conduct pain. Schematically, neuromodulation includes neurostimulation with epidural electrodes and the inhibition, by means of radiofrequency, of the ganglion of the dorsal root of the diseased sensitive root.

In a specialized manner, the principal pain treatment centres can also use specific programmes with combined interventions on the part of several practitioners (for example, physical medicine, rehabilitation, psychology, psychiatry, anaesthesiology, etc.) so as to improve the physical, psychological and social dimensions of the quality of life of the patient suffering from severe neuropathic pain.

The various therapies needed to treat neuropathic pain are presented in **Table 3** on the following page.

TABLE 3: Treatment options for chronic neuropathic pain

## TREATMENT OPTIONS FOR CHRONIC NEUROPATHIC PAIN

### PHYSICAL

Normal physical activities

Swimming, physical activity

Passive and active occupational therapy

Stretching

Training

Weight loss

Massage and acupuncture

Physical rehabilitation

Physical re-education

| PSYCHOLOGICAL | INVASIVE INTERVENTIONS |
|---|---|
| Psychotherapy | Steroids |
| Stress management and reduction | Injections |
| Behaviour therapy | Sympathetic block |
| Cognitive therapies | Nervous and plexic blocks |
| Mirror imaging | Therapeutic epidurals |
| Reprogramming | Specific rhizotomy by means of radiofrequency or cryotherapy |
| Specific individual and group therapies | Implementation of central and peripheral spinal stimulation |
| Family therapy | Spinal injection of opiates in a closed circuit |
| | Nerve decompression surgery |

### PHARMACOLOGICAL

Canadian and Quebec pharmacological treatment for neuropathic pain

## GOALS OF THE BEST THERAPY

**The goals of the best therapies for patients suffering from neuropathic pain are as follows:**
- The greatest evidence of effectiveness;
- The most readily available;
- The least costly;
- The one with the fewest secondary or harmful effects;
- The least painful therapy.

# 10. ALGORITHM OF THE TREATMENT OF NEUROPATHIC PAIN*

* The right to reproduce the pain algorithm provided on page 17 of this chapter was granted by its publisher. This algorithm was first published in *Cahiers MedActuel dpc*, in the May 7 and May 14 2008 editions of *L'actualité médicale*.

**Figure 1** presents the neuropathic pain treatment algorithm as developed by consensus by the special Quebec forum.

First-, second-, third- and fourth-line medications are proposed in it. Once the diagnosis has been determined, administering a first-line agent, to be used alone, is recommended. When the pain is intense, opiates or short-acting tramadol can be combined with the first-line medications in order to ensure better pain relief for the patient while waiting for the titration of the first-line agents to be complete. If, however, the pain is less intense, opiates or tramadol can be used as second-line medications either alone or in combination with other medications.

Generally, a small dosage of the first-line agent is prescribed, which can then be increased gradually depending on the patient's reaction and the undesirable effects. If the first agent selected is not effective in therapeutic dosages or is poorly tolerated by the patient, it can be replaced by another first-line agent from another class.

If these medications provide only partial relief, they can be combined with a second agent proposed as a first-line medication that operates on a different site. If adding a new agent does not provide relief, the patient can be taken off that medication and the treatment can be continued with second-, third- and fourth-line agents. **Figure 1** and **Tables III**, **IV** and **V** present the suggested treatment algorithm, the indications and the contraindications, the costs, warnings, undesirable effects, the dosage, and a list of medications that are not covered by the Quebec health insurance plan (RAMQ).

(Editor's note: **Tables IV** and **V** of the neuropathic pain treatment algorithm were presented in the second part of this article, namely in the May 14, 2008 issue.)

FIGURE 1: Algorithm of the treatment of neuropathic pain

### 1st line

**Gabapentinoids**
Pregabalin
Gabapentin

**Tricyclic or tetracyclic antidepressants**$^\alpha$
Tertiary amines:
Amitriptyline
Clomipramine
Imipramine
Secondary amines:
Nortriptyline
Desipramine
Tetracyclic amines:
Maprolitine

**Local anaesthetic**
Topical lidocaine 10%$^\beta$

### 2nd line

**SNRI**$^\chi$
Venlafaxine
Duloxetine

**Cannabinoids**
Dronabinol
Nabilone
THC/CBD orally

### 3rd line

**SSRI**
Citalopram
Paroxetine

**Other antidepressant**
Bupropion

**Other anticonvulsants**
Topiramate
Carbamazepine
Levetiracetam
Lamotrigine

### 4th line

Methadone
Ketamine
Mexiletine
Baclofen
Clonidine
Clonazepam

**Not advised:**
Meperidine
Phenytoin

**Opiates or tramadol**

Use short-action medications as first-line treatment in combination with other first-line agents in the presence of the following situations:
- Rapid relief during the titration of first-line agents (up to the effective dosage);
- Episodes of serious exacerbation of pain;
- Acute neuropathic pain;
- Neuropathic pain

Use as second-line treatments either on their own or in combination with other agents (when long-term use is considered, encourage the administration of long-acting agents).

**LEGEND**: Figure 1 and Table III
CNS: central nervous system
COPD: chronic obstructive pulmonary disease
ECG: electrocardiogram
MAOI: monoamine oxidase inhibitors
QT interval: measure of the time between the start of the Q wave and the end of the T wave in the heart's electrical cycle

SNRI: serotonin–norepinephrine reuptake inhibitors
SSRI: selective serotonin reuptake inhibitors
THC/CBD: tetrahydrocannabinol/cannabinol

FIGURE 1: Algorithm of the treatment of neuropathic pain (cont'd)

α   Indicated for use in first-line treatment in the case of patients under the age of 60. For patients who are 60 years old or older, avoid the tertiary amines in the tricyclic class as a result of their anticholinergic effects. Nortriptyline and desipramine can be prescribed with caution, in low dosages.

β   Indicated in the case of peripheral pain and allodynia. Do not apply on a surface exceeding 300 cm$^2$ (namely the equivalent of half a sheet) as a result of the dangers related to systemic absorption. Lidocaine can be used along with all classes of medication. Nevertheless, the associations most commonly cited in the medical documentation are lidocaine and anticonvulsants, and lidocaine and antidepressants.

χ   There is no advantage to prescribing SNRIs if the tricyclic or tetracyclic anti-depressants administered in the optimal dosages are ineffective. Nevertheless, SNRIs are indicated for first-line treatment in the presence of a major depression, intolerance to tricyclic and tetracyclic anti-depressants or a contraindication of these latter medications.

## Particular cases

• **Kidney failure:** avoid or decrease the dosage of medications that are principally eliminated through the kidneys (ex.: gabapentinoids, SNRIs, tramadol, levetiracetam, topiramate) or for which the active metabolites are excreted by the kidneys (ex.: morphine).
• **Obesity/diabetes:** topiramate can be an interesting agent as a result of the potential weight loss.

TABLE III: Medication for neuropathic pain | First line

| MEDICATIONS | OFFICIAL INDICATIONS | WARNINGS |
|---|---|---|
| **FIRST LINE** | | |
| **Gabapentinoids**<br>Pregabalin | ➜ Neuropathic pain associated with peripheral diabetic neuropathy or post herpes zoster neuralgia and neuropathic pain of a central origin in adults<br><br>➜ Adjuvant treatment of epilepsy | *Class effects:*<br>Adjust the dosage in the presence of kidney failure<br>Caution in the presence of Class **III** or **IV** heart failure |
| Gabapentin | ➜ Antiacid solutions can hinder gabapentine absorption | |
| **Tricyclic or tetracyclic antidepressants**<br><br>Amitriptyline<br>Clomipramine<br>Imipramine<br>Nortriptyline<br>Desipramine<br>Maprolitine | Depression | *Class effects:*<br>Heart problems, central effects, glaucoma, risk of suicide, blurred vision, urinary retention, dry mouth<br><br>Possibility of serotoninergic syndrome if associated with other antidepressants or tramadol |
| **Topical cream**<br>Lidocaine, 10% | | Skin damaged, inflamed; results in increased cutaneous penetration |
| **Opiates**<br>Oxycodone<br>Morphine<br>Hydromorphone<br>Fentanyl<br>Codeine | Pain relief | *Class effects:*<br>History of drug abuse, COPD, sleep apnea, risk of suicide, kidney failure (principally for morphine) |
| **Opioid analgesic**<br>Tramadol | Analgesic | Adjust dosage in the presence of kidney failure<br>Possibility of serotoninergic syndrome and convulsions if associated with certain antidepressants<br><br>Total acetaminophen dosage must be taken into account in the case of patients who use it and for whom Tramacet (tramadol and acetaminophen) is prescribed |

\* All of the medications are contraindicated in the presence of signs of hypersensitivy to the principal active agent or any other ingredient or in the case of pregnant or breastfeeding patients.
Nevertheless, tricyclic antidepressants seem to be safer than other options for pregnant women.

\*\* Cost of an average dosage according to the RAMQ's February 2008 list or the purchase cost for the community pharmacist (excluding the pharmacist's fees).

$ = less than $50 per month; $$: between $50 and $100 per month; $$$: more than $100 per month

**(Cont'd on next page)**

**TABLE III (cont'd): Medication for treating neuropathic pain** | First line

| CONTRAINDICATIONS * | UNDESIRABLE EFFECTS | DRUG INTERACTIONS | COST** |
|---|---|---|---|
| **FIRST LINE** | | | |
| | *Class effects:* Dizziness, drowsiness, peripheral oedema, confusion, dry mouth, blurred vision, ataxia, headache, nausea, weight gain, myoclonus, dystonia, asterixis | → None known <br> → Antacids hinder the absorption of gabapentin | $$-$$$ |
| *Class effects:* Left bundle branch block, bifascicular block, extended QT interval, moderate or serious ischemic disorder (taking Class 1 anti-arrhythmic medications at the same time increases the risk of death), heart failure, recent heart attack, closed-angle glaucoma | *Class effects:* Central: fatigue, sedation, decreased vigilance, confusion, anxiety <br><br> Peripheral: blurred vision, constipation, dysuria, shaking, weight gain, hypotension, sexual dysfontion | *Class effects:* • Numerous drug interactions, Class **Ia** anti-arrhythmic medications, flumazenil, MAOI, pimozide <br> • Association with bupropion reduces the convulsion threshold <br> • The risk of orthostatic hypotension increases if tricyclic antidepressants are associated with clonidine | $-$$ |
| | Risk of toxicity to local anaesthetics if used on a large area | | $-$$$ |
| | *Class effects:* Nausea, vomiting, drowsiness, dizziness, constipation, diaphoresis, pruritus, myoclonus, depression, respiratory, hyperalgesia to opioids, hypogonadism | Codeine and oxycodone are metabolized in part by CYP4052D6 <br><br> Fentanyl is metabolized by CYP4503A4 | Others: $-$$$ |
| Contraindicated in association with MAOIs. Slow release formulas are contraindicated in the case of patients suffering from serious kidney failure. For short-acting formulas, do not exceed 2 tablets/12 hours if ClCr < 30 mL/min | Dizziness, nausea, vomiting, constipation, drowsiness | Tramadol is metabolized in part by CYP450 2D6 <br><br> Shorter half-life in association with a CYP3A4 inducer | $$$ |

TABLE III (cont'd): Medication for treating neuropathic pain | Second line, Third line

| MEDICATIONS | OFFICIAL INDICATIONS | WARNINGS |
|---|---|---|
| **SECOND LINE** | | |
| **SNRI** Venlafaxine | → Depression, generalized anxiety, social anxiety, panic disorder | → Dosages must be adjusted in the presence of kidney failure |
| Duloxetine | → Major depressive disorder, pain associated with a peripheral diabetic neuropathy | → An increase in the concentration of liver enzymes has been reported. Dosages must be adjusted in the presence of kidney failure |
| **Cannabinoids** Dronabinol | → Nausea and vomiting induced by chemotherapy and anorexia (AIDS) | *Class effects:* Hypotension, CNS effects, psychiatric history |
| Nabilone | → Nausea and vomiting induced by chemotherapy | |
| THC/CBD orally | → Treatment of pain in the case of patients suffering from multiple sclerosis and cancer | N.B.: Urine tests are positive for cannabis in the case of patients taking dronabinol and THC/CBD orally |
| **THIRD LINE** | | |
| **SNRI** Citalopram Paroxetine **Other antidepressants** Bupropion | Citalopram and paroxetine: depression, obsessive-compulsive disorder, panic disorder, social phobia, generalized anxiety, post-traumatic stress syndrome<br><br>Bupropion: depression, cessation of smoking | Paroxetine must be used cautiously in the case of patients with liver or kidney failure |
| **Other anticonvulsants** Carbamazepine | → Epilepsy, trigeminal nerve neuralgia, treatment of acute mania, prevention of bipolar disorders | Lamotrigine: allergies, central effects, skin reaction, including Stevens-Johnson syndrome |
| Topiramate Levetiracetam | → Epilepsy, migraines → Adjuvant treatment of epilepsy | Carbamazepine: hepatitis, Stevens-Johnson syndrome, suppression of bone marrow |
| Lamotrigine | → Epilepsy | Exercise close clinical supervision and perform laboratory tests throughout the treatment |

TABLE III (cont'd): Medication for treating neuropathic pain | Second line, Third line

| CONTRAINDICATIONS * | UNDESIRABLE EFFECTS | DRUG INTERACTIONS | COST** |
|---|---|---|---|
| **SECOND LINE** | | | |
| → Contraindicated in association with an MAOI | → Headaches, nausea, sedation, sweating, sexual dysfunction, hypertension, convulsions | *Class effects:*<br>• Numerous drug interactions: phenothiazines, triptans, Class Ia antiarrhythmics, droperidol, flecainide, pimozide, sibutramine, sotalol, stimulants/anorexigens | $$-$$$ |
| → Contraindicated in the case of patients suffering from a liver disease causing liver failure and in the case of patients who consume substantial amounts of alcohol. Contraindicated in association with an MAOI | → Nausea, dizziness, headache, constipation, fatigue, drowsiness | | $$-$$$ |
| *Class effects:*<br>Allergy to marijuana, history of a psychotic disorder | *Class effects:*<br>Decreased concentration, hypotension, dry mouth, dizziness | *Class effects:*<br>Potentiates the sedative effects of other CNS depressants | $-$$ |
| | Mouth irritation | | |
| **THIRD LINE** | | | |
| | Dizziness, drowsiness, anticholinergic effects, nausea, headaches | • Citalopram, paroxetine and bupropion: MAOIs over the course of the 14 previous days<br>• Citalopram and paroxetine: pimozide<br>• Paroxetine and bupropion: thioridazine<br>• Associating bupropion with tricyclic antidepressants lowers the convulsion threshold | $$<br>$$<br>$ |
| Bupropion: convulsive disorders, eating disorder, withdrawal from alcohol or sedatives | | | |
| Carbamazepine: liver disease, history of intermittent, acute porphyria, serious blood disorders, history of bone marrow deficiency | *Class effects:*<br>Nausea, fatigue, drowsiness | • Taking an MAOI during the course of the 14 previous days or the 14 following days (class effect)<br>• Carbamazepine: MAOI associated with numerous other drug interactions. Before prescribing another medication, it is suggested that you verify with a reference work or consult a pharmacist<br>• Lamotrigine: carbamazepine, oxcarbazepine, phenytoin, valproic acid | $<br><br>$$$<br>$$$<br><br>$$$ |

**(Cont'd on next page)**

* All of the medications are contraindicated in the presence of signs of hypersensitivy to the principal active agent or any other ingredient or in the case of pregnant or breastfeeding patients.
Nevertheless, tricyclic antidepressants seem to be safer than other options for pregnant women.

** Cost of an average dosage according to the RAMQ's February 2008 list or the purchase cost for the community pharmacist (excluding the pharmacist's fees).

$ = less than $50 per month; $$: between $50 and $100 per month; $$$: more than $100 per month

**TABLE III (cont'd): Medication for treating neuropathic pain | Fourth line**

| MEDICATIONS | OFFICIAL INDICATIONS | WARNINGS |
|---|---|---|
| **FOURTH LINE** | | |
| **Opioid and NMDA blocker**<br>Methadone | Drug abuse, analgesic | The equianalgesic equivalencies are not linear with the other opioids; they vary in keeping with the dosage used |
| **NMDAR blockers**<br>Ketamine | Anaesthetic for diagnostic and surgical operations | Dissociative central effects |
| **GABA-ergic action**<br>Clonazepam | ➜ Convulsive disorders | |
| Baclofen | ➜ Spasticity caused by multiple sclerosis or a medullar disease | ➜ During withdrawal, the dosage must be reduced progressively by 5-10 mg per week |
| **Alpha-adrenergic and antiarrythmic agonists**<br>Clonidine | ➜ Hypertension | ➜ An evaluation of the risk of orthostatic hypotension is recommended when clonidine is prescribed |
| Tizanidine | ➜ Spasticity | ➜ Liver function may be affected when tizanidine is used. Blood tests should be performed at 1, 3 and 6 months |
| Mexiletine | ➜ Arrhythmia | ➜ An ECG and eventually a consultation with a cardiologist is recommended before starting mexiletine |

TABLE III (cont'd): **Medications for treating neuropathic pain** | Fourth line

| CONTRAINDICATIONS * | UNDESIRABLE EFFECTS | DRUG INTERACTIONS | COST** |
|---|---|---|---|
| FOURTH LINE | | | |
| | See opioids | Drug interactions possible with several agents, primarily those that are metabolized by CYP450 3A4 | $-$$ |
| Patients with a cardiovascular history | Drowsiness, hallucinations | Potentiates the action of certain neuromuscular blockers | $$-$$$ |
| → Acute angle closure glaucoma, serious liver disease, serious myasthenia, serious respiratory difficulty | → Drowsiness, dependency | *Class effects:* Potentiates the effects of certain CNS depressants | $ |
| | → Drowsiness, dizziness, weakness, headache, constipation, vertigo, ataxy, hypotension | | $ |
| → Patient suffering from serious bradycardia secondary to a sinus problem or an atrioventricular (AV block) | *Class effects:* Orthostatic hypotension Mexiletine: arrhythmia | → MAOI, mirtazapine, tizanidine | $ |
| | | → Fluvoxamine, cyclofloxacine | $-$$ |
| | | → Clozapine, flecainide, pimozide, tizanidine, tricyclic antidepressants | $$-$$$ |

\*   All of the medications are contraindicated in the presence of signs of hypersensitivy to the principal active agent or any other ingredient or in the case of pregnant or breastfeeding patients.
Nevertheless, tricyclic antidepressants seem to be safer than other options for pregnant women.

\*\*  Cost of an average dosage according to the RAMQ's February 2008 list or the purchase cost for the community pharmacist (excluding the pharmacist's fees).

$ = less than $50 per month; $$: between $50 and $100 per month; $$$: more than $100 per month

# MY LIFE WITH CHRONIC PAIN!

Line Brochu, CAdm, Quebec City, Quebec, Canada

I was 9 years old and I'd been having abdominal pain for some time, but I still went to school. One day, the pain was too much for me to go to school and I stayed home with my sister, who had chicken pox. In the afternoon, my mother told me, "This evening we'll see the doctor and if there's nothing wrong you'll go back to school tomorrow morning." I knew that I had pains, but I wondered if there was anything to prove it. I was afraid… I couldn't go back to school.

I saw the doctor… and went to the hospital immediately. The doctor thought I was pregnant since I had a lump as large as a child's head in my abdomen. The final diagnosis was an invasive, abdominal "ganglioneuroma" (benign tumour). Normally, a ganglioneuroma is easy to remove with surgery, but sometimes it isn't as a result of the complexity of the nervous system.

I had a first operation and immediately after the surgery the surgeon told my parents he gave me three months to live, if I woke up. I managed to leave the hospital. We celebrated my tenth birthday and I was given more presents than ever. All my classmates came to see me and brought gifts. The next day, I went into St. Justine's hospital (Montreal, Quebec) for three months. A surgeon spent seven hours removing the portion of the ganglioneuroma that went to the liver. He treated me until I was 21 years old and saw me again at the age of 33 to refer me to another surgeon. I was hospitalized every year from the age of 9 to 21. Following this, I was treated as an out-patient, but in addition to this, I was hospitalized again and underwent surgery.

It's not only doctors who can help us. We can work on self-management of pain. When I returned to school, the year after my second surgery, I was allowed to be absent from school on Wednesdays. I never used that permission. I wanted to be like others. I always wanted to be like others. I think that's what allowed me to get through my suffering. We must observe children: they know they are sick, but they act as if they were not.

Even after many operations, I still live with the same problem. The ganglioneuroma has invaded my abdomen, a large part of my spinal column and has penetrated the sacral plexus, where all the nerves are located at the base of the spinal column. It penetrated inside and the nerve roots became very painful. It was only through the use of a strong medication as well as the efforts of an excellent family physician and anaesthesiologist, that I managed to reduce the pain. But, even though the surgeons managed to remove a few pieces of the ganglioneuroma two times out of six, it kept coming back stronger than ever and changed direction.

Since 1964, I have experienced suffering and that suffering affected my morale as well. For that reason, about ten years ago, I had a major depression. I had to see psychologists who also helped me get through this. When we suffer mentally as well, we think that there is no more hope, but there always is. I often thought that it was the end and I would get back on my feet with an injection and a new medication. You always have to start over but you shouldn't get discouraged.

We always have to have hope because there are better days and we have to trust in life. Research, doctors, specialists and the large pharmaceutical companies are making a great deal of progress. We must think about these people who are working for us every day and, as result, feel encouraged, if only for a few hours.

Medication takes first place in the treatment of my chronic pain. At the beginning, when they prescribed anxiolytics or anti-depressants for me, I wasn't very happy. But I read a lot and I learned that they are part of the medication arsenal that works against pain. Of course, several medications have side effects, but the best medication is only found through trial and error. You can't get discouraged if, in a few months or years, that medication doesn't work in the same way because there will be other medications. You can be sure of that. Moreover, it is certain that when you change your medication you have to deal with the side effects. However, even if a medication may have certain side effects that doesn't necessarily mean you will feel them.

Apart from the medications, I've taken my life in hand, I've taken therapy, therapies such as hypnosis, yoga, walking, meditation, relaxation, acupuncture, etc. For me, relaxation can be very beneficial. I want to help other people and be a part of the care team since I know that is good for me and I'm convinced my experience can be used to help others. I have an extraordinary family physician. He's my orchestra conductor, who maintains the link between me and the specialists. The family physician is the one who coordinates everything with the other professionals such as the physiotherapist, the occupational therapist, the psychologist, etc. I think it's essential for people to have a conductor but it wasn't always like that and I know that not everyone has a good one.

I have to mention something that people in pain often find difficult, namely when people are rude to them. We know that it's not easy to keep a smile on your face all the time, that the hospital employees also have their own problems. But when we have to go to hospitals regularly and someone is rude to us, it's as if everything comes crashing down! Tears come easily to us… and we can feel so misunderstood.

# COMPLEX REGIONAL
# PAIN SYNDROME (CRPS)

**Dat-Nhut Nguyen** MD, anaesthesiologist,
**Josée Boucher** PRT
Centre de Santé et des Services Sociaux de Rouyn-Noranda, Rouyn-Noranda, Quebec, Canada

http://maladieschroniques@uqat.ca (in French only)

Read by **Harry FL Pollett** MD, FRCPC
Director, Pollett Pain Services, Northside General Hospital, North Sydney, Nova Scotia, Director,
Cape Breton Island Pain Clinic, Cape Breton, Nova Scotia, Canada

## ABSTRACT

One of the most painful diseases treated in our clinics is CRPS, complex regional pain syndrome. Following in the footsteps of recent developments in the neurosciences, researchers have developed more effective treatments for this still mysterious disease. In this chapter, we will provide an overview of current medical knowledge, as well as a description of the treatment programme used in our facility.

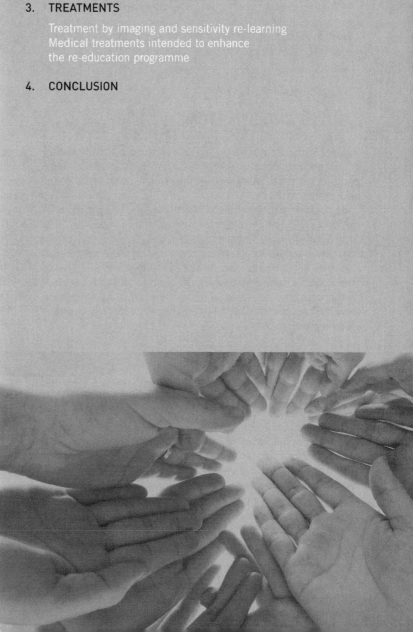

# 1. INTRODUCTION

Complex regional pain syndrome (CRPS) was, until very recently, a disease (pathology) about which very little was known. It can be caused by a trauma, a fracture, a heart attack, etc. Occasionally, it is even impossible to determine any cause. This pathology has gone by different names in different periods of time and in different countries (algodystrophy, reflex sympathetic dystrophy, Sudeck's atrophy, causalgia, shoulder-hand syndrome). Thus, in order to simplify the nomenclature and encourage the establishment of more standard diagnostics, a panel of specialists from the International Association for the Study of Pain (IASP) established a series of diagnostic criteria in 1993 and settled on a single name: **complex regional pain syndrome**. Until then, it was a disease that was described as very serious, rare and mysterious. Fortunately, since the turn of the century, new research studies and progress in our knowledge in the field have enabled us to understand this syndrome and its treatments.

In this chapter, we will explore the most recent data on CRPS, from a point of view focused on patient rehabilitation and autonomy.

More specifically, we will describe:
· CRPS symptoms and what science currently understands about these symptoms;
· Treatment using imaging and sensory re-education; and
· Medical treatments intended to promote re-education.

**N.B.:**
**If you get an urge to research this subject on the Internet (particularly on CRPS support group sites and on YouTube), it is possible that you will be shocked to find a much more pessimistic viewpoint, and one that is focused on passive treatments that are of little use.**

FIGURE 1: CRPS in the left hand

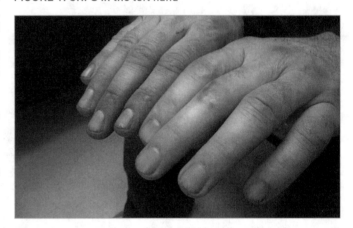

# 2. SIGNS AND SYMPTOMS

CRPS is defined, among other things, as a painful condition secondary to a trauma, most often to an extremity, for which the clinical manifestations and the duration are **disproportionate** with respect to the initial trauma.

We would like to draw your attention to the term "disproportionate" used in the definition. In order to better illustrate our comments, let us consider the example of a sprained ankle, which hurts to such an extent that it limits walking for anywhere from a few days to a week. But if, after two weeks, the pain increases, this is disproportionate. The health professionals' job is to detect the possible complications and treat them: infection, fracture, torn tendons. Unfortunately, 1 to 2 people out of every 1000 will not have any infection, fracture or torn tendons; they will have developed CRPS.[1]

Pain is the predominant symptom of CRPS:
· Pain when resting, continuous, intense;
· The skin is sensitive, brushing fabric against the skin is painful (allodynia);
· Small, simple movements become painful;
· The pain extends to other parts of the body that were initially intact: for example, the patient injured his/her thumb, but progressively the other fingers of the hand become painful and stiff;
· The pain may be experienced as a burn, an electrical discharge, thousands of needles sensation, stinging, tingling; the affected limb may become very sensitive to temperature changes. "A little cold" may be experienced as "painfully icy" (thermal hyperalgesia).

These manifestations are probably related to important changes in the nervous system. These include changes in the transmission of painful information, of course, but also in the transmission of information pertaining to the control of temperature, the control of movements and fine tactile sensitivity (for example, recognizing the type of fabric by touch). Major changes are also observed in the information integration, and movement planning and recognition zones in our body.

These changes in the nervous system also produce unusual symptoms, which are so different from the symptoms for other painful diseases that the patients are sometimes treated as liars and fakers:
· Feeling that the affected limb is very swollen whereas the limb is only visibly a little swollen;
· Feeling that the limb is longer, shorter, larger, smaller than it actually is;
· Having difficulty imagining performing a simple movement with the affected limb (or simply imagining the movement already hurts);
· Feeling that the affected limb does not belong to one (the patient speaks about his/her limb saying "this hand", "this thing" rather than "my hand");
· Losing fine touch and feeling numbness, pins-and-needles, tingling, and/or pain in parts of the body that were not injured during the initial accident (sometimes throughout the arm in the case of CRPS affecting a hand, sometimes even in the face or throughout half of the body);
· Developing tremors, stiffness, abnormal positioning of the affected limb, particularly during voluntary movements and during periods of stress. These movement anomalies decrease when the patient is distracted or relaxed.

FIGURE 2: The patient FEELS as if his/her hand is deformed and swollen, although it does not appear to be so. He/she has difficulty feeling his/her fingers and occasionally mixes them up.

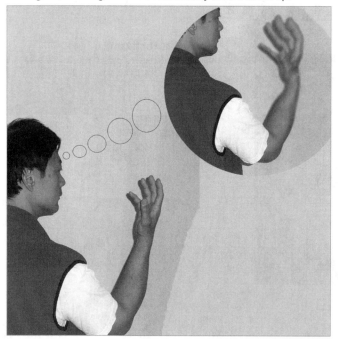

FIGURE 3: Neurogenic inflammation and disorders of the sympathetic nervous system

### NEUROGENIC INFLAMMATION

With each injury, inflammation is a normal process that protects the part of the body that has been injured and provides comfort to the repair cells in order to cause healing. Unfortunately, in the case of certain diseases (including CRPS), this process becomes deregulated. Neurogenic means that the inflammation is not caused by the infection, the cancer, or the arthritis but by a deregulation of the nervous system that regulates inflammation.

### SYMPATHETIC SYSTEM

Our nervous system controls several functions that are related to maintaining the homoeostasis of the body, namely maintaining the stability of temperature, water, blood sugar levels, etc. through the involvement of the sympathetic system, among other things. This system helps regulate skin temperature, perspiration and blood circulation. This system also prepares our body for stress so that we can face external dangers.

Patients with CRPS also have various signs and symptoms related to neurogenic inflammation and disorders of the sympathetic nervous system:
- Redness, heat, oedema (swelling) that extends beyond the part that was initially injured;
- Or, the opposite, namely a bluish, purplish or white colour to the skin, accompanied by coldness. Sometimes, this coldness can even alternate with episodes of redness, heat and oedema. These symptoms (hot, cold, red, purple, blue, marbled) often fluctuate. They increase and decrease during the course of the day, over weeks and months. They increase when the patient takes part in painful activities or exceeds certain limits;
- Sweating may become abnormal, increasing or decreasing, in the part of the body that is affected and even beyond it;
- In the region affected, the skin, nails, and hair become dry, thin, irregular, cracked, and fragile. The tissues under the skin may also become hardened, thick, and less supple.

In addition to the specific symptoms indicated above, the patients also experience symptoms common to most types of chronic pain:
- Sleep disorders;
- Stress related to the difficulties of doing daily household chores;
- Stress related to employment, possible disputes with paying organizations;
- Stress related to the uncertainty caused by the disease, the difficulties of finding resources for treatment;
- Stress related to the continuous pain, but above all to the lack of means for controlling it;
- Major side effects caused by medication (particularly when medication is used in high dosages);
- Unavoidable family and personal problems, as a result of major losses, which require difficult adjustments; and
- Psychological problems (anxiety, depression, anger, etc.) that occur when the stress becomes too much.

## 3. TREATMENTS

Since the exact cause of the disease is unknown, science has been unable to offer (even as recently as 2009) any specific treatment intended to cure CRPS.

Until recently, medicine had few effective treatments to offer and most of the patients diagnosed were stuck with severe pain and handicaps in daily activities.

However, studies conducted at the beginning of this century have indicated that doing exercises that provoke pain on a repetitive basis activates the neuromatrix of pain.[2] See **Figure 4**, next page.

FIGURE 4: Neuromatrix of pain

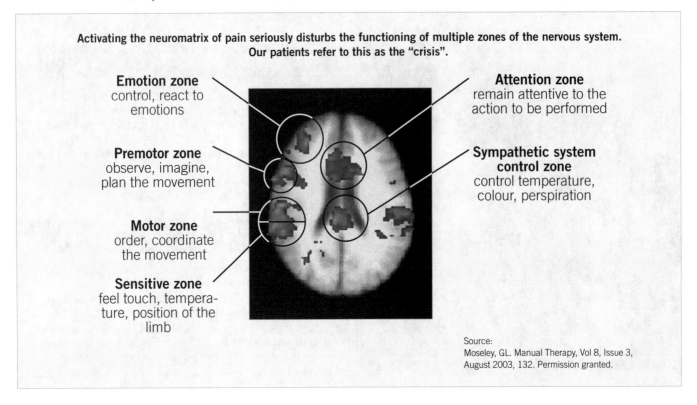

**Activating the neuromatrix of pain seriously disturbs the functioning of multiple zones of the nervous system. Our patients refer to this as the "crisis".**

**Emotion zone**
control, react to emotions

**Premotor zone**
observe, imagine, plan the movement

**Motor zone**
order, coordinate the movement

**Sensitive zone**
feel touch, temperature, position of the limb

**Attention zone**
remain attentive to the action to be performed

**Sympathetic system control zone**
control temperature, colour, perspiration

Source:
Moseley, GL. Manual Therapy, Vol 8, Issue 3, August 2003, 132. Permission granted.

Today, we have a better understanding of the downward spiral into CRPS. See **Figure 5**.

FIGURE 5: Downward spiral into CRPS

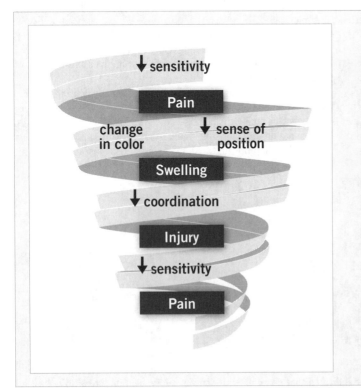

↓ sensitivity

Pain

change in color    ↓ sense of position

Swelling

↓ coordination

Injury

↓ sensitivity

Pain

The patient continues to "push" (or is pushed), doing exercises that are too demanding for the condition, which causes a great deal of pain.

The pain results in swelling, change in colour, change in temperature, and disturbances in the nervous system (numbness, loss of sensation, imprecise movements, and disturbed sense of position, etc.) In turn, these disturbances cause movements to be imprecise, causing other injuries, other pains.

And the vicious circle starts all over again.

This led researchers Moseley[3] and Pleger[4] to design a treatment intended to rehabilitate these disturbances, a treatment based on daily exercises.

This treatment is based on three important principles:

- Re-education, in steps, for each of the functions altered by CRPS through daily exercises;
- So as to avoid provoking a crisis (pain, swelling, heat, redness, coldness), the patient must go through the steps slowly, patiently, one step at a time. It is important to follow one treatment at a time, one exercise programme planned by one person at a time (to avoid contradictory explanations and exercises that go in different directions);
- The person with CRPS must also learn to be patient in daily life, so as not to provoke a crisis outside the exercise programme (it would be illogical to spend 20 minutes per day imaging movements without moving so as to avoid provoking a crisis and then carry wood for two hours and provoke a crisis of pain, swelling, etc.).

These techniques revolutionized the treatment of CRPS. As the patient recovers his/her sense of fine touch, the ability to imagine the movement and the ability to move, the pain decreases, the swelling disappears and the temperature of the limb returns to normal.

This programme has been in use in our hospital since 2004. It is also available in certain hospitals (going by the name of imaging rehabilitation programme, motor imaging, and graded motor imagery. Today, with a regular exercise programme, most patients regain a good quality of life, and most return to work with the necessary adjustments. Unfortunately, a minority of patients still have a severe handicap and have to take medication on a long-term basis to stabilize their condition.

One of the inconveniences of this programme is that most health professionals still do not know about it. It is possible that you will encounter difficulty during follow-up with certain professionals who order you to endure more pain, to surpass your limits, to be more active immediately.

## TREATMENT BY IMAGING AND SENSITIVITY RE-LEARNING

In this section, we will describe the principles and provide examples of exercises used in the rehabilitation programme. For a complete description or to obtain the tools that are available (CD, DVD, photos, protocols), we suggest you consult our internet site (http://www. maladieschroniques@uqat.ca).

**We divide the treatment into six phases.**

### Phase 1: Right-left recognition, sensory re-education, WITHOUT PAIN (about two weeks)

**This is the crucial step. The primary objective of this phase is to learn to manage the exercises and daily life in order to minimize the "crises".**

### Imaging exercises
**Recognizing left from right, either with the CD, or with a deck of cards (the two versions are available on our Internet site).** You can practise identifying whether the hand (or the foot) presented is the right or the left. The exercise is intended to activate the premotor zone (zone where movement is planned), which must turn and manipulate the image of your own hand in your body diagram in order to identify each image presented. The exercise is repeated for a few minutes at a time at the start, three times per day. Then, if that is comfortable, you can gradually increase to 10 minutes, three times per day, six days per week. Throughout the programme, it is important to be attentive to the signs of pain, changes in colour, swelling, and deterioration. These signs are your guides with respect to reducing, or adjusting the duration or the difficulty of the exercises.

**The hands (or feet) must remain immobile while you practise exercising left and right.**

**If you use the deck of cards, handle the cards with your healthy hand.**

**If some of the images cause particular difficulties, continue with the exercise, but drop the "problematic" images. After a few sessions, try the "problematic" images again.**

### Exercises for improving the sense of touch and temperature
In the case of CRPS, during crises, the nervous system tends to disconnect from the affected limb. To reverse this tendency, you use cotton batting, a soft brush, fabric, or just the heat of your hand to gently pinch, without causing pain, the skin of the affected limb. The purpose is to pay attention to these sensations in order to re-educate the nervous system.

In the case of the exercise for re-learning the sense of touch, two bowls of water are placed in front of you, one containing slightly warm water and the other containing slightly cool water. Dip the affected limb in the buckets, alternating from one to the other and pay attention to re-learning to discern changes in temperature.

**PHASE 1** (CONT'D) : **Right-left recognition, sensory re-education, WITHOUT PAIN (about two weeks)**

**Learning to manage daily activities so as to minimize crises**

Have you ever seen an animal (dog, cat) with an injured foot? It holds the injured foot close to its body and does not use it until it has healed. This effective strategy is more difficult to use in the case of human beings. Learning to function in daily life (walking, shopping for groceries, cooking, washing, etc.) without provoking pain or a crisis is a major challenge. In this respect, we suggest that you read **Chapter 23**.

Analgesic medication (pain killers) can be of use to certain patients on a short-term basis.

FIGURE 6: Examples of exercises to improve sensitivity

**Proceed with your eyes closed.**

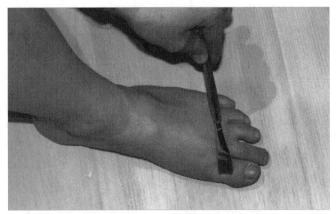

Re-learning the sense of touch with a soft brush

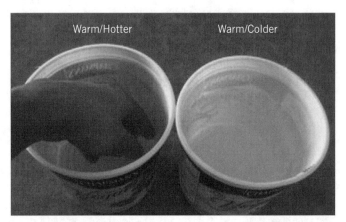

Re-learning to sense temperature

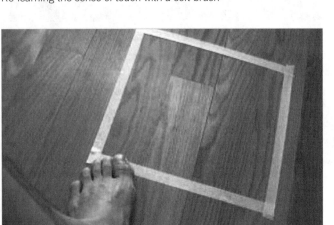

Following the tape on the floor

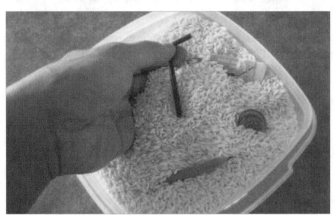

Finding objects in a bowl of rice

**PHASE 2: Re-learning to prepare, to imagine simultaneous movements of both hands (or both feet) in the mirror, to improve fine touch, to specify, and distinguish small differences in temperature WITHOUT PAIN (approximately two weeks)**

**Preparing the movement**

We suggest you try this experience: take time for a quiet moment, standing (or sitting), close your eyes, take the time to make sure you are balanced, and feel your weight in the middle of your feet (or your hips). When you are ready, lift both arms in front of you. Feel your weight shift slightly backwards (toward your heels or tail bone). Do this several times, making sure you can feel the shift in your centre of gravity.

Now, imagine that you are moving both arms forward without actually moving them. You will probably feel your weight shift slightly to the back as well.

This experience illustrates an essential mechanism: just before initiating a movement, our nervous system must construct the sequence of the movement, shift the centre of gravity, position the supporting joints, and stabilize them. All of this work is done without our knowledge by the premotor zone in our brain. And this zone is altered by CRPS.

In phase 2, you will imagine the movement WITHOUT MOVING, specifically in order to activate the premotor zone in order to re-learn to prepare the movement adequately.

**Imaging exercises**

Hold a stable mirror with two hands (or both feet) so as to hide the affected hand (or the foot). During the exercise, position yourself so that you can see your healthy hand and the reflection of the healthy hand (which creates the illusion of seeing the affected hand).

The exercise involves imagining the **simultaneous** movements of both hands (or feet). In **Figure 7**, the patient is looking at examples of movements that appear on the computer. If you want to use the same software, you can download the CD from the Internet site. The exercise can also be done with picture cards (also available on the Internet site).

The objective is to do the exercise for 10 minutes, three times per day, 6 days per week, for two weeks. This requires patience and perseverance.

FIGURE 7: Position for the exercises in the mirror

**Positioning (phases 2, 3 and 4)**

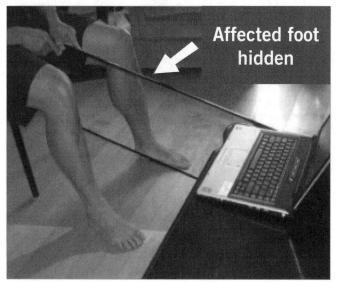

Lower limb

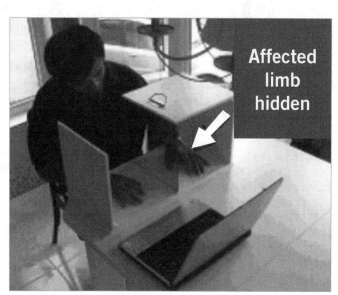

Upper limb

## Exercises for improving the sense of touch and temperature

These are the same exercises as for Phase 1. Proceed slowly, stimulating the skin with brushes with hairs that are a little harder (or a toothbrush), and with rougher fabric.

To proceed with the re-education process for the sense of temperature, use buckets of water that are closer and closer in temperature.

To re-learn the sense of position, with your eyes closed, use the index finger on the healthy hand to gently touch each of the fingers on the affected hand (or each toe on the affected foot). If someone in your family can help you, ask them to gently touch your fingers (or your toes) and you identify which toes or fingers are touched, without looking.

## Learning to manage daily activities

Managing more and more of your daily activities without triggering crises involves negotiating, delegating and refusing to do certain tasks. We suggest that you continue to integrate the information provided in **Chapter 24**.

At the end of Phase 2, pain while resting is usually well controlled. The imaging exercises are comfortable, and do not trigger any symptoms. Finally, episodes of colour changes, and swelling have been reduced significantly.

---

### PHASE 3: Moving the healthy side, WITHOUT PAIN (approximately two weeks)

#### Imaging exercises

Same set up as for the Phase 2 exercise using the mirror. This exercise involves starting the movements using only the healthy side while observing the image of your healthy hand in the mirror. Slowly, gently.

For certain patients, the Phase 3 imaging exercise is particularly easy (namely, no discomfort, no increase in symptoms). Thus they move on to the Phase 4 imaging exercise immediately.

#### Exercises to improve the sense of touch and temperature

Same exercises as for Phase 2; proceed slowly and surely.

Another exercise involves placing various objects on a table and learning to recognize them by touch, without looking. (For a foot that is affected, it involves recognizing different types of surfaces by touching them with your bare foot: wood, carpet, rubber, etc.).

#### Learning to manage daily activities

Same tasks as for Phase 2; proceed slowly and surely.

DANGER: The risk is that you will want to return to your normal life immediately because you feel better.

---

### PHASE 4: Re-learning to do simultaneous movements with both hands (or both feet) in the mirror; re-learning fine, precise gesture, WITHOUT PAIN (approximately two to four weeks)

#### Imaging exercises

Same set-up as for the mirror exercise for Phases 2 and 3. This exercise involves starting simultaneous movements with both hands (or both feet) while observing the image of your healthy hand (or foot) in the mirror. The objective is: slowness, precision, comfort. Strength and flexibility will be covered in the next phase.

#### Exercises to improve the sense of touch and temperature

In this phase, you will start to handle small, light objects (beach ball, plastic glass, large puzzle pieces, etc.). Then, move on to exercises that require more skill (stacking blocks with your eyes closed, putting together a four-piece puzzle with your eyes closed, and so on). In the case of CRPS affecting a foot, the exercise is to explore different ways of transferring some of the weight to the affected foot WITHOUT causing pain.

The objective is: slowness, precision, comfort. Strength and flexibility will be analyzed in the next phase.

**Bowls of water**: once you have learned to distinguish small differences in temperature, the next step is to teach your limb to manage larger contrasts. This exercise involves using a bowl of slightly cold water and another of slightly hot water and dipping the limb alternatively in the two bowls. As the contrasts become more comfortable, increase the temperature differences.

#### Learning to manage daily activities

At this stage, several patients are tempted to increase their level of activity quickly… and they get worse each time. It is very important to continue to progress very slowly and cautiously.

## PHASE 5: Re-learning to perform every day gestures fluidly and precisely

Usually, after Phase 4, the pain is well controlled, the "crises" are more spaced out and you can perform small movements with the affected limb comfortably. In Phase 5, the objective of the programme is to:
- Re-learn the "normal" sequence rhythm and coordination of the actions performed in everyday life. "Normal" means that the action is supple, fluid, with no catching, no cracking, comfortable, easy and effective. This may involve re-learning to balance the arms while walking or re-learning to lift an object fluidly and efficiently. An example of one exercise is provided in **chapter 23**;
- Gradually increasing muscle strength, the flexibility of joints through "conventional" exercises (weight bearing, lifting small weights, stretching, gentle aerobic exercises);

- When the gestures of daily life become easy, you will move on to re-learning the gestures you will perform (or currently do perform) at work. It is important that you respect the rules of biomechanics and ergonomics (See **Chapter 24.**)

### Imaging exercises
The imaging exercises are normally completed by this phase. However, if certain exercises remain difficult and/or a serious crisis has occurred, it is important to return to the imaging exercises, respecting the order of the phases (1, then 2, 3, 4). The speed with which you move on from one phase to another is adjusted in keeping with the success you experience with the exercises.

## PHASE 6: Managing a relapse

**Carole had successfully completed the imaging and sensory re-education programme. She had returned to her work and her normal life. Approximately one year later, she called me and told me that she had re-built her patio and that the symptoms of CRPS had reappeared. She got her CD out and re-started the treatment programme from the beginning. Within a week her arm was once again functional.**

Almost all CRPS patients will experience a relapse. For a certain amount of time, the nervous system seems to remain "fragile". The changes in the nervous system have a tendency to reappear when an injury occurs, during demanding work, or following surgery. Certain patients have to continue paying attention to the actions they

perform with the affected limb. Others continue to do exercises and play games in order to improve their skill and precision.

In the event of a relapse, you should start the programme over from the beginning:
- Imaging exercises;
- Exercises to improve the sense of touch and temperature; and
- Managing daily activities.

The speed at which you progress from one phase to another is adjusted in keeping with the success you achieve with the exercises and the changes in your symptoms.

**Don't forget: slow and easy.**

## MEDICAL TREATMENTS INTENDED TO ENHANCE THE RE-EDUCATION PROGRAMME

Various medical means can be used to support the re-education programme. These means are particularly useful on a short-term basis. They can cause complications on a long-term basis.

### Pain medications (see chapter 30)
- **Gabapentin and pregabalin** are medications used to treat epilepsy and are useful for controlling pain;
- **Acetaminophen** is a mild analgesic, with very few side effects;
- **Anti-inflammatories** (naprosen, ibuprofen, etc.) are mild analgesics. As a result of the side effects, avoid taking these medications for more than three weeks. Gastro-intestinal distress, bleeding and other side effects may restrict the use of these drugs to a brief course of treatment reducing their value in the management of a chronic condition.
- **Opiates** (narcotics, morphine, codeine, hydromorphone, oxycodone, etc.): are powerful analgesics; the side effects are primarily sleepiness and, above all constipation. The long-lasting formulas (ex.: morphine contin, hydromorph contin, oxy contin, duragesic, etc.) are particularly useful for this type of continuous pain;

- **Amytriptiline** (an anti-depressant) helps patients sleep, in small doses.
- Your doctor may occasionally suggest medications that are used to treat osteoporosis (demineralization of the bones).
- Rarely, when the swelling and redness are significant, a brief cortisone treatment may be used (one to four weeks).
- Certain patients may benefit from sympathetic blocks and vein blocks. With these techniques, the anaesthesiologist uses one or more needles to inject medications to temporarily block the sympathetic nerves of the affected limb. These techniques are repeated 6 to 10 times and temporarily relieve the pain and swelling of certain patients.

### Other treatments
- **Sympathectomy**: With these techniques, the anaesthesiologist or the surgeon destroys the sympathetic nerves of the affected limb. The effectiveness of sympathectomy has never been proven and the operations can result in a lot of complications (phantom sensations, increased pain). Even when successful, the duration of pain relief may last only a few months.

A small minority of patients do not progress well: the rehabilitation programme does not progress, and the pain is significant despite the treatment. These patients will continue to experience severe handicaps and long-term medications will be necessary to control the pain.

A few rare patients will receive invasive palliative treatment to control the pain. With neurostimulators and epidural catheters, the neurosurgeon or the anaesthesiologist implants catheters (small tubes) close to the spine. (See **Chapter 34**). These are very powerful medical means for blocking the pain signals, but they are also the most dangerous.

## 4. CONCLUSION

In this chapter, we have explored CRPS, a painful disease with unusual symptoms for which the exact cause is still unknown. Our objective was also to help you better understand and use the treatment that has been the most effective to date:

- Managing activities so as to avoid triggering a "crisis";
- Using progressive exercises to re-educate the nervous system to overcome the alterations that occur;
- Re-learning to do daily and work activities without triggering a "crisis".

It is not possible to describe all of the details of the programme and the tools in this chapter. We suggest that you visit our Internet site at http://maladieschroniques@uqat.ca.

Unfortunately the road to rehabilitation is littered with stumbling blocks: the lack of understanding on the part of certain professionals, certain paying organizations, the lack of resources, and aid. There will be moments of anger, rebellion and discouragement. There will be other moments when you feel like going far too fast and skipping steps. Our experience with CRPS patients has been: three steps ahead, two steps back, three steps ahead, one step back... and that's normal.

The road to recovery requires courage, perseverance and patience. **Fortunately, improvement is definitely possible and attainable.**

## REFERENCES

1. De Mos M (2008). Medical history and the onset of Complex Regional Pain Syndrome (CRPS). Pain, 139, 458-466.
2. Moseley G.L. (2003). A pain neuromatrix approach to patients with chronic pain. Manual Therapy (2003) 8(3), 130-140.
3. Moseley G.L. (2004). Graded motor imagery is effective for long-standing complex regional pain syndrome: a randomised controlled trial. Pain 108 (2004), 192-198.
4. Burkhard Pleger, MD (2005). Sensorimotor Returning in Complex Regional Pain Syndrome Parallels Pain Reduction. Annals of Neurology Vol. 57 No 3, 425-428.

# FIBROMYALGIA:
## PAIN WITHOUT END!

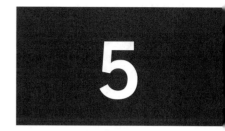

**5**

Pierre Arsenault PhD, MD, CPI, Sherbrooke, Quebec, Canada
Alain Béland MSc, MD, FRCPc, Roberval, Quebec, Canada

## ABSTRACT

Fibromyalgia is one of the painful clinical conditions about which the clinical world knows the least. The increase in the number of patients with this condition has given rise to many questions and both the scientific community and the political authorities must resolve them in order to identify the causes, the mechanisms and the treatments. For some patients suffering from this condition, the psychosocial consequences can be many: isolation, lack of understanding, stigmatization, abandonment, divorce, eviction from work. Physical pain is experienced along with emotional pain and even profound existential questions: why so much pain?

For society, extreme cases mean inestimable losses: absenteeism from work, disruption of family activities and domestic chores, multiplication of consultations and examinations, not to mention the astronomical costs they generate.

As a result of recent scientific inroads, new hypotheses have been developed, generating hope that effective treatments will be developed in a not too distant future. This chapter will review current knowledge about the mechanisms identified to date to explain this syndrome, etiological hypotheses and treatments.

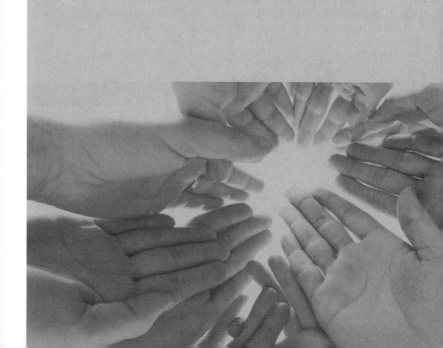

# 1. WHAT EXACTLY IS FIBROMYALGIA?

Fibromyalgia is a clinical syndrome characterized by diffuse pain, affecting the four quadrants of the body (**Figure 1**), which is experienced daily, 24 hours a day. This pain must have existed for at least three months in an uninterrupted manner to be recognized as such. The level of the pain is variable, but generally high, ranging from hyperalgesia (increased pain response to a painful stimulus) to allodynia (pain caused by stimulation that is normally not painful). It fluctuates in keeping with physiological and emotional stress. It is experienced mainly in the muscles, joints and skin, but is also often accompanied by visceral pain (for example, intestinal and bladder pain) and occasionally migraines. It occurs during sleep and results in intense fatigue when the individual gets up in the morning (**Figure 2**). It does not prevent the individual from moving, walking and occasionally taking part in more intense activities, but it leads to early muscle fatigue and reduced physical

resistance. These clinical manifestations are accompanied by a variety of symptoms that vary from one patient to another, in terms of quantity, quality and intensity. Therefore, it is difficult to categorize people with fibromyalgia in a single group. Some authors, moreover, refer to the potential existence of sub-groups (de Souza JB & coll 2009 a,b, Müller W & coll 2007, Giesecke T & coll 2003,Rehm SE & coll 2010). We are of the opinion that it is more appropriate to speak of a "continuum" in the severity of the clinical manifestations than of specific sub-groups (**Figure 3**, page **37**). This continuum, moreover, explains why people with fibromyalgia should not compare themselves to one another. Even if they may be similar in certain respects, they do not have the same pain thresholds, the same constellations of symptoms or the same response to treatments.

FIGURE 1 : Body-wide pain of fibromyalgia

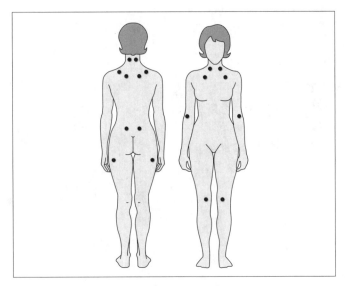

The pain affects all four quadrants of the body (upper and lower limbs, trunk and para-spinal regions). Specific points (18 tender points) are more sensitive than in the general population (red points).

FIGURE 2 : Repercussions of the pain of fibromyalgia on the various spheres of human activity

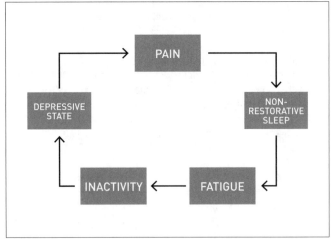

Pain disrupts sleep. A lack of sleeps disrupts tissue repairs and increases fatigue. Fatigue reduces motivation and the ability to initiate a physical activity programme. Inactivity, whether it is associated with a loss of social function or not, occasionally leads to depressives states. Depression affects pain thresholds.

## 2. WHAT FIBROMYALGIA IS NOT

**Fibromyalgia is not a muscular pain caused by "fibrosis".** The word "fibromyalgia" is a poorly chosen term. Almost all of the studies done on muscle biopsies have never confirmed a structural anomaly specific to people with fibromyalgia. The anomalies identified in terms of muscular fibres and collagen (present in the muscle fibres) are also observed in healthy but sedentary individuals (Arsenault P & coll 2007).

**Fibromyalgia is not a depression as some clinicians have tried to lead us to believe.** It is true that a significant number of people with fibromyalgia (approximately 40%) develop a depression sooner or later during the course of their life, but this should not lead us to conclude that fibromyalgia is synonymous with depression.

**Fibromyalgia must not be confused with other psychiatric diagnoses such as psychosomatization.** According to the DSM-IV (psychiatric diagnostic guide), psychosomatization is the expression in the physical body of psychological disturbances. Even if it is true that most people with fibromyalgia are subjected to significant psychological stresses, this does not mean that the physical symptoms they report are not physically real! Recent work by Goffaux & coll. (2007) have clearly demonstrated that definite physiological phenomena are disturbed in the spines of people with fibromyalgia.

**Fibromyalgia is not a personality disorder.** All of the studies that have verified this hypothesis have reached the same conclusions: there is no fibromyalgic personality disorder or personality, but simply just more common personality traits. The tendency to experience anxiety or to catastrophize is included among the most frequently identified traits. When such traits are present, it is important to identify them since their consequences cannot be underestimated (See **Figure 4** on page **34**). In fact, catastrophization encourages hyper-vigilance and leads patients into a spiral that merely amplifies the symptoms.

FIGURE 3: Continuum of clinical presentation in fibromyalgia (theoretical models)

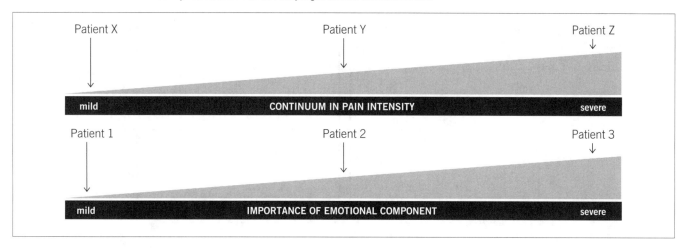

The profiles of three patients (X, Y, and Z) are indicated in the continuum of pain intensity. Those of three other patients (1, 2 and 3) highlight the importance of the physiological and psychological components of pain. The respective positions of these patients are not necessarily fixed in time, but bilateral shifts are possible.

FIGURE 4 : Two directions in the pain experience: that of depression and disability or that of recovery

**ALGORITHM**

### Two directions in the pain experience

On the left side, the pain experience evolves in keeping with the emotional reaction that is associated with it. With catastrophization, a fear of movement, a state of hyper-vigilance and a need for flight develops. These reactions lead to depression and disability, which merely amplify the pain. On the other hand (on the right side), adequate management of fear and exposure to activities is clearly more realistic and part of the road to recovery.

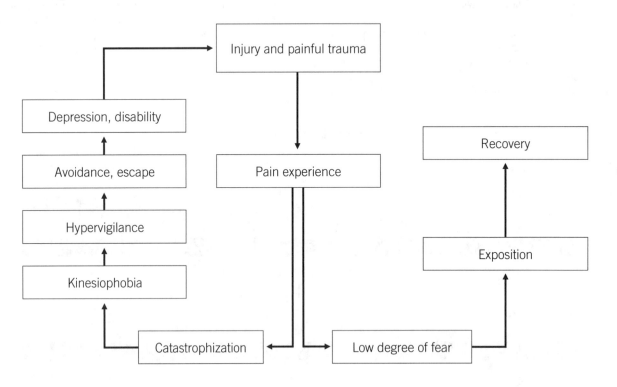

Vlaeyen JWS, Kole-Snijders AMJ, Boeren RGB, van EEK H. Fear of movement/(re)injury in chronic low back pain and its relation to behavioral performance. PAIN 1995 Sept; 62(3): 363-372. This figure has been reproduced with permission of the International Association for the Study of Pain® (IASP®). The figure may not be reproduced for any other purpose without permission.

# 3. CURRENT HYPOTHESES FOR EXPLAINING FIBROMYALGIA

## INCREASED PAIN: WHEN THE ACCELERATOR IS STUCK!

Patients with fibromyalgia often report an **amplification of their sensory perceptions** (touch, odour, hearing, taste, smell). This amplification varies from patient to patient in terms of means and intensity. It is not uncommon to hear someone with fibromyalgia state that they feel more pain throughout their body when inhaling the odour of a cleaning product or the cashier's perfume in a store. Similar phenomena are also reported by people who have had strokes (Taylor JB 2008). This hypersensitivity is also tactile. A small tap of encouragement on a shoulder and a firm handshake in greeting are often major sources of pain for people with fibromyalgia to the great surprise of the person initiating such a gesture. The hyperexcitability of the skin, muscles and other structures, as peripheral as it may seem, results from physiological and biochemical modifications in the central nervous system. It is, in particular, the spine and the brain that coordinate and regulate the information contained in pain. Researchers interested in studying these centres have recently identified anomalies for each of these centres that provide a somewhat better understanding of the phenomena of the perceptual amplification of pain.

## Anomalies in superior centre activity

One the most recently identified anomalies is that of atrophy of the gray matter in the brain. A team of researchers at McGill University demonstrated that the loss of gray matter is accelerated in patients with fibromyalgia as compared to healthy subjects (Kuchinad A & coll 2007). It is possible that the disruptions in certain cognitive functions (concentration and memory above all) reported by people with fibromyalgia are related to this cortical atrophy. However, this discovery is not specific to fibromyalgia since it has also been observed in patients suffering from major depressions and those with serious hip pain (Dotson VM & coll 2009, Frodi TS & coll 2008, Rodriguez-Raecke R & coll 2009). It is, moreover, comforting to know that when the pain (or the depression) is controlled in these groups of patients, the gray matter recovers its initial properties (Rodriguez-Raecke R & coll 2009). Therefore, it is not a matter of degeneration but rather a phenomenon of "cerebral plasticity" in which the brain re-arranges its own structure under certain conditions (Begley S 2008, Doidge N 2007).

Other teams of researchers have, moreover, demonstrated that blood circulation to the centres involved in the management of emotions (thalamus, basal ganglia) was reduced in the case of people with fibromyalgia (Kwiatek R & coll 2000, Chen JJ & coll 2007). This hypovascularization could also affect the cerebral cortex (and the gray matter) and account for the phenomenon described in the previous paragraph.

This phenomenon also contributes to the understanding of common observations concerning those with fibromyalgia: depressive states, palpitations, dizziness when changing position, sleep disorder, excessive sweating, etc. The thalamus is in fact at the centre of an extraordinary set of sensory and motor functions while working closely with other cerebral nerve structures such as the hypothalamus and the pituitary gland, which are involved with the two principal systems that control the internal balance of the body: the automatic nervous system (which includes the sympathetic and the parasympathetic nervous systems) and the endocrine system (which concerns the various hormones, including the growth hormone, the thyroid hormone or thyroxin, the adrenal hormones including cortisone, etc.).

## Anomaly in spinal cord activity

In the case of animal models of diffuse pain, it has been demonstrated on numerous occasions that the spinal cord undergoes structural and chemical changes. Certain nerve cells atrophy whereas others multiply or transform in an aberrant manner (D'Mello R & Dickenson AH 2008, Ikeda H & coll 2009, Inoue K & Tsuda M 2009). The activities of certain excitatory substances and their receptors become increasingly significant. This is the case of glutamate and one of its receptors, known as the NMDA receptor (for N-Methyl-D-Aspartate).

In the case of people with fibromyalgia, it is impossible to confirm such observations directly for an obvious reason: we cannot access the nerve tissue without the risk of permanent consequences. Nevertheless, using indirect means, researchers have been able to demonstrate that an identical phenomenon should exist in the case of these people. Blocking NMDA receptors, for example, (by injecting ketamine close to the spine) relieved the pain significantly. Recourse to approaches based on psychophysical principles (temporal summation of pain) has also led to the same conclusions (Price DD & coll 2002, Staud R & coll 2007).

## PAIN THAT IS NOT SLOWED DOWN: DYSFUNCTION OF THE ENDOGEN MECHANISMS OF INHIBITION

The human body is composed of opposing mechanisms that maintain an internal balance. There are many examples. Insulin and glucagon work in opposing manners to find a balance and adjust blood sugar levels. The sympathetic and parasympathetic nervous systems (called the "autonomic nervous system" because they function autonomously in the body, without requiring conscious effort) act in a synchronous manner and their efforts are opposite. Pain is not different. Nature has provided mechanisms that both promote pain (for the purpose of protecting against dangerous injuries) and others that strive to neutralize it. These latter are called "diffuse noxious inhibitory controls" or DNIC. We have known about them only since the end of the 1970s (Besson JM & coll 1975). Increasingly, it is believed that "accelerator" and "inhibitor" systems are in constant equilibrium in the healthy person but that the patient with fibromyalgia suffers from a lack of balance with respect to these two mechanisms (**Figure 5**). This lack of balance could be caused by an increase in the pain information that is sent to the brain and/or a reduction in the response of the mechanisms normally involved in neutralizing such information, the DNICs.

FIGURE 5 : Theoretical model explaining the pain of fibromyalgia

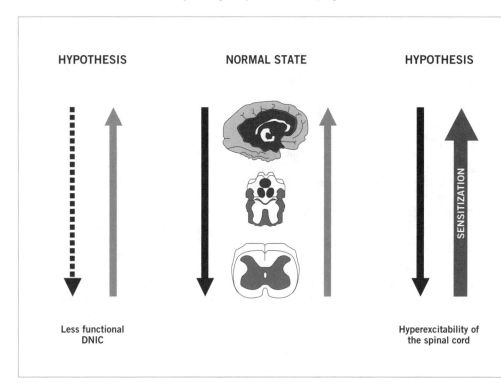

HYPOTHESIS        NORMAL STATE        HYPOTHESIS

SENSITIZATION

Less functional
DNIC

Hyperexcitability of
the spinal cord

Two hypothetical mechanisms. In the centre, during the normal state, the pain information that is sent to the brain is controlled by equivalent inhibiting responses from the superior centres. No pain is perceptible. In the case of a dysfunction of the DNICs (left hypothesis), and/or the presence of a hyperexcitation of the spinal cord (right hypothesis), the balance is broken and the pain information is predominant.

The DNICs are located at the top of the cervical spinal cord (under the nerve centres of the brain) in the region called the brainstem. They produce chemical substances that slow pain, specifically serotonin, noradrenalin, and dopamine. The circulating levels (in the liquid that bathes the central nervous system or the cerebrospinal fluid, or even the blood) of these substances are almost systematically reduced in the case of people with fibromyalgia (Russell IJ & coll 1992, Russell IJ 1998). The decrease of these substances in the biological liquids reflects decreases in concentrations in the nervous system as well. A shortage of one or more of these substances will certainly disrupt the inhibitory functions of the central nervous system. Finally, recent studies that were also based on psychophysical principles have also confirmed the inability of the central inhibitory systems to reduce the pain of patients with fibromyalgia (Julien N & coll 2005, Goffaux P & coll 2009).

If we were to caricaturize the situation experienced by patients with fibromyalgia based on recent discoveries, we would say that the pain of fibromyalgia is like a car that is racing out of control: the accelerator is stuck and the brakes don't work adequately!

# 4. ETIOLOGICAL HYPOTHESES

Humans are beings that reason. They try to understand the phenomena that concern them and their environment. When they do not understand, they become anxious, concerned and start to look for explanations. In the case of fibromyalgia, complete and precise explanations are still to come. We still have not identified the series of cellular and infracellular anomalies of the nervous system, which is an important step if we want to be able to offer a specific, more targeted treatment some day. And as if that were not enough, the individual with fibromyalgia must also deal with the resistance of certain health professionals who still have doubts with respect to the existence of such a clinical problem. Therefore, it is just as important to take stock of our knowledge concerning the causes that may be involved in fibromyalgia. Nevertheless, we must admit that the causes indicated in this chapter are only possibilities. No solid scientific proof has ever established any of the hypotheses. Moreover, in the case of self-administered questionnaires, no cause is identifiable in the case of more than 55% of the patients.

## Genetics

When the families of people with fibromyalgia are studied, researchers never identify more than 10% of the first-line descendents as having fibromyalgia (Arsenault P & coll 2007, Stisi S & coll 2008, Williams DA & Clauw DJ 2009, Bradley LA 2009). This observation confirms that fibromyalgia is not transmitted by only one gene. As a result, it does not follow the transmission mode described by Gregor Mendel (recessive gene, dominant gene). If genetic baggage is involved, it must also include several genes and it follows the polygenic mode of transmission.

To date, a few potential genes have presented anomalies that seem specific to the fibromyalgic population. These genes are related to the neurotransmitters already cited and are involved in the inhibition of pain (serotonin, noradrenalin and dopamine).

A first gene, which appears to be involved, takes part in the production of an enzyme that is involved in the transformation of dopamine and noradrenalin, COMT (Carbamyl-O-Methyl-Transferase). A second gene (5HTTPR) is involved with a protein that carries serotonin. A third gene (DRD3Ser9Gly), which was discovered recently, is related to a dopaminergic function. And a final gene, 5HTR2A, also plays a role in the metabolism of serotonin. Other genes will probably be added to this list since genetic work on fibromyalgia is just beginning (Cohen H & coll 2009, Potvin S & coll 2009, Tander B & coll 2008).

## A physical injury

Many patients with fibromyalgia claim that their condition developed following an accident or a major physical injury. Others report slight, but repeated, injuries. Injuries to the cervical spine, particularly whiplash, are among the most frequently identified to date (Buskila D et Neumann L 2000, Banic B et coll 2004, McLean SA et coll 2005). Proof of a direct link is still to be made since recent studies do not always show this causal association (Shir Y & coll 2006, Tishler M & coll 2010).

When they are asked questions about their pain history, many patients with fibromyalgia report an initial traumatic event and a localized injury. This injury either resisted the therapeutic interventions offered or took a long time to be treated. The phenomenon has also been reported by various specialists (dentist, gynaecologist, gastroenterologist, etc.). It appears increasingly obvious that, in the case of certain individuals, unrelieved pain quickly becomes a threat for the central nervous system, and there is a major risk of sensitization and even chronicity.

## An infection

Sometimes fibromyalgia appears following an infection. For these patients, the clinical characteristics of fibromyalgia are no different than those observed in the presence of other suspected etiologies. The potential infections identified include: viral infections (parvovirus, Epstein-Barr virus, hepatitis B virus, hepatitis C virus, HIV, etc.), bacterial infections (mycoplasma, chlamydia, etc.) and parasitic infections (Lyme disease in particular). Researchers are still studying the possibility that, in the case of these patients, the immune system suffered certain disturbances following such infections. Since many immune cells are anchored in the nervous structures (in particular the glial cells), certain authors believe that their own groups of hormones stimulate the nervous system, and make it hyperexcitable (Inoue K & coll 2009, Vallejo R & coll 2010). In the case of rodents, when immune factors such as interleukin-6 (which is produced by the immune cells) are administered, pain states appear and resemble those experienced by people with fibromyalgia in many respects (Dina OA et coll 2008).

## An "emotional" injury

In clinical settings, a certain proportion of people with fibromyalgia denies any physical trauma, but confirms that they have experienced serious emotional stresses at one or more times during their lives. The most frequently documented emotional stresses include: sexual abuse during childhood or adolescence, major losses (death of parents, etc.), major depression (unique or recurring), etc. Science is not yet capable of explaining all the repercussions such injuries have on the central nervous system, but it has been established that sensory and emotional experiences restructure the brain either favourably or unfavourably (Begley S 2006, Doidge N 2008). The other side of the coin in the case of cerebral plasticity may well be pain.

## Sleep disorders

Since people with fibromyalgia generally report sleep that does not restore them and serious daytime fatigue, many clinicians attribute the development of the pain condition to the sleep disorders. Various research models have demonstrated that serious sleep disorders increase the perception of pain that is induced experimentally (Lavigne GJ 2010). Dr. Moldofsky (1975), one of the defenders of this theory was, moreover, one of the first to demonstrate that, during the deep sleep phase (delta waves or Phase IV waves), alpha waves (waking waves) have been found in people with fibromyalgia. The chemical substances that repair tissues, specifically muscles, are released during the deep sleep phase. These substances include the growth hormone and the insulin-like growth factor 1 (ILGF-1). These deficiencies could be responsible for multiple changes in both muscles and cerebral structures and result in the pain symptoms of people with fibromyalgia.

## 5. DIAGNOSTIC APPROACHES

At present, there are no infallible diagnostic methods for confirming the existence of fibromyalgia. There is no blood or urine marker that would prove its existence. The same applies to x-ray tests. The levels of certain substances do appear to be modified by fibromyalgia (increase of substance P in the cerebrospinal fluid (CSF), increase of nerve growth factor (NGF) in the blood, decrease of the insulin-like growth factor or ILGF-1 in the blood and the CSF, decrease in levels of serotonin and noradrenalin in the CSF, etc.), but none can be verified in hospital laboratories. Moreover, there is still no certainty that such chemical variations occur exclusively in the case of people with fibromyalgia.

The diagnosis is based on the symptoms reported by the patients, the physical examination and certain blood tests that serve to exclude other medical conditions associated with pain (thyroid problems, diabetes, lupus erythematosus, rheumatoid arthritis, etc.). Generally, the diagnosis is established by means of a simple questionnaire, and the physical examination and blood tests can often be omitted.

### Diagnostic criteria in the medical questionnaire

The criteria required for considering a diagnosis of fibromyalgia include:
- Diffuse pain in all four quadrants of the body as well as the notochord (**Figure 1**, page 36);
- Constant pain lasting at least three months. As a result, pain that comes and goes cannot be retained for establishing the diagnosis.

Fibromyalgia is often accompanied by other clinical symptoms such as abdominal pain (intestinal or vesical), headaches, troubles with concentration and memory (the renowned fibro fog), whitish discoloration and pain of the extremities in response to cold (Raynaud's syndrome, etc.). Although these symptoms are not necessary to make a diagnosis, they are very common in the case of people with fibromyalgia.

### Criteria for the clinical examination

During the clinical examination, the physician will make a painstaking physical evaluation of the patient. He/she will make sure there are no clinical signs indicating another disease that would explain the patient's pain (such as inflamed joints and thickening of the synovial membranes for rheumatoid arthritis, an increase in the volume of the thyroid gland for hypothyroidism, problems with reflexes, etc.).

Then the physician will examine the sensitive of various tender spots (18 specific locations in the musculature). By using his/her thumb to apply pressure not exceeding 4kg per cm$^2$ in area (until the base of a fingernail turns white) on each of the tender spots, the clinician counts the number of painful spots. The American Rheumatism Association has indicated that 11 out of the 18 points must be sensitive in order to confirm the diagnosis. Although this examination is still done in clinics, its pertinence is now being questioned (Baldry P 2007, Harth M & Nielson WR 2007, Wilke WS 2009). Clinicians are waiting for new guidelines for confirming the diagnosis of fibromyalgia.

### Laboratory blood tests

The blood tests requested in case of doubt to eliminate diseases other than fibromyalgia include: complete blood count (count of the various types of blood cells), the sedimentation rate of red blood cells and the level of C-reactive proteins (these proteins confirm or discount the presence of inflammation), blood sugar level (to eliminate diabetes), TSH (thyroid stimulating hormone; bloods levels increase in the case of hypothyroidism), and rheumatoid factor (that may occur in the presence of rheumatoid arthritis).

The practitioner generally completes the assessment with an evaluation of mineral levels (sodium, potassium, calcium, phosphorus), liver enzymes (AST, ALT), the amount of creatine kinase (CPK), a muscular enzyme, and through a verification of kidney function (creatinine level of the blood, urea, and a urine analysis).

Although all these diagnostic steps are always recommended during medical consultations, fibromyalgia can often be easily identified by means of simple medical questioning. Repeated blood tests and x-rays are not recommended if the clinical situation of the patients remains stable. However, physicians should avoid diagnosing fibromyalgia for every little hurt and pain, and neglect investigating new symptoms that present potential risks (bleeding, fever, significant weight loss, unusual and serious pain, etc.)! People with fibromyalgia may suffer new clinical problems just like any other patient, and must discuss them with their physicians, regardless of the welcome they receive.

## 6. THERAPEUTIC APPROACHES

### PHARMACOLOGICAL APPROACHES

### Stimulating the body's braking system

For several years, the pharmacological treatment of fibromyalgia was based on tricyclic antidepressants (called that as a result of their three cycle molecular structure) and muscular relaxants. Since the few clinical tests were concentrated on these molecules, the therapeutic options were rather limited. The improvement in the clinical condition of the patients treated in this manner suggested that once the "depressive" component was targeted and treated, the pain could be controlled.

In recent years, as a result of new knowledge about fibromyalgia (central sensitization and inhibition dysfunction), new avenues have been explored (Arsenault P & Potvin S 2007, Arsenault P & Thiffault R 2010a,b).

By targeting the neurotransmitters involved in the inhibition of pain, therapeutic tests have been conducted using pharmacological agonists to imitate (or optimize) the DNICs (the famous natural internal braking system). The thinking was that increasing serotonin or noradrenalin in the central nervous system could help optimize the pain inhibition mechanisms (**Figure 6**, p. 43).

FIGURE 6 : Theoretical model of a "lack of endogen inhibition" (DNIC dysfunction) in fibromyalgia and some of the appropriate medications

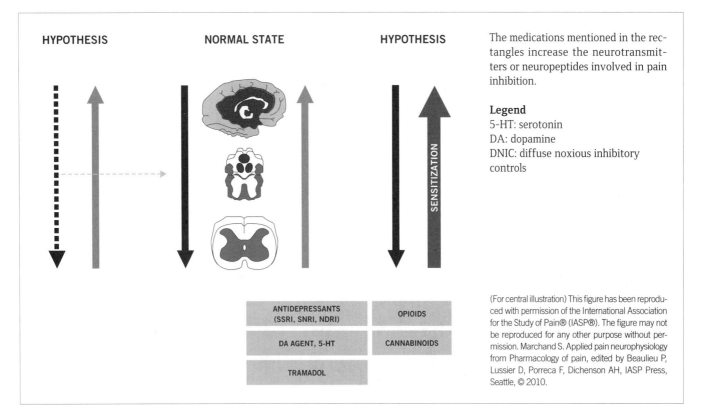

HYPOTHESIS        NORMAL STATE        HYPOTHESIS

SENSITIZATION

ANTIDEPRESSANTS (SSRI, SNRI, NDRI)

DA AGENT, 5-HT

TRAMADOL

OPIOIDS

CANNABINOIDS

The medications mentioned in the rectangles increase the neurotransmitters or neuropeptides involved in pain inhibition.

**Legend**
5-HT: serotonin
DA: dopamine
DNIC: diffuse noxious inhibitory controls

(For central illustration) This figure has been reproduced with permission of the International Association for the Study of Pain® (IASP®). The figure may not be reproduced for any other purpose without permission. Marchand S. Applied pain neurophysiology from Pharmacology of pain, edited by Beaulieu P, Lussier D, Porreca F, Dichenson AH, IASP Press, Seattle, © 2010.

In order to increase the levels of serotonin or noradrenalin, antidepressants belonging to one or the following classes must be used: selective serotonin reuptake inhibitors (SSRIs), serotonin and noradrenalin reuptake inhibitors (SNRIs) and the norepinephrine-dopamine reuptake inhibitors (NDRIs). The potential therapeutic options are presented in **Figure 7** (page 45) and **Table 1** (page 44). Of all these inhibitors, the only one which, according to Health Canada, is officially indicated for the treatment of fibromyalgia, is duloxetine. Venlafaxine, which acts on the same neurotransmitters (serotonin and noradrenalin), but at higher doses, has been the object of "open" studies, but there have been no solid clinical trials to date. As for all the other antidepressants, and particularly serotonin reuptake inhibitors, only citalopram, paroxetine and fluoxetine seem to demonstrate certain analgesic virtues for people with fibromyalgia.

TABLE 1 : Medications that are likely to optimize the "braking" activity in the response to pain in people suffering
from fibromyalgia and their side effects

| Medication | Dosage (initial - maximum) | Undesirable effects | |
|---|---|---|---|
| **Selective serotonin reuptake inhibitors (SSRIs)** | | | |
| Fluoxetine | • 10 mg – 40 mg (1X/day) | • Anxiety and nervousness<br>• Decreased appetite<br>• Diarrhea<br>• Fatigue or weakness<br>• Headaches | • Nausea<br>• Drowsiness<br>• Hyperhidrosis<br>• Shaking<br>• Sleep disorders |
| Citalopram | • 10 mg – 40 mg (1X/day) | • Fatigue<br>• Drowsiness<br>• Dry mouth<br>• Hyperhidrosis<br>• Shaking | • Headaches<br>• Vertigo<br>• Sleep disorders<br>• Nausea and vomiting<br>• Diarrhea |
| **Selective noradrenaline reuptake inhibitors (SNRIs)** | | | |
| Duloxetine | • 30 mg – 120 mg (1X/day) | • Nausea<br>• Dry mouth<br>• Constipation<br>• Decreased appetite | • Fatigue<br>• Drowsiness<br>• Sweating |
| Venlafaxine | • 37.5 mg – 300 mg (1X/day) | • Headaches<br>• Nausea<br>• Dizziness<br>• Insomnia | • Dry mouth<br>• Decreased libido<br>• Hyperhidrosis |
| **Other antidepressants** | | | |
| Bupropion | • 100 mg – 300 mg (1X/day) | • Dry mouth<br>• Nausea and vomiting<br>• Abdominal pain | • Constipation<br>• Insomnia<br>• Headaches |
| **Cannabinoids** | | | |
| Nabilone | • 0.25 mg – 5 mg (from 1X/day at bedtime to 2X/day) | • Clumsiness<br>• Headaches<br>• Dry mouth | • Drowsiness<br>• Dizziness |
| **Dopamine agonists** | | | |
| Pramipexole | • 0.25 mg – 5 mg (from 1X/day at bedtime to 2X/day) | • Nausea<br>• Hallucinations<br>• Dizziness<br>• Drowsiness | • Headaches<br>• Confusion<br>• Weakness<br>• Constipation |

**Legend**
1X/day: once a day

Arsenault P, Thiffault R. La fibromyalgie II – Aider le système nerveux à « appliquer les freins ». Le Médecin du Québec 2010; 45 (4): 65-7. ©FMOQ. Reproduction rights granted by editor.

Another option for stimulating the braking function, which is less popular and subject to controversy, is recourse to opioids (morphine, to a certain extent) and cannabinoids (molecules similar to cannabis). Since the central nervous system produces endorphin and cannabinoids, it would seem logical to assume that administering one or the other of these substances should activate the body's braking system. Unfortunately, scientific proof of such behaviour is poor and even lacking. There are no articles demonstrating the analgesic effects of cannabinoids (in particular nabilone), and reports of the effectiveness of opioids are anecdotal. Moreover, in the case of opioids, certain clinicians have stressed the potential complications of long-term use: tolerance, increasing doses, dependency, decline in sexual hormones, and even the possibility of provoking a reaction opposite to the one sought, namely an increase in pain (referred to as "hyperalgia" that is induced by the opioids). As a result, clinicians tend to use opioids only in the case of extreme pain that cannot be controlled by other analgesic molecules.

Despite this knowledge, it is surprising to note that Europeans have been using a medication that exercises "serotoninergic", "noradrenigeric" and opioid activities with success for over 20 years. This medication is tramadol.

## Reducing the excitement of the central nervous system: releasing the accelerator

The molecules that exercise a stabilizing (or tranquilizing) function on the central nervous system belong principally to five classes of medication: anticonvulsants, "tricyclic" and tetracyclic antidepressants, antiarrhythmics and NMDA-receptor antagonists (N-methyl-D-Aspartate) (**Figure 7**, **Tables 2** and **3**, pages 46 and 47). Despite the stabilizing potential of opioids and cannabinoids, we tend to consider them as agents that act above all on the braking system rather than the nerve network that carries painful stimuli to the brain.

FIGURE 7 : Theoretical model of the "hyperexcitability of the central nervous system" in fibromyalgia and some of the appropriate medications

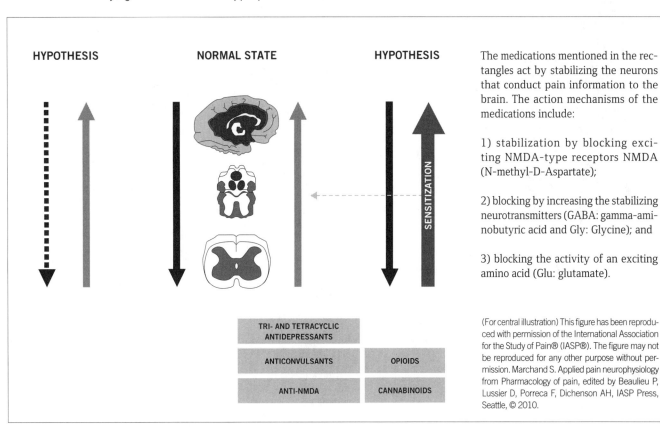

The medications mentioned in the rectangles act by stabilizing the neurons that conduct pain information to the brain. The action mechanisms of the medications include:

1) stabilization by blocking exciting NMDA-type receptors NMDA (N-methyl-D-Aspartate);

2) blocking by increasing the stabilizing neurotransmitters (GABA: gamma-aminobutyric acid and Gly: Glycine); and

3) blocking the activity of an exciting amino acid (Glu: glutamate).

(For central illustration) This figure has been reproduced with permission of the International Association for the Study of Pain® (IASP®). The figure may not be reproduced for any other purpose without permission. Marchand S. Applied pain neurophysiology from Pharmacology of pain, edited by Beaulieu P, Lussier D, Porreca F, Dichenson AH, IASP Press, Seattle, © 2010.

TABLE 2 : Anticonvulsants used in the treatment of fibromyalgia and their side effects

## ANTICONVULSANTS USED IN THE TREATMENT OF FIBROMYALGIA AND THEIR SIDE EFFECTS

| Medication | Dosage<br>• Initial<br>• Usual<br>• Maximum | Most common<br>undesirable effects | Precautions |
|---|---|---|---|
| Pregabalin | • 25 mg at bedtime<br>• 75 mg, 2X/day<br>• 300 mg, 2X/day | • Dizziness<br>• Drowsiness<br>• Weight gain<br>• Peripheral oedema<br>• Infections | In case of:<br>• Class III or IV heart failure<br>• kidney failure<br>• Concomitant use of thiazolidinediones |
| Gabapentin | • 100 mg at bedtime<br>• 300 mg, 3X/day + 600 mg at bedtime<br>• 3600 mg per day, 3X or 4X per day | • Drowsiness<br>• Vertigo<br>• Heart failure<br>• Blurred vision<br>• Muscle cramps<br>• Peripheral oedema<br>• Shaking<br>• Fatigue and weakness | In case of:<br>• Class III or IV heart failure<br>• kidney failure |
| Topiramate | • 25 mg at bedtime<br>• 50 mg – 100 mg, 2X/day<br>• 200 mg, 2X/day | • Distal paresthesia of the limbs<br>• Vertigo and dizziness<br>• Drowsiness<br>• Asthenia<br>• Anorexia<br>• Various neuropsychic disorders (anxiety, etc.)<br>• Blurred vision (reversible)<br>• Metabolic acidosis | Increased risk in case of:<br>• non-anion gap metabolic acidosis<br>• urinary lithiasis<br><br>In case of:<br>• kidney or liver failure |
| Lamotrigine | • 25 mg<br>• 50 mg – 100 mg<br>• 100 mg, 2X/day | • Drowsiness<br>• Dizziness<br>• Vertigo<br>• Ataxia<br>• Asthenia<br>• Headaches<br>• Blurred vision (reversible)<br>• Double vision<br>• Skin rashes | • Initial dosage of 25 mg to be increased very slowly<br>• In case of kidney failure<br>• Stevens-Johnson syndrome reported (vigilance required) |
| Levetiracetam | • 250 mg at bedtime<br>• 500 mg, 2X/day<br>• 1500 mg, 2X/day | • Drowsiness<br>• Asthenia<br>• Vomiting<br>• Headaches<br>• Urinary symptoms<br>• Ataxia<br>• Weakness<br>• Dizziness<br>• Infections<br>• Disrupted thinking<br>• Amnesia<br>• Anxiety | • In case of kidney failure<br>• Risk of a reduction in the number of various cell lines (check complete blood count) |

**Legend**
1X/day: once a day

Arsenault P, Thiffault R. La fibromyalgie – Aider le système nerveux à « lever le pied ». Le Médecin du Québec 2010; 45 (3): 61-4. ©FMOQ. Reproduction rights granted by editor.

TABLE 3: Tricyclic and tetracyclic antidepressants used in the treatment of fibromyalgia and their side effects

## TRICYCLIC AND TETRACYCLIC ANTIDEPRESSANTS USED IN THE TREATMENT OF FIBROMYALGIA AND THEIR SIDE EFFECTS

| Medication | Dosage • Initial • Usual • Maximum | Most common undesirable effects | Precautions |
|---|---|---|---|
| Amitriptyline | • 10 mg at bedtime • 25 mg – 50 mg at bedtime • 300 mg at bedtime | • Drowsiness • Dry mucous membranes • Dizziness • Orthostatic hypotension | To be avoided in case of: • glaucoma • prostatism • arrhythmia |
| Desipramine | • 10 mg at bedtime • 25 mg – 50 mg • 300 mg | • Drowsiness • Dry mucous membranes • Constipation • Dizziness • Orthostatic hypotension | To be avoided in case of: • glaucoma • prostatism • arrhythmia |
| Mirtazapine | • 15 mg at bedtime • 15 mg – 30 mg at bedtime • 30 mg – 45 mg at bedtime | • Drowsiness • Increased appetite • Weight gain • Dry mouth • Constipation • Asthenia • Dizziness | • In case of kidney or liver failure • Caution is the presence of arrhythmia |
| Trazodone | • 25 mg at bedtime • 50 mg – 100 mg per day, 2X/day • 400 mg per day, 2X or 3X per day | • Drowsiness • Dizziness • Dry mouth • Headache • Blurred vision • Nausea or vomiting • Fatigue • Constipation | To be avoided in case of: • glaucoma • prostatism • arrhythmia |

**Legend**
1X/day: once a day

Arsenault P, Thiffault R. La fibromyalgie – Aider le système nerveux à « lever le pied ». Le Médecin du Québec 2010; 45 (3): 61-4. ©FMOQ. Reproduction rights granted by editor.

Anticonvulsants reduce the reactions of the neurons that result in the conduction of the nervous messages (or "nervous influx"). To simply this, let us say that the neurons can be stabilized by various mechanisms that act on a cellular level, and that anticonvulsants are classified according to the mechanism(s) they use (**Figure 8**).

Anticonvulsants stabilize the neurons of the central nervous system, by blocking the ion channels (calcium or sodium), increasing the level of certain inhibiting neuropeptides (gamma-aminobutyric acid or GABA and glycine or GLY), or by inhibiting the transmission of glutamate (glutamate: an exciting amino acid). The action mechanisms of the medications are illustrated in this figure.

FIGURE 8 : Anticonvulsant action mechanisms

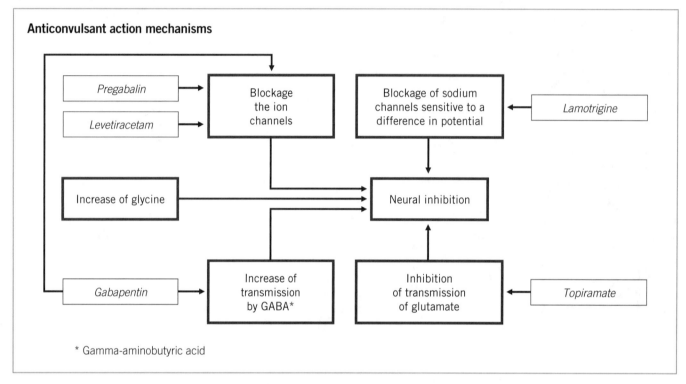

Arsenault P, Thiffault R. La fibromyalgie – Aider le système nerveux à « lever le pied ». Le Médecin du Québec 2010; 45 (3): 61-4. ©FMOQ. Reproduction rights granted by editor.

The anticonvulsants that are frequently used in fibromyalgia include: pregabalin and gabapentin (the "gabapentenoids"), topiramate and lamotrigine. Of all these substances, the only one that is recognized by Canadian regulatory organizations (Health Canada) is pregabalin. The antalgic, anxiolytic and sedative effects of pregabalin make it a weapon of choice in the treatment of fibromyalgia.

The tricyclic antidepressants (amitryptiline, nortryptiline) are without question the oldest molecules used to treat the pain of fibromyalgia. These are the drugs that have been the object of the largest number of clinical studies. Unfortunately, they are not without side effects (dry mouth, constipation, urinary retention, etc.), and should be avoided in the presence of glaucoma, urinary problems and cardiac arrhythmia. The tetracyclic antidepressants (mirtazapine), which appeared at the beginning of this century, have effects similar to the tricyclic antidepressants and a similar side effect profile. Few studies have been conducted but they are occasionally used by certain clinicians on an empirical basis.

The antiarrhythmics, which are interesting on a "theoretical" basis, are of no interest for the treatment of fibromyalgia at present. The side effects of these medications and their contraindications (table) limit their use considerably. Moreover, scientific reports on their effect on people with fibromyalgia are rare.

The most frequently-used NMDA-receptor antagonists include ketamine, methadone and dextromethorphan (contained in cough syrups!). In order to block NMDA receptors using dextromethorphan, the subjects would have to take such large quantities that they would not be able to tolerate the side effects. As a result, dextromethorphan is not used. Ketamine blocks NMDA receptors quite well, but causes serious sedation and there is a risk of hallucinations. There are no publications supporting its use for fibromyalgia. Finally, methadone, which exercises anti-NMDA activities as well as opioid activities, has never been evaluated in therapeutic studies and could cause the inconveniences explained previously.

## NON-PHARMACOLOGICAL APPROACHES

The non-pharmacological approaches include all of the means of intervention that do not involve the use of medication. Some of these approaches that are prescribed by physicians and others belong to a vast field of approaches referred to as complementary and alternative medicine (CAM). The non-pharmacological approaches that are not considered complementary and alternative medicine and that are no longer used to treat fibromyalgia belong to two large groups: physical approaches and psychotherapy.

### Physical approaches

One of the greatest certainties when it comes to people with fibromyalgia is the benefits of physical exercise. There are hundreds of references to the benefits of exercise in the scientific literature. No additional proof is required. But what type of exercise should we focus on? The answer is easy: medium or long-term aerobic exercise! Caution and patience are required. After several months of inactivity, why subject your body to energy demands that it is no longer used to responding to! It is recommended that you start with a physical activity you like and a programme that takes several months that will enable you to increase your pace slowly. Certain patients will choose walking, for example, starting with a few minutes a day and then progressing until they can walk at a rapid pace (or even run) for 30 to 40 minutes at the end of three to six months. It is important to note that relapses are possible and you should not get discouraged. Some days will be more difficult than others. You will step back and move ahead. But the benefits are well worth it! Physical exercise improves general circulation, stimulates the production of several hormones, improves sleep quality, acts as an antidepressant and has numerous other beneficial effects that it would take too long to list here.

The other physical approaches that are not considered part of complementary and alternative medicine (CAM) include physiotherapy and occupational therapy. We are of the opinion that these approaches should only be used for very specific purposes: providing an exercise programme that is adapted to the clinical condition of the patients as well as the tools needed to launch such programmes. There is no point in trying to treat a specific musculoskeletal structure unless, of course, it has caused an additional injury. People with fibromyalgia will never find themselves in wheelchairs unless they have another illness or handicap or unless they want to.

### Psychotherapy

People with fibromyalgia are often surprised to find their physician referring them to a psychologist or a mental health professional. They often have the impression that their doctor considers their problem to be imaginary, namely created in their head. In actual fact, the purpose of most of these referrals is often to highlight false beliefs, poor means for managing pain cognitively and/or emotionally, even in terms of social relations. They are also intended to give patients the psychological tools they need to face their pain in the most intense times. Numerous articles published about pain in the last decade have clearly indicated that the perception of pain and its "management" are inevitably handled by cerebral and psychic mechanisms and it is possible reduce pain through certain mental activities. The psychotherapeutic approach the most often studied is that of cognitive-behaviour therapy (Thieme K & Gracely RH 2009, Häuser W & coll 2010). This approach has proven very effective for several people with fibromyalgia.

# 7. CONCLUSION

Fibromyalgia has been the subject of numerous documents and many web pages in recent years. While many of these sources of information are based on reliable references, others are based on simple reports of isolated cases and should be interpreted with caution. The data provided in this article is the most prevalent at this stage in the development of our knowledge and is based on excellent scientific proof. A growing number of studies throughout the world is progressively changing the way in which we view this syndrome and will indicate the best means for dealing with it. Research teams located around the world are working on trying to understand what goes on in the person with fibromyalgia, "from cellular interactions to social interactions". For the time being, the best approaches for relieving a given patient must be determined through trial and error. Pluridisciplinary interventions have the advantage of addressing the various dimensions of the human experience. As a result, they are given preference. Once the biological markers are identified, it will be easier to specifically target the interventions that will be effective. We believe that, with the courage and patience of patients and clinicians, we will vanquish fibromyalgia one day!

# REFERENCES

- Arsenault P, Marchand S. Synthèse des mécanismes impliqués dans un syndrome douloureux complexe : la fibromyalgie. Douleur et Analgésie 20(4) : 200-212. 2007.
- Arsenault P, Potvin S. Interventions pharmacologiques chez le patient fibromyalgique : par ou commencer? Douleur et Analgésie 20(4) : 227- 233. 2007.
- Arsenault P, Thiffault R. La fibromyalgie : aider le système nerveux à « Lever le pied ». Le Médecin du Québec 45(3) : 61-64. 2010a.
- Arsenault, P, Thiffault R. La fibromyalgie-II. Aider le système nerveux à « appliquer les freins ». Le Médecin du Québec 45(4) : 65-67. 2010b.
- Baldry P. Large tender areas, not discrete points, observed in patients with fibromyalgia. Acupunct Med 25(4) : 203. 2007.
- Banic B, Petersen-Felix S, Andersen OK, Radanov BP, Villiger PM, Arendt-Nielsen L, Curatolo M. Evidence for spinal cord hypersensitivity in chronic pain after whiplash injury and in fibromyalgia. Pain 107(1-2) : 7-15. 2004.
- Begley Sharon. Entrainer votre cerveau. Transformer votre cerveau. Ariane Edition Inc. 2008.
- Besson JM, Guibaud G, Le Bars D. Descending inhibitory influences exerted by the brain stem upon the activities of dorsal horn lamina V cells induced by intra-arterial injection of bradykinin into the limbs. J Physiol 248(3) : 725-739. 1975.
- Bradley LA. Pathophysiology of fibromyalgia . Am J Med 122(12 Suppl) : S22-S30. 2009.
- Buskila D, Neumann L. Musculoskeletal injury as a trigger for fibromyalgia/posttraumatic fibromyalgia. Curr Rheumatol Rep 2(2) : 104-108. 2000.
- Chen JJ, Wang JY, Chang YM, Su SY, Chang CT, Sun SS, Kao CH, Lee CC. Regional cerebral blood flow between primary and concomitant fibromyalgia patients : a possible way to differentiate concomitant fibromyalgia from the primary disease. Scan J Rheumatol 36(3) : 226-232. 2007.
- Cohen H, Neumann L, Glazer Y, Ebstein RP, Buskila D. The relationship between a common catechol-O-methyltransferase (COMT) polymorphism val(158) met and fibromyalgia. Clin Exp Rheumatol 27(5 Suppl 56) : S51-S56. 2009.
- de Souza JB, Potvin S, Goffaux P, Charest J, Marchand S. The deficit of pain inhibition in fibromyalgia is more pronounced in patients with comorbid depressive symptoms. Clin J Pain 25(2) : 123-127. 2009a.
- de Souza JB, Goffaux P, Julien N, Potvin S, Charest J, Marchand S. Fibromyalgia subgroups : profiling distinct subgroups using the Fibromyalgia Impact Questionnaire. A preliminary study. Rheumatol Int 29(5) : 509-515. 2009b.
- Dina OA, Green PG, Levine JD. Role of interleukin-6 in chronic muscle hyperalgesic priming. Neuroscience 152(2) : 521-525. 2008.
- D'Mello R, Dickenson AH. Spinal cord mechanism of pain. Br J Anaesth 101(1) : 8-16. 2008.
- Doidge Norman. Les étonnants pouvoirs de transformation du cerveau. Guérir grâce à la neuroplasticité. Edition Belfond. 2007.
- Dotson VM, Davatzikos C, Kraut MA, Resnick SM. Depressive symptoms and brain volumes in older adults : a longitudinal magnetic resonance imaging study. J Psychiatry neurosci 3495) : 367-375. 2009.
- Frodi TS, Koutsouleris N, Bottlender R, Born C, Jäger M, Scupin I, Reiser M, Möller HJ, Meisenzahl EM. Depression-related variation in brain morphology over 3 years : effect of stress? Arch Gen Psychiatry 65(10) : 1156-1165. 2008.
- Giesecke T, Williams DA, Harris RE, Cupps TR, Tian X, Tian TX, Gracely RH, Clauw DJ. Subgrouping of fibromyalgia patients on the basis of pressure-pain thresholds and psychological factors. Arthritis Rheum 48(10) : 2916-2922. 2003.
- Goffaux P, Redmond WJ, Rainville P, Marchand S. Descending analgesia- when the spine echoes what the brain expects. Pain 130(1-2) : 137-143. 2007.
- Hart M, Nielson WR. The fibromyalgia tender points : use them or lose them? A brief review of the controversy. J Rheumatol 34(5) : 914-922. 2007
- Häuser W, Thieme K, Turk DC. Guidelines on the management of fibromyalgia syndrome - a systematic review. Eur J Pain 14(1) : 5-10. 2010.
- Ikeda H, Kiritoshi T, Murase K. Synaptic plasticity in the spinal dorsal horn. Neurosci Res 64(2) : 133-136.2009.
- Inoue K, Tsuda M. Microglia and neuropathic pain. Glia 57(14) : 1469-1479. 2009.
- Julien N, Goffaux P, Arsenault P, Marchand S. Widespread pain in fibromyalgia is related to a deficit of endogenous pain inhibition. Pain 114(1-2) : 295-302. 2005.
- Kuchinad A, Schweinhardt P, Seminowicz DA, Wood PB, Chizh BA, Bushnell MC. Accelerated brain gray matter loss in fibromyalgia patients : premature aging of the brain? J Neurosci 27(15) : 4004-4007. 2007.
- Kwiatek R, Barnden L, Tedman R, Jarrett R, Chew J, Rowe C, Pile K. Regional cerebral blood flow in fibromyalgia : single-photon-emission computed tomography evidence of reduction in the pontine tegmentum and thalami. Arthritis Rheum 43(12) : 2823-2833. 2000.
- Lavigne GJ. Effect of sleep restriction on pain perception : towards greater attention! Pain 148(1) : 6-7. 2010.
- Marchand S. Applied pain neurophysiology from Pharmacology of pain, edited by Beaulieu P, Lussier D, Porreca F, Dichenson AH, IASP Press, Seattle, ©2010.
- McLean SA, Clauw DJ, Abelson JL, Liberzon I. The development of persistent pain and psychological morbidity after motor vehicle collision : integrating the potential role of stress response systems into a biopsychosocial model. Psychosom Med 67(5) : 783-790. 2005.
- Moldofsky H, Scarisbrick P, England R, Smythe H. Musculoskeletal symptoms and non-REM sleep disturbance in patients with «fibrositis syndrome» and healthy subjects. Psychosom med 37(4) : 341-351. 1975.
- Müller W, Schneider M, Joos T, Hsu HY, Stratz T. Subgroups of fibromyalgia. Schmerz 21(5) : 424-429. 2007.
- Potvin S, Larouche A, Normand E, de Souza JB, Gaumond I, Grignon S, Marchand S. DRD3 Ser9Gly polymorphism is related to thermal pain perception and modulation in chronic widespread pain patients and healthy controls. J Pain 10(9) : 969-975. 2009.
- Price DD, Staud R, Robinson ME, Mauderli AP, Cannon R, Vierck CJ. Enhanced temporal summation of second pain and its central modulation in fibromyalgia patients. Pain 99(1-2) : 49-59. 2002.
- Rehm SE, Koroschetz J, Gockel U, Brosz M, Freynhagen R, Tölle TR, Baron R. A cross-sectional survey of 3035 patients with fibromyalgia : subgroups of patients with typical comorbidities and sensory symptom profiles. Rheumatology (Oxford) Mar 17 2010. (Impression à venir).
- Rodriguez-Raecke R, Niemeier A, Lhle K, Ruether W, May A. Brain matter decrease in chronic pain is the consequence and not the cause of pain. J Neurosci 29(44) : 13746-13750. 2009.

- Russell IJ. Advances in fibromyalgia: possible role for central neurochemicals. Am J Med Sci 315(6): 377-384. 1998.
- Russell IJ, Vaeroy H, Javors M, Nyberg F. Cerebrospinal biogenic amine metabolites in fibromyalgia/fibrositis syndrome and rheumatoid arthritis. Arthritis Rheum 35(5): 550-556. 1992.
- Shir Y, Pereira JX, Fitcharles MA. Whiplash and fibromyalgia: an ever-widening gap. J Rheumatol 33(6): 1045-1047. 2006.
- Staud R, Koo E, Robinson ME, Price DD. Temporal summation of second pain and its maintenance are useful for characterizing widespread central sensitization of fibromyalgia patients. J Pain 8(11): 893-901. 2007
- Tander B, Gunes S, Boke O, Alayli G, Kara N, Bagci H, Canturk F. Polymorphisms of the serotonin-2A receptor and catechol-O-methyltransferas genes: a study on fibromyalgia susceptibility. Rheumatol Int 28(7): 685-691. 2008.
- Taylor JB. Voyage au-delà de mon cerveau. Une neuro-anatomiste victime d'un accident cérébral raconte ses incroyables découvertes. JC Lattès Ed. 2008.
- Thieme K, Gracely RH. Are psychological treatments effective for fibromyalgia pain? Curr Rheumatol Rep 11(6): 443-450. 2009
- Tishler M, Levy O, Amit-Vazina M. Can fibromyalgia be associated with whiplash injury: A 3-year follow-up study. Rheumatol 2010 (impression à venir).
- Vallejo R, Tilley DM, Vogel L, Benyamin R. The Role of Glia and the Immune System in the Development and Maintenance of Neuropathic Pain. Pain Pract 2010. (Impression à venir.)
- Vlaeyen JWS, Kole-Snijders AMJ, Boeren RGB, van EEK H. Fear of movement/(re)injury in low back pain and its relation to behavioral performance. PAIN 1995 Sept; 62(3): 363-372.
- Wilke WS. New developments in the diagnosis of fibromyalgia syndrome: say goodbye to tender points? Cleve Clin J Med 76(6): 345-352. 2009.
- Williams DA, Clauw DJ. Understanding fibromyalgia: lessons from the broader pain research community. J Pain 10(8): 777-791. 2009.

# FIBROMYALGIA:
# A STORY FOR CHILDREN

**Christine Fogl,** Montreal, Quebec, Canada (illustrations)
**Lucie Bouvrette-Leblanc**, BSc OT, MAP (candidate), Montreal, Quebec, Canada (text)

**ABSTRACT**

Fibromyalgia affects between 2% and 5% of the population. The majority, approximately 80%, are women.

The principal symptoms of fibromyalgia are pain, fatigue and sleeping disorders. Several other symptoms can also be associated with fibromyalgia. **This story was written to help parents affected by fibromyalgia tell their children about this syndrome.**

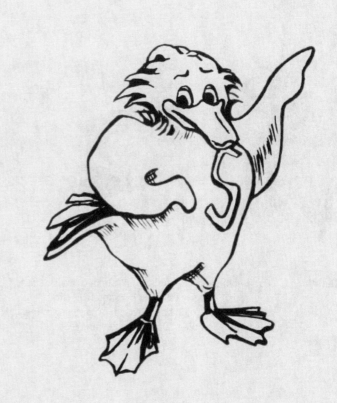

**FIBROMYALGIA**
by
Superduck

**Claudia**    - Hey there, Rick!

**Rick**    - Hey, Claudia!

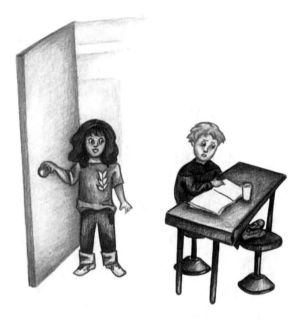

**Claudia**    - Can I come and play with you? Mommy doesn't feel
well today. She says she's in pain and feels tired. I just
don't get it! She didn't hurt herself.  And she even feels
tired in the morning.  Do you understand it?

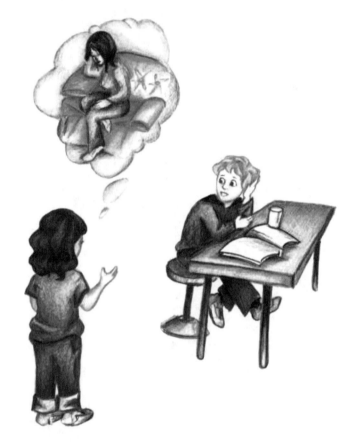

**Rick**    - Mom told me she has fibromyalgia.

**Claudia**    - But what's fibromyalgia?

**Rick**    - I don't know what fibromyalgia is either.

**Claudia**    - Maybe we can ask Superduck!

**Rick**    - Superduck? Who's Superduck?

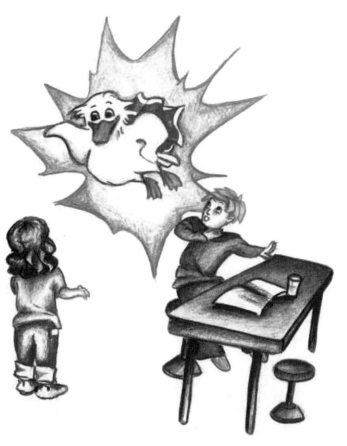

**Superduck** - Superduck to the rescue! QUACK! QUACK!

- Let me introduce myself! I'm Superduck, the magic duck! With my magic cape, I appear whenever you have a question! Tell me, what do you want to know? Quack! Quack!

**Rick** - Our mother has fibromyalgia, and we'd like to know what that is.

**Superduck** - Of course! Quack! Quack! People with fibromyalgia are often in pain; they feel tired and they have trouble sleeping. These symptoms can vary from one day to the next, and from one person to another.

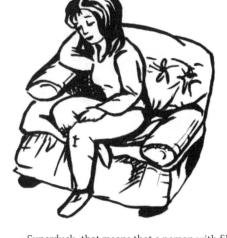

**Rick** - Superduck, that means that a person with fibromyalgia will feel pain and be tired and not sleep as well!

**Superduck** - That's right, Rick!

**Rick** - That explains why Mommy is often tired...

**Superduck** - You're right, Rick. People with fibromyalgia are often tired because they don't get enough deep sleep. If you sleep lightly at night, you'll feel tired the next day. Someone who is tired will find it harder to concentrate, and their fatigue might affect their mood.

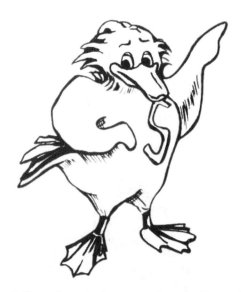

**Claudia**   - Tell me, Superduck, can we do something to help
Mommy?

**Superduck**   - Of course you can! First of all it's important to talk. You can't guess what your mother needs. And she needs to know what you need, too. Sometimes, she may need a little help setting the table, washing the dishes or doing the housework. It's important to ask your Mom how you can help her. Other times, you may need help, or to talk to your Mom. Your Mom also needs time for herself before going to bed so that she can start to wind down. That will help her sleep better.

She also needs to take regular breaks so she can "charge her batteries". If your Mom tells you that she needs to take a break, but you want to play with her, you have to respect her need for a break. Maybe she can play with you after her break, or at some other time. You can also ask your Dad, a friend or your brother or sister to play with you.

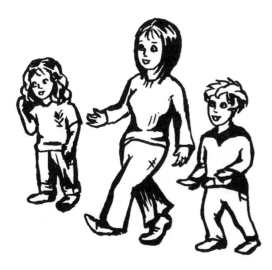

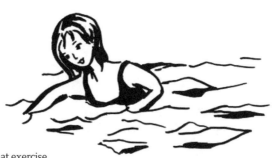

**Superduck** - Another thing your mother needs to know is that exercise is a good way to help her feel better. For example, you can both go for a walk, or you can go swimming with her.

**Claudia** - What can Mom do to feel better?

**Superduck** - The following elements are also important for helping your Mom feel better.

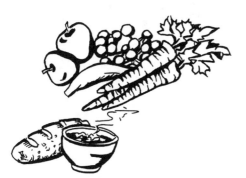

1. Nutrition: It is important to eat well. Fruits and vegetables are healthy foods. Do you know any other healthy foods?

3. She has to manage her level of energy. It's important to plan, set priorities, adopt good posture and take breaks on a regular basis.

4. Stress management: It's important to manage stress. Managing stress helps manage pain and improve sleep.

5. Do you remember, kids? I mentioned another means to you. What was that? Exactly! It was exercise!

6. People also have to have a good routine before they go to bed: they should always go to bed at the same time, not drink coffee, tea or chocolate during the evening, keep a notepad next to the bed to write down things they don't want to forget once they've gone to bed… and relax.

**Superduck** - There are various techniques for relaxing. I'll show you how to use breathing to relax. Look, Claudia! You can breathe in deeply through your nose, and exhale slowly through your mouth.

**Claudia** - Like this, Superduck?

**Superduck** - That's perfect, Claudia! You're good at this! Rick, can you take deep breaths through your nose, and exhale slowly through your mouth?

**Rick** - Like this?

**Superduck** - Perfect, Rick! Your Mom can also use this relaxation technique if she wants to.

**Claudia** - I'll tell her that and show her what to do.

**Superduck** - There are other ways to relax as well. Like taking a bath, going for a walk in the woods, listening to music, laughing, taking part in pleasant activities, etc. What do you do to relax?

**Claudia** - I like to draw.

**Rick** - I like to make things.

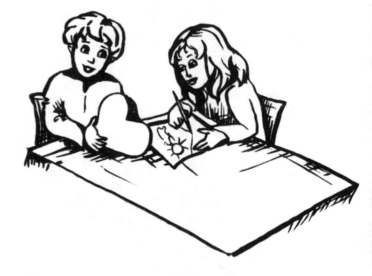

**Superduck** - You can ask your mother how she likes to relax.

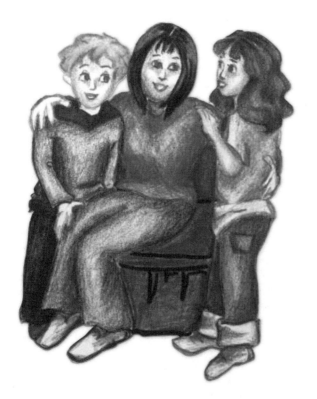

**Rick** - But it's important to talk about it and to express our emotions.

**Superduck** - That's it, kids! And don't forget the most important thing!

**Rick** - What's that, Superduck?

**Superduck** - Your Mom loves you!

**Claudia** - That's true, Superduck!

**Rick** - We love our Mom too!

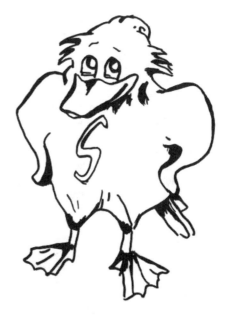

**Claudia** - But, Superduck, when we feel powerless and we feel all kinds of emotions because our mother is not well, what can we do?

**Superduck** - The important thing is to express your emotions and find something enjoyable to do. You can draw pictures or write poetry to express your emotions. You can also sing or play sports that you enjoy. It's important for you not to keep your emotions inside. You have to talk about what you feel.

Do you understand what fibromyalgia is now?

**Claudia** - Yes, Superduck! It's a condition that Mom has to manage every day, and sometimes she has ups and downs.

**Superduck** - Don't forget, fibromyalgia doesn't affect your mother's love for you!

Until next time, kids!

# MY STORY

**Helen Tupper,** Dartmouth, Nova Scotia, Canada

Helen Tupper joined the North American Chronic Pain Association of Canada (NACPAC) in 1993, then was President of the association from 1998 to 2001. *Having retired from NACPAC, Helen Tupper and Celeste Johnston ( who was then president of the Canadian Pain Society - CPS) formed the Canadian Pain Coalition (CPC) in 2002. Helen Tupper was president of the CPC from 2004 to 2008, and past president for two years. She speaks to associations or symposiums occasionally.*

(See other testimonial, page 76.)

I was working one evening as a registered nurse when I injured my back lifting a patient who had fallen out of bed. That was the beginning of the rest of my life, and it was never the same again. I was hospitalized for two weeks, hoping that bed rest would bring improvement. It didn't, and I had a discotomy. The pain in my leg was gone, and I felt much improved. I had been working for just under two years when the injury occurred. Certainly not the way I had planned things in the idealistic mind of a 23-year old.

I recovered quite well from the surgery and was without pain. We then moved to another city, then to Nova Scotia. We had our first child. The delivery was difficult. I experienced acute pain in my right leg during the delivery, and following it as well. It lasted for several weeks and gradually subsided to a nagging, less acute pain. That pain has been with me ever since, to varying degrees. Because of these difficulties, and in order to avoid more problems, we decided to adopt our second child. Our son being 19 months-old at the time, we had 2 toddlers under the age of 2. I was very busy for the next few years, and I remember them as being red-hot pain filled days. The bending and lifting of children was difficult. I saw a couple of doctors who told me I just needed to learn to live with it, and perhaps get a hobby to take my mind off it. Looking after the children and running the home took all my time and energy, how could I fit a hobby in? This comment made me really angry because I felt he was not taking my pain seriously, and dismissed me as a whining complainer. This was in 1971, when little was known about chronic pain. I carried on as best I could, but often found it very difficult.

Later on, after an abdominal surgery, my back was injured again when I was being lifted off an operating room table to a stretcher. From that point on, it was obvious I had to be my own advocate. I finally was able to start swimming again, and to exercise 3 times a week, which helped to strengthen my back and legs, and helped with the pain as well. Things were looking up! In 1975, we were in a head on collision with a dump truck. The children and my husband were fine, but I suffered a dislocated collarbone and a whiplash, which I felt in my neck and lower back. Following the accident, my back pain had increased considerably, and I had constant headaches. My joints were all very painful, and I hurt all over. My doctor sent me for x-rays, and nothing abnormal was found. He referred me to a physiotherapist that I saw for weeks, and as long as I was having the therapy it helped, but as soon as I stopped it, the pain returned with a vengeance. I struggled to carry on, not able to go to the gym because the exercises hurt too much to do them. I got steroid injections in the occipital nerve in my neck, and this helped to relieve the headaches for a while. They would return about three months later. Finally, my doctor admitted me to the hospital for seven weeks, where I had physiotherapy, pool therapy in the hydro pool, and rest. My children were placed with family during this time, and it was a very long, lonely, scary seven weeks. Then my doctor suggested I see a psychiatrist. I agreed, because I would do anything to get rid of the pain.

The psychiatrist felt that I was depressed and suggested I take some medication to relieve it. I told him that I wouldn't take the antidepressants, because I knew if they could relieve the pain, the depression would go away with it.

So it was back home to struggle on, the best way that I could. Meanwhile, my husband was working very hard to set up his own business, and build a practice. I required help with the housework, and looking after the children. I was often in bed. I hated that and I felt guilty that I couldn't do my share to look after the home and children.

A year later, in Toronto, I was diagnosed with fibromyalgia. To the best of my knowledge, I was the first person to be diagnosed with fibromyalgia in Nova Scotia. I knew there had been something wrong, and it wasn't all in my head. However he told me there was no cure or treatment at this time. It was now 1977. I returned to Nova Scotia thrilled to have a diagnosis, and I waved it in front of my doctor telling him I was not crazy, nor had I imagined my symptoms. He was almost as excited as I was, because he truly cared and wanted to know what I had. He then wrote an article in the medical journal about me, and described this "new" condition.

I began to realize that all was not solved. I had to accept that there was no cure for this, and they didn't know how to treat it. I had to figure out how to help myself.

My doctor referred me to the pain clinic that had just recently opened. I was met by people who accepted that I had pain and treated me well. They treated me with acupuncture, and I returned to an exercise program again, and tried to balance my life and look after myself all at the same time. Meanwhile, the back and leg pain continued to get worse, along with the joint and all-over pain of fibromyalgia.

My children learned to become very independent, which was a good thing most of the time. I felt guilty that I couldn't spend more time with them, and do more things with them. Like skiing, and skating like the other moms. They developed a very caring attitude, and helped around the house with things I couldn't do, without too much pain and discomfort. My husband was very caring. My illness taught them that not everyone had good health, and they were most grateful for the health and freedom that they had. They just accepted it as the way things were.

In 1980, I had a spinal fusion, and was out of bed the next day and discharged in ten days. My children were now teen-agers, and quite helpful around the house. Friends came along to help. Gradually, I got stronger. Three months later, my surgeon said he wanted me walking four miles a day. I did it, and I felt great. I thought I was healed, and that all the pain was behind me. However, I was not so lucky!

In about a year or year and a half, the pain returned to my right leg. Gradually, the back pain returned, but not the same as it had been before the surgery. The fibromyalgia was still there, and there were times when it was horrible. The worst has always been the pain around my torso, or ribs. It felt like I was in a vice. Pain drained my energy, and some days,

I couldn't do much. I always tried to have supper at the table with my family because I felt it was important to sit down together each night to eat, and share our days. I tried to have interesting things to say, because I didn't want to discuss my pain or disability. I tried to hide it even from my family. At the pain clinic, I had more acupuncture and physiotherapy, which fortunately helped once more.

One day in the summer in 1986, I injured my leg again, when the lawn chair I was sitting on collapsed. The pain was excruciating. I was admitted to the hospital where I was once again referred to the pain clinic. I had 12 series of nerve blocks in my back. The blocks brought relief for some time, and I felt better. There was still the fibromyalgia pain, but the back pain seemed less sharp. During the 13th set of blocks, the doctor hit the spinal canal by accident, which causes horrific headaches. A blood patch was done to correct this, but the side effects were horrible for about five months.

I then learned that I had "arachnoiditis" in my back which caused inflammation that continued to affect the durra of my spinal column, as it spread down my back. So now I had failed back surgery, fibroymyalgia from the car accident, arachnoiditis as a result of the myleograms, and sciatic pain due to the damage to my spine. What was wrong with me? Take your pick.

Some of the doctors I saw didn't understand or believe that the fibromyalgia was as bad as I said it was. In fact some doctors don't believe that it exists. I have met many kinds of doctors over the years, and it is very difficult to be polite with the ones who don't believe you or suspect that you are making things up. Sometimes I wonder why I should be polite to them, when they are not to me. However, for the past 18 years, I have had an excellent family doctor who understands pain, fibromyalgia, and that I live with both conditions.

# MIGRAINES AND CHRONIC
## DAILY HEADACHES

Stéphanie Jacques MD, FRCPC, neurologist, Rouyn-Noranda, Quebec, Canada

## ABSTRACT

Once considered an episodic illness, migraines are now viewed as a chronic illness that can result in cerebral and physical changes. Comorbidities are numerous, complicating both diagnosis and treatment. The treatment of these other affections must also be included in the treatment for chronic migraines. Treatment is more effective when the patients become experts in their disease. They must understand the physiopathology in order to be able to work on healing with their doctors.

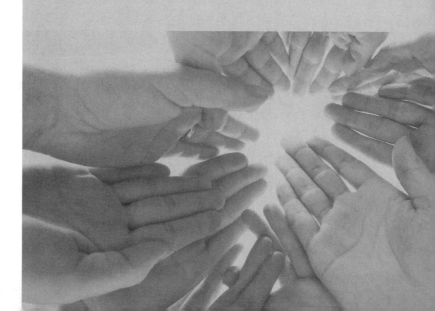

# 1. INTRODUCTION

Migraine is a particular disease. Most often it does not give any warning. It appears suddenly, at the worst time, overwhelming its victim for anywhere from a few hours to a few days. Time stands still. The victim can no longer function.

Most people simply cannot understand this invisible disease. How can a headache prevent someone from functioning? Even worse, how can someone have a headache every day? How can people let themselves go like that? You simply have to make an effort and get up!

According to the World Health Organization, migraine ranks 19th in terms of years of quality of life lost. And migraine ranks in 8th place if you consider only neuropsychiatric diseases. Daily headaches upset family, social and work relationships. Since 4% of adults and 2% of children suffer from daily headaches, this is a problem that must be treated to the best of our ability.

This chapter will discuss new discoveries and hypotheses concerning chronic headaches, including risk factors and the mechanisms of chronicization. This chapter will also provide a brief discussion of the means for controlling and treating this disease.

# 2. MIGRAINE, AN EVOLVING CONCEPT

Since the turn of the century, the concept of migraine has evolved. Once considered an episodic disease, distinct from other more chronic forms of headaches, migraine is now considered a chronic disease with episodic manifestations which, in certain people, can be progressive. This way of looking at migraine stresses the importance of recognizing the risk factors for the progression and chronicization of this disease.

The risk factors must be identified before headaches become a daily occurrence. The associated conditions must be treated in order to maximize the chances of remission.

# 3. PAIN MECHANISM AND HYPOTHESES CONCERNING THE CHRONICIZATION OF MIGRAINE HEADACHES

Chronic migraine is, in fact, a transformed episodic migraine. There is a progressive increase in the frequency of the painful attacks. Then the individual will experience more days with pain than days without pain. This transformation takes place in an insidious manner until the individual notes that he/she is functioning poorly on a daily basis. Often, it is only at this point that the individual will consult a physician, and occasionally, several years will have already been spent in pain.

Neurological changes will have already occurred by this time. A decrease in sensitivity thresholds will become manifest through an abnormal sensitivity of the skin to touch, allodynia. Modifications will also take place in the cerebral pain circuits. In certain cases, anatomical changes will take place in the brain in the form of small strokes, anomalies in the white matter and iron deposits in the periacqueductal region of the brainstem. These findings suggest that repeated migraine attacks are associated with neuron damage that will result in an abnormal modulation of pain, and consequently, resistance to treatment.

Chronic migraines also have systemic consequences. People who suffer from these attacks have an increased risk of cardio-vascular disease. This is possibly related to the inflammatory states induced by chronic migraines. There also appears to be a common genetic risk for chronic migraines, hypertension and dyslipidemia. The physiological modifications caused by migraines seem, therefore, to be more extensive than once believed. However, little has been done yet in these areas of research, and caution must be exercised before clinical applications can be deduced.

# 4. DEMOGRAPHICS

Women are more subject to chronic headaches than men by a factor of two to one. The same applies to adolescents. A low socio-economic status is a risk factor and ensures a poor prognosis. Finally, married people are at less risk for chronic headaches.

# 5. DIFFERENCE DEPENDING ON TIME OF DEVELOPMENT AND INDIVIDUAL'S AGE: CHILDHOOD, ADOLESCENCE, ADULTHOOD AND ADVANCED AGE

As migraines become chronic, there is a change in the ways they manifest. The associated symptoms, such as nausea, vomiting, sensitivity to light and sound, are less frequent. The pain resembles that of tension headaches. Several patients complain of pain in their necks, and will already have consulted a physician about that, without success. Adolescents will have a greater tendency to extended migraine crises, separated by days without symptoms. In the case of adults, the typical migraine episodes will be clearly less frequent. Another important difference concerning the adult population is the use of more over-the-counter medications. As a result, headaches caused by the over-use of medication are more common in this group.

# 6. COMORBIDITIES OF CHRONIC HEADACHE

Comorbidities are conditions associated with a disease without necessarily being the cause. Obesity, snoring, sleep disorders, head or neck injuries, chronic pain, major life events, smoking, consumption of caffeine, and the use of analgesic medication are comorbidities that have been found in epidemiological studies.

All of these comorbidities cannot necessarily be changed and, in certain cases, controlling them does not necessarily relieve the pain.

## OBESITY

A body mass index greater than 30 increases the risk of chronic headache by a factor of 5. However, no study has yet demonstrated that losing weight improves the chances of remission. On the other hand, losing weight serves to reduce snoring and improve sleep, and these two factors have an impact on chronic headaches.

## SNORING

This problem increases the risk of chronic headaches by a factor of 3. This risk is independent of other snoring risks such as obesity, sleep apnea, age or gender.

Controlling snoring starts with stopping smoking, reducing the consumption of alcohol or any sedative or muscle relaxant. A reduction in weight, no matter how minimal, can also make a difference.

Patients at risk must be screened for sleep apnea. People who suffer from sleep apnea will need a CPAP (continuous positive airway pressure) machine.

Dental prosthetists are also occasionally used in the case of individuals with a particular anatomy of their upper respiratory passages. A change in sleeping position is useful for people who only snore when lying on their backs. Also, patients will be tested for the presence of an allergy that could cause a nasal obstruction.

## INSOMNIA AND SLEEP DISORDERS

Insomnia affects two-thirds of the people who suffer from headaches. Initial insomnia is defined as being awake for more than 30 minutes in bed before falling asleep or waking up after less than 30 minutes of sleep. This type of insomnia is common in the case of people suffering from anxiety disorders.

Terminal insomnia, namely the inability to fall back to sleep after waking up in the early morning, is associated with mood disorders. Screening for anxiety and mood disorders must be part of the initial investigation into insomnia, and must be included in the questionnaire for chronic headaches.

**Restless leg syndrome** in which the individual experiences an irresistible need to move just as he/she falls asleep is also a frequent cause of sleep disorder. This problem is often described as leg pain, but is rather a discomfort that cannot be defined. Restless leg syndrome has a genetic incidence, and is associated with the secondary pain of peripheral nerve diseases such as those experienced by diabetics. Restless leg syndrome is accompanied by both initial insomnia and difficulty falling back to sleep after waking at night. Treatment with dopaminergic agents easily relieves this discomfort, and it is important to screen for this common problem.

## CHRONIC PAIN

Epidemiological studies have demonstrated that people who experience daily chronic headaches are four times more at risk of suffering from other painful syndromes. The central sensitization process is common to both conditions and probably accounts for the association.

## NECK AND HEAD INJURIES

It is estimated that 20% of men suffering from chronic headaches report having had a neck or head injury in the past year. This connection is not significant in the case of women. It is interesting to note that a neck or head injury at any point in an individual's life is also a risk factor for the development of chronic headaches. However, in my clinical experience, very few patients obtain a remission from their symptoms through massage therapy, physiotherapy or any other treatment targeted for the neck.

## MAJOR LIFE EVENTS

Major life events include: moving, the death of a loved one, the change in a couple's status, and the persistence of a daily stress factor such as difficulties at work or at home. In the case of adolescents, family stresses are risk factors for chronic headaches.

## CAFFEINE AND TOBACCO USE

Although caffeine is the only substance which a randomized control-led trial has demonstrated will cause a headache when withdrawn, its chronic use seems to have a modest association with chronic headaches. Therefore, in my practice, I suggest that patients who drink several cups of coffee each day reduce their consumption without necessarily completely stopping. A few studies have also established a link between chronic headaches and smoking. Stopping smoking may have an impact on the chronicity of the painful syndrome.

## OVER-USE OF PAIN MEDICATION

Daily headaches induced by the over-use of medication usually occur when medication is taken more than three days per week. The total quantity of medication seems to be less important than the fact that medication is taken on a habitual basis.

In other words, the number of days on which medication is taken is more important than the total quantity taken in a week. Therefore, it is recommended that patients limit their use of medication to three days per week which, unfortunately, is difficult in a situation of chronic pain. The most commonly used medications are acetaminophen, triptans and opiates. It is rare, however, that simply stopping the medication for more than eight weeks will completely cure chronic headache. It seems that there are other associated factors.

## 7. TREATING CHRONIC HEADACHES

The treatment for chronic headaches starts with painstaking research into all of the precipitants and factors associated with the disease. In my practice, I systematically look for anxiety disorders, mood disorders, and the over-use of analgesic medications.

I treat psychiatric disorders aggressively since it is rare that the patients I treat experience remission unless these problems are controlled. I have noted this tendency regardless of whether the mood disorder caused the pain or vice versa.

Often, the associated sleep disorders also correct themselves, and the headache has less impact on concentration and fatigue. Then I apply the traditional algorithms for treating chronic headaches. Obviously, life habits must also be changed. I suggest starting with the factor that causes the most suffering, or the habit that will be the easiest to change, depending on the patient's choice and personality.

## 8. CONCLUSION

Chronic headache is an insidious disease. It develops over a period of several years and takes on multiple forms. There are multiple comorbidities, which complicate both the diagnosis and the treatment. The pain is real, and prevents the individual from functioning.

With experience, I have noted that the treatment is more effective when the patient becomes an expert with respect to his/her own disease. I spend a lot of time explaining the physiopathology and the mechanisms behind the appearance of pain. The patient then guides me in his/her treatment, and we form a team that plans the therapeutic steps together. Unfortunately, this practice is not always applicable in all practices, and the patient must then have recourse to books that provide information about his/her disease.

## REFERENCES

- Lipton RB, Pan J. Is migraine a progressive brain disease? JAMA 2004 Jan 28; 291(4): 493-4.
- Bradley LA, PhD. Pathophysiologic mechanisms of fibromyagia and its related disorders, J Clin Psychiatry 2008; 69 Suppl 2: 6-13.
- Penzien Donald B., PhD, and Jeannetta C. Rains, PhD ; Richard B. Lipton, MD, Editors. The Chronification of Headaches: Mechanism, Risk Factors and Behavioral Strategies Aimed at Primary and Secondary Prevention of Chronic Headache. Headache 2008, Vol 48, no 1, 1-58.

# CHRONIC LOW
# **BACK PAIN**

Multifactorial management of patients with low back pain due to spinal degeneration:
psychosocial factors predictive of chronicity and quality of life, means of assessment and protocols

Benoît Lavignolle MD, PhD, Bordeaux, France

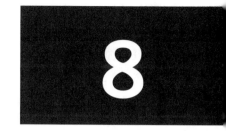

**8**

## ABSTRACT

According to various epidemiological studies, the pre-valence and incidence of lower back pain are high, with a pseudo-epidemic exponential increase that remains unexplained (four-fold increase over two decades). As a result, it is important to consider factors other than just medical ones. The medicosocioeconomic cost (direct and indirect) is considerable. Lower back pain is the primary cause of disability among adults under the age of 45 as well as disruption of employment. Low back pain is multifactorial. The somatic, psychosocial, occupational and medicolegal factors need to be assessed, and early management needs to be proposed.

The goals of a study into the psychological factors of lower back pain (Koleck-Mazaux) were to find predic-tive psychosocial factors in patients with a high risk of developing chronicity. Four transactional strategies were isolated with significant predisposing factors.

Assessment of low back pain should be comprehensive, physical, psychological and functional with a physical examination, pain assessment, psychological assessment, social/professional assessment, medicolegal assessment, and quantified muscle assessment.

People with lower back pain often experience muscle loss leading to reduced performance (maximum strength and endurance) and a cardiovascular mismatch during exertion. The physical deconditioning syndrome is global. There is often fear of movement with inadequate motor control, which perpetuates the symptoms.

With respect to the treatment protocol, we prefer a mul-tidisciplinary and multifactorial program (Chenard JR, Charest J, Marchand S) for a four- to five-week period presented in this chapter.

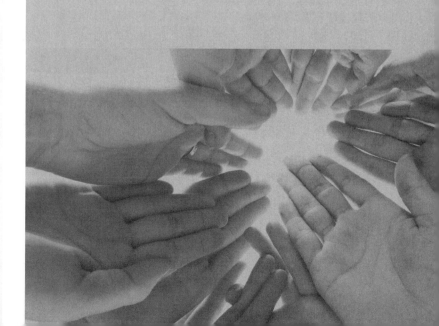

# 1. EPIDEMIOLOGY, COSTS AND RISK FACTORS

With a cumulative incidence of 70% and a mean annual prevalence of 35%, low back pain is a factor of chronic debilitating pain and poor quality of life in the adult population, and had disastrous public health effects in the 20th century with a 5-fold increase in socio-medical expenditures in the last 30 years (Waddell G 1998). Time plays a major role since acute and subacute low back pain evolves favourably in 80 to 90% of cases, whatever the treatment (Andersson GBJ 1999). Common low back pain has no specific etiology, and it is impossible to identify any particular anatomical structure in 99% of subjects (Québec Task Force 1987).

## SNAPSHOT OF THE SITUATION

- Low back pain lasting over 3 months is considered chronic (Duquesnay 1994), and is the single most important source of disability and health care expenditures, with 7 to 10% of chronic cases accounting for 75% of socio-medical costs (Rossignol 1988, Maezel 2002).
- To this should be added the indirect burden of daily allowances, disability benefit and loss of production and employment (Valat 1998, Van Tulder 1995, Underwood 1998, Bolten 1998, Waddell 1998).
- Nevertheless, only 5 to 10% of patients need to stop work as a result of low back pain, and the average time off work rarely exceeds 7 days, with only 6 to 10% of patients seeking care.
- The likelihood to resume work is 50% after 6 months and less than 10% at 2 years (Waddell 1998). The current guidelines are to keep sufferers active during the acute and sub-acute phases (Anaes 2000).
- The direct costs attributable to low back pain represent 5% of the healthcare budget, and vary from country to country. About 1.4 billion euros is spent each year by France, the United Kingdom and Holland, while the figure is 4-fold greater for the U.S. Of these costs, 75% are devoted to the prolonged absenteeism and healthcare provided to chronic sufferers.
- The socioeconomic impact of the disorder represents 7% of all time off work, 12 million working days lost per year, a duration off work exceeding 30 days in 11% of women and 22% of men, 10% of all medical consultations (second most frequent cause), 3% of prescriptions, 9% of medical imaging and 30% of physiotherapy sessions. It is the third leading cause of disability in the general population and the first in subjects over 45 years of age.
- The disorder accounts for 13% of work-related accidents, with a mean time off work of 33 days, an annual loss of 3.6 million working days, and a low mean permanent partial disability between 5 and 8%.
- In France, the indirect costs amount to 4.5 billion per year. Prevention of chronic low back pain is a major goal, and the reasons why and when pain becomes chronic need to be sought. Some authors underline the need for early management from the first month (Atlas SJ 1996).

Briefly, there is a high prevalence and incidence of low back pain that is increasing exponentially in a pseudo-epidemic manner (4-fold increase in 20 years). Since this is difficult to explain, it is important to investigate factors other than medical ones. The considerable medicosocioeconomic cost, both direct and indirect, amounts to 6 billion euros per year in France, of which 75% is accounted for by only 7 to 10% of all low back pain sufferers. It is the main cause of disability in the under-45 group, and is the leading cause of absenteeism for illness (3.6 million working days per year). Just a 1% reduction in the number of chronic sufferers would lead to annual savings of 100 million euros.

The current objectives of France's healthcare system are as follows:
- Detect patients at risk of becoming chronic;
- Validate and assess the therapeutic options.

The options are to develop indices for assessing physical, professional, psychosocial and medicolegal factors, and to offer early management starting five weeks following diagnosis.

# 2. RISK FACTORS

Low back pain is a complex multifactorial process that is so highly dependent upon somatic psychological and environmental factors that the classic linear medical approach is frequently unable to prevent the shift to the chronic state. Waddell (1987) explains chronic low back pain by a biopsychosocial model.

## SOMATIC FACTORS

In France, somatic medicine signifies physical medicine.

The somatic factors in chronic low back pain are well known and not determinant.

Poor physical condition and inadequate muscular strength in the trunk are consequences of low back pain rather than the cause. Physical training can prevent relapses, but it is not predictive of the absence of chronicity (Cady 1979, Leino 1993). Low back pain is twice as frequent in high-level athletes as in people who do not practise sport.

There is no direct relationship between chronic low back pain and spinal degeneration, as evidenced by imagery (Carragee 2005). (Degeneration of our spinal column starts in our 30s. However, for most of us, it is not painful.) Back pain occurs in 42 to 58% of adolescents with repetitive spinal microtrauma or in those who practise too much sport in the prepubertal period (Balagué 1988, Salminen 1992, Sward L 1992, Erikentalo 1995, Kujala 1996, Troussier 1997). The prevalence of chronic low back pain in adolescents is 3% (Taimela 1997). Moreover, many chronic adult sufferers were already affected at 15 years of age, so primary prevention at school and in sports clubs is important (Salminen 1999).

## OCCUPATIONAL FACTORS

The occupational risk factors of low back pain are present for people who perform arduous physical work, must maintain prolonged stressful working positions, and are exposed to vibration. Some occupational factors are associated with low back pain, such as work that is monotonous, repetitive and stressful, and that provides little satisfaction or prestige. Precarious, poorly paid work requiring a low level of qualification is also detrimental, as are poor relations with colleagues and management. All these occupational factors are highly associated with chronic back pain (Waddell 2000).

## PSYCHOSOCIAL FACTORS

Psychosocial factors have little impact in acute low back pain, but are heavily involved in chronic pain (Truchon 2000). Previous studies have shown that psychosocial factors are more important in lumbar disability related to biomechanical and medical factors (Carragee 2005, Linton 2000, Waddell 1998). Some of the social determinants include family influence, underprivileged social background, low level of education and poor professional integration (Pope MH 1989, Symonds TL 1996, Vällfors 1985, Waddell 2000). Medicolegal disputes also worsen disability and increase the risk of chronicity. The CES-D (Center for Epidemiologic Study Depression scale) and BDI (Beck Depression Index) are good predictors of patient dissatisfaction with surgery for low back pain (Sorensen 1987, Schade 1999, Hoffmann 1993, Junge 1995, De Groot 1997, Coskin 2000, Hagg 2003).

## PSYCHOLOGICAL FACTORS

Among the psychological factors, anxiety and depression are the most prevalent (Polatin 1993, Kessler 1996, Schermelleh-Engel 1997, Clauw 1999, Epping-Jordan 1998, Fisher 1998, Pincus 2002, Duplan 2005, Lequesne 1973, Marty 1952, Deburge 1998).

Very few mentally ill subjects suffer from low back pain (psychiatric treatment is required only in 5%), and such patients tend to be managed by health psychologists in order to assess their cognitive and emotional organization.

Cognitive factors in pain with the fear of moving and low psychological adjustment to pain or the inability to cope with pain are related to pain and physical disability in individuals with level A pain and disability (Linton 2000).

Fear of moving (kinesiophobia) is associated with chronicity of low back pain (Fritz 2001, Gatchel 1995, George 2003).

Catastrophism and passive "hope and pray" fatalism are related to the negative aspects of chronic low back pain (intensity of pain, disability and fragile emotional state), while cognitive restructuring and pain control are associated with favourable progression (Tuttle 1991, Dozois 1996, Kröner-Herwig 1996, Lin and Ward 1996, Robinson 1997, Mc Craken 1998, Riley 1999, Hyathornthwaite 1998, Lewandowski 2004). However, all the abovementioned investigations were retrospective crossover studies.

In the prospective studies, catastrophism and fear of movement were the most predictive factors of pain and disability (Hasembring 1994, Burton 1995, Klenerman 1995, Linton and Hallden 1998, Picavet 2002). Passive psychological adjustment to pain or coping (Potter and Jones 1992), hoping and praying (Burton 1995) and self-perception of the evolution of pain and disability (Hazard 1997, Linton and Hallden 1998) are predictive of disability one year after diagnosis.

While these studies examined the level of pain and functional criteria (disability, return to work and quality of life), the relationships between functional and emotional criteria have received little attention.

## 3. A PROSPECTIVE STUDY IN CLINICAL PSYCHOLOGY (KOLECK, MAZAUX 2006) CONDUCTED AT THE CENTRE HOSPITALIER UNIVERSITAIRE (CHU) DE BORDEAUX

### INTRODUCTION TO THE STUDY

A prospective study in clinical psychology conducted at the CHU de Bordeaux (Koleck, Mazaux 2006) aimed to identify the emotional and functional interactions in acute low back pain suffers who were progressing toward chronicity. One year after the initial episode, 67% of 99 patients had improved and 33% had chronic pain.

During this study, patients were asked to complete initial and final psychological and functional assessment questionnaires.

See Appendix 1, page 72.

The question was to know how low back pain patients react to pain.

Four transactional strategies were identified with significant predisposing factors (gender, number of children, level of education, income, obesity, reduced activity, poor quality of life, history of low back pain in the last two years, trauma for more than one year, anxiety, depression, locus of control and job satisfaction).

- **Hoping and praying (HP)** (20%): passive attitude in daily life, fatalism, irrational attitude, concentrating on something other than pain, adjustment to pain by praying, dependency, hypokinesia, avoidance strategy, fear of moving, low income, job dissatisfaction and history of low back pain.

### STUDY RESULTS

No significant difference was noted between chronic and non-chronic low back pain patients with regard to anxiety or depression in the study, but a principal components analysis demonstrated two factors of non-adjustment (70.8% of total variance) in chronic subjects: functional (37.5%) and emotional (33.3%).

- **Helplessness/hopelessness (HH)** (17.4%): negative emotions, anxiety and depression, catastrophism, dramatizing, hopelessness about getting better, highly deteriorated quality of life, high income.
- **Cognitive restructuring (CR)** (15.3%): reinterpreting pain, ignorance, stoicism, denial of pain, quality of life maintained, external control, hyperactivity.
- **Perceived control (PC)** (13.7%): control of perception of pain, attributing medical cause, actively participating in care, high level of education and integration, excellent quality of life.

HP and HH evolved chronically indicating the inability to cope with low back pain. HP had a direct effect on functional adjustment and HH had an effect on emotional adjustment. However, CR and PC had a satisfactory course without any decline into chronicity.

### STUDY CONCLUSIONS

Low back pain is therefore a multifactorial problem and multidimensional studies have demonstrated that chronic evolution may be predicted by analyzing its social and psychosocial parameters (Hasembring 1994). Physical and psychological treatment alone, for example cognitive-behavioural therapy, cannot prevent chronic back pain. Functional rehabilitation programs are now recognized as having an impact on low back pain because they reduce the patient's disability while increasing their physical ability (Brady 1994, Curtis 1994, Mayer 1994). At the same time, they have been found to provide psychological support in studies where a cognitive strategy of coping with pain was compared to a control group not receiving such training. The experimental groups were less affected by catastrophism and hypokinesia (Chaory 2004, Jousset 2004, Kole-Snidjers 1999, Spinhoven 2004).

## 4. MEANS OF ASSESSMENT AND PROTOCOL

**Randomized study:**
A randomized study is the study of a new treatment where participants are randomly divided into a control group and an experimental group.

Among the more than 25,000 studies on treatment for low back pain, only 1,000 have been randomized (see definition above) or controlled.

Most of the medical treatments or surgical procedures recommended in the acute phase are ineffective in chronic sufferers. On the other hand, there is substantial evidence that in chronic low back pain patients (level A), manual therapy, back school (*École interactionnelle du dos*) and combined physical and psychological treatment involving cognitive-behavioural therapy are efficient in relieving pain (Nachemson, Van Tulder, Goossens, Waddell 2000).

## ASSESSMENT METHODS

See Appendix 2, page 72.

Assessment should be all-encompassing, physical, functional and psychological, and comprise various assessments or exam: routine somatic medical exam; and psychological, pain, quality of life, socioprofessional, medicolegal and muscular assessment.

In low back pain sufferers, the loss of muscle capacity leads to decreased performance (maximal strength and endurance) and cardiovascular deficiency on exertion. This in turn leads to inappropriate perception of the requirements of exercising with the anarchical recruitment of muscle groups, especially the peripheral group, by the deficiency of the axial group. The syndrome of physical deconditioning is both muscular and central (involving gestures and proprioception) and impacts professional movement. Kinesiophobia and maladapted motor control often make the symptoms chronic.

## MULTIDISCIPLINARY PROGRAMME

A low back pain patient may be included in a multidisciplinary programme only if they are committed to making the considerable effort required of them in order for the programme to work. It is not possible to include the rare psychiatric patients nor those who are unable to accept the constraints that working in a rehabilitation group places on them. Nor can one include those who are waiting for reclassification or disability. However, the assessment process is subject to bias because there will always be patients who cannot be treated owing to psychosocial factors.

The multidisciplinary approach in managing programme participants demonstrated that when several healthcare professionals of different skills are involved in the same medical problem with the aim to continuously improve the quality of care and patient satisfaction, it leads to benefits for healthcare professionals and savings in the field of public health.

There are several multidisciplinary teams in France and throughout the world that include physicians and/or rheumatologists trained in spinal rehabilitation, a psychiatrist or psychologist, physiotherapist, occupational therapist, psychometrician, dietician and social assistant. These teams are in frequent contact with occupational doctors, medical examiners and France's technical commission for professional reclassification and career counselling (COTOREP) and its equivalent in other countries.

The objectives of the multifactorial programme are to control and manage pain, improve functional capacity, treat psychological disorders, and help sufferers cope with pain and resume their socio-professional activity.

The four- to five-week program includes the following:

- Pain management (with or without medication)
- Rehabilitation, balneotherapy, posture training, stretching and muscle reinforcement
- Occupational training and relearning the gestures of professional and daily life
- Psychological management (antidepressants, refocusing on existential problems, stress management, behavioural therapy, relaxation)
- Pedagogy, dietetics, ergonomics and *École interactionnelle du dos* (Charest J, Chenard JR, Lavignolle B, Marchand S.: *Lombalgies; école interactionnelle du dos*. Masson 1996)
- Professional training and reclassification

The team is co-ordinated in review meetings where the improvement in physical progress and psychological behaviour of patients is assessed. It is not always easy to objectively quantify a patient's progress. Post-rehabilitation follow-up includes social, medical and psychological monitoring accompanied by physical self-evaluation.

## MULTIFACTORIAL MANAGEMENT RESULTS

In most studies on rehabilitation, the outcome is favourable (Alaranta 1994, Frost 1995, Hazard 1989, Järviloski 1993, Lindström 1992, Manniche 1990, Mannion 1999, Mayer 1994) with a more rapid return to work, improved mobility and muscle strength at 3, 6 and 12 months after multifactorial management, and subjective improvement of physical and cardiovascular capacity.

The type of physical programme seems to have little influence on the outcome, whether it is isometric, dynamic or isokinetic. The most important point is to recover flexibility, muscle strength and endurance, and to learn how to cope with pain by using coping strategies.

In a series of 194 patients seen one year after following a rehabilitation programme at the Centre de réadaptation Tour de Gassies (rehabilitation centre) in Bruges (Bordeaux, France) (Ravaud, De Mounico 2001), EVA assessment decreased from 50 to 30 mm, quality of daily life improved 50%, professional life improved 60%, social life 80%, and there was a 70% decrease in depression and anxiety. Of all the patients, 85% were keeping up with their exercise routine, and 77% had returned to work. A prospective longitudinal study focused on psychosocial factors (Koleck and Gouverneur 2005) with assessment of body image (Bruchon-Schweitzer), cognitive coping strategies (Rosentiel), behavioural coping strategies (Jensen), EVA assessment, the Dallas Pain Questionnaire or the DRAD and the short version of the SF36 or MOS confirmed the physical and psychological benefit of this form of multifactorial management.

## 5. CONCLUSION

The multifactorial management of chronic low back pain sufferers is complex and calls upon the expertise of several trained experts. The aim of treatment is to wean the patient off of medication, dedramatize their suffering, make them accountable and motivate them so that they can play an active role in their own rehabilitation. As Watzlavick says, the situation may seem hopeless but it is not serious. However, if one does not use one's back, one becomes deconditioned. "Use it or lose it" has never been a truer adage. The activities of daily life and work are beneficial for low back pain sufferers.

For patients who cannot be included in such programmes, it is possible to offer them adapted and reduced routines aimed at improving their daily lives, even if they are unable to return to work. Moreover, it is essential to begin combined psychosocial and physical rehabilitation early, to prevent chronicity. The slippery slope into chronic pain is only favoured in situations where the patient keeps their old habits, if prolonged time off work and rest are prescribed, medication (especially morphinic drugs) is given without any objective signs calling for its use, and loses contact with his/her place of work (Nordin, Abenhaïm, Rossignol, Bortz, Buckwalter).

A state of permanent disability is a good choice neither for the patient nor for the healthcare system. Indeed, there is much scope for developing ancillary patient-oriented services that do not fall within the realm of traditional medicine, but that meet the psychosocial and professional needs of patients.

## APPENDIX 1

### Psychological questionnaires
Psychological questionnaires used during this study investigated the predisposing psychological state and the transactional state of anxiety (STAI, Spielberger 1983), depression (CESD, Radloff 1977), locus of control (LCS, Lumpkin 1985), job satisfaction and social state (PSSS), and coping with pain (CSQ, Rosentiel and Keefe 1983).

### Functional questionnaires
Functional criteria were assessed by the following: EVA, quality of life (MOS short form of the SF 36, Ware and Sherbourne 1992), functional limitation (NHP, Bucquet 1990), duration of time off work and number of consultations. Multiple regression analysis was performed on all the data with the SPSS package.

## APPENDIX 2

### Methods for assessing low back pain
- Routine **osteoarticular neurological medical work-up** with full imaging data. Search for medical contraindications to physical rehabilitation (cardiovascular).
- **Psychological assessment:** anxiety, depression, coping strategies with anxiety questionnaires (STAI, Spielberger 1983), depression (CESD, Radloff 1977), locus of control (LCS, Lumpkin 1985), job satisfaction, social state (PSSS) and coping with pain (CSQ, Rosentiel and Keefe 1983).
- **Pain assessment:** EVA and drawing pain and disability (Dessin de la douleur et de l'incapacité, EIFEL Québec, Echelle d'incapacité fonctionnelle d'évaluation des lombalgiques du Québec)

- **Quality of life:** DRAD or Dallas Pain Questionnaire MOS short version of SF36 the NHP(Nottingham Health profile) for the assessment of perceived health with the concept of health associated with real, objective and subjective morbidity
- **Socioprofessional assessment** (level of education, family status, degree of mechanical constraints at workstation, level of job satisfaction)
- **Medicolegal assessment** (accidents at work, occupational conflicts)

- **Muscle evaluation** is the pillar of any spinal functional rehabilitation programme.
  - Muscle extensibility: hand-floor distance in spine flexion
  - Overall mobility of spine (goniometry, measurement of spine mobility, electronic goniometry)
  - Measurement of isometric strength: endurance of flexors (Ito, Querido), normal values in females = 1.5 Nm, in males = 3 Nm, endurance of extensors (Biering-Sorensen), normal value = 2 Nm
  - Measurement of isokinetic strength: concentric and eccentric strength of flexors and extensors as a function of speed of trunk movement 30°/s, 60°/s, 90°/s and 120°/s. Extensor/flexor ratio
  - Variations between devices (6 machines) may range from 0 to 3.8%, and readings may vary between position seated and standing
  - Mean isokinetic concentric strength vales according to age (20–45 years) with gender variations of 60% according to age and a 30–40% decrease after 30 years (Langrana 1984, Matheson 1992, Mandell 1993, Mayer 1995, Salanon 1998)

| 30°/s: | F (flexion): | 130 Nm | E (extension): 190 Nm | ratio E/F = 150% |
| 60°/s: | F (flexion): | 200 Nm | E (extension): 240 Nm | ratio E/F = 140% |
| 90°/s: | F (flexion): | 130 Nm | E (extension): 160 Nm | ratio E/F = 110% |

(only values < 120°/s are isokinetic)

In most chronic sufferers tested, strength decreased on average by 40% in the extensors and by 20% in the flexors. The E/F ratio was inverted. The decrease in strength was greater as the speeds increased. The drawbacks were the reproducibility of measurements from one device to another, their cost, the test duration (one hour), the number of parameters and the fact that the extensors, flexors and rotators are analyzed indiscriminately.

Currently, a distinction is drawn between the role of the axial muscles of the trunk (multifidus, psoas, tranversus abdominalis, rectus) and the peripheral muscles (longissimus, iliocostalis, internal and external obliques, quadratus lumborum) (Danneels 2000). The axial group plays a static role in the spine while the peripheral group is dynamic.

It is therefore possible to make simple isometric measurements with the Biering-Sorensen test for the extensor muscles and to use the Querido-Ito tests for the flexor muscles. EMG coupled with dynamic testing (Sivhonen) demonstrates overuse of the peripheral extensors of the trunk during flexion and an absence of relaxation during the fatigue test. Thus, the multifidus, gluteus maximus and axial muscles tire more quickly.

The endurance test demonstrates the patient's aptitude to lift a load 4 times in 20 seconds from ground level to a height of 50 cm. The weight increments are 5 kg for men and 2.5 kg for women. The maximal load normally raised is around 45 to 55% of body weight.

# BIBLIOGRAPHY (FOR SECTIONS 1, 2 AND 3 OF CHAPTER)

- ANDERSSON, GBJ. Epidemiological features of chronic low back pain, Lancet, [s.I], [s.n], 1999, 354, 581-585.
- BALAGUE F., G. Dutoit et M. Walburger. Low back pain in school children an epidemiologic study, Scand J Rehab Med, 1988, 20: 175-179.
- BALAGUE F., M. Nordin, ML Skovron et al. Non specific low back pain among school children; a field survey with analysis of some associated factors. J. Spinal Disord, 1994, 7: 374-379.
- BRADY S, Mayer T. et RJ Gatchel. Physical progress and residual impairment quantification after functional restoration. Part II: Isokinetic trunk strength, Spine, 1994, 19(4): 395-400.
- BUCQUET, D. et al. The french version of Nottingham Health Profile. A comparison of items weights with of the source version. Soc Sci med, 1990, 30 (7): 829-835.
- BURTON, AK et al. Psychosocial predictors of outcome in acute and subchronic low back trouble, Spine, 1995, 20 (6): 722-728.
- CADY, L., D. Bischoff et E. O'Connell, Strength and fitness and subsequent back injuries in firefighters. Journal of Occupational Medicine, 1979, 21: 269-272.
- CARRAGEE EJ, T. Alamin, JL Miller et al. Discographic, MRI and psychosocial determinants of low back pain disability and remission: a prospective study in subjects with persistent back pain. [s.I], The Spine Journal, 2005, 5: 24-35.
- CHAORY, K., M. Revel, S. Poiraudeau et al. Impact of functional restoration programs on fears, avoidance and beliefs in chronic low back pain patients. [s.I], Ann Readapt Med Phys, 2004, 47( 3): 93-97.
- CLAUW, DJ et al. Pain sensitivity as a correlate of clinical status in individuals with chronic low back pain. [s.I], Spine, 1999, 24 (19): 2036-2041.
- CHENARD, JR, J. Charest, B. Lavignolle et S. Marchand. Lombalgies chroniques: du modèle médical au paradigme multifactoriel. [s.I], Sciences et comportement, 1988, 18: 250-281.
- CHENARD, JR, B. Lavignolle et J. Charest. Lombalgie, dix étapes sur les chemins de la guérison. [s.I], Masson, 1991.
- CHAREST J., JR Chenard, B. Lavignolle et S. Marchand. Lombalgie: école interactionnelle du dos. [s.I], Masson, 1996.
- COSKUN E., T. Suzer et O. Topuz et al. Relationship between epidural fibrosis pain, disability and psychological factors after lumbar disc surgery. [s.I], Spine, 2000, 9: 218-223.
- CURTIS L., T. Mayer et RJ Gatchel. Physical progress and residual impairment quantification after functional restauration. Part III: Isokinetic and isoinertial lift capacity. [s.I], Spine, 1994, 19(4): 401-405.
- DEBURGE, Anne. Approche du traitement psychodynamique de la lombalgie par un analyste. [s.I], Cahier de la SOFCOT: lombalgies et lombosciatiques, Expansion Scientifique, [s.d]
- DE GROOT, K., S. Boecke, H. Dozois, DKA et al. A predictive utility of CSQ in low back pain: individual vs composite measures. [s.I], Pain, 1996, 66: 171-180.

- DUPLAN, B., B. Lavignolle, M. Rossignol, B. Troussier et JF Roche. Lombalgies chroniques et écoles du dos, Aix-les-Bains, Table ronde 4011, semaine de Rhumatologie. Rhumatologie, 1994, (4§), (8): 209-256.
- DUPLAN, B., A. Lambert., P. Bernard, A. Martin et JF Roche. Prise en charge multidisciplinaire des lombalgiques chroniques. Rhumatologie, 1994, 46 (8): 215-220.
- DUPLAN, B. La douleur: un affect à partager. Contribution à l'étude du mal au dos, à la métapsychologie de l'affect. Master humanités et sciences humaines «psychologie clinique», 2005, Université Lumière, Lyon 2.
- DUQUESNOY, B. Définition de la lombalgie chronique. Rev Rhum, 1994, 61 (4 bis), 9-10.
- EPPING-JORDAN, JE et al. Transition to chronic pain in men with low back pain: predictive relationships among pain intensity, disability and depressive symptoms. Health Psychol, 1998, 17 (5): 421-427.
- FISHER, K. et M. Johnston. Emotional distress and control cognitions as mediators of the impact of chronic pain on disability. Br J Health Psycho, 1998, 3: 225-236.
- FRITZ, JM, SZ George et A. Delitto. The role of fear-avoidance beliefs in acute low back pain: relationships with current and future disability and work status. Pain, 2001, 94 (1): 7-15.
- GATCHEL, RJ, PB Polatin et TG Mayer. The dominant role of psychosocial risk factors in the development of chronic back pain disability. Spine, 1995, 20 (24): 2702-2709.
- GEORGE, S.Z, JM Fritz et al. The effect of fear-avoidance based physical therapy intervention for patients with acute low back pain: results of a randomized trial. Spine, 2003, 28, 23: 2551-2560.
- HAGG, O., P. Fritzell, L. Ekselius et al. A predictors of outcome in fusion surgery for chronic back pain. A report from the Swedish Lumbar. Spine Eur, Spine, 2003, 12: 22-33.
- HASEMBRING M. et al. Risk factors of chronicity in lumbar disc patients. A prospective investigation of biologic, psychological and social predictors of therapy outcome. Spine, 1994, 19, 24: 2759-2765.
- HAZARD, RG et al. Early prediction of chronic disability after occupational low back injury. Spine, 1996, 21: 945-951.
- HOFFMAN, RM, KJ Wheeler et RA Deyo. Surgery for herniated lumbar discs: a literature synthesis. J Gen Intern Med 1993, 8: 487-496.
- HYATHORNTHWAITE, JA et al. Pain coping strategies predict perceived control over pain. Pain, 1998, 77: 33-39.
- KESSLER, M. et al. Depressive symptoms and disability in acute and chronic back pain patients. Int J Behav Med, 1996, 3,2: 91-103.
- JUNGE, A, M. Frolich, S. Ahrens et al. Predictors of bad and good outcome of lumbar spine surgery. Spine,1996, 21: 1056-1065.
- JOUSSET, N., S. Fanello, L. Bontoux et al. Effects of functional restauration versus 3 hours per week of physical therapy: a randomized controlled study. Spine, 2004, 29, 5: 487-493.
- KLENERMAN, L. et al. The prediction of chronicity in patients with an acute attack of low back pain in a general pratice setting. Spine, 1995, 20, 4: 478-484.
- KOLE-SNIDJERS, AM et al. Chronic low back pain: what does cognitive coping skills training add to operant behavioral treatment? Results of randomize clinical trial. J Consult Clin, 1999, 67, 6: 931-934.
- KOLECK, M. Rôle de certains facteurs psychosociaux dans le profil évolutif des lombalgies communes. In: Bruchon-Schweitzer M, Quintard B ed., Personnalité et maladies, Dunod, Paris, 2001.
- KOLECK, M. Rôle de certains facteurs psychosociaux dans l'évolution des lombalgies communes: Étude semi-prospective en psychologie de la santé. Thèse Doctorat Psychologie, 2000, Université Bordeaux, France.
- KOLECK M., JM Mazaux, N. Rascle et M. Bruchon-Schweitzer. Psychosocial factors and coping strategies as predictors of chronic evolution and quality of life in patients with low back pain: a prospective study. European Journal of Pain, 2006, 10: 1-11.
- KRÖNER-HERWIG, B. et al. Predicting subjective disability in chronic pain patients. Int J Behav Med, 1996, 31, 1, 30-40.
- KUJALA, UM, S. Taimela, M. Erikentalo et al. Low back pain in adolescent athletes. Med. Sci Sports Exerc 1996, 28, 2, 165-170.
- LEQUESNE, M. ret M. Gourevitch. Le préalable psychiatrique à l'indication d'arthrodèse lombaire. Rev Rhum, 1973, 29: 1-7.
- LEWANDOWSKI, W. Psychological factors in chronic pain: a worthwhile undertaking for nursing? Arch Psychiatr Nurs, 2004, 18, 3: 97-105.
- LIN, CC et SE Ward. Perceived self-efficacy and outcome expectancies in coping with chronic low back pain. Res Nurs Health, 1996, 19, 199-310.
- LINTON, SJ et K. Hallden. Can we screen for problematic back pain? A screening questionnaire for predicting outcome in acute and subacute back pain. Clin J Pain, 1998, 14, 209-215.
- LINTON, SJ. A review of psychological risk factors in back and neck pain. Spine 2000, 25, 9, 1148-1156.
- LUMPKIN, JR. Validity of a brief Locus of Control Scale for survey research. Psychol Rep, 1985, 57, 655-659.
- MAEZEL, A., L. Li. The economic burden of low back pain; a review of studies published between 1996 and 2001. Best Pract Res Clin Rhumatol, 2002, 16 (1), 23-30.
- MARTY, P. et M. Fain, Contribution à l'étude des rachialgiques. Évolution Psychiatrique, 1952, 1, 95-121.
- MAYER, T., J. Tabor, E. Bovasso et al. Physical progress and residual impairment quantification after functional restauration, Part I, Lumbar mobility. Spine, 1994, 19, 4, 389-394.
- McCRACKEN, LM et al. Coping with pain produced by physical activity in persons with chronic back pain: immediate assessment following a specific pain event. Behav Med, 1998, 24, 29-34.
- PICAVET, HS et al. Pain catastrophizing and kinesiophobia: predictors of chronic low back pain, Am J Epidemiol, 2002; 156, 11, 1028-1034.
- PINCUS T., AK Burton, S. Vogel et al. A systematic review of psychological factors as predictors of chronicity/disability in prospective cohorts of low back pain. Spine, 2002, 27, 5, 109-120.
- POLATIN PB et al. Psychiatric illness and chronic low back pain.: the mind and the spine –Which goes first? Spine, 1993, 18,1, 66-71.
- POPE, MH. Risk indicators in low back pain. Ann Med 1989; 21, 387-392.
- Quebec task force on spinal disorders. Spine 1987, 12, 1-59.
- Groupe de travail québecois sur les aspects cliniques des affections vertébrales chez les travailleurs. Rev clinique et expérimentale, 1987, 10, 1-57.
- RADLOFF, LS. The CES-D Scale, a self-report depression scale for research in the general population. Applied Psychological measurement, 1977, 1, 385-401.
- LEINO, PL. Does leisure time physical prevent low back disorders? Spine, 1993, 18, 863-871.
- RILEY, JL et al, Empirical subgroups of the Coping Strategies Questionnaire – Revised: A multisample study. Clin J Pain, 1999, 15, 11-116.
- ROBINSON, ME et al. The Coping Strategies Questionnaire: a large sample, item level factor analysis. Clin J Pain, 1997; 13, 43-49.
- Rossignol M., S. Suissa et L. Abenhaim. Working disability due to occupational back pain: three-year follow of 2300 compensated workers in Quebec. J Occup Med. 1988; 30: 502-505.

- ROSENTIEL, AK et FJ Keefe. The use of coping strategies in chronic low back pain patients : relationship to patient characteristics and current adjustment. Pain, 1983, 17, 33-44.
- SALMINEN, J., M. Erikentalo, M. Laine et al. Low back pain in the young. A prospective three-year follow-up study of subjects with and without low back pain. Spine, 1995, 20, 2101-2108.
- SALMINEN, J., M. Erikentalo, J. Pentti et al. Recurrent low back pain and early disc degeneration in the young. Spine, 1999, 24, 13, 1316-1321.
- SCHADE, V., N. Semmer, C. Main et al. The impact of clinical, morphological, psychosocial and work-related factors on the outcome of lumbar discectomy. Pain, 1999, 80, 239-249.
- SCHERMELLEH-ENGEL, K. et al. Perceived competence and trait anxiety as determinants of pain coping strategies. Person Indiv Diff, 1997, 22, 1, 1-10.
- SORENSEN, LV, O. Mors et O. Skovlund. A prospective study of the importance of psychological and social factors for the outcome after surgery in patients with slipped disk operated upon for the first time. Acta Neurochir, 1987, 88, 119-125 .
- SPIELBERGER, CD et al. Manual for the State-Trait Inventory (STAI) Form Y. Palo Alto. Consulting Psychologists Press, 1983.
- BRUCHON-SCHWEITZER M. et cal. L'inventaire anxiété-trait et d'anxiété-état : adaptation française et validation du STAI −Y de Spielberger. Paris, Éditions du Centre de Psychologie Appliquée, 1993.
- SPINHOVEN, P. et al. Pain coping strategies in a Dutch population of chronic low back pain patients. Pain, 1989, 45, 29-24.
- SPINHOVEN, P. et al. Catastrophizing and internal pain control as mediators of outcome in a multidisciplinary treatment of chronic low back pain. Eur J Pain, 2004, 8, 3, 211-219.
- SWARD, L. The thoracolumbar spine in young elite athletes, Current concepts on the effects of physical training. Sports med, 1992, 13, 5, 357-364.
- SYMONDS, TL, AK Burton, KM Tillotson et al. Do attitudes and beliefs influence work loss due to low back trouble. Occup Med, 1996, 46, 1, 25-32.
- TROUSSIER, B., F. Balagué et X. Phelip. Lombalgies non spécifiques de l'enfant et de l'adolescent: facteurs de risque. Rev Rhum, 1998, 65, 49-57.
- TRUCHON, M. et L. Fillion, Biopsychosocial determinants of chronic disability and low back pain: a review. J Occup Rehabil, 2000, 10, 2, 117-142.
- TUTTLE, DH et al. Empirical dimensions of copping in chronic pain patients : a factorial analysis. Rehabilitation Psychology, 1991, 36, 3, 179-188.
- VÄLLFORS, B. Acute, Subacute and chronic low back pain : clinical symptoms, absenteeism and working environment. Scand J Rehab Med, 1985, 11, 1-98.
- WADDELL, G., H. Waddell. A review of social influences on neck and back pain and disability, In: Neck and back pain, The scientific evidence, chapter 2, 13-55. Nachemson A., Jonsson E., Lipincott, Willimas & Wilkin ed. 2000.
- Waddell G. The back pain revolution. Churchill Livingstone, ed., 1998, 438 pages.
- Ware, JE, CD Scherbourne, The MOS 36-item Short-Form Health survey (SF36), Conceptual framework and item selection. Med Care, 1992, 2, 30, 473-483.

## BIBLIOGRAPHY (FOR SECTION 4 OF CHAPTER)

- ABENHAÏM, L., M. ROSSIGNOL et S. SCOTTS. The prognostic consequences in the making of the initial medical diagnosis of work-related back injuries. Spine 1995, 20, 791-795.
- ALARANTA, H. et al. Intensive physical and psychosocial training program for patients with chronic low back pain, A controlled clinical trial. Spine, 1994, 19, 1339-1349.
- COLLE, F., S. POIRAUDEAU et M. REVEL. Exercices physiques et lombalgies chroniques : à la recherche de l'évidence. Ann Readaptation Med Phys, 2001, 44, 393-6.
- BENDIX, AF, T. BENDIX et al. Functionnal restoration for chronic low back pain, Two-year follow-up of two randomized clinical trials. Spine, 1998, 23, 717-725.
- DANNEELS, LA, GG VANDERSTRAETEN, DC CAMBIER et al. CT imaging of trink muscles in chronic, Low back pain patients and healthy control subjects. Eur Spine J, 2000, 9, 266-272.
- FROST, H. et al. Randomised controlled trial for evaluation of fitness programme for patients with chronic low back pain. Br Med J, 1995, 310, 151-154.
- HAZARD, RG et al. Functionnal restoration with behavioral support, A one-year prospective study of patients with chronic low back pain. Spine, 1989, 14, 157-161.
- JÄRVILOSKI, AA et al. Outcome of two multimodal back treatment programs with and without intensive physical training. J Spinal Disord, 1993, 6, 93-98.
- LINDSTRÖM, I. et al. Mobility, strength and fitness after a graded activity program for patients with subacute low back pain. Spine, 1992, 17, 641-649.
- MANNION, A.F., L. KASER, E. WEBER et al. Influence of age and duration of symptoms on fibre type distribution and size of back muscles in chronic low back pain patients. Eur Spine J, 2000, 9, 273-281.
- MANNICHE C. et al. Intensive dynamic back exercises for chronic low back pain: a clinical trial. Pain, 1991, 47, 53-63.
- MANNION, A.F. et al. A randomized clinical trial of three active therapies for chronic low back pain. Spine, 1999, 24, 2435-2448.
- MAYER, T, V. MOONEY et R. GATCHEL. Contemporary conservative care for painful spinal disorders, Phildelphia, Lea & Fibiger ed., 1991.
- MAYER, T. Physical progress and residual impairment quantification after functional restoration, Part II: isokinetic trunk strength. Spine, 1994, 19, 395-400.
- NORDIN, M. Restauration fonctionnelle et reconditionnement musculaire. Revue de Médecine vertébrale 2001, 3, 4-9 (60 références).
- RAVAUD, C. et R. De MUNICO. Une approche interdisciplinaire de la lombalgie chronique: expérience de la Tour de Gassies, résultats à un an. Ann Readaptation Med Phys, 2001, 44, 395.
- SALANON, L. Évaluation des valeurs normales au niveau du rachis lombaire par la méthode isocinétique. Thèse, 1998, Université libre de Bruxelles−Erasme, (88 références).
- SIVHONEN, T. et al. Averaged surface EMG in testing back function. Electromyogr Clin Neurophysiol, 1988, 28, 335-339.
- SIVHONEN, T. Exercise therapy effects on functional radiographic findings and segmental electromyographic activity in lumbar spine instability. Arch Phys med Rehab, 1993, 74, 933-939.
- VAN TULDER, MW, M. GOOSSENS, G. WADDELL et A. NACHEMSON. Conservative treatment of chronic back pain. In: A. NACHEMSON, E. JONSSON. Lippincott Williams & Wilkins ed., 2000, Neck and back pain, the scientific evidence of causes, diagnosis and treatment.

# MY STORY

Helen Tupper, Dartmouth, Nova Scotia, Canada

Helen Tupper joined the North American Chronic Pain Association of Canada (NACPAC) in 1993, then was President of the association from 1998 to 2001. Having retired from NACPAC, Helen Tupper and Celeste Johnston ( who was then president of the Canadian Pain Society - CPS) formed the Canadian Pain Coalition (CPC) in 2002. Helen Tupper was president of the CPC from 2004 to 2008, and past president for two years. She speaks to associations or symposiums occasionally.

(See other testimonial, page 60.)

I have learned a great deal over the years about pain and doctors, also about nurses. I am sad to say not a lot has changed with some nurses. Those who take the time to learn, and attend workshops and conferences, do learn and try to educate others. But as with any other profession there will always be those who just don't care.

My pain will never go away. The day I made the admission to myself I realized I was in this for the long haul, and I could do it hard or easy. We all have choices to make, and I chose to try to make the best of it. I didn't want to become a complaining woman who people would avoid because I was so negative. I wanted my friends to continue to be friends, so I have tried not to complain or even talk about my pain. I try not to bother my husband either. But he knows me so well he can just look at me to know what kind of day I had. He still supports me after 42 years, and we have been fortunate in many ways. My son told me when he was just about ten years old that one day when he was walking home from school he decided that he could either be happy or sad. He liked being happy better, so he made the decision to be happy. I have tried to adopt the same attitude. I believe that when we are sad, or down, we make those around us sad too. It rubs off on people and that isn't a good thing. But happiness also rubs off, and that is a good thing. Even though we hurt we can still contribute. It may not be the way we thought we would when we were planning our lives. In fact I expect most people, with or without pain find that to be the case.

We must be our own advocates, because no one knows our problems better. We have to learn how to explain ourselves, and not to complain while doing it. Doctors get very tired of hearing a lot of complaints. We can express ourselves about pain without being negative all the time. When it is horrific, I believe perhaps then we are allowed to talk about it. We need help then, so we have to ask for it.

What I have learned is this. Accept that chronic pain is going to be with you for the rest of your life. Learn to live around it the best you can. Rest when you have to, and you will most likely have to rest daily. Give up the idea you can do what everyone else can do, you can't. Chronic pain limits our abilities, but it doesn't remove them. Just learn to work with what you have and do your chores in stages. Take days instead of hours. Learn to divert your attention by getting interested in something else. I mean something you like to do, that might take your mind off the pain. I paint, and scrap book. Both things I love to do, but can only do for limited times because the pain takes over. I had to learn how to pace myself, and that is a never-ending process. I am always learning what I can and can't do. I still end up flat on my back because I have over done it. But most of the time the pain goes down again and I can cope with it.

Try to find a doctor who will treat you kindly and with compassion as well as understanding. Some doctors just don't get it, and if you run into one of those, try to move on. You have the choice to find the right doctor for you. But remember try not to complain too much, because they get tired of hearing the same thing all the time. Save the complaints for when you are really bad.

If you have a spouse or partner, let them know if you are in a lot of pain and ask them to please excuse you while you lie down for a while. It is far better to do this than to try to push on and become grumpy and not be able to do what it was you started to do. They have to live with us, so let us try to make ourselves likeable rather than grumpy and unhappy. It rubs off.

Try not to be hard on yourself. When the pain comes and you find it really difficult to do what you are trying to do, don't beat yourself up and try to push yourself through it. Perhaps it is time to stop and rest. There is nothing wrong with that. Resting gives our body time to get the pain under control, and we can then function much better and more successfully. It isn't just platitudes, it does work.

The last thing I will say is this. No one deserves pain, and it isn't given to make particular people suffer. It just happens, and those who get it just have to learn how to cope with it. Don't blame yourself or others, it isn't going to help. When one door closes, another one opens. Sometimes our pain allows us to see things we didn't see before, or might never have seen if we didn't have pain and been slowed down. Keep your eyes open and be observant. Encourage others who have chronic pain, especially if they have not had it as long as you have. It helps to hear from others who have it, and are living with it. And remember pain won't kill us, just test our patience along the way. Make the best of it if you can and try to be in charge, don't let the pain take over.

Presently I still take narcotics, and have accepted that I will probably have to take them the rest of my life. I can't do the things I would like to do, but have modified my life so that I do as much as possible between the rests and down times. I always have books beside my bed for when I have to rest. I love to read and it really helps to pass the time.

Choose your favourite things to do, and eliminate those that don't really matter as much. If you can afford to have help with your housework, then do it. Save your energy for something more important. If you can't then don't try to do it all in one day. Break it up into small segments, so that it won't send you to bed for days. Just try to remember that while chronic pain does hurt, and does change our lives, it doesn't need to destroy them. The old cliché of make lemon aid out of the lemons applies big time. Learn to turn the difficult into something doable.

**Don't give up.**

# A BETTER UNDERSTANDING
## OF OROFACIAL PAIN

# 9

Jean-Paul Goulet DDS, MSD, FRCD(c), specialist in oral medicine, Quebec, Quebec, Canada
Professor, Faculty of Dentistry, Université Laval, Quebec, Canada

## ABSTRACT

The orofacial region is no different than the other parts of the body when it comes to chronic pain. Pain can take different forms in different faces. Some patients will experience burning sensations in their mouths, others will have toothaches, and still others will feel pain in the face and the jaw, with the inconveniences this causes in everyday life. The challenge involves identifying the cause. Yet, despite scientific progress, we are sometimes unable to find an answer or a definitive solution. This section discusses the most common types of orofacial pain so that people suffering with this type of pain can have a better understanding of their torment. Advice will be given to help them clearly understand their condition so as to avoid useless actions and manage to make the most of the therapeutic approaches currently available.

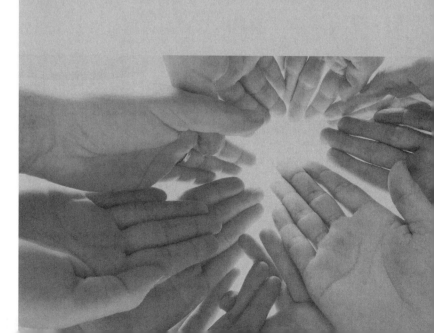

# 1. INTRODUCTION

The orofacial region is no different than the other parts of the body when it comes to chronic pain. Pain can take various forms. Some patients will experience burning sensations in their mouths, others will have toothaches, and still others will feel pain in the face and the jaw, not to mention the constellation of secondary symptoms that often accompany chronic pain. Since the orofacial region is the centre of several functions that are closely related to the pleasures of life and communication, particular attention is paid to it, all the more so since it provides a multitude of starting points as a source of pain, beginning with the teeth and the sinuses. Many types of pain will be fleeting, but those that become chronic are accompanied by their own share of anguish and concern and, once pain is chronic, the cognitive, emotional and motivational components will give a very personal dimension to this unpleasant experience, which remains very subjective.

# 2. PRESENTATION OF THE CASE STUDIES OF THREE INDIVIDUALS WITH CHRONIC OROFACIAL PAIN

In order to place the topic of this chapter in context, I think it is interesting to share the experiences of a few patients who have already consulted medical professionals for chronic orofacial pain. The purpose is to better understand what most people with such problems have in common. The rest of this chapter will focus on the types of chronic orofacial pain we usually encounter in clinical practice so as to help those who suffer from such pain better understand their condition and make better decisions, while avoiding pointless actions.

## MRS. *Y*'S CASE

Mrs. *Y*, a baby-boomer, came in for a consultation, declaring "My mouth hurts, but I can't tell if it's my teeth or my gums; my left ear hurts and I hear cracking sounds more often in my left ear than in the right ear." Then she went on to say that her discomfort and her pain started about a year ago "following a surgery to the maxillary sinuses for an ear infection," and for a feeling of pressure and a plugged ear on the left side. The surgery went well and, although the ear symptoms went away, the pain persisted. However, since the operation, her jaw no longer feels like it did before. The way her jaws close is uncomfortable. Moreover, her upper left teeth hurt and she experiences pressure on her gums that changes place. The otorhinolaryngologist (ORL) who performed the operation confirmed that her sinuses are normal, and that there is nothing in her ear to account for the remaining symptoms. Moreover, he recommended that she be seen by her dentist since he feels that it is a problem of "dental occlusion". Mrs. *Y* saw her dentist who told her, following a clinical examination and x-rays of her jaws, that everything is normal, but that an occlusal splint could provide some relief since her problem might be related to the clenching and grinding of teeth.

She was referred to an oral and maxillo-facial surgeon who prescribed a muscle relaxant to be taken at bedtime. She stopped taking the medication because she was too sleepy when waking the morning after. Her dentist made a mandibular occlusal splint for her that she wore while sleeping for about six weeks. It relieved the pain a little. Mrs. *Y* then consulted a physiotherapist and, following that, an osteopath who treated her for "tension in the cervical region". These treatments had no beneficial effects on the pain in her ear and teeth. She started to wear her mandibular splint more regularly at night and during the day when she had an opportunity to do so. After a few weeks, she noted that she experienced less pain when she wore her mandibular splint during the day. However, this had no effect on the pain in her ear. Searching for a solution, Mrs. *Y* saw an auriculotherapist. An initial treatment that involved placing "magnets along the edge of the ear" caused the pain to disappear completely for a few days. However, the pain returned following the second treatment, and since then, Mrs. *Y* wonders if her occlusion is responsible for her symptoms.

## MRS. *Z*'S CASE

The second case is that of Mrs. *Z*, who has been retired for several years. She was referred by her dentist for "pain in her gums, ear and eye on the right side" which appeared with no apparent cause three years ago. The pain, described as a "toothache that extends up to the eye and the eyebrow", is shooting and the epicentre is located on the lower right jaw where she is missing teeth. Initially, her ear was very painful and her right eye seemed to be "wet all the time". She consulted her physician who ordered a brain scan, which turned out to be normal. Then she saw an otorhinolaryngologist (ORL) who examined her ear and concluded that it was normal. When the ORL saw the missing teeth in the lower jaw, he indicated that her symptoms were probably related to the lack of posterior teeth, which caused the temporomandibular joint (TMJ) problem, with referred pain to the ear. Mrs. *Z* saw her dentist who restored the toothless space with implant-borne crowns. Since the treatment was completed

## MRS. Z CASE (SUITE)

two years ago, Mrs. Z has noticed no change in her state. The site of the pain was re-examined and x-rays were taken, but no anomaly was noted. The pain she has to deal with on a daily basis has no pulsing, stabbing or electrical character. The pain is remittent (comes and goes) and is generally present at night when she goes to bed, but she does not wake up at night. Mrs. Z can chew on the side where the pain occurs and this does not change anything. Pressing her teeth together, pressing or rubbing her cheek provides some relief. Two treatments with an orthotherapist resulted in pain-free periods lasting three to four days after which it returned as before. Her physician suggested that she take an antidepressant to relieve her pain, which Mrs. Z refused since she said she was not at all depressed and did not see how an antidepressant could help her.

## MRS. B'S CASE

The third case is about Mrs. B, a patient in her early 50s who has been complaining of "burning sensations in her mouth" for a year and a half. She recalled that the sensations started during a trip, for no apparent reason. During the first year, the burning sensations came, and then disappeared after one or two weeks before returning later. Periods without burning sensations varied, but for the last six months it has been there all the time. They start a few hours after she wakes up, hit a plateau and last all day long until she goes to bed. The burning sensations affect her tongue, palate and the inside of her lips. When she eats or drinks she experiences no burning sensation. Also, she always has a bottle of icy water within reach, and she drinks frequently.

## WHAT ELSE THE CASES OF MRS. Y, MRS. Z AND MRS. B REVEAL

These three cases have a certain number of things in common that can be used as references for most people who have chronic orofacial pain. Regardless of the context and the circumstances, pain is a personal and subjective experience. Its presence is acknowledged based on what the patient says and feels. Clearly, these three women experience chronic pain since, in each of the three cases, the pain has persisted for at least three months. Chronic pain may be continuous, meaning it is there all the time, or remittent, meaning it comes and goes for days or weeks before reappearing again. At the beginning, Mrs. B's burning sensations were remittent, and they are now continuous, although they may once again become remittent. Whether the pain is continuous or remittent, the intensity may remain the same or vary over time, with peaks of greater intensity and periods of calm.

As is the case with Mrs. Y and Mrs. Z, patients with chronic orofacial pain are likely to consult several health professionals. This is not surprising since the orofacial region is very complex and contains various organs with specialized functions. Think of the eyes, ears, nose, throat, sinuses, neck, blood vessels and other intracranial structures, as well as the oral cavity and the jaws. Beside the fact that the innervation of all these structures is complex, their proximity is also a frequent source of projected or referred pain. Thus, the expertise of various specialists is often required in an attempt to elucidate the source of the pain, considering the number of conditions that could affect the orofacial region. The coexistence of several conditions must also be taken into account.

For Mrs. Y and Mrs. Z, dental occlusion was identified as possibly responsible for the persistence of the orofacial pain based on the fact that all the examination and investigation results were within normal limits. Unfortunately, dental occlusion is all too often the scapegoat when no other cause is found to account for a chronic orofacial pain problem. This reinforces the false belief that occlusion results in a temporomandibular disorder (TMD) through the harmful effects it has on the masticatory muscles and/or the temporomandibular joints (TMJ), which are the source of chronic orofacial pain. Those advocating this point of view refer to the vertical dimension of the occlusion, the displacement of the articular condyles and the lower jaw (the mandible), the occlusal disharmonies and the neuromuscular imbalance of the masticatory muscles to justify rehabilitation treatments that are complex and very expensive. Patients with chronic orofacial pain must understand that this type of treatment will not solve their problem. There have been no well controlled clinical studies showing that chronic orofacial pain attributed to a temporomandibular disorder is relieved by modifying the way teeth come together or the position of the articular condyles in the fossa. People should also not conclude that the occlusion was the source of the pain when their jaw or joint pain decreases after wearing an occlusal splint. There are many other factors that need to be taken into account to explain such relief, particularly since the chronic orofacial pain associated with TMDs also affects subjects with a normal occlusion, and they do benefit from wearing an occlusal splint.

Mrs. B's case history is similar to Mrs. Z's in the sense that no particular event was associated with the onset of the pain, which is the opposite of the pain experiences we may have had in the past. Most of the time when pain occurs, we can identify a potential cause such as an infection of the upper respiratory tract, an oral-dental problem, some sort of trauma to the face, or a recent intervention by a dentist. Usually our healing mechanisms take over, and the pain will be relieved with an appropriate treatment. However, when pain constantly comes back or persists, and becomes overwhelming, we are concerned and discouraged because we cannot find a valid explanation. Such a scenario is not in keeping with the traditional model of pain as playing a protective biological role, as an alarm signal following an injury or some sort of physical damage. When chronic pain has no protective biological role, it should be seen as a dysfunctional state of the peripheral and or the central nervous system involving the transmission, the modulation and the perception pain pathways. Thus, unless a cause can be identified that would enable us to eliminate a chronic pain state, we look for strategies that can act on the pain perception pathways so that we have a better understanding of the underlying mechanisms. Headaches such as tension headaches and migraines clearly illustrate the concept of "chronic pain devoid of any biological role" for which the mechanisms and events that lead to pain are better known than the causes themselves.

The cases of Mrs. *Y*, Mrs. *Z* and Mrs. *B* are good examples of chronic orofacial pain that plays no protective biological role. Regarding Mrs. *Y*'s case, there is a plausible temporal relationship between the intervention performed on the sinuses and the pain and discomfort she is still experiencing. This suggests an iatrogenic type of pain caused by trauma to the nerve responsible for the innervation of the upper back teeth that could have occurred during the surgery.

A majority of patients with chronic orofacial pain suffer from musculo-skeletal pain and, more specifically, pain associated with temporomandibular disorders, which will be discussed later. However, Mrs. *Y*, Mrs. *Z* and Mrs. *B* are good examples of neuropathic orofacial

pain, based on examination findings and diagnostic investigations. This represents the second most common cause of chronic orofacial pain. Burning mouth syndrome and atypical odontalgia belong to this group and will also be discussed later. Chronic neuropathic orofacial pain often remains unexplained, but most people acknowledge that it is usually the result of some kind of dysfunction of the nervous system combined with other predisposing factors. When there is no identifiable cause, we call it idiopathic. Neuropathic orofacial pain can also occur following a trauma or as a result of the compression of a nerve path, after an accident or a surgical procedure. The treatment for neuropathic orofacial pain is above all pharmacological and is similar to neuropathic pain observed in other parts of the body. Since most chronic pain state has its share of psychosocial impacts, psychological assessment and interventions should be considered soon and not only when years have gone by and prior treatments have failed to improve the patient's condition. Finally, there are other types of chronic orofacial pain that are encountered less frequently in the clinical setting, such as vascular pain (a type of migraine), which must be taken into consideration when a patient consults for chronic orofacial pain.

## 3. HOW THE PATIENT CAN CONTRIBUTE TO THE DIAGNOSIS

Pain as an unpleasant subjective experience can only be assessed through the information the patient provides to the health professional. That will help the professional to better understand the patient's suffering. The history of the pain experienced remains one of the major elements of the diagnostic process, which is why the questions asked by the health professional during the interview are so important.

From the outset, the first question will concern the site of the pain, and this information will guide the clinical examination, which is intended to determine if the source, namely the origin of the pain, is really at the site where the patient experiences the pain. Knowing if the pain is clearly localized or diffuse will also help the health professional. It is important to determine both the site and the source of the pain for the diagnosis and treatment. For example, a patient may experience pain in the teeth in his/her upper jaw, yet the teeth may not be the cause if he/she is suffering from a maxillary sinusitis. Treating the sinusitis and not the teeth will relieve the pain. Frequently, the pain is not confined to the immediate region corresponding to its source, but may also extend beyond that site and occasionally even be projected to distant structures. A good example is that of patients suffering from angina. Most often they experience retrosternal pain that is projected

to their arms, yet the pain may also be referred and experienced only in the lower jaw. In this case, we have a pain of cardiac origin that is projected to an anatomical site, the jaw, which has nothing at all to do with the cause.

This clearly illustrates why we must avoid falling into the trap of focusing solely on the site of the pain. Information pertaining to the onset, the character of the pain (if any), the intensity, the duration, the absences, the time of day, what triggers it, aggravates it and relieves it, as well as its effect on sleep can also be of assistance to the health professional.

The impact the pain has on the patient's activities and quality of life in general is another important aspect to be explored. Numerous researchers have shown that chronic pain has a negative effect on mood, attitude, behaviour and sleep. Apart from their concern, patients generally wind up consulting health professionals because the pain is sustained, frequent and severe. But pain also interferes with daily activities, work, leisure activities and relations with loved ones (spouses, children, relatives, friends). Information about these changes can be used to adjust the intervention plan accordingly in order to promote a return to normal.

## 4. CHRONIC PAIN IN THE JAW AND JOINTS

Temporomandibular disorders (TMDs) are a frequent cause of pain and jaw dysfunction that affect the masticatory system. The pain associated with these disorders occurs in 10-12% of the Quebec population, predominantly in women between the ages of 20 and 45. For several patients, the symptoms disappear spontaneously, but approximately half of the patients seek out treatment for moderate to intense pain that interferes with their quality of life.

TMDs are musculoskeletal disorders such as those found in other parts of the body and they include a set of rather heterogeneous conditions involving the masticating muscles, primarily those used for closing the mouth and moving the jaw joints, namely the temporomandibular joints

(TMJs) and associated structures (ligaments, capsule, joint disk, condyle, eminence). Of all the TMDs, myofascial pain of the masticatory muscles is the most frequent cause of chronic musculoskeletal pain of the jaws, followed by arthralgia, namely pain from the temporomandibular joints.

Most of the time, the onset of myofascial pain of the masticatory muscles is insidious and for no apparent reason only on one side. Initially the pain is episodic, and then it can either stay that way or become daily and persistent. Over time, the patient sees basically the same symptoms appear on the opposite side of his/her face, although they are frequently not as severe. The intensity of the pain tends to increase as the day progresses, and it is aggravated by jaw movement and chewing. Patients usually complain of a deep, dull and aching pain, that limits mastication and the opening of the mouth. The pain arising from the masticatory muscles can be projected to the teeth, the temporomandibular joint and the forehead. Other less specific symptoms are frequently reported: headaches, a sensation of blocked or plugged ears, tinnitus, vertigo, neck pain, sensations of swelling. A diagnosis of myofascial pain is based on the patient's history and a positive clinical examination for masticatory muscles tender to palpation that reproduce the patient's symptoms, and cannot be attributed to any other conditions.

Pain from the temporomandibular joint is usually well localized and felt just in front of or inside the ear. It is sharper than myofascial pain. Often, patients think that they have an ear infection, which explains why they initially go to see their physician or an ORL. As in the case of myofascial pain, temporomandibular joint pain is aggravated by mastication, yawning and hyperextensions that occur when the mouth is opened. Patients generally avoid opening their mouths wide and eating food that needs too much chewing. Sometimes the pain is so serious that patients abstain from singing or playing a musical instrument (ex.: violin, saxophone). Those who chew gum cannot do so without experiencing more pain. Temporomandibular joint pain can be idiopathic, caused by a disc displacement problem, osteoarthritis, rheumatoid arthritis or an auto-immune disease of the connective tissues. Apart from the patient's history and the clinical examination, the diagnosis of temporomandibular joint pain is mainly based on imaging of the joint, and a medical work-up.

There is still a great deal of controversy concerning the causes and treatment of chronic pain associated with TMDs. The assumption that an occlusal disharmony can be held responsible for muscular and joint pain is not supported by any scientific data. Despite this, complex occlusal rehabilitation treatments are still offered, and, when the symptoms recur, these patients become candidates for even more invasive treatments including surgery to the temporomandibular joints. Unfortunately, all unanswered questions regarding the etiology of chronic pain associated with the TMDs benefit those who support mechanistic occlusal treatment or similar procedures since, regardless of the treatment used, the average success rate is always around 70%.

The current consensus is that a biopsychosocial model can best explain the chronicization of jaw and face pain associated with a temporomandibular disorder. A combination of genetic, behavioural, emotional and social factors provides a realistic explanation for a dysfunction of the pain regulating systems. Such a biopsychosocial model is moving away from mechanical interventions that focus solely on the occlusion and the position of the jaw to take advantage of strategies used in physical and behavioural medicine. The therapeutic approach is therefore conservative, reversible and not invasive, focusing primarily on management strategies tailored to the coping abilities of the individual for the best control of the pain and dysfunction. As with other types of chronic pain state, the aim is not so much to find a cure but rather to manage the patient's condition with a more realistic approach.

Depending on the nature of the factors that lead to, trigger and perpetuate the pain (ex.: clenching and grinding of teeth, bad habits, trauma, emotional tension, anxiety, depression, hormonal factors, an underlying medical condition, etc.), the therapy will usually start by educating the patient, raising his/her awareness about the parafunctional habits to be avoided, and modifying the patient's diet to rest the jaw muscles and joints. The treatment is then personalized by adding one or more of the following: stress and behavioural management, medication (anti-inflammatories, myorelaxants, antidepressants), physical therapy (heat, cold, jaw mobilization exercises), occlusal splint and trigger point injections. The use of muscular injections of botulinum toxin (Botox) to treat chronic refractory TMD pain is controversial, although it has been reported that a few patients may benefit from it.

## 5. CHRONIC TOOTH PAIN

As the saying goes, there is nothing worse than a toothache, and fortunately the dentist is there to help by providing the appropriate treatment, depending on whether the patient has a cavity, a defective filling, an abscess, or a loose tooth. There are, however, patients that complain of constant pain from a tooth that presents no problem. The clinical examination and the x-ray are within normal limits; there is no cavity or defective filling. There is no abnormal contact on the tooth that hurts, and tests checking the integrity of the tooth nerve are normal. Exasperated patients will end up having the tooth pulled when all of the treatments intended to relieve their pain have failed. Paradoxically, the pain continues where the tooth was, even after the extraction site has healed completely, giving rise to the expression "phantom tooth pain".

A certain number of conditions should be taken into account when dealing with a patient with pain coming from a tooth that is otherwise normal. For example, trigeminal neuralgia, also called "painful tic", can mimic a true toothache, but the pain has a rather unique character and is usually described as an electrical discharge. Piercing and stabbing are other descriptors. When a patient consults for a sustained tooth pain that has no apparent cause, a diagnosis of idiopathic, atypical odontalgia is very likely after the possibility of referred pain or a root fracture is excluded. The site, the character, the history and the temporal pattern of the toothache can alert the clinician to suspect a diagnosis of idiopathic atypical odontalgia. It should be noted that odontalgia simply means toothache. "Idiopathic" means that the cause of the pain is undetermined or unknown. Idiopathic atypical odontalgia is a frustrating condition for those who suffer from it, as well as for the dentist who happens to investigate such cases.

# 6. IDIOPATHIC ATYPICAL ODONTALGIA

Idiopathic atypical odontalgia is mainly seen in patients over 40 years old, and is more frequent among women. The teeth most frequently affected are the upper teeth (upper maxillary), and more specifically the bicuspids and the molars. The pain is described as throbbing and continuous, lasting all day long with peaks of more severe pain. Some patients avoid eating on the painful side since the pressure of chewing increases the pain, or because the gum around the tooth is more sensitive. The patient often associates the onset of the pain with a dental treatment. The fact that the pain is localized may make people think that the cause is dental, related to an inflammation, an infection of the nerve or a root fracture, that may lead to treatments (redoing a filling, root canal, apicoectomy, extraction) that will turn out to be useless. The fact that a treatment is occasionally followed by a brief period of relief gives false hope and encourages patients to continue with procedures that are often more invasive. But the pain comes back and often the surrounding teeth start to hurt. With atypical odontalgia, patients must understand that they can have persistent pain from a particular tooth without that tooth being the cause. Moreover, treatment to the tooth will not solve the problem and there is a risk that the pain will worsen following an invasive treatment.

Idiopathic atypical odontalgia is considered by most to be a neuropathic pain. The treatment is pharmacological, and most patients will usually benefit from taking medication. Low doses of tricyclic antidepressants and membrane stabilizers that act on nerve conduction are the most used medications. Unless contraindicated, there is no rule of thumb regarding which medication should be used first. Since pain relief will differ from one patient to another, the medication should be used for a few weeks and the dosage adjusted before one can tell if it can help. The most frequently asked question with respect to pharmacological treatment is: "Will I have to take the medication forever?" Several factors ought to be taken into account but, generally speaking, once the pain has been under control for weeks or months, the dosage of the drug is reduced gradually over several weeks so that the patient can eventually stop taking it. If the pain returns at some point, the medication is adjusted to the smallest dosage that ensures satisfactory pain relief.

# 7. CHRONIC PAIN OF ORAL MUCOUS MEMBRANES

At one point or another, everyone has had one or more canker sores in their mouth, especially the lips, the cheeks or under the tongue. These usually heal after a week or so, and do not lead to chronic mouth pain. Instead, it is a persistent burning sensation that is most often responsible for chronic oral mucosal pain (ex.: Mrs. *B*'s case).

Several reasons can account for a burning sensation in the mouth: the most common would be ingesting spicy food, a fleeting experience

in which the enjoyment of the delicacy is momentarily replaced by an unpleasant sensation. In the end, people deal with this type of situation well. Now, let's imagine that such sensations last for weeks, months, even years, and no cause can be found after all the relevant investigations and examinations have been done. This corresponds to a diagnosis, by means of exclusion, of a "burning mouth syndrome".

# 8. BURNING MOUTH SYNDROME

The burning sensations experienced by patients suffering from burning mouth syndrome are not really different from those that are secondary to canker sores or dryness of the mouth and associated with a drug intake or a medical problem. This is why patients should see their dentist for a full head, neck and mouth examination with special attention to the sites where the burning sensations are experienced. This is the only way to make sure that the oral cavity is well lubricated and looks otherwise normal at the site of the burning sensations. Patients who are concerned about cancer of the mouth will then be reassured by their dentist. At the same time, a review of the patient's health history will help in assessing the possible contribution of a medical problem and drug intake. This type of investigation to refute or confirm suspicions that a local condition or medical problem is the potential source of the burning sensations is best handled by a dentist who specializes in oral medicine or oral pathology and who will work with the patient's physician if necessary. The general dentist can refer the patient to one of these specialists, who are listed on the internet site of the *Ordre des dentistes du Québec* (www.odq.qc.ca).

People dealing with burning mouth syndrome experience their symptoms on the dorsum and side of the tongue, but the anterior aspect of the palate, inside the lips and cheeks are other intraoral sites that can be affected. Moreover, patients may complain of dry mouth

and an altered taste sensation. This syndrome, which is rather rare in men, is observed primarily in women in the years just before and after menopause. The symptoms usually start suddenly and for no apparent reason although, in retrospect, patients may sometimes attribute the onset to a recent illness or life event which could be a pure coincidence.

When questioned about their burning sensations, nine out of ten patients claim that it is present daily and, for a majority, the burning starts when they wake up and lasts throughout the day. For others, the burning sensations appear slowly later in the day and peak in severity in the evening. Approximately one-third of patients continue to have symptoms at night and, as a result, find it hard to fall asleep. Interestingly, the burning sensations are not present when eating and drinking, or when the patient's attention is diverted. Spicy food and acidic drinks will, however, make it worse. For patients wearing upper dentures, the burning sensation experienced in the palate becomes less and less tolerable as the day progresses. Removing the dentures provides a certain amount of relief, but does not cause the burning to disappear completely.

As soon as patients are informed that everything in their mouths is normal, two questions come to mind: "Is it possible that this is all in my head and I'm imagining it?" and "Will I feel these sensations for the rest of my life?" Despite the absence of clinical signs, the burning sensations are quite real and not the fruit of the patient's imagination. Certain psychiatric disorders can be accompanied by orofacial pain, but the pain will be vague, diffuse and not specific. Population studies have not demonstrated that patients with burning mouth syndrome have a greater tendency to have psychiatric problems. The concern about the expected duration of the burning mouth sensations is quite legitimate as a result of the discomfort the patient has to endure. A good number of patients see their burning mouth syndrome disappear within a few years. There are also cases of spontaneous remission that occur shortly after the onset of the syndrome. As we will see, patients with burning mouth syndrome can generally benefit from pharmacological support treatment.

The scientific community is making a great deal of effort to elucidate the why and how of burning mouth syndrome. One of the proposed mechanisms has to do with an abnormal interaction between the impulses generated by the branches of two cranial nerves, one of which is responsible for the taste sensations of the tongue (the chorda tympani branch of the VIIth cranial pair), and the other responsible for the sensation of pain (the lingual branch of the Vth cranial pair). As a result, a path would be opened to intensify the painful sensations through the receptors responsible for burning sensations. The most recent hypothesis suggests that the hormonal changes related to menopause apparently reduce the neuroprotective effects of the endogenous steroids, resulting in the degeneration of small nerve fibres. These changes could also account for the dry mouth sensation and the taste alterations often observed in the case of burning mouth syndrome.

The therapeutic approach for burning mouth syndrome initially involves avoiding anything that could make the burning sensations more unbearable. First, patients must increase their liquid intake, while avoiding acidic or astringent drinks. The best solution is to drink water to relieve the dry mouth sensation. If hypofunctioning of the salivary glands is documented using appropriate tests, medication can be prescribed to stimulate the production of saliva. With respect to the burning sensations caused by this syndrome, the treatment is still symptomatic (there is no cure), and it is based primarily on medication. The medications used include first-generation antidepressants taken in small dosages for their pain relief effects, anticonvulsants, anxiolytics and other medications that are known to act on the receptors involved in the modulation of the pain message. More recently, the use of antioxidants has been shown to be beneficial for certain patients. It should be noted that the response to these treatments varies from one patient to another and, when faced with a mitigated result or a failure after the dosages have been properly adjusted, it is reasonable to test another molecule. Finally, it is important that patients with burning mouth syndrome understand their condition and that they feel comfortable seeing a psychologist if they receive little support from those around them, tend to feel discouraged and have few special activities.

## 9. CONCLUSION

As the reader may have realized, the problem of chronic orofacial pain is complex. It is easy to get lost in conjecture since we are still far from understanding all of the mechanisms that give rise to such pain, without any structural or physical cause. Despite the limits that science places on us, there are pharmacological treatments and cognitive and behavioural strategies that can help people with chronic orofacial pain relieve their suffering on a daily basis. It is important for these people to see a generalized or specialized dentist who is qualified to evaluate the structures of the mouth cavity as well as the jaw muscles and joints before they start treatment. Finally, we must stop thinking that chronic pain can only be healed through physical and mechanical interventions that target the mouth cavity, jaws and occlusion. Unfortunately, this view fails to take into account the emotional dimensions of chronic pain when it is time to choose a therapeutic approach.

# PAIN, MY JAILER

Louise O'Donnell-Jasmin, BEd, Laval, Quebec, Canada

(See other testimonials, pages 266 and 328. See Chapter 1, page 3.)

*«I don't have time to waste». That was my motto before. Now, I give myself the right to waste time. Nothing is urgent anymore. I've survived. Now, I'm living my new life. I've had brushes with death so many times already that now I focus only on life.*

*Taking the road back to health and happiness has become my priority. Once again, I focus on love, love to be given, love to offer and self-love. Pleasing others, doing things that are filled with love for my family, doing everything to make sure they feel cherished, nurtured, overwhelmed with love. Taking pleasure in activities that were within my reach during the worst years of the pain was something I had to learn to do. My life before pain had always been focused on the people I loved, often to my own detriment. I had to learn to feel alive again: to dream, to feel emotions, to plan, to draw, to fill notebooks with ideas and clippings. Very simple gestures that filled my days of solitude and isolation. Then, one day, I was able to start writing again, to write about my journey through the desert of pain. I wrote until I felt that I was once again taking my place in everyday life, that I was writing exactly what I felt when it was too painful to say it out loud.*

*The text* **Pain, my jailer** *was written after a particularly difficult episode in my journey through pain. I didn't know that I would find the key to my prison of pain in that text, the key I dreamed of finding, without ever saying so. Life often holds extraordinary surprises in store for us...*

## Pain, my jailer

Pain, my jailer, had taken everything away from me. All my life, all my treasures, all that I was. I had been dispossessed by pain. It left me there without any boundary or limit to my sorrow, without any escape route from the hell inside my body, in a world that no longer recognized me. Its grip was so strong on me that many people thought I would never get through. So many others acted as though I had died, from the very first month on. Gradually, pain crawled under my skin, like a deep burn. Every opportunity it had to invade my freedom or my life a bit more, it did.

My personality had become pain. I spoke pain. My very existence was pain. Humanity is a thin layer of the spirit that envelops the body. In peaks of pain, I was no longer human. I was a body that had capitulated to pain, that was aggressed by pain. Did my desire to survive take precedence over my desire not to suffer anymore? I no longer had any desire to go on living. I was just a body for months, and many years. I walked beside my body like a zombie. My humanity surfaced now and again through the maelstrom that was now my life. I held a hand out to my loved ones, to touch their love for me once more, time and time again... never enough.

How can pain become a jailer? By building walls around us, from our greatest strengths as well as our weaknesses. Our first experiences with pain are being jailed in by loneliness, isolation, doubt, fear to identify ourselves to pain and confrontation with the fear of dying that so many of us try to silence.

So many questions come forth. Who was I before pain? (I don't remember.) Who am I now? Why me? How can my family tolerate my moods, my blackness, my pain crises? Why is there so much ignorance about pain? Why are lives wasted, futures uprooted, friendships lost — why so much pain? There comes a day when we have to stop asking ourselves questions and turn to finding a new meaning to our lives. Hence the great difficulty of taking that very step.

Pain has long been part of my body. I have lived with my tormentor, and my jailer. My pain was deep inside me. It was a product of my brain that had forgotten how to fight it. What a horrifying thought: I created the beast that was hurting me; I invented my prison and my jailer because my brain could no longer resist pain.

Pain had once turned everything I loved into stone, and the stones had become my prison walls. But I always hung on to the dream of pulling through. Eventually, others joined me. I found the will to live again, and to forget, a little more each day, the horrors of pain. I finally found the key to the prison door. And I walked out.

What if pain invaded your life? Your landmarks would no longer exist. You'd want to live as before — just live — but you wouldn't be able to do so any longer. Who would you be without your job or your career? Who would you be if you could no longer tolerate the pain, knowing you don't have the choice? What would you do? What would your future hold?

**So many of us are lost in pain. Together, we can reach out to those who are isolated in a prison of pain. One day, we will open each prison door and keep the jailer far away. Together, we can do it.**

# THE ROLE PLAYED BY THE DENTIST
## IN CHRONIC OROFACIAL PAIN

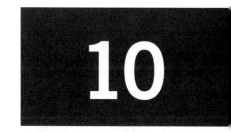

Éric Lessard DMD, FAAHD, Fellow AAOP, Diplomate ABOP, Diplomate ABOM, Diplomate ABSCD, Assistant Professor, Faculty of Dentistry, McGill University Health Centre (MUHC), Montreal General Hospital, Montreal, Quebec, Canada

## ABSTRACT

Despite the fact that people are often afraid of dentists, these health professionals spend their time constantly trying to relieve pain. Obviously, they are essentially concerned with oral and maxillofacial pain. Certain dentists that specialize in oral medicine have received special training on recognizing and treating chronic and acute pain of the orofacial region. One of the worst types of pain a human being has to endure occurs in the face: trigeminal neuralgia. This chapter will discuss this condition and several others.

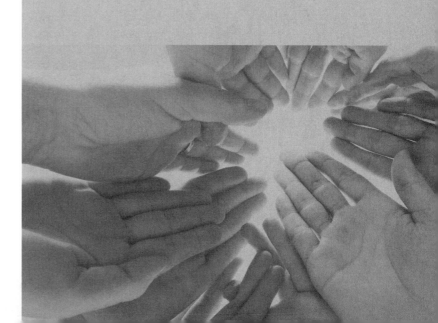

# 1. INTRODUCTION

I have met people who experience pain in various locations. And I ask these patients the following question: if I could take away one kind of pain, which one would you choose? Without hesitating, they tell me mouth and face pain. Since there are few experts in this kind of pain, patients suffer for a long time before they consult a professional for help. The training provided for dental students in North America has drastically changed for the better over the years. Quebec is no exception. We have focused on improving medical knowledge while continuing to concentrate on the mouth and the maxillo-facial complex. This includes pain. Therefore, the tendency is to improve the abilities of our future generation of dentists to diagnose and manage mouth and face pain.

# 2. SCOPE OF THE PROBLEM

Who has not experienced or still feels pain somewhere in their face? According to a study by Lipton, 22% of the general public experienced a painful sensation in their face or their head in the six months prior to the study[1]. This represents a major sociodemographic problem since it leads to absenteeism from work and many visits to health professionals, resulting in a high bill for a system such as ours. Apart from the financial aspect of the problem, people's suffering is legendary and deserves our attention.

# 3. PHYSIOLOGY OF THE TRANSMISSION OF PAIN BY THE TRIGEMINAL SYSTEM[2-3]

The innervation of the head and face is very complex. The trigeminal nerve is the fifth of 12 cranial nerves that run from the brain stem to the lower part of the brain. The trigeminal nerve is responsible for the sensory innervation of all the structures of the face, the mouth, and a part of the ear up to the top of the head. The peripheral structures are connected to an initial nerve fibre called the first order fibre (**Figure 1**). This fibre connects to another fibre in the central nervous system, the second order fibre. This second fibre runs to the superior centres of the brain. Therefore, the painful information moves from the periphery by way of the first order fibre, moves on to the second order fibre, and then on to the superior centres to be modulated and analyzed.

FIGURE 1: Neuron paths of pain

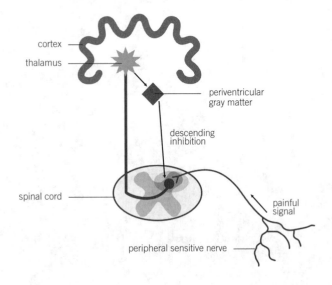

cortex
thalamus
periventricular gray matter
descending inhibition
spinal cord
painful signal
peripheral sensitive nerve

There are two types of first order sensitive fibres, the C and A delta (A$\delta$) fibres. The major difference between the two is the presence of insulating material: myelin. This substance serves to insulate the fibre, allowing information to be transmitted faster. The A$\delta$ fibres are myelinated whereas the C fibres are not. Another difference that makes the A$\delta$ fibres transmit information faster is that they are larger. The first order fibres of the trigeminal system are mostly A$\delta$ fibres, which means that pain in this system generally is transmitted faster than elsewhere in the body.

After the second order neuron, the information is relayed in a structure called the thalamus, and then directed to the somatosensory cortex, where the pain is perceived (character, intensity, localization), and towards the limbic system, where the cognitive, behavioural and emotional component is experienced. Therefore, in addition to the actual sensation of pain, pain also has an emotional or psychological component. This component will be a very important element to be taken into consideration when discussing treatment.

Pain is modulated when it travels through the system. A very efficient one is the descending inhibition system. It originates in the limbic system structures and descends, via a structure called the periaqueductal gray matter, to the first order and second order neurone connection to activate an interneuron that is responsible for releasing endorphins (opiates manufactured by the neuron itself). It takes two important substances to activate the interneuron: neurotransmitters known as noradrenaline and serotonin. This information is important for the discussion of pharmacological therapeutic options.

One problem that lies at the heart of treating chronic pain, including orofacial pain, is the notion of central sensitization. This extremely complex phenomenon can be summarized in a few lines and deserves attention. When the second order neuron is bombarded with pain messages for an extended period of time, it becomes hypersensitive, and its activation threshold is lowered. It even acquires the capacity to transmit information without a peripheral contribution. This results in spontaneous neuron activity, an expansion of the receptive field, and pain references at locations other than the source of the pain. It is easy to understand that this must be avoided at all costs since pain is consolidated in this manner. One study has demonstrated that we start to see manifestations of central hypersensitization after two weeks of continuous pain[4]. It is a myth that enduring pain eventually leads to a reduction in the pain perceived because you get used to it. Enduring pain is not desirable, but since pain is a subjective phenomena, what one individual perceives as a simple discomfort that does not require treatment can be unbearable pain for another. This must, obviously, be taken into consideration.

# 4. CONTRIBUTION OF THE NECK

It is now known that there is a dynamic interaction between the structures of the neck and the orofacial structures. The nociceptive fibres of the C1-C2 region deep structures have connections in the sensory nucleus of the trigeminal nerve, and vice versa for the dorsal horn of the spinal chord at C1-C2. Therefore, when treating maxillo-facial musculoskeletal pain, this cervical contribution must be taken into consideration. Important factors in the history of the pain complaint include motor vehicle accidents (particularly those involving whiplash), the type of work, and whether the individual has an ergonomic work station or not. Occasionally, the pain may disappear only after changes have been made in the work position[5].

# 5. DIAGNOSTIC PROCEDURE[1-3]

The procedure for gathering data from a patient with orofacial pain does not differ very much from that for other types of pain. Since this has already been discussed in other sections of this book, I will stick to the basic notions. The notions of localization, intensity, progression over time, the circumstances under which the pain appeared, characteristics, and elements that aggravate or alleviate the pain are the same as for other types of pain. One important element to be noted is the notion of parafunction. Parafunctions are habits that lead to the overstressing of the structures in the mastication system and include, for example, chewing gum, chewing the lips or cheeks, biting one's fingernails or cuticles (onychophagia), grinding one's teeth (bruxism), and clenching one's teeth.

The purpose of this diagnostic procedure is to classify the patient's pain in one of the three following categories:
- Musculoskeletal pain;
- Neurovascular pain; and
- Neuropathic pain.

The diagnostic approach may include imaging to evaluate the structures of the temporomandibular joint, the skull, the facial bones or the brain. Usually, for viewing calcified tissues such as bones, we use conventional x-rays and tomography. In order to look at soft tissues, we use magnetic resonance. The big difference between these methods is that we use x-rays to see bones, and a magnetic field to see soft tissues. Therefore, magnetic resonance does not use radiation.

## THE DIAGNOSTIC APPROACH FOR MUSCULOSKELETAL PAIN (TEMPOROMANDIBULAR DYSFUNCTION) [1-3, 6-8]

The diagnostic approach for musculoskeletal pain (temporomandibular dysfunctions) will be presented in two phases: internal capsular disturbance and muscular pain.

## THE DIAGNOSTIC APPROACH FOR INTERNAL CAPSULAR DISTURBANCES

The diagnostic approach for internal capsular disturbances will be discussed for capsulitis/synovitis and disk displacements.

### Capsulitis/synovitis
Capsulitis/synovitis is an inflammation of the articular capsule. This condition can be caused by a chronic process, such as in the case of arthritis/parafunctions, or an acute phenomenon, such as a trauma to the joint (a blow to the face).

The pain of capsulitis/synovitis is usually described as a piercing pressure in the region just in front of the tragus of the ear. The pain can be either continuous or intermittent, and increases when the individual speaks, chews or yawns. There may or may not be swelling; opening the mouth is generally restricted.

Upon examination, palpation of the joint generates acute pain that even cause the individual to withdraw. If the capsulitis is caused by arthritis, a crackling sound will be heard during auscultation of the temporomandibular joint.

The treatment for capsulitis/synovitis includes non-steroidal anti-inflammatory drugs such as ibuprofen, naproxen and diclofenac. A soft diet is also recommended so as to allow the joint to rest and, above all, the parafunctions must be stopped. If oedema is present, the patient is advised to apply ice. Occasionally, the dentist will recommend gentle exercises to maintain the mobility of the structures and the fluidity of the synovial fluid. Capsulitis/synovitis can be eliminated quite easily if the individual follows the practitioner's instructions to the letter. If the condition has settled in as a result of arthritis, a procedure such as arthrocentesis may be considered. This involves inserting an entrance needle and an exit needle into the joint in order to circulate saline solution. The movement of the solution cleans out the inflammatory products, after which a long-acting corticosteroid can be administered. This intervention can be repeated several times over the course of a year, but the corticosteroid cannot be administered more than twice a year[10].

## Disk displacements

The articular disk can move in any direction. However, in most cases, it moves forward and inwards[6]. When the condyle moves forward to open the mouth, it comes into contact with the rear part of the disk, which forms an obstacle (partial or total) for the movement of the condyle. As the movement continues, if the disk has not moved too far forward and allows the condyle to move, that latter will slip under the disk in a single movement, with a sound like the clicking of a joint. At this point, the mandible shifts to the side of the click, but then returns to the centre. In the event that the disk has moved too far forward, and the condyle cannot advance, the opening of the mouth will be restricted, and the clicking will disappear. The exact reason the disk becomes displaced is still being debated in the literature. Some authors say that parafunctions cause this by increasing the pressure on the joint and pulling the structures forwards (biting one's fingernails). Others say that the position of the teeth plays a predominant role and suggest interventions such as orthodontal work, grinding teeth contact, or the installation of crowns. They use analytical devices that are not accepted unanimously in the scientific world. These techniques were not supported by scientific research at the time this chapter was written. Although certain patients do obtain relief through these treatments, others find themselves paying thousands of dollars, and obtaining no relief[6, 8, 12]. However, there are non-invasive treatments that are much less costly, and do have a very high success rate[13]. Another reported cause is an increase in the viscosity of the synovial fluid as a result of parafunctions.

Disk displacements are often accompanied by pain that is usually described as a pressure that increases with function. The pain eventually disappears, and the disk displacements are, in the long run, rarely the cause of joint pain[6, 8, 12].

The treatments for disk displacements that do not cause pain include preventive recommendations such as restricting the opening of the mouth to a comfort zone, stopping parafunctions, and avoiding trauma to the joint structures as much as possible (martial arts, boxing, contact sports) by using a mouth protector. It should be noted that, in the case of the structures that are responsible for keeping the joint disk in place, when the ligaments have been stretched, the elongation of the ligaments is irreversible. In adults, the ligaments lose their elasticity and remain stretched.

In the case of a disk displacement without reduction (the disk doesn't return to its anatomical position) and with a restriction of the opening, an experienced physiotherapist can remedy the problem in most cases. As a result, the patients are once again able to open their mouths almost to the same extent as before. Capsulitis may accompany the disk displacement. The treatment for this condition was discussed earlier.

## THE DIAGNOSTIC APPROACH FOR MUSCULAR PAIN

The diagnostic approach for muscular pain will be discussed in terms of myogenic pain.

## Myogenic pain

Myogenic pain is pain of muscular origin. It is more resistant to treatment than joint pain. The masticating muscles are the ones most often affected and this includes the temporal, masseter and pterygoid muscles. The pain is usually described as a pressure, a tension or a heaviness accompanied by a sensation of weakness or fatigue when speaking or eating. The pain may be experienced on both sides, but is usually felt on just one side. In all likelihood, the function increases the pain, and hampers mastication significantly. This pain is usually related to an overload involving an extended contraction of the muscular fibres, and leading to the production of metabolic waste that accumulates in the muscle[14].

The most frequent forms of muscular pain are myalgia resulting from overstressing and myofascial pain. The two conditions are similar with respect to their presentation with the exception that the second one involves the presence of tender spots. These spots are hyperirritable spots in a muscle cluster. Fibres that are contracted on a permanent basis and are very tense generate a great deal of pain upon palpation; they are associated with characteristic reference models, depending on the muscle involved. This myofascial pain can be continuous or intermittent, but it is persistent. Myofascial pain involves the presence of central hypersensitization as discussed earlier[14].

The prevalence (percentage of patients suffering from a disease in a given population) of myofascial face pain varies from 4 to 19%[15]. People do not generally realize that the masticatory muscles can be chronically overstressed, since these muscles are in the face. Apparently, we perform actions automatically without realizing that we are doing them. The literature is divided with respect to the role of parafunctional habits as a cause for temporomandibular dysfunctions (TMD) but, in practice, it seems that stopping these habits helps improve the symptoms to a certain extent[16, 17]. Therefore, it is a good idea to develop an awareness of these habits and concentrate on stopping parafunctions. According to a study published by John[18], if you experience pain elsewhere, you have more chances of developing a TMD.

## TEMPOROMANDIBULAR DYSFUNCTIONS AND MOOD DISORDERS

Several studies have demonstrated a link between pain in general and mood disorders (anxiety and depression). This is also true for temporomandibular disorders (TMD). The presence of traumatic stressors such as being attacked, a serious traffic accident, the death of a loved one, witnessing a murder or a war are all risk factors for developing a TMD in the future[19]. The presence of a post-traumatic syndrome is also a risk factor [20]. It should be noted that pain is not necessarily caused by these conditions, but the groundwork has been laid for triggering pain through the overloading of a muscle. It appears that this combination is problematic.

When the practitioner recommends that the patient see a psychologist for his/her pain, this does not mean that the patient's pain is imaginary but rather that this intervention is an inherent part of the overall management of the pain in keeping with a biopsychosocial mode. With this model, pain is approached by considering the biological cause in the individual's psychosocial context[1-3].

## PAIN AND SLEEP[21]

Sleep hygiene is a sine qua non condition for improving pain. An individual whose sleep is disrupted suffers much more and much longer than another individual with the same conditions. The pioneering work done by Dr. Gilles Lavigne of the *Université de Montréal* (Quebec, Canada) has made an enormous contribution to our understanding of the link between pain and sleep. It appears that stress and anxiety lead to hypervigilance and this causes an alteration in the normal sleep cycles. This alteration in the quality of sleep leads to a reduction in the pain threshold. Improving sleep, therefore, is a critical step in managing pain. A sleep study to determine the cause of the sleep disorder may be indicated. This study may confirm a parafunction such as bruxism or sleep apnea, for example. Sleep apnea can lead to major health problems, including high blood pressure as well as an increased risk of heart disease and stroke.

## TREATMENT[1-3, 6-8]

As indicated earlier, the therapeutic approach used for orofacial pain must be global and in keeping with the biopsychosocial model. From a physical point of view, the patient's dentist can prescribe pharmacological agents such as muscle relaxants and anti-inflammatories.

In the presence of orofacial pain, it is important for the patient to stop all parafunctions and become aware of them. Here are a few recommendations that can be of help:
- A soft diet;
- Applying heat to muscles;
- Keeping the jaw relaxed, with a space between the upper and lower teeth; and
- Stopping parafunctions.

It is important to determine if the patient has any sleep parafunctions since, if that is the case, his/her dentist can make a device called an occlusal stabilisation appliance to be worn while sleeping. This device maintains a space between the teeth, protecting them from premature wear. It is also thought that the prosthesis may cause the masticatory muscles to relax, but this has not been demonstrated in clinical studies. We still do not know how these devices work, although several patients report benefits. Since these prostheses are not invasive, it is reasonable to recommend them[22].

In the case of dental occlusion (the manner in which the upper teeth come into contact with the lower teeth), if there is slippage between the first dental contact when the mouth is closed and the position of the mandible where the contacts are at a maximum, this can constitute a factor that contributes to instability, and may require more in-depth analysis.

Involving a physiotherapist who is experienced in treating the neck and the facial bones can be very effective. In addition to the treatment, the physiotherapist will propose an exercise program to relax the tense muscles and reduce pain.

As for sleep, it must be optimized and the individual must wake up as rested as possible. The sleeping position is also important. People who sleep on their stomachs apply pressure to the mandible and neck in general. Their sleeping position must be modified so that they sleep on their backs or one of their sides, if their overall health status allows for this. Obviously, people with back problems will find it hard to sleep on their backs. They should check with their physicians to confirm the best sleeping position. Physicians may, if they think this is necessary, prescribe medications such as zopiclone or trazodone to help with sleep. No one likes to take medication; for this reason patients must decide if putting up with the pain is preferable to taking medication. One thing is certain, altered sleep will perpetuate pain in most patients[21].

The psychosocial aspect includes psychotherapy (cognitive-behavioural therapy seems to be particularly effective), with a specific focus on learning stress management techniques. It is important to understand that this does not at any time mean the individual's pain is imaginary, but rather that there is a perpetuation factor that must be addressed if we want to reduce the pain as much as possible. The therapist must be familiar with managing chronic pain[1-3, 6-8].

# 6. NEUROPATHIC PAIN

As already indicated in **Chapter 3** of this book, neuropathy is defined by the International Association for the Study of Pain (IASP) as a disturbance of function or pathological change in a peripheral or central nerve. This can lead to negative symptoms (loss of sensation on the reception field of the nerve) or positive symptoms (formication, pain). Neuropathic pain is usually described as a burning or an electrical discharge. The intensity of the pain varies from one individual to the next. This pain can be classified as episodic or continuous.

## EPISODIC NEUROPATHIC PAIN

The most common types of episodic neuropathic facial pain are trigeminal neuralgia and occipital neuralgia.

### Trigeminal neuralgia[1-3, 6-8]

The pain caused by trigeminal neuralgia is one of the worst types of suffering a human being can experience. In the Middle Ages, people suffering from this kind of pain committed suicide or were burned alive, since people suspected them of being possessed by demons during the episodic pain crises. The discovery of carbamazepine in 1953 dramatically improved the quality of life of people dealing with this disease, and will be discussed later.

The typical patient is over the age of 50 (although trigeminal neuralgia can occur at any age), and in 90% of the cases a blood vessel is compressing the trigeminal nerve root. This is referred to as the classical form. In other cases, trigeminal neuralgia is a symptom of another disease and is referred to as symptomatic. The associated diseases include: a tumour, an aneurysm or a demyelinating disease such as multiple sclerosis.

In the case of trigeminal neuralgia, the pain is experienced in the face and follows a route corresponding to one or more of the three branches of the nerve. The pain is only felt on one side (although multiple sclerosis can cause pain on both sides), and is perceived as very sharp and extremely intense electrical discharges (or piercing pain). It is rare for people with this kind of pain to have sensory deficits in their face or mouth, except in the case of symptomatic neuralgia. The duration of the attacks ranges from a few seconds to two or three minutes. The episodes are caused by the stimulation of regions known as **tender spots** which may be located anywhere within the territory of the affected nerve. Therefore, brushing one's teeth, eating or speaking, touching or even a light breeze on the face can trigger pain.

### Pharmacological or surgical treatment of trigeminal neuralgia

Pharmacological treatment involves prescribing medications classified as antiepileptic drugs such as carbamazepine (Tegretol®), oxcarbazepine (Trileptal®), gabapentin (Neurontin®) and pregabalin (Lyrica®). These medications have side effects that vary from one individual to another. They include, but are not limited to: attention problems, memory problems, skin rashes, oedema, weight gain, headaches or dizziness. Patients should note that, after a certain number of years, the medications lose their effectiveness and they must be replaced periodically[9, 23, 24]. Surgical treatment involves the following options[24]: microvascular decompression, radiosurgery with a gamma knife, rhizotomy by thermolesion, partial rhizotomy, microcompression with balloon and cryotherapy. (See **Chapter 34.**)

**Microvascular decompression** involves placing a small teflon sponge between the blood vessel and the trigeminal nerve root to decompress the nerve. This technique is very successful and has a success rate of 93% and a rate of 1 to 10% for neurological complications[25]. The neurosurgeon makes an opening at the back of the skull, under general anaesthesia to reach the site of the nerve. Based on our experience, the operation requires hospitalization for approximately five days, and convalescence of about four weeks. The possible complications include: a cerebrospinal fluid leak, stroke, facial paralysis, increased pain, loss of sensation, haemorrhage, infection and death (0.3 %)[26].

**Radiosurgery with a gamma knife** involves administering radiotherapy to the nerve to prevent it from functioning. The effect is not instantaneous, and it usually takes several weeks for the patient to enjoy the benefits. The only place in Quebec where this operation is performed is at the *Centre hospitalier universitaire de Sherbrooke*. The side effects include loss of sensation, and the long-term possibility of a brain tumour later in life. This is an interesting alternative for patients who are not candidates for decompression surgery because of a high risk of complications.

**Rhizotomy by thermolesion** involves radiofrequency to destroy the nerve. It is very effective, relieving pain immediately in 90% of the patients. However, 27% suffer a relapse, and most experience a loss of sensitivity (which can be just as bad as the pain) along with an increase or a transformation of their pain.

**Partial rhizotomy** involves a partial surgical sectioning of the trigeminal nerve (20 to 70%). This technique is indicated if vascular decompression and radiosurgery with a gamma knife have failed. The success rate ranges from 48 to 86%. The relapse rate is 17 to 42% at one year and 2% per year after that. The rate for major sensory deficits is about 18%. Other possible complications include stroke, a leak of cerebrospinal liquid and deafness.

**Microcompression using a balloon** involves inserting a microcatheter and inflating slowly in order to compress the trigeminal ganglion and render it non-functional. This is easier to do than radiofrequency, and has a similar success rate (95%). The relapse rate at five years is 20 to 30%. Possible complications include: haemorrhage and double vision, which is usually temporary and lasts less than five months. This option is to be considered particularly if the patient is too old for vascular decompression.

**Cryotherapy** involves the surgical exposure of the peripheral branch of the trigeminal nerve in question, and then freezing the nerve directly with a cryoprobe. This procedure is temporary, and may be repeated as needed to give the patient a period of time so that he/she can make a decision concerning a definitive treatment. The success rate is excellent (almost 100%), but the pain is relieved on average for 6 to12 months. There is a possibility that the pain will move to another nerve.

These are the most common techniques used; patients who wish to know more should consult their physician and neurosurgeon.

### Occipital neuralgia[1]

Occipital neuralgia is pain that is experienced at the back of the head. It is closely related to posture. The pain is perceived as a pressure on the back portion of the head with occasional electrical discharges. Some people will also experience formication and pain when they brush their hair. The pain is caused by a muscular compression of the occipital nerve at the base of the skull. The treatment involves postural re-education, including provision of an ergonomic workstation, and the use of anti-inflammatories, antiepileptics, anaesthetic blocks with or without cortisone, BOTOX®[25] injections and, ultimately, the implantation of a neurostimulator. The results of these therapies are very good and lasting.

### CONTINUOUS NEUROPATHIC PAIN

The most common types of continuous neuropathic pain include atypical odontalgia or deafferentation pain, traumatic neuroma, post-herpetic neuralgia and stomatopyrosis (burning mouth syndrome).

### Atypical odontalgia or deafferation pain[1-3, 26]

Atypical odontalgia or deafferation pain has been called by many names. The experts have had difficulty agreeing on a definitive name. This is a phantom pain that occurs following dental treatments, or following trauma to the dental-bone structures. If the region of the tooth was painful before the intervention, the risks increase. The typical patient is over the age of 50, and describes the pain as a pressure that may include a burning and pulsing component. The pain is continuous and present for more than four months. The intensity of the pain varies from moderate to severe and applying local anaesthetic to the region does not completely eliminate the pain. The pain is the consequence of trauma caused to a nerve during a dental treatment. The pain also causes hypersensitivity of the central nervous system. The pain is usually persistent, and can last for several years.

The treatments for atypical odontalgia include medications such as tricyclic antidepressants, selective noradrenaline inhibitors and antiepileptics. It is important for the patient to stop all elective dental treatments until the pain is controlled, since additional treatments multiply the chances that the pain will increase and irradiate.

### Traumatic neuroma[1-3, 27]

In the case of traumatic neuroma, a small mass of peripheral nerve tissue is formed after a nerve is cut. This injury is very unstable and is described as a burning sensation with pulsing and small shocks, provoked by touching of or pressure on the affected zone. Any surgical procedure can cause this condition. The treatments for traumatic neuroma include cortisone injections and pharmaclogical options such as antidepressants.

### Postherpetic neuralgia[1-3, 28]

Post-herpes neuralgia is continuous pain that occurs following an episodic reactivation of the herpes simplex and varicella-zoster virus (herpes zoster or shingles). When it reactivates, the virus destroys the nerve endings in the skin and causes a functional anomaly. The pain is described as burning and shooting. Individuals with this condition have sensory deficits limited to the branch of the trigeminal nerve affected by the disease. Postherpetic neuralgia is very difficult to treat. It may respond to topical anaesthetics and antidepressants. The risk factors for developing this kind of pain include the severity of the lesions, the severity of the pain felt during the herpetic reactivation and advanced age.

### Stomatopyrosis (burning mouth syndrome)[1-3, 29, 30]

Stomatopyrosis (burning mouth syndrome) is relatively frequent, affecting 0.6 to 15% of the population. The vast majority of people affected are menopausal women. The symptoms include a burning sensation that is almost absent upon waking, and starts shortly after breakfast, reaching a peak at the end of the day, without the presence of oral lesions. The condition may be associated with a change in taste or a dry mouth sensation. It is important to note that this dryness is subjective since examination reveals that the secretion of saliva is normal. Although all of the tissues in the mouth may be affected, the front and the sides of the tongue are affected most often by far. Upon examination, the dentist is unable to identify a cause for stomatopyrosis. The treatment may be triggered by a dental treatment, the use of new dental prosthetics, an intense psychological event, and diseases such as Sjogren's syndrome or diabetes. Sometimes, there is no identifiable cause. Although the exact cause is unknown, it appears that a taste dysfunction may be behind the problem.

The treatment for stomatopyrosis involves reassuring the patient, and explaining that the condition is benign. The pharmacological options include benzodiazepines, antidepressants and antiepileptics. Non-pharmacological treatments include sessions with a psychologist who specializes in the treatment of pain, or with an acupuncturist.

The application of capsaicin (an active ingredient in jalapeno peppers) may also be considered. The pain tends to persist, varies from one individual to another, and can last for years.

## 7. CONCLUSION

This chapter has provided a brief description of various orofacial disorders and identified treatments and practitioners, particularly the dentist, that may be of help to people suffering from this kind of pain. Since pain causes us to change the way in which we think, it is important to note that catastrophic thinking increases and perpetuates pain.

For this reason, we must keep the psychological component of pain in mind; it is far too often neglected by health professionals or denied by patients. The therapeutic results are far more favourable when pain is treated in a global manner. People suffering with pain have the option of going to the pain centres in various hospitals throughout Quebec, which is a major advantage as a result of the multidisciplinary approach to managing pain.

All of the conditions described in this chapter can refer pain to the teeth or the neighbouring structures. In all likelihood, the first thing the dentist should do is try to find an oral-dental cause for the pain using the various tests and diagnostic aids available. If this cause is eliminated, he/she will have to look elsewhere since treating a patient without first making a diagnosis could lead to treatments that are not necessary, and could even increase or consolidate the pain.

# REFERENCES

1. DE LEEUW, Reny. Orofacial Pain: Guidelines for Assessment, Diagnosis, and Management, 4th edition, Quintessence

2. SHARAV, Yair, and Rafael Benoliel. Orofacial Pain and Headache. Mosby, 2008

3. LUND, James P, Gilles J. Lavigne, Ronald Dubner, and Barry J, Sessle. Orofacial Pain: From Basic Science to Clinical Management. 2nd edition, quintessence, 2008

4. JUHL, GI, P. Svensson, SE Norholt and TS Jensen. Long-lasting mechanical sensitization following third molar surgery. J Orofac Pain. 2006 Winter; 20(1):59-73

5. HU T, J.W., K.-Q. Sun, H. Vernon, and B.J. Sessle. Craniofacial inputs to upper cervical dorsal horn: Implications for somatosensory information processing, Brain Research 1044 (2005) 93-106

6. LASKIN, DM, CS Greene, and WL Hylander. Temporomandibular Disorders: An Evidence-Based Approach to Diagnosis and Treatment, Quintessence, 2007

7. OKESON, JP. Management of Temporomandibular Disorders and Occlusion, 6th edition, Mosby

8. MURPHY, E. Managing Orofacial Pain in Practice, Quintessentials of Dental Practice, 2008

9. ZAKRZEWSKA, Joanna M. and S. D. Harrison, Assessment and Management of Orofacial Pain, Elsevier

10. ÖNDER, ME, HH Tüz, D. Kocyigit and RS Kisnisci, Long-term results of arthrocentesis in degenerative, Oral Surg Oral Med Oral Pathol Oral Radiol Endod 2009;107:e1-e5

11. MANOLOPOULOS, L, PV Vlastarakos, I LG Giotakis, A. Loizos, and TP Nikolopoulos. Myofascial pain syndromes in the maxillofacial area: a common but underdiagnosed cause of head and neck pain, Int. J. Oral Maxillofac. Surg. 2008; 37:975–984

12. GONZALEZ, YM, CS Greene, and ND Mohl, Technological Devices in the Diagnosis of Temporomandibular Disorders, Oral Maxillofacial Surg Clin N Am 20 (2008) 211–220

13. TRUELOVE, E, KH Huggins, L. Manc L, and SF Dworkin. The efficacy of traditional, low-cost and nonsplint therapies for temporomandibular disorder: A randomized controlled trial, J Am Dent Assoc 2006;137;1099-1107

14. TRAVELL, JG, and DG Simmons. Myofascial Pain and Dysfunction: The Trigger Point Manual, vol.1, Lippincott Williams & Wilkins, 1998

15. ARKLUND, S, and A. Wänman, Incidence and prevalence of myofascial pain in the jaw-face region. A one-year prospective study on dental students, Acta Odontol Scand. 2008 Apr; 66(2):113-21

16. MIYAKE, R, R. Ohkubo, J. Takehara, and M. Morita. Oral parafunctions and association with symptoms of temporomandibular disorders in Japanese university students, J Oral Rehabil. 2004 Jun; 31(6):518-23

17. VAN SELMS, MK, F. Lobbezoo, CM Visscher, and M. Naeije. Myofascial temporomandibular disorder pain, parafunctions and psychological stress J Oral Rehabil. 2008 Jan; 35(1):45-52

18. JOHN, MT, DL Miglioretti, L. LeResche, M. Von Korff, and CW Critchlow. Widespread pain as a risk factor for dysfunctional temporomandibular disorder pain. Pain. 2003 Apr; 102(3):257-63

19. DE LEEUW, R., E. Bertoli, JE Schmidt, and CR Carlson. Prevalence of traumatic stressors in patients with temporomandibular disorders, Journal of Oral & Maxillofacial Surgery. 63(1):42-50, 2005 Jan

20. DE LEEUW, R. E. Bertoli, JE Schmidt and CR Carlson. Prevalence of post-traumatic stress disorder symptoms in orofacial pain patients, Oral Surg Oral Med Oral Pathol Oral Radiol Endod 2005;99:558-68

21. LAVIGNE, G, BJ Sessle, M. Choiniere, and P. Soja. Sleep and Pain. Seattle, Wash: International Association for the Study of Pain; 2007

22. DAO, T.T., and GJ Lavigne, Oral Splints: the Crutches for Temporomandibular Disorders and Bruxism? Critical Reviews in Oral Biology & Medicine, Jan 1998; vol. 9: pp. 345-361

23. GRONSETH, G., G. Cruccu, J. Alksne, C. Argoff, M. Brainin, K. Burchiel, T. Nurmikko, and J. M. Zakrzewska. Practice Parameter: The diagnostic evaluation and treatment of trigeminal neuralgia (an evidence-based review): Report of the Quality Standards Subcommittee of the American Academy of Neurology and the European Federation of Neurological Societies, Neurology 2008;71;1183-1190

24. KATSUHIRO, Toda. Operative treatment of trigeminal neuralgia: review of current techniques, Oral Surg Oral Med Oral Pathol Oral Radiol Endod 2008;106:788-805

25. OLSON, S, L. Atkinson, and M. Weidmann, Microvascular decompression for trigeminal neuralgia: recurrences and complications, Journal of Clinical Neuroscience (2005) 12(7), 787–789

26. TAYLOR, M, S. Silva, and C. Cottrell. Botulinum toxin type-A (BOTOX) in the treatment of occipital neuralgia: a pilot study. Headache 2008;48:1476-1481

27. RAM, S, A. Teruel, SKS Kumar, and G. Clark. Clinical Characteristics and Diagnosis of Atypical Odontalgia: Implications for Dentists, J Am Dent Assoc 2009;140;223-228

28. RASMUSSEN, OC, Painful traumatic: neuromas in the oral cavity, oral surg oral med oral path, Volume 49, Number 3, March, 1980

29. FIELDS, HL, M. Rowbotham, and R. Baron. Postherpetic Neuralgia: Irritable Nociceptors and Deafferentation, Neurobiology of Disease 5, 209–227 (1998)

30. KLASSER, GD, DJ. Fischer, and JB Epstein. Burning Mouth Syndrome: Recognition, Understanding, and Management, Oral Maxillofacial Surg Clin N Am 20 (2008) 255–271

31. ABETZ LM and NW Savage. Burning mouth syndrome and psychological disorders, Australian Dental Journal 2009; 54: 84–93

# UNDERSTANDING AND MANAGING THE INTERACTION BETWEEN SLEEP AND PAIN:
## AN UPDATE FOR THE DENTIST

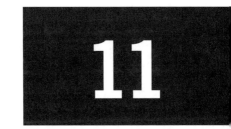

**Maryse Brousseau** DMD, MSc, Montreal, Quebec, Canada
**Christiane Manzini**, Montreal, Quebec, Canada
**Norman Thie** BSc, MSc, DDS, Diplomat ABOP, Fellow AAOM, Edmonton, Alberta, Canada
**Gilles Lavigne** DMD, MSc, FRCD(C), Montreal, Quebec, Canada

## ABSTRACT

Pain is a symptom well known to disrupt numerous aspects of normal physical and psychological life, including work, social activities and sleep. In daily practice, general dentists and specialists are frequently confronted with issues concerning pain, as their patients seek management that integrates oral health with overall well-being. An example of a dental condition involving pain is temporomandibular disorder, which is one of the most common sources of chronic orofacial pain and which shares similarities with back pain in terms of intensity, persistence and psychosocial impact. The objective of this paper is to inform and aid the general dentist and the specialist concerned with the sleep quality of patients with orofacial pain.

**MeSH Key Words:**
Words: facial pain/complications; sleep/physiology; temporomandibular joint disorders/physiopathology

Reprinted with the permission of the Canadian Dental Association.
Originally published as J Can Dent Assoc 2003;69(7):437-42.
This article has been peer reviewed.

ABSTRACT

1. PAIN

2. SLEEP

3. CLINICAL GUIDELINES

   Step 1: Evaluation for primary sleep disorder
   Steps 2 and 3: Sleep hygiene and behavioural and cognitive strategies
   Step 4: Pharmacological interventions

4. CONCLUSIONS

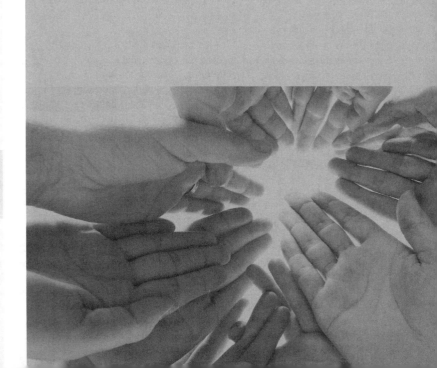

Pain disrupts numerous aspects of physical and psychological life, including sleep, and dental problems, such as temporomandibular disorder, are often sources of chronic pain that can alter sleep patterns. The objective of this paper is to inform and aid the general dentist and the specialist concerned with the sleep quality of patients with orofacial pain.

# 1. PAIN

Pain creates behavioural states that allow the conscious individual to react to noxious threats. It is characterized by the integration of sensory (e.g., intensity), emotional (e.g., unpleasant) and motivational (e.g., running for survival) experiences.[1] The behavioural and cognitive aspects of pain perception are complex; clinicians need to understand this complexity when treating patients who complain of pain. For example, when a clinician asks a patient about pain relief, the patient is invited to compare what he or she is currently feeling with feelings that prompted a prior visit. In addition, a person's memory of chronic pain is known to increase the intensity of current reported pain, which can complicate a clinician's understanding of the signs and symptoms of pain.[2]

Diffuse musculoskeletal pain is often associated with complaints of poor sleep and fatigue.[3-6] Brain imaging studies have revealed that "emotional" brain areas (e.g., the cingulate cortex, the prefrontal cortex and the hypothalamus) have a direct role in pain perception and that subjects reporting the most severe pain may have fewer binding sites for brain opioids (e.g., brain morphine, known as endorphin).[6,7] These observations could account for some of the high variability in measured pain perception and efficacy of analgesics. Moreover, in recent years, the placebo effect has been rediscovered as a powerful factor influencing pain behaviour, pain reporting and use of medication.[8,9]

Pain is reported by approximately 15% of the general population and by over 50% of older people. With aging, pain perception either remains relatively constant or decreases.[10,11] Interestingly, even though older patients use more medications (because of an increased prevalence of various diseases and disorders), in general they are better able to cope with the effect of pain on their quality of life than middle-aged adults.[12,13] This could be because older patients accept and understand pain as an unpleasant companion of age, whereas younger patients may feel that pain threatens their capacity for life and productivity.

If a conscious person interprets a potentially harmful sensory input

as painful, he or she reacts accordingly to protect bodily integrity and physiological homeostasis. In the absence of consciousness (e.g., under general anesthesia or hypnosis and, to a certain degree, during sleep), the brain retains the ability to detect painful input, thereby maintaining some protective reactivity.[14] The processing of pain from the periphery toward the brain, in particular toward the cortex, involves a complex sequence of events. First, specific receptors (e.g., free nerve endings) are activated; then, relay neurons in the spinal cord and thalamus change their firing patterns, and finally, information about the noxious stimulant reaches the sensory motor and emotional brain areas. The autonomic nervous system is also activated when pain is perceived: the heart rate increases, respiration is faster, and sudation is frequently present. A rise in cyclooxygenase-2, commonly recognized in the periphery, has also been observed recently in the spinal cord and brain neurons, which suggests that analgesic medications (e.g., rofecoxib and celecoxib) do not act exclusively in the periphery.[15,16] More recently, a third cyclooxygenase has been found in the heart and brain, which supports a role for the analgesic acetaminophen.[17]

Pain can be either acute and transient or chronic and persistent (more than 1 to 6 months, depending on the condition). Acute pain is common after dental surgery and endodontic treatments. Chronic pain, which can last for years, often affects quality of life and may persist long after an injury has apparently healed. Chronic pain is frequently associated with permanent modifications of central nervous system processes, such as chemical overexpression due to gene induction; lack of enzymatic chemical degradation (e.g., of inflammatory or pain mediators); nerve overactivity associated with aberrant connections (e.g., nerves or cells in the spinal cord that normally respond only to touch now respond to painful stimuli); a damaged dental nerve that sprouts and makes unusual connections to bone, mucosa, periodontal ligament, blood vessels and other tissues.[15,16]

# 2. SLEEP

Sleep is a regular process within the 24-hour cycle; humans typically have approximately 16 hours of wakefulness and 8 hours of sleep. Each night's sleep is divided into two main types of sleep periods: non-rapid eye movement (REM) periods (which have a sequence of light sleep [stages 1 and 2 non-REM] and deep sleep [stages 3 and 4 non-REM, responsible for restorative function]) and REM periods (also named paradoxical sleep, characterized by muscle atonia and paralysis). Humans dream during various sleep stages, but the dreams of REM sleep are, in general, more vivid, creative and fantastical. The dreams of patients with chronic pain encompass pain experiences from several body sites, including the head and neck regions.[18,19] Patients with chronic pain can be encouraged to keep a journal of their dreams (with instruction about avoiding overinterpretation), which may improve their understanding of the causes (e.g., a traumatic event) and consequences (e.g., mood alteration, familial roles, avoidance of social activities) of the pain.

Sleep is a behavioural and physiological state that is generally resistant

to nonmeaningful external stimuli.[20] In the general population, the proportion of people reporting insomnia (either a long delay in sleep onset or no return to sleep if awakened) increases from 20% among people 15 to 24 years of age to 36% after the age of 75. Anxiety is an important factor in insomnia and poor sleep,[21,22] and patients with chronic pain are at high risk of insomnia.[22-24]

In most (50% to 90%) patients with acute pain, the occurrence of pain generally precedes complaints of poor sleep.[22,24] However, studies of patients with burn pain or chronic pain have indicated bidirectional influences: a night of poor sleep may be followed by greater pain the next day, and a day with high pain levels is often followed by a night of poor sleep.[25,26]

In general, the percentage of time spent in each sleep stage is not markedly different between patients with chronic pain and control subjects. However, in patients with chronic pain and other poor sleepers, sleep is often more fragmented than that of "normal" healthy adults (i.e., the overall sleep period is broken down into several brief periods of sleep). This fragmented sleep is characterized by subtle changes, including frequent micro-arousals (3 to 10 seconds long, involving transient brain, heart and muscle activations), awakenings (activations lasting longer than 10 to 15 seconds, with possible consciousness), shifts in sleep stage (e.g., from a deeper to a lighter sleep stage) or body movements (or some combination of these characteristics).These subtle changes may occur in clusters, repeating every 20 to 40 seconds, accompanied by rapid alpha cortical waves (known as alpha wave intrusions) and increases in heart rate and muscle tone. These changes are collectively termed cyclic alternating pattern (CAP), and when CAP occurs too frequently, it can lead to poor sleep.[27,28] Interestingly, a recent report indicates that patients with fibromyalgia do not display the reduction in heart rate that is usually observed during the deeper restorative sleep stages (i.e., stages 3 and 4 of non-REM sleep).[29] Thus, if the brain is overactive during sleep (i.e., an excessive frequency of CAP), with heart rate remaining at daytime levels, sleep could be nonrefreshing. This might account for complaints of poor sleep, daytime fatigue, lack of concentration, memory dysfunction and increased risk of motor vehicle crashes and workplace accidents.[30-33] These findings might also explain the interrelationship between poor sleep and other manifestations of pain, including fatigue and irritability. These observations merit consideration when planning both basic research and clinical assessments of pain management strategies.

The pain perceived during an unconscious or unresponsive state, such as sleep or general anesthesia, is termed nociception.[34] During sleep, nociception remains active to protect bodily integrity. In light sleep (stages 1 and 2 non-REM) and in REM sleep, the body can react rapidly to meaningful external stimuli (e.g., the sound of a telephone, an alarm or a crying baby).[35,36] However, in deep sleep (stages 3 and 4 non-REM), this responsiveness is partially suppressed to protect sleep continuity. To better understand how the brain processes sensory pain information, the authors used young, healthy subjects in a laboratory setting to compare intramuscular injection of noxious hypertonic saline solutions with injection of non-noxious solutions and vibrotactile stimulation during sleep. Patients experiencing pain were not included in these studies since it would have been difficult to isolate sleep fragmentation variables from the influence of medications, mood alteration, poor sleep and other factors. The results revealed that experimental pain stimulations triggered awakenings and shifts in sleep stage over all sleep stages, including the usually less responsive deep sleep and REM sleep.[37] This novel finding suggests that management strategies should focus on all sleep stages to maintain the best sleep quality. Additional studies are now underway to determine whether these responses explain the poor sleep, fatigue (e.g., low restorative effect) and lower cognitive function reported by patients with chronic pain.[38]

## 3. CLINICAL GUIDELINES

The assessment and treatment of sleep problems among patients with chronic pain can be approached in four steps (see below and **Table 1**). Management of pain and sleep may include the use of behavioural strategies with or without medications that improve sleep by reducing microarousal or CAP activation and thereby decrease persistent autonomic–cardiac activation (e.g., strategies that improve the parasympathetic drive during deep sleep). Because a higher quality of life is important for all patients, it is considered necessary to prevent the effects of sleepiness on important cognitive functions (e.g., memory and driving). This paper does not address the use of oral splint appliances and physical therapy in the management of orofacial pain; reviews of these subjects can be found elsewhere.[39,40]

### STEP 1: EVALUATION FOR PRIMARY SLEEP DISORDER

Before pharmacological approaches are considered, it is important to obtain a complete history of the patient's sleep habits and to determine if he or she has a primary sleep disorder (e.g., a disorder that affects breathing, such as snoring or apnea, periodic limb movement syndrome, sleep bruxism or insomnia). For this, a screening questionnaire[41] can be invaluable. If a primary sleep disorder is suspected, the patient needs to consult the family physician for possible referral to a sleep centre.

## STEPS 2 AND 3: SLEEP HYGIENE AND BEHAVIOURAL AND COGNITIVE STRATEGIES

If a primary sleep disorder is not suspected, the patient's sleep hygiene is then reviewed. This review includes questions about the sleep environment, such as whether a baby sleeps in the same bedroom, whether the bedroom is also used as an office (with or without a computer) and the level of outside traffic noise. For optimal sleep, the bedroom should be a quiet "oasis," not an area for work and negotiation. The patient should be asked whether he or she has a regular daily schedule (i.e., a regular 24-hour sleep–wake cycle on both weekdays and weekends). Furthermore, lifestyle issues should be assessed, including evening habits (e.g., caffeine intake, smoking, alcohol consumption or intense exercise late in the evening); such habits are to be discouraged, since this time should be reserved for relaxing before sleep.

Several well-defined behavioural and relaxation methods are available for stress management in relation to the interaction of sleep and pain.[42-44] These techniques include progressive muscle relaxation (sequential relaxation of major muscle groups), meditation, imagery training and hypnosis. Although relaxation techniques differ in philosophical approach, they share two main components: repetition of a specific activity, such as words, sounds, prayers, phrases, body sensations or muscular activity; and a passive attitude toward intruding thoughts, which should result in a return of focus. These techniques are intended to induce a common set of physiological changes, such as decreased metabolic activity, heart rate and muscle tone. Relaxation methods require training motivation and daily practice, but the patient can anticipate long-term effects if compliant. Professional guidance from a psychologist or a physical therapist is often necessary during the initial stages of treatment to help patients master the selected technique.

Meditation techniques do not involve suggestion; rather, the individual is trained to passively attend to a bodily process, a word or a stimulus. The goal of "mindful meditation" is the development of nonjudgemental awareness of bodily sensations and mental activities occurring in the present moment.

Medical hypnotic techniques induce a state of selective attention in which the subject isolates himself or herself from his or her thoughts. It is often combined with enhanced imagery. Patients may also learn autohypnosis, a relaxation technique in which thinking is directed toward pleasant images. People vary widely in their "hypnotic susceptibility" and "suggestibility," although the reasons for these differences are not clearly understood.

### Stimulus control and sleep hygiene

Improvement of sleep quality through changes in sleep hygiene proves beneficial for many patients. For example, the patient may be instructed to go to bed only when sleepy, to get out of bed when unable to sleep, to rise at the same time every morning and to take only brief naps during the day (20 to 30 minutes or less before 3 p.m. is thought to not significantly alter nighttime sleep). Patients should avoid caffeinated beverages after dinner and smoking around bedtime and upon nighttime waking, and should either reduce or avoid alcohol consumption in the evening. Patients should also avoid intense exercise before bedtime and should minimize bedroom noise, light and extreme temperatures.[45]

### Cognitive strategies

Cognitive–behavioural therapy attempts to reorient patterns of negative thoughts and dysfunctional attitudes toward a focus on healthy adaptive thoughts, emotions and actions. Patients must be reminded to keep expectations realistic and to avoid blaming insomnia for all of life's difficulties. In addition, patients should avoid catastrophic attitudes (exaggerated negative orientation toward experiences) after a poor night's sleep.[46]

## STEP 4: PHARMALOGICAL INTERVENTIONS

If poor sleep persists during or after institution of steps 1 to 3, the dentist, in consultation with a physician, may consider pharmacotherapy.

### Pharmacological strategies for short-term and mild conditions

Among the pharmacological agents available, analgesics alone or in combination with a mild muscle relaxant, administered in the evening, can be tried (see **Table 1**). A low dose of cyclobenzaprine or clonazepam, taken in the evening, either alone or with an analgesic (e.g., acetaminophen or ibuprofen), may promote muscle relaxation, reduce pain and produce light sedation. Sleep facilitators, such as zaleplon, triazolam, temazepam and zopiclone, may also prove helpful for short periods, but they are not recommended in very young or older patients. In the presence of sleep-disordered breathing (e.g., sleep apnea), zaleplon or zopiclone is preferred. For refractory cases, physicians may prescribe low-dose amitriptyline (with slowly increasing doses), trazodone or nefazodone before sleep. These medications may have the secondary effect of improving mood and altering the experience of pain. Gabapentin, codeine and morphine are sometimes used for severe pain, but these drugs are known to interfere with sleep quality. Caution is advised in prescribing selective serotonin reuptake inhibitors such as fluoxetine, sertraline, and paroxetine, since these medications can trigger or aggravate movement during sleep, including periodic limb movement and sleep bruxism. The use of cardioactive medications for pain management (e.g., propranolol) is associated with increased risk of sleep apnea and nightmares.[47]

### "Natural" and herbal products

Herbal medicines are widely used in the treatment of pain and to aid sleep, but most lack evidence to support these uses. Examples include St. John's wort (for depression), valerian (for sedation and sleep),[48,49] lavender (for sleep),[49,50] kava (for anxiety and sleep),[51] glucosamine sulfate (for arthritis)[52,53] and even cannabis. Nonetheless, given their growing popularity, dentists should ask patients whether they are using any of these products before contemplating the prescription of a more conventional medication that might have an additive sedative action or that might cause an adverse drug interaction.[48] Most natural medicines have the potential to produce interaction effects with conventional medications.

TABLE 1 : Essential sleep management issues to be addressed in patients with orofacial pain

## ESSENTIAL SLEEP MANAGEMENT ISSUES TO BE ADDRESSED IN PATIENTS WITH OROFACIAL PAIN

| STEP OF ASSESSMENT AND TREATMENT | COMMENTS |
|---|---|
| Step 1<br>Evaluation for primarysleep disorder | Examples: insomnia, sleep-disordered breathing, primary snoring, daytime fatigue or sleepiness. Consult physician if necessary. |
| Step 2<br>Review of sleep hygiene | Evaluate :<br>· Sleep environment (e.g., bedroom dark, cool and quiet)<br>· Wake–sleep cycle (e.g., consistent bedtime and morning awakening)<br>· Lifestyle habits (e.g., intense exercise, smoking or alcohol intake at night) |
| Step 3[a]<br>Behavioural and cognitive strategies | Examples: establish regular routines for evening relaxation, avoid intense or troubling evening discussions |
| Step 4[a,b]<br>Pharmacological interventions[c] | **Short-term therapy**<br>Analgesic, either alone or combined with a muscle relaxant, administered in the evening:<br>· ibuprofen (Advil©, Motrin), acetylsalicylic acid (ASA, Aspirin) or acetamino-phen (Tylenol)<br>· acetaminophen with chlorzoxazone (Tylenol Aches and Strains)<br>· methocarbamol with either acetaminophen (Robaxacet) or ASA (Robaxisal)<br><br>**Mild condition**<br>Muscle relaxant or sedative *(in early evening, to reduce morning dizziness)*<br>· low-dose cyclobenzaprine (Flexeril, half or full 10-mg tablet)<br>· clonazepam (Rivotril 0.5 mg short term because of risk dependence)<br>· analgesics such as acetaminophen, ibuprofen or ASA can be taken with cyclobenzaprine and clonazepam if the pain is too great<br><br>**Sleep facilitator**<br>· triazolam (Halcion 0.125 to 0.250 mg)<br>· temazepam (Restoril 10 to 20 mg)<br>· zopiclone (Imovane 5 to 7.5 mg)<br>· zolpidem (Ambien 5 to 10 mg); not currently available in Canada<br>· zaleplon (Starnoc, 10 to 20 mg)[d] — very short acting, useful for middle of the night or late-night wakefulness or insomnia<br><br>**More severe or persistent cases (physician consultation recommended)**<br>· low-dose amitriptyline (Elavil 5 to 50 mg, in increasing doses if required) in the evening<br>· trazodone (Desyrel 50 mg)<br>· nefazodone (Serzone)<br>· gabapentin (Neurontin), codeine (Codeine Contin) + morphine (MS Contin)<br><br>**Others:**<br>· valerian<br>· lavender<br>· glucosamine sulphate<br>· kava |

[a] *For steps 3 and 4, combined strategies could be considered but only on a case-by-case basis.*
[b] *Patients should be forewarned of potential side effects associated with the medications listed; these may include daytime sleepiness and dizziness. Patients should avoid driving in the morning and they should use caution in operating any potentially hazardous tool.*
[c] *Brand names are included only as examples and not to promote any one product. The manufacturers are as follows: Advil, Whitehall-Robins; Motrin, McNeil Consumer Healthcare; Aspirin, Bayer Consumer; Tylenol and Tylenol Aches and Strains, McNeil Consumer Healthcare; Robaxacet and Robaxisal, Whitehall-Robins; Flexeril, Alza; Rivotril, Roche; Halcion, Pharmacia; Restoril, Novartis Pharmaceuticals; Imovane, Aventis Pharma; Ambien, Sanofi-Syn-thelabo Inc.; Starnoc, Servier; Elavil, Merck Frosst; Desyrel, Bristol; Serzone, Bristol-Myers Squibb; Neurontin, Pfizer; Codeine Contin and MS Contin, Purdue Pharma.*
[d] *Ideal for patients with sleep apnea.*

## 4. CONCLUSIONS

Dentists play an important role in relieving orofacial pain and are front-line managers of temporary sleep disturbances associated with pain.[41] Given the increasing popularity of herbal and other alternative medicines, the risks of adverse interactions with more conventional medications need to be assessed for each patient. Three Web sites are suggested as sources of additional information: Saskatoon Health Region (www.sdh. sk.ca), National Center for Complementary and Alternative Medicine (www.nccam. nih.gov) and Réseau Proteus (www.reseauproteus.net/ 1001solutions).

**Acknowledgments:** The authors' research is supported by the Canadian Institutes of Health Research and the Quebec Health Research Fund (FRSQ). This paper was presented in part at the "Sleep in older person" symposium held at the Faculty of Medicine, University of Toronto, March 2002, and at the Canadian Pain Society meeting held in Winnipeg, May 2002.

Dr. Brousseau recently completed an MSc in biomedical sciences. She is a part-time clinician at the faculty of dentistry, University of Montreal, Quebec.

Ms. Manzini is research assistant, faculties of dentistry and medicine, University of Montreal, Departments of stomatology and pneumology, CHUM – Hôtel-Dieu de Montréal, and Research centre on sleep, Hôpital du Sacré-Cœur de Montréal, Montreal, Quebec

Dr. Thie is director of the Temporomandibular Disorder/Orofacial Pain Clinic and clinical associate professor, faculty of medicine and dentistry, University of Alberta, Edmonton, Alberta.

Dr. Lavigne is professor, faculties of dentistry and medicine, University of Montreal, Department of stomatology, CHUM – Hôtel-Dieu de Montréal, and Research centre on sleep, Hôpital du Sacré-Cœur de Montréal, Montreal, Quebec.

The authors have no declared financial interests in any company manufacturing the types of products mentioned in this article

## REFERENCES

1. Price DD. Psychological and neural mechanisms of the affective dimension of pain. Science 2000; 288(5472):1769–72.
2. Feine JS, Lavigne GJ, Dao TT, Morin C, Lund JP. Memories of chronic pain and perception of relief. Pain 1998; 77(2):137–41.
3. Craig JC, Rollman GB. Somesthesis. Annu Rev Psychol 1999; 50:305–31.
4. Kosek E, Hansson P. Modulatory influence on somatosensory perception from vibration and heterotopic noxious conditioning stimulation (HNCS) in fibromyalgia patients and healthy subjects. Pain 1997; 70(1):41–51.
5. Washington LL, Gibson SJ, Helme RD. Age-related differences in the endogenous analgesic response to repeated cold water immersion in human volunteers. Pain 2000; 89(1):89–96.
6. Edwards RR, Fillingim RB. Effects of age on temporal summation and habituation of thermal pain: clinical relevance in healthy older and younger adults. J Pain 2001; 2(6):307–17.
7. Zubieta JK, Smith YR, Bueller JA, Xu Y, Kilbourn MR, Jewett DM, and others. Regional Mu opioid receptor regulation of sensory and affective dimensions of pain. Science 2001; 293(5528):311–5.
8. Pollo A, Amanzio M, Arslanian A, Casadio C, Maggi G, Benedetti F. Response expectancies in placebo analgesia and their clinical relevance. Pain 2001; 93(1):77–84.
9. Kleinman A, Guess HA, Wilentz JS. An overview. In: Guess HA, Kleinman A, Kusek JW, Engel LW, editors. The science of the placebo toward an interdisciplinary research agenda. London: BMJ; 2002. p. 1–32.
10. Meh D, Denislic M. Quantitative assessment of thermal and pain sensitivity. J Neurol Sci 1994; 127(2):164–9.
11. Kaasalainen S, Molloy W. Pain and aging. J Can Geriatr Soc 2001(Feb):32–7.
12. Harkins SW, Price DD, and Martelli M. Effects of age on pain perception: thermonociception. J Gerontol 1986; 41(1):58–63.
13. Riley JL, Wade JB, Robinson ME, Price DD. The stages of pain processing across the adult lifespan. J Pain 2000; 1(2):162–70.
14. Lavigne GJ, Brousseau M, Montplaisir J, Mayer P. Pain and sleep disturbances. In: Lund JP, Lavigne GJ, Dubner R, Sessle BJ, editors. Orofacial pain: from basic science to clinical management. Illinois: Quintessence; 2001. p. 139–50.
15. Julius D, Basbaum AI. Molecular mechanisms of nociception. Nature 2001; 413:203–10.
16. Woolf CJ, Salter MW. Neuronal plasticity: increasing the gain in pain. Science 2000; 288(5472):1765–9.
17. Chandrasekharan NV, Dai H, Roos KL, Evanson NK, Tomsik J, Elton TS, and other. COX-3, a cyclooxygenase-1 variant inhibited by acetaminophen and other analgesic/antipyretic drugs: cloning, structure, and expression. Proc Natl Acad Sci USA 2002; 99(21):13926–31.
18. Zadra AL, Nielsen TA, Germain A, Lavigne GJ, Donderi DC. The nature and prevalence of pain in dreams. Pain Res Manage 1998; 3(3):155–61.
19. Raymond I, Nielsen TA, Lavigne GJ, Choinière M. Incorporation of pain in dreams of hospitalized burn victims. Sleep 2002; 25(7):765–70.
20. Carskadon MA, Dement WC. Normal human sleep: an overview. In: Kryger MH, Roth T, Dement WC, editors. Principles and practice of sleep medicine. 3rd ed. Philadelphia: W.B. Saunders Co.; 2000. p. 15–25.
21. Moldofsky H. Sleep and pain. Sleep Med Rev 2001; 5(5):387–96.
22. Morin CM, Gibson D, Wade J. Self-reported sleep and mood disturbance in chronic pain patients. Clin J Pain 1998; 14(4):311–4.
23. Sutton DA, Moldofsky H, Badley EM. Insomnia and health problems

in Canadians. Sleep 2001; 24(6):665–70.

24. Smith MT, Perlis ML, Smith MS, Giles DE, Carmody TP. Sleep quality and presleep arousal in chronic pain. J Behav Med 2000; 23(1):1–13.

25. Affleck G, Urrows S, Tennen H, Higgins P, Abeles M. Sequential daily relations of sleep, pain intensity, and attention to pain among women with fibromyalgia. Pain 1996; 68(2-3):363–8.

26. Raymond I, Nielsen TA, Lavigne GJ, Manzini C, Choinière M. Quality of sleep and its daily relationship to pain intensity in hospitalized adult burn patients. Pain 2001; 92(3):381–8.

27. Terzano MG, Parrino L, Sherieri A, Chervin R, Chokroverty S, Guilleminault C, and others. Atlas, rules, and recording techniques for the scoring of cyclic alternating pattern (CAP) in human sleep. Sleep Med 2001; 2:537–53.

28. Parrino L, Smerieri A, Rossi M, Terzano MG. Relationship of slow and rapid EEG components of CAP to ASDA arousals in normal sleep. Sleep 2001; 24(8):881–5.

29. Martinez-Lavín M, Hermosillo AG, Rosas M, Soto M-E. Circadian studies of autonomic nervous balance in patients with fibromyalgia: a heart rate variability analysis. Arthritis Rheum 1998; 41(11):1966–71.

30. Mahowald ML, Mahowald MW. Nighttime sleep and daytime functioning (sleepiness and fatigue) in well-defined chronic rheumatic diseases. Sleep Medicine 2000; 1(3):179–93.

31. Kewman DG, Vaishampayan N, Zald D, Han B. Cognitive impairment in musculoskeletal pain patients. Int J Psychiatry Med 1991; 21(3):253–62.

32. Côté KA, Moldofsky H. Sleep, daytime symptoms, and cognitive performance in patients with fibromyalgia. J Rheumatol 1997; 24(10):2014–23.

33. Grace GM, Nielson WR, Hopkins M, Berg MA. Concentration and memory deficits in patients with fibromyalgia syndrome. J Clin Exp Neuropsychol 1999; 21(4):477–87.

34. Bromm B. Consciousness, pain, and cortical activity. In: Bromm B, Desmedt JE, editors. Pain and the brain: from nociception to cognition. New-York: Raven Press; 1995. p. 35–59.

35. Langford GW, Meddis R, Pearson AJ. Awakening latency from sleep for meaningful and non-meaningful stimuli. Psychophysiology 1974; 11(1):1–5.

36. Perrin F, García-Larrea L, Maugière F, Bastuji H. A differential brain response to the subject's own name persists during sleep. Clin Neurophysiol 1999; 110(12):2153–64.

37. Brousseau M, Kato T, Mayer P, Manzini C, Guitard F, Montplaisir J. Effect of experimental innocuous and noxious stimuli on sleep for normal subjects. IASP Abstr 2002; 10:498-No.1491.

38. Bonnet MH. Sleep deprivation. In: Kryger MH, Roth T, Dement WC, editors. Principles and practice of sleep medicine. 3rd ed. Philadelphia: W.B. Saunders; 2000. p. 53–71.

39. Dao TT, Lavigne GJ. Oral splints: the crutches for temporomandibular disorders and bruxism? Crit Rev Oral Biol Med 1998; 9(3):345–61.

40. Feine JS, Lund JP. An assessment of the efficacy of physical therapy and physical modalities for the control of chronic musculoskeletal pain. Pain 1997; 71(1):5–23.

41. Lavigne GJ, Goulet JP, Zucconi M, Morrison F, Lobbezoo F. Sleep disorders and the dental patients: an overview. Oral Surg Oral Med Oral Pathol Oral Radiol Endod 1999; 88(3):257–72.

42. NIH technology assessment panel. Integration of behavioral and relaxation approaches into the treatment of chronic pain and insomnia. JAMA 1996; 276(4):313–8.

43. Stepanski EJ. Behavioral therapy for insomnia. In: Kryger MH, Roth T, Dement WC, editors. Principles and practice of sleep medicine. 3rd ed. Philadelphia: W.B. Saunders Co.; 2000. p. 647–56.

44. Morin CM, Blais F, Savard J. Are changes in beliefs and attitudes about sleep related to sleep improvements in the treatment of insomnia? Behav Res Ther 2002; 40(7):741–52.

45. Zarcone VP. Sleep hygiene. In: Kryger MH, Roth T, Dement WC, editors. Principles and practice of sleep medicine. 3rd ed. Philadelphia: Saunders, W.B. Co.; 2000. p. 657–61.

46. Sullivan MJ, Stanish W, Waite H, Sullivan M, Tripp DA. Catastrophizing, pain, and disability in patients with soft-tissue injuries. Pain 1998; 77(3):253–60.

47. Lavigne GJ, Manzini C. Sleep bruxism and concomitant motor activity. In: Kryger MH, Roth T, Dement WC, editors. Principles and practice of sleep medicine. 3rd ed. Philadelphia: W.B. Saunders; 2000. p. 773–85.

48. Gyllenhaal C, Merritt SL, Peterson SD, Block KI, Gochenour T. Efficacy and safety of herbal stimulants and sedatives in sleep disorders. Sleep Med Rev 2000; 4(3):229–51.

49. Schultz V, Hansel R, Tyler VE. Rationale phototherapy. Berlin: Springer; 1998.

50. Buchbauer G, Jirovetz L, Jager W. Aromatherapy: evidence for sedative effects of lavender oil. Bull Inst Physiol 1970; 8:69–76. 51. Lehmann E, Klieser E, Klimke A, Krach H, Spatz R. The efficacy of Cavain in patients suffering from anxiety. Pharmacopsychiatry 1989; 22(6):258–62.

51. Lehmann E, Klieser E, Klimke A, Krach H, Spatz R. The efficacy of Cavain in patients suffering from anxiety. Pharmacopsychiatry 1989; 22(6):258–62.

52. Parkman CA. Alternative therapies for osteoarthritis. Case Manager 2001; 12(3):34–6.

53. Thie NM, Prasad NG, Major PW. Evaluation of glucosamine sulfate compared to ibuprofen for the treatment of temporomandibular joint osteoarthritis: a randomized double blind controlled 3 month clinical trial. J Rheumatol 2001; 28(6):1347–55.

# MORRIS' STORY

**Morris K.**, Montreal, Quebec, Canada

(See other testimonials, pages 246, 300, 310, 372 and 382.)

I was born in 1941, but on June 24, I celebrated my 22nd birthday! How can that be, you ask. As you can imagine, it's a long story. My journey started on a fishing trip. We were flying to a fishing camp in a remote area of the Laurentians. Unfortunately, our plane crashed at midday, in the middle of nowhere. I was unconscious for about one hour. If you believe that we all have a predetermined time, then I guess that my number was not yet up. I regained consciousness in the middle of the wilderness. I quickly realized that the pilot and my three companions had died. The two-way radio was not working. I could not bear weight on my right leg. The pain in my ankle was excruciating when I tried to stand. I was able to crawl a little with great effort and get to a large tree about 20 feet away, so that I could use it as a backrest. I had no way of knowing if there was an automatic device that sends out a distress signal. I was exhausted.

Looking back, I can now see that I subconsciously went into survival mode to stay calm. I was using relaxation techniques that I had learned 10 years earlier. Time passes very slowly when you can hear the sounds of motorboats and trucks, but cannot see them or get to them. I was unable to crawl the distance to the road or water, so I felt it was wise to conserve my energy and rest and hope for a miracle of some sorts. I also heard airplanes flying over, and I could often see them. On what I counted as one plane's ninth time making the circle, I saw that the door was open. On the next pass, two parachutists dropped from the plane and I saw a large red maple leaf in the centre of the white parachute. That was the most beautiful sight imaginable. Once they had landed, I called out so that they would know that I was alive. I was rescued within the last bits of daylight.

I was taken by ambulance helicopter to a hospital in La Tuque (Quebec), then to Quebec City, and then later on to a Montreal hospital. I had a broken jaw, a broken ankle and a CT scan showed multiple levels of compression fractures of the spine. In doctor speak, "A compression fracture occurs when the normal vertebral body of the spine is squished, or compressed, to a smaller height." In layman's terms, the spine collapses over itself. This injury tends to happen to people who are involved in traumatic accidents. "When a load placed on the vertebrae exceeds its stability, it may collapse. This is commonly seen after a fall." I believe that the airplane crash qualifies as a fall. Before these events I was five foot eight and a half inches. I am now five foot five inches. I actually shrank three and a half inches.

I spent about a month in hospital and about 11 months at home in recovery mode. It changed my life going forward forever. I adapted to a new life style. I am most fortunate for my wife's support from day one and throughout this ordeal. I am the luckiest guy in the world to have my wife's continued support for my entire new life span of 22 and a half years now as I write my story. I have been travelling on rocky roads for a long time.

As we pass through the four seasons in Montreal, spring brings with it new potholes in the roads. Potholes mean bumps as we drive along, and bumps annoy my spine. Sure as anything, my spine will send out messages letting me know that it is not pleased. Reality says that I cannot avoid everything that will bring on new pain messages. The best that I can do is try to be vigilant. I can be aware, but life must go on. That means that I will work with my team of pain doctors to find ways to minimize my pain level and maximize all the activities I can fit back into my life.

# CHRONIC PAIN IN
# CHILDREN AND ADOLESCENTS

**Christina Rosmus** RN, MSc, Montreal, Quebec, Canada
**Céleste Johnson** RN, DEd, FCAHS, Halifax, Nova Scotia, Canada

CHAPTER

**12**

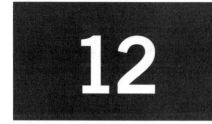

## ABSTRACT

To see one's child in pain is possibly one of the most difficult experiences a parent goes through. Pain in children and adolescents has many consequences for them, for their family and the social network in which they interact. However, important progress has been made to treat and alleviate chronic pain in children and adolescents. A great proportion among them goes on to lead a productive future with no other incidents of chronic pain. Some will have recurrent pain, but often they will have acquired skills and knowledge to help them get through further episodes in a less disruptive way. Few will need continuous services as they reach adulthood.

In recent decades, chronic pain in children and adolescents has been given more attention in the scientific world. Therefore, knowledge to guide the recognition, assessment and treatment of chronic pain in children and adolescents is increasing. Looking for information is often a useful way of coping and learning in difficult situations. However, the quality of the information is an important element to be considered. Parents and their children often look to the Internet, and find sites that may or may not give appropriate information. Most are based on adult experience, which is often very different in children and adolescents. Such resources can enlighten, but may also lead to confusion and misconceptions.

This chapter aims to help the reader become more familiar with the important concepts related to the chronic pain experience of children and adolescents, what it means and what are some consequences for them and their family, how it compares with the adult experience, and what are some treatments and approaches commonly used. It is by no means a complete overview of the subject, but provides some information and understanding of the basic principles that help children and adolescents with chronic pain regain a normal life.

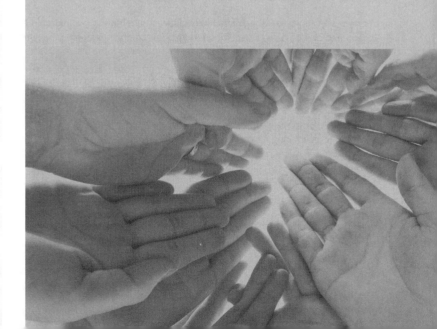

# 1. WHAT IS CHRONIC PAIN IN CHILDREN AND ADOLESCENTS?

What is considered chronic pain in children and adolescents? First and foremost, "it is what the experiencing person says it is." This definition was proposed many years ago by McCaffery and Beebe (1989), and is the one that has the most appropriate value when trying to get at children's and adolescents' experience. Pain is a very individual experience, and results from the combination of many factors. These factors originate from the pain transmission system, interrelated psychological elements, social impacts, and the parent's and their child's environment. Components of the pain experience have been identified to include its intensity, and its sensory and affective aspects. Intensity is experienced as the degree of severity ranging from mild to severe. The sensory aspect refers to the type of sensation felt, for example throbbing, pounding, burning etc. The affective component has to do with the emotions elicited by the pain such as depression, frustration, distress, etc.

Pain is defined as chronic once it has persisted for three months or more. Although this is considered the standard, most children who receive a diagnosis of chronic pain unfortunately have had pain for much longer.

Most of us are more familiar with the concept of acute pain where pain occurs for some known reason (e.g. appendicitis), signals a problem or a danger (massive infection), or goes away with healing (surgery and convalescence). Acute pain is often associated with anxiety or fear because it happens suddenly, and requires immediate attention. Chronic pain, on the other hand, does not usually signal a danger or serve such a purpose, but can, as in adults, exist on its own or in relation to a chronic disease or medical condition. Examples of this would be children who have arthritis, migraine headaches or different problems with their bones and muscles. This kind of pain is often associated with depression and frustration because it comes back at times, and is a reminder of the chronic disease or condition the child has.

Children and adolescents can also have a type of pain called neuropathic pain. This is pain related to nerve damage, compression or conduction problems. It may be temporary or long-lasting, and in this case is considered a type of chronic pain.

The pain transmission system that helps explain the way in which chronic pain develops is the same as in adult chronic pain and other chapters of this book offer a more detailed explanation. A simplified explanation will be given here, as it may be beneficial to help children understand what is happening in their body. After the body or body part has been exposed to pain for a long time, the pain system sometimes goes into a type of "short-circuit." The reason for the pain is gone and sometimes will never be identified, but the pain system has become oversensitized, and keeps sending pain messages to the brain. Even a more normal pain — for example, hitting your toe on a piece of furniture — will stimulate this oversensitized pain system, making it feel differently than it would normally have. When a pain message arrives in the brain, the brain reacts by sending different messages back to calm down the pain. These messages could be something like a logical thought ("This pain is not dangerous!") or some physical action such as relaxation techniques or muscle stretching. These messages will help reduce the pain, or make it go away. Because the system is in "short-circuit," it is thought that the system by which the brain sends messages back down to calm the pain is also having trouble.

Another scientific finding that helps us understand children's and adolescents' pain comes from studies that looked at pictures of the brain. Studies have shown that the centres for pain and emotion sit side by side in the brain, and have the capacity to interrelate or respond to each other. This helps us understand why the pain can trigger negative emotions and, conversely, why the negative emotions can trigger an increase in pain, or why positive emotions have a beneficial impact on pain. Children and adolescents experience emotions according to their level of development. This will also impact on how they experience pain in relation to emotion, and how they experience emotion related to pain.

Though the mechanism of chronic pain transmission for children and adolescents can be similar to that of adults, the experience can be very different for them and for their family. The factors involved are very different for a child or an adolescent compared to an adult, and neither is to be considered a miniature adult. One of the most important differences between adult and pediatric chronic pain is that the prognosis or recovery is much better in children and adolescents. When living with chronic pain, they are often otherwise healthy, and their psychological outlook is such that their motivation and abilities for physical activities result in most of their chronic pain being treated with good outcomes.

The types of chronic pain in children and adolescents are often different than in adults as well. Back pain is the most frequent adult problem, mostly due to occupational issues. Back pain is as frequent a problem in children and adolescents, and when seen is usually related to an injury or medical condition.

**Children and adolescents are more likely to have the following chronic pain problems: chronic daily headaches, recurrent abdominal pain, widespread diffuse pain, musculoskeletal pain or complex regional pain syndrome.**

In all cases, the first step is to make sure that there is no other underlying problem or cause that will respond to its corresponding treatment to resolve the pain. In this process, families may go from physician to physician and undergo many investigations to try to find the cause of the pain. This can sometimes become a long journey, and though this process eliminates serious problems, families can become very frustrated in this search and fixate on finding the cause.

In the end, the good news is that there is nothing serious or dangerous in their child's condition. However, the pain problem remains unattended to, and families become fearful that something has been missed, or that no one is able to offer their child much needed help. Family life continues to be disrupted and disorganized. The child or adolescent, on the other hand, may get the impression that they are not being believed about their pain and that is it "all in their head." This feeling is well illustrated in the following quotations of children being interviewed before their visit to a pain clinic.

**On not being believed...**

"The worst thing is when they don't see my pain, it makes them think that I am not in pain."

"Just because I smile, the doctors don't believe me. They say, 'Oh, he must be fine. See, he is smiling.'"

"They think I am faking my pain."

Source: Dell'Api, Rennick & Rosmus, Journal of Child Healthcare, 2000.

## EXPRESSION OF PAIN

Expression of pain is one of the indicators used when assessing children's and adolescents' pain. The expression of pain is usually more specific in acute pain where facial grimacing, vocalizations, guarding motions and distress are present to a degree. However, in chronic pain, these expressions lessen as they habituate to living with the pain. Therefore, they can sometimes be maintaining activities such as school attendance, and present a normal facial expression with few signs of being in pain. However, if given the opportunity to tell about their pain, they may give high scores of pain and describe their experience with intense words that illustrate the negative impact of their pain on their life.

Some very good tools have been developed to assess pain in children and adolescents, but they are mostly best suited to acute pain. Contrary to acute pain measures in which repeated assessments help monitor progress, in chronic pain the emphasis is on function and quality of life.

The trajectory of recovery from chronic pain occurs over time. Sometimes the pain does not abate at first, but the child and adolescent will start demonstrating an increase in activity and function. This in itself will boost confidence, and have positive psychological repercussions. All pain is multidimensional in nature, which is why a multimodal approach usually gives the best results.

FIGURE 1 : Expression of a ten-year-old's headache

A. Pain in my head

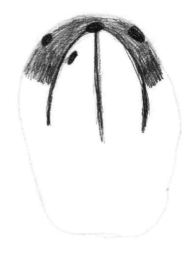

B. Pain on my head

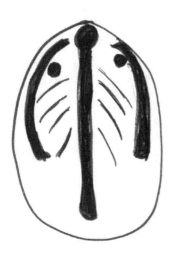

## 2. WHAT ARE SOME EFFECTS OF CHRONIC PAIN IN CHILDREN AND ADOLESCENTS?

The impact of chronic pain in children and adolescents has repercussions in many domains of daily life. It affects the emotional, relational, social and financial aspects of family life. Their chronic pain can lead to disorganization and turmoil in daily life. The goal is to return to normal daily patterns, or keep them as orderly as possible. However, this challenge is often not possible until the child's pain has been recognized and treatment has begun.

## PARENTAL EMOTIONS

Parents are the pillars of children's lives. However, parenting a child in pain presents a demanding and emotional challenge. Parental support is essential. Yet parents often face difficult emotions, and struggle themselves as they try to help their child with a pain problem. One mother, speaking of her feelings and those of other parents, said, "You just want to make that pain go away." It is a very difficult experience for a parent to go through. "I wish I could take his pain away, and make it mine." In their need to express how much they want to help their child, parents will verbalize how much they identify with their child's pain, and that they wish they could take their child's pain as their own. They live with a terrible feeling of not knowing how to help their child in pain.

The process of getting help for their child becomes a primary mission for parents. After having waited a given time to see if this pain would go away on its own, the next step is to seek medical advice as to the cause and treatment of the pain. In looking for the cause of the pain, several tests and investigations may be ordered, and a number of specialists consulted in that process. In certain cases, a cause may be identified especially in children and adolescents who already suffer from another chronic condition. But, most often, the test results will come back as "normal" as physicians try to eliminate any problems from the perspective of their speciality area. Although it only took a few lines to describe the process above, in reality this process may take weeks, months, or sometimes a year or two. In the meantime, parents' anxiety may increase as they travel through this path without finding the cause of their child's pain, and not getting effective pain control. Frustration and helplessness develop as time goes by and parents and children start feeling like this pain will last forever.

It is important for parents to acknowledge these feelings, and to find healthy ways to deal with them. Although most parents try to remain encouraging to their child, it is not always easy to hide true feelings. Children and adolescents are very good at picking up cues from their parents, and when they sense their parents' anxiety and frustration, this then causes them to become more anxious and worried. Talking to other adults or healthcare professionals can help to keep a positive attitude. Talking with knowledgeable and supportive others, goes a long way in helping parents cope with the difficult experience of having a child with pain. This can help parents to continue being effectively supportive to their child. Expressing thoughts and emotions with adult friends and family can be a source of strength and comfort, which can in turn benefit the child who needs parental support.

## CHILDREN AND ADOLESCENT EMOTIONS

As mentioned earlier in the chapter, **one of children's greatest fears is not being believed**. This thought creates a sense of isolation in which children and adolescents feel alone with their pain, and grows into a fear that no one can help. Often, despair can set in when they see their limitations, and how this negatively affects their daily quality of life. When parents become solicitous by frequently attending to pain symptoms and allowing avoidance of regular activities, their children's feelings of despair or depression are reinforced, as they interpret their situation as hopeless, and that life is forever altered. Therefore, it is important to keep normal daily routines as much as possible. Modifying an activity to make it attainable and rewarding children or adolescents for maintaining these activities, helps to create a positive frame of mind, and is far preferable to allowing complete avoidance.

Anger at the situation is also a common emotion felt by children and adolescents. "Why me?" Unless related to another illness, the answer to this question does not exist. Guilt of having done something to produce this pain may be present for some children and adolescents. As part of the explanation of how chronic pain can exist on its own, reassurance that there is nothing they have done to cause their pain can help alleviate this feeling of guilt.

A common attitude once children and adolescents begin treatment, especially physiotherapy, is fear of experiencing more pain. This fearfulness can become a barrier for them, and impair their ability to become fully co-operative and involved in the recovery process. Parental support and encouragement is vital to help overcome this fear. In some cases, this fear can also be addressed concurrently through psychological intervention to assist in moving them forward along the therapeutic plan. A good psychological or nursing assessment would be warranted, and other resources brought in.

Keeping children and adolescents motivated through the course of treatment is a joint effort of the parents and treating team. Parents know what can create this motivation and can share this information with members of the team, which can help reinforce the motivating factors.

The younger the children, the lesser understanding they have of the complexity of a chronic pain syndrome. Understanding, as discussed earlier, affects emotions. It is important to make sure that children understand as much as they can, and in a language that promotes this understanding. This in itself is a major factor in engaging them, and sets the tone for keeping a positive attitude.

Stress and anxiety related to the pain need to be tackled, as they also have a negative effect on recovery. Children and adolescents may need encouragement to actively participate in the psychological work required to deal with these emotions in a healthy way.

## RELATIONSHIPS

Having a child with pain in the family also affects how people relate to each other around this pain. As with any chronic condition, siblings may feel that a lot of the parental attention and energy is directed at the child with pain. Family life disruptions can lead to conflicts and increased tension at home contributes to a negative climate. For example, if a parent feels a child must be carried because he or she cannot walk, the amount of energy and number of times this occurs in a day can heavily impact the daily routine. Also, family activities may be curtailed to suit the child with pain, or because the burden of maintaining a given activity is too great. Disorganization sets in and everyone becomes affected in one way or another. Soliciting everyone's co-operation including the child with pain, to help temporarily reorganize until things go back to normal, can serve to stabilize the family.

Socialization is an essential part of children's and adolescents' lives, and is required for healthy development. Children and adolescents with chronic pain can become challenged in this respect. Friends and peers play an important role, and facilitating their involvement should be included in every child or adolescent's life. However, pain can limit activities. Friends who share activities develop a bond, but very often the group of friends may not remain as close or involved if participation in the activity is curtailed. For example, this is especially frequent when friends have been made through a sports activity that the child in pain cannot continue. For that same reason, getting children and adolescents back to school if they have not been attending, is part of the treatment plan. Even if they are not ready for full academic commitment, a gradual return may serve the purpose of reintegrating them to socialization, which provides support and validation of being part of a group of friends.

Modifying activities due to chronic pain also alters the ability to keep up with peers. Some children and adolescents will decide on their own to isolate themselves because they cannot keep up, whereas in other cases the friends begin to not include the one with pain, as they continue their normal course of activities. The most helpful friends are the ones who will continue including the child or adolescent with pain, and modify some activities to allow him or her to be part of their plans. The negative consequence of the loss of social connections is its contribution to depression and sadness. This may also affect motivation, and bring it back to a full circle of emotions affecting thoughts, and then behaviour.

School is the most formative activity for children and adolescents. School attendance is a priority, and should be reintegrated into or maintained. The school environment can be supportive, and enlisting their collaboration can also help them get through the weeks or months toward recovery. School staff may have been understanding, and accommodated their needs in the context of returning to normalcy, knowing that a treatment plan is in place. However, the school may not have informed of the child or adolescent's condition. This may result in ill consequences as he or she is trying to do their best, and receiving negative feedback from teachers and/or other students. At times, a progressive reintegration is a good approach for both academic and socialization reasons. The emphasis is then more on the attendance as such rather than on academic performance, which will follow once the recovery process moves forward. Gym class is sometimes an area of difficulty, but most children can do some if left to pace the exercises to their capabilities, or to use this time to do their physiotherapy exercises. Most parents can negotiate suitable arrangements with the school, but engaging health professionals in the process may be a helpful avenue in this vital goal if necessary.

Little attention has been paid to the financial burden of attending to the needs of a child or adolescent with chronic pain. Probably the fact that healthcare in Canada is provided for, and that no cost is usually attached to it, may explain the lack of attention to this aspect of the burden of having a child with chronic pain. Coming to appointments means taking time off work, and is one of the burdens that parents must endure. Employers have different conditions, and not all provide relief time for health reasons. As well, not everyone has a plan to help support the cost of medications and modalities not covered otherwise. So families must incur these costs in addition to the usual expenses of their monthly budget. In some circumstances, employment has been an issue. Financial burdens have been increased due to mothers or fathers either stopping work or reducing their hours considerably, to have more time and energy to deal with the issues presented by their child's pain. This is an unfortunate situation as it reduces family income, and also gives the message to the child with pain that the situation is desperate, and has consequences that require drastic measures. On the other hand, compassion must be felt for families who get to this point of burnout, and resort to these types of strategies to be able to survive with such a situation. An alarm signal must be recognized, and resources pulled in to assist in reducing the impact of this pain condition.

## 3. WHAT CAN BE DONE FOR A CHILD OR AN ADOLESCENT'S CHRONIC PAIN?

Pain is a multidimensional experience and therefore better tackled in a multimodal way. Multidisciplinary teams working together with patients and families usually achieve the best results. These teams offer specific medical, physical, and/or psychological modalities along with support, co-ordination and continuity of care. In cases where these teams are not available, a physician with an interest or a subspeciality in pain who can refer to other allied health professionals, can provide an array of services that can help with the many issues that pain brings about.

### MEDICATIONS

Medications used for the treatment of chronic pain in children and adolescents are mostly the same as used in adults. The pharmacological properties of these medications are discussed in **chapters 30, 31** and **32**, and also apply to them. The most commonly used medications are listed in **Table 1** (next page) with their commercial name followed by the generic one.

TABLE 1 : Most commonly used medications in pediatric chronic pain management

| MOST COMMONLY USED MEDICATIONS IN PEDIATRIC CHRONIC PAIN MANAGEMENT | | |
|---|---|---|
| | **Commercial name** | **Generic name** |
| **Anticonvulsants** | Neurontin<br>Lyrica | gabapentin<br>pregabalin |
| **Antidepressant** | Elavil | amitriptyline |
| **NSAIDS (non-steroidal anti-inflammatory medications)** | Advil, Motrin<br>Naprosyn<br>Voltaren | ibuprofen<br>naproxen<br>diclofenac |
| **General analgesics** | Tylenol | acetaminophen |
| **Opioids** | | codeine<br>hydromorphone |

Although the medications for chronic pain in children and adolescents are similar to those used in adults, they are used differently and according to developmental needs. The dose and method of administration are important to consider. The dose is usually adjusted to both weight and response. Children and adolescents are intolerant of feeling bad or feeling "weird." With good explanations and support from healthcare professionals and parents, they are better equipped to deal with this but, generally speaking, it is best to start these medications gradually to avoid side-effects and "weird feelings." Also, most medications used in chronic pain do not act immediately. They can take weeks to build up in the bloodstream before they reach an effect. It is therefore very important for children or adolescents, and their parents, to make sure they understand this, and continue taking the medication even when they themselves feel "it is not doing anything." A lot of patients and families will ask: "At what dose will this medication work?" Often it is a question of attaining the dose that will work for the child or the adolescent, which can be different from one person to another. Sometimes one medication may not have the desired effect and, after a good trial with one medication, it is sometimes better to move on to another one, which again may take some time to work. Opioids are sometimes used in chronic pain but are not usually the first choice because most types of chronic pain do not necessarily respond well to them.

Medication is only one of the factors that can help; they can be made more effective in combination with other approaches. The search for the "magic pill" is sometimes an expectation of children or adolescents and/or their family. This poses a problem as such a magic pill does not exist, and continuing to seek it builds frustration and creates a barrier to other modalities that can make a more important contribution to recovery.

There are some issues specific to children and adolescents taking medication. Some medications can be broken up into smaller pieces, or exist in liquid form to easily accommodate smaller pediatric doses, but not all. Getting them to take the medication may involve choosing a liquid or soft food such as yogurt to help them swallow the pill. The medication schedule may or may not involve the school. Negotiating an arrangement with the school may help or in some cases add a complicating factor. Discussing this issue with the pain physician or the pain nurse may help to set up a more suitable schedule for the child or adolescent, which might avoid having to take medications during school hours. Giving responsibility for taking the medication independently is part of parental decisions about their child's maturity and abilities. Before adolescence, it is usually preferable for the parents to keep this responsibility, and distribute the medications themselves. Adolescents can often take on the responsibility themselves, though they may need some supervision and reminders. To lessen the verbal reminders by parents, a different strategy may be developed such as putting the medication in a familiar place or with an object used on a daily basis. It is also always important to keep medications in safe places, so that younger children cannot access them.

In contrast to adults, there are fewer situations in children or adolescents that lend themselves to the use of "nerve blocks." In some cases, such as in the condition called complex regional pain syndrome (CRPS), which used to be called reflex sympathetic dystrophy (RSD), a block may have to be administered to enable the child to do physiotherapy. A block consists of an injection of local anaesthetic medication in the epidural space found around the spinal cord. The goal is to calm the pain system and lower the pain to enable the child to do physiotherapy, the main modality to treat this condition. In children and adolescents, these blocks are usually administered under sedation. As with other types of chronic pain in children and adolescents compared to adults, the prognosis and recovery from CRPS are better.

## PHYSIOTHERAPY

Physiotherapy is a modality frequently used to treat chronic pain. Chronic pain often sets up a cycle, in which, in order to keep from hurting, children and adolescents will guard their posture or stop moving the body part that hurts. In doing so, compensatory movements are adopted that in themselves become a problem, and often contribute to more pain. An example would be a child who has pain in a hip, and starts using the other hip more to compensate. Soon after, the child or adolescent will also experience pain in the overtaxed compensatory hip, and possibly also in his or her back due to postural changes. In a pain system that is already hypersensitized, this results in greater pain. The physiotherapist's goal is to decrease the pain, increase function and return the child or adolescent to normal daily activities. The education component of physiotherapy is also very important, where children and adolescents learn which exercises will gradually help them to move normally again. An intense period of physiotherapy over two to three weeks gives the possibility to adjust, and readjust, what works best for each of them, and often gives the best results to get over that first difficult period of facing the hurt, in order to begin moving and strengthening the painful part(s) of the body.

Some home exercises may be given and become a tool children and adolescents can use to lower or prevent pain in many cases. Parental support and guidance may be required for younger children, but adolescents need to take control of these tools themselves as they progress to recovery. The recovery time varies, but a positive attitude is the key to keeping children or adolescents motivated. Parents and therapists are often better able to see the small changes as they cumulate to make a difference, and they can use these observations to give positive feedback. Children and adolescents often have a harder time seeing the smaller improvements, because they tend to see the world more in terms of "black and white" or look for major differences rather than more subtle nuances. This is one area where the parents' support can be made very concretely. As the physiotherapy program progresses, medications may be adjusted accordingly. The other modality that contributes to better outcomes is psychology.

## PSYCHOLOGY

The role of psychology in chronic pain management is far-reaching, and is part of all other modalities of treatment. Some principles of pain psychology are used by most professionals involved in chronic pain management. As discussed in the earlier section on mechanisms, one of the first goals is to deal with the emotions triggered by the pain. Stress, anxiety, depression, anger, discouragement and feelings of helplessness are all areas of psychological work that need to be incorporated into an overall treatment program both for children or adolescents and their family. The goals are to regain control of one's life beyond the pain and normalize life as much and as soon as possible.

Several techniques are helpful in reaching these goals. To maintain a sense of control, getting information to guide one's thinking can be a useful strategy to try and make sense of what is happening. Nowadays, there is a lot of information available especially with electronic databases that are widely accessible. Knowing what information is accurate is more difficult. Healthcare professionals and reputable associations can usually identify good resources and sources of information. As mentioned earlier, much less information addresses chronic pain in children than in adults. Some of it can be extrapolated to children's pain but certainly the experience and the impact can be quite different.

The Internet is probably the source most used by many parents and children to access information and guidance. For example, for children and adolescent, chat rooms and experiential Web sites can serve to comfort them and decrease their sense of isolation. However, in using these, parental guidance is important to ensure that the child's sense of security is maintained. There was this case of a child who had complex regional pain syndrome, and found a chat room where adults who had this same condition, and were extremely debilitated for many health reasons, chatted together. The adults told stories of how this all started for them, which the child thought resembled her situation. She became very fearful that she would become as debilitated as they were, but did not share this with anyone. Her emotional distress affected her attitude, and she became less co-operative and more apprehensive when doing her physiotherapy work, which slowed her recovery. Once her mother discovered that she was chatting with other patients, she and the treating team were able to reassure her of her progress and her ability to recover from her pain. Her hope restored, she went on to gradual improvements and full recovery.

Cognitive behavioural therapy (CBT) is usually incorporated in the use of most modalities, and by all members of the team to some degree. This consists of helping children and family to use different thoughts about the situation, which will then influence emotions and subsequently, behaviour. Behaviour, in turn, influences thoughts and emotions and so forth, to ultimately make an important contribution to the recovery from pain. The classic example of this would be the ability to think of the glass being half full, as opposed to half empty. For instance, the idea is that instead of focusing on the fact that the child cannot play soccer at this time, the attention to the fact that the child is now able to use the stairs, and that this is a wonderful accomplishment is a positive thought. This positive thought then translates into a feeling of hope and reassurance, which serves to motivate the child to persevere and continue improving.

Other techniques offered by the psychologist are the identification and practice of relaxation techniques, visualization and specific coping strategies. Biofeedback, which can be learned and practised by the child, can help regain a sense of control in some cases by lowering the pain, preventing the pain or becoming better able to cope while the other modalities come into effect. Often, sleep problems become part of the pain problem, and in themselves, contribute to the pain. Working on sleep hygiene can be added to the other strategies that help normalize quality of life, and have a positive impact on the pain, and emotions related to sleep difficulties.

One of the common barriers encountered when working on psychological issues, is the reluctance to get involved with a psychologist or psychiatrist because of the misbelief that people who do are considered "crazy." Another barrier, is that it is not an easy process to confront one's emotions and thoughts, especially for children or adolescents who need to express themselves to someone who they may feel at first is a stranger. The value of such work cannot be underrated, as the quality of the outcome is usually much better achieved with the accompaniment of such a process. Parents play a key role in encouraging their child to do this, and to keep them motivated. Parents' concerns need to be addressed as well, and bringing them forth with the treating professionals is important, as a better understanding of the issues and goals of the treatment plan enables parents to learn how to best support their child or adolescent.

## NURSING

The role of nurses may vary depending on the context of how, where and when the pain care is being delivered. However, most pain nurses have extensive knowledge in the experience of chronic pain for children and families. They are often the easiest professional to reach. Their knowledge and experience is a valuable resource that can sustain children and families through the process of recovery. Nurses can answer questions, offer education, provide safe monito-

ring of medications and other modalities, help with coping strategies and parenting skills, support the efforts and the journey, become a sounding board, and suggest an array of resources and liaise with the other professionals or non-professionals involved in the daily life of children or adolescents and families. As well, nurses assess quality of life and collaborate in integrating patients' goals and aspirations, within realistic expectations of how the process unfolds. Nurses assist in the way of living that can bring families and children or adolescents to successful outcomes of the multidimensional approaches in which they are involved. Although the above describes in a succinct manner the nursing interventions that contribute to the recovery from chronic pain, the contact and time spent with nurses usually leads to the greatest knowledge of the children or adolescents' and families' daily struggles, and how they fair through this difficult experience. Nurses are helpful in identifying strengths and barriers to the recovery process. They are instrumental in helping to capitalize on strengths, and in finding ways to minimize the barriers. Nurses' advocacy allows a voice with other professionals and non-professionals, which helps individualize the plan and ensures that a continuity and reality check are offered to the patients and caregivers.

## ALISSA

This is the story of Alissa (not actual name of patient), eight years old, who from objective observations by the team and her parents, had recovered from her pain. However, she was still reporting pain and at times showing behaviours of pain. The parents had shared the task of bringing her to appointments, so that one or the other came with Alissa. As the nurse was meeting with them independently to assess how the daily reality was evolving, father and mother were reporting some tension and marital difficulties. It turned out that by trying to link pain and family events, it was recognized that Alissa had caught on to the fact that her parents rallied when she had a pain crisis. As committed parents, they allied together to help her and come up with mutual ways to deal with her pain situation. Therefore, in her eight-year-old way of looking at the world, she concluded that her pain had the benefit of making her parents co-operate with each other. Through problem-solving discussions with the parents, they accepted a referral for marital counselling. By telling Alissa that they were getting help to get along better, and as the climate at home improved, she abandoned her behaviours, and returned to her normal life.

The above example can also serve to briefly discuss the issue of "secondary gain." Some children and adolescents may derive secondary gains from their pain. In many cases, as in Alissa's, this process is mostly subconscious, and becomes a way of coping with some perceived lack. Regardless, an understanding of the factors leading to this situation can help put in place some remedial measures, which can result in a normalization of behaviour. The most frequent reason for secondary gain is increased attention of one or both parents. This is usually addressed by having the parent give attention for non-pain-related behaviours, and setting up pain-related activities that are not dependent on a parent's attention. In some cases, the intervention of a psychologist and a nurse is key in solving the issue.

## 4. CONCLUSION

Much can be done to alleviate chronic pain in children and adolescents. The partnership between the child or adolescent, their family and healthcare professionals, is crucial in attaining good outcomes, and returning life to normal function. Gradual recovery requires tenacity and a positive attitude. Tools such as coping strategies can help through the recovery process, and should be discussed on an on-going basis, with the professionals caring for the child or adolescent and his or

her family. As well, expectations need to be kept realistic, and match the stage at which progress is being made. Entering the journey of tackling this pain is best accomplished with an open mind, rather than fixed expectations. Each journey will present its own challenges and characteristics, but with confidence in scientific knowledge and the human spirit, children and adolescents with chronic pain can go on to normalcy, and quality life with their family and friends.

# GERIATRICS AND
## PAIN MANAGEMENT

**Yvon A. Beauchamp** MD, CCFP, Montreal, Quebec, Canada
Palliative Care Unit and Consultant for the Pain Clinic at the Hôpital Sacré-Cœur de Montréal,
Assistant Professor (clinic), Université de Montreal, Quebec, Canada

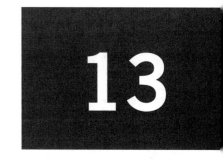

**13**

## ABSTRACT

People are growing older and surviving longer; this is a relatively new situation. As a result of this fact, the science of the study of aging is young. Over the years, more and more syndromes appear, and they often have a common element: pain. Geriatrics is a young field and knowledge about the pain experienced by elderly people (geralgia) is even younger.

In the case of elderly people, pain, whether it is chronic or not, is more difficult to identify, diagnose and treat when practising a humane and attentive form of medicine. It is becoming a major medical challenge for a clientele that is often fragile and in great need of assistance.

This chapter explores the various aspects of chronic pain in geriatrics. First, we cover the issue of pain management in the case of elderly people, by analyzing the socio-demographic aspect and the prevalence of pain in geriatrics. By defining pain next, the chapter concentrates on the physiological aging process, and makes a link with the clinical treatment of pain. The perception of pain and the psychological factors are important aspects that are discussed next. The comorbidities with pain and the major pain symptoms in geriatrics are described in order to provide an evaluation of chronic pain in geriatrics, an exploration of the various tools and instruments available to the physicians and finally, pharmacological treatment.

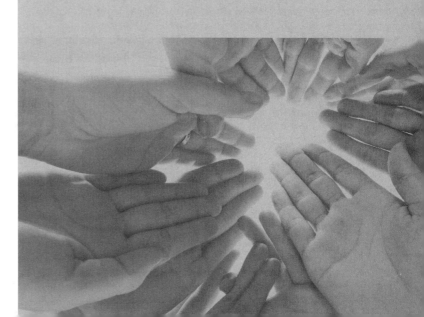

# 1. INTRODUCTION

In another millennium (1971), when I received my medical degree, medical ultrasounds were not used yet as clinical diagnostic application; neither did imaging, as used in magnetic resonance imaging and positron emission imaging.

The medical term "geriatrics" appeared and came into use in Quebec with the publication of *"Précis pratique de gériatrie"* by Arcand-Hébert in 1987. Life expectancy was 70 years. At that time, geriatric specialists were just starting to graduate from various specialized schools and beginning to take an interest in this segment of the population at the top of the demographic pyramid, a pyramid that was starting to invert under the growing number of elderly people and the decreasing and more limited number of young people.

Alzheimer's disease was recognized as a histopathological entity and was diagnosed through autopsy. Today, as a result of genetic research, it is now possible to conceive of developing a kit to screen for this chemical disease of the brain for current and future generations. A treatment based on very new chemical molecules that can slow the disease is now available.

Between the end of the 1970s and the start of the 1980s, acquired immunodeficiency syndrome (AIDS) was officially named. As our understanding of the mechanisms that invade and destroy immune defences grew, pharmacological treatments were developed to extend the life expectancy of people with AIDS, until such time as a vaccine is marketed and we enter into a prevention period.

Between 1970 and 1975, an international association of health professionals focusing on the field of pain was founded: the International Association for the Study of Pain (IASP). Created in the United States, this major association is now present in more than 80 countries. The IASP includes researchers in the fundamental sciences, such as pharmacologists, geneticists, chemists, and physiologists, as well as clinicians in medicine, nursing, and psychology, among others, all of whom are professionals with an interest in pain.

So many new developments during the course of a medical career! Therefore, geriatrics and pain as subjects of study are relatively recent arrivals in modern science. Progress, however, has been rapid and the body of knowledge accumulated on these two topics in recent decades is impressive. In this chapter, we will discuss aging and pain and will explore the characteristics that make them different and unique topics when handled together. As a result, we will discuss "gerialgia" or "presbyalgesia", pain in the elderly.

# 2. THE SOCIO-DEMOCRATIC ASPECT OF GERIATRICS

When are we considered old? Are we old when we retire from work? Are we old when we become grandparents? There are as many clichés and definitions as there are specialists in geriatrics and pain. For the clinicians who deal with older people, physiological aging is not necessarily the same as chronological aging, and vice versa.

A major shift in the age distribution in the world population is taking place. In developed countries, the percentage of the population between the ages of 65 and 80 will increase 17.5%, to 36.3% between 2006 and 2050. During this same period, the number of people over the age of 80 will more than triple[1].

In 1987, Kergoat and Lebel[2] divided all of the people over the age of 65 into two groups: "the young elderly", those between the ages of 65 and 79, and the "old elderly", those 80 years and older. In subsequent years, the authors of the most specialized medical literature concerning pain in geriatrics felt a need to divide the elderly into three groups rather than two: those aged from 65 to 74 (1), from 75 to 84 (2) and those over 85 (3). This geriatric algological distinction grew out of the conclusions of clinical studies concerning certain segments of the population but also, as a corollary, as a result of the absence of clinical studies concerning people over the age of 85.

The phenomenon of the aging of the population is associated with a much greater prevalence of persistent pain, ranging from 25% to 65% in the population living in the community and 80% of the population living in institutions. [1-9] Are the differences noted with respect to pain among these three groups exclusively the result of physiological, demographic, clinical-diagnostic or pharmacological criteria or even new criteria such as the notion of intellectual ability or disability? [3] It is my opinion that all of these criteria make gerialgia a completely different kind of pain. The elderly are not a homogenous group. They share a physiology that is not homogenous, related to a different amount of wear time for each of them, non-homogenous heredity, intellectual capacity that ranges from complete ability to complete disability, with progressive intermediary states. The physical and intellectual state of each individual is subject to comorbidities that inevitably accumulate over the years, disrupting the various physiological systems. These factors influence both the perception of pain and the treatments and have an impact on the functionality and socialization of the elderly.

As if all this demographic heterogeneity were not enough, researchers are now making a distinction between "aging" and "late life".[4] We are starting to talk about another phase in life that occurs when the aging processes have been completed. While the **aging** period is characterized by deterioration in the capacity to survive and procreate, the expression **late life** is characterized by the cessation of deterioration related to age; this new approach attempts to find an explanation through demographic heterogeneity throughout life as well as part of the theory of evolution based on the strength of natural selection. Will we have to sub-divide our group of elderly people yet again?

Studies on **geriatric pain** in the literature are still too few. In 2000, of the 4,000 articles found in the medical literature on pain, barely 1% dealt with pain in geriatrics. And by medical literature, we mean the medical journals that publish research results on the issue of pain and old age. Therefore, there is little research specifically focused on pain in geriatrics. Yet, older people have the highest rate of surgical procedures and the highest rate of painful diseases. The prevalence of persistent pain increases continuously up to the seventh decade of life, often exceeding 50% in samples of people living in their community and 80% of people living in institutions[5].

Whether it is acute, such as after a surgical procedure, or persistent, such as in the case of chronic diseases, geriatric pain becomes **an urgent problem** and its relief is just as **urgent**. Unfortunately, the few studies published make us realize just how little interest health care professional have in the issue of pain and pain relief in the case of elderly people who are cognitively intact and that the situation is even worse when the patient is unable to verbalize with respect to his/her pain in a coherent manner and ask for relief.

## 3. PREVALENCE OF GERIATRIC PAIN AND ITS INTEREST

Morrison[6] has reported conclusions that are rather disturbing and even shocking. When elderly people who are cognitively intact are compared, in the same study, to senile elderly people who have broken a hip and undergone surgery, the following facts were noted. Of the 59 cognitively intact patients, 44% reported pain that was deemed severe to very severe before the surgery; 42% of them also reported the same severe pain after the operation and 22% of them received inadequate pain relief. The 38 patients, who were handicapped by senile dementia who also suffered a broken hip and had less ability to speak and, thus, a very reduced ability to make requests, received 66% less pain relief than the cognitively intact patients (who in turn had received little). Only 24% of them received a prescription for pain relief when they left the operating room, and 76% of them received a prescription for pain relief only when their behaviour showed signs of obvious pain. This example, taken from a large university hospital in the United States, demonstrates the scope of the problem on many levels: the interest in the operation phase and a lack of interest in the pre- and post-surgery phases; possibly the lack of knowledge about pain and its relief and stubborn prejudices about pain relief. **What is even worse, medical students cannot acquire the knowledge they were not given during their practical training, which merely serves to perpetuate the serious shortcomings from one generation of doctors to another.**

**Is there a solution?** It is obvious that, in all spheres of knowledge, there are few interesting topics; there are only the topics that we are interested in! **When will more doctors take an interest in pain and its treatment?** I am tempted to answer "when the medical schools include this topic in the obligatory programme for fundamental sciences". The knowledge acquired in this manner by future doctors will appear natural and not threatening to them. Patients with pain will not be enigmatic or bothersome; the treatments that are still subject to a world of prejudice will lose their aura of inaccessibility. Patience is necessary. The future is full of promise.

## 4. PAIN AND ITS DEFINITION

The experts of the IASP had to meet many times in order to agree on a definition which, even today, is accepted by consensus in the medical world. **Pain is an "unpleasant sensory and emotional experience associated with actual or potential tissue damage, or described in terms of such damage".**

A visible injury may cause pain and the absence of an injury does not eliminate pain. An open fracture of the leg causes pain that is clearly visible and accepted by those around you; an amputated leg which has a painful phantom limb is much harder to accept because the pain is not visible and it is difficult to explain.

**What accounts for the difference in the pain felt by a younger person and that felt by an older one?** Yet, the definition is the same, regardless of whether the person is young, not so young or elderly. We can look to psychology and inquire about the normal changes of aging. Generally we can accept the fact that the aging process is a characteristic specific to complex biological systems. The changes in the individual are dependent on modifications in our genetic material, modifications on a molecular level and the loss of certain regenerative capacities in the cells; organic deficiencies appear in certain systems along with neuroendocrine deficiencies, which have difficulty maintaining homeostasis.

# 5. THE PHYSIOLOGICAL AGING PROCESS

The human being is a complex entity formed by various biological systems that are totally unrelated, but totally integrated and which, when combined, form a complicated and delicate being. These systems, regardless of whether they have a neurological, hepatic, gastric or renal function, help one another whenever there is a break-down in one of the modules that make up the human being. Throughout life, there will be episodes during which cellular breakdowns, chemical or electrical defects, or infectious attacks will occur, with particular consequences that will affect overall functioning of the organism. In addition to the normal and expected episodes of disease, and independently of functional damage to the various systems, there is the outrage of time and biological wear from which no one can escape. Certain systems are more involved in the case of the pain experience and the relief of pain. When these systems age what can we expect? What changes occur in the nervous system for the transmission and perception of pain, in our digestive system, which is responsible for assimilating medication, and in our system for eliminating medications through the kidneys?

The aging of the nervous system results in a loss of motor, intellectual and cognitive ability to adapt. Past experiences are very important in psychomotor performance. The brain has so few cells that are subject to mitosis (cell division) or regeneration that the majority of the non-divisible cells leads, in the aging process, to a progressive reduction in the number of cells, particularly in the frontal and temporal regions, as well as in the cerebellum and the hippocampus, namely in the regions which are responsible for good memory, good fine motor control and adequate behaviour. In the case of people between the ages of 20 and 85, the brain loses 7 to 8% of its mass and 10 to 15% of its volume. These electrical, cerebral regions all have an integrated role in the handling and retention of sensitive painful information and in the preparation of an adaptive motor and psychological response following a painful process.

## THE AGING OF THE CENTRAL AND PERIPHERAL NERVOUS SYSTEM[7]

A particular, major problem in geriatrics is the loss of cognitive abilities, of which the memory is one of the essential parameters. This damage to thinking and judgement is striking down more and more people as they grow older. How can senile patients handle the information they receive from their senses correctly, compare it to past experiences stored in their memory of life, or interpret a primary emotion that will become a sentiment, and how will they use their brain to analyze the damage they experience, the part of the body that is injured and the intensity of the assault? The atrophy of the cerebral parenchyma has been well documented in people in the case of the aging process. This atrophy is visible in the gray matter in several regions involved in managing pain. These regions are important and particular (insula, cingulate cortex, parietal and somatosensory cortex, basal nuclei, etc.). **Is this atrophy significant? What are the functional consequences?**

Does supraspinal modulation decrease as people age? [8] **Compared to the elderly, young adults have less chronic pain.**

## THE SLOWING OF MOTOR AND SENSORY CONDUCTION

A slowing of the conduction speed of the motor nerves and sensitive nerves has been observed in elderly people; demyelination (loss of the insulation between the neurons) is responsible for this. If demyelination is significant, the anti-pain response is slower and the voluntary motor response in reaction to the painful process will also be slower.

## THE AGING OF THE GASTRO-INTESTINAL SYSTEM[7]

The gastro-intestinal system is of interest since, in geriatric algologia, **it serves as the gateway for medication, and is responsible for the absorption of medication**. Moreover our detoxification plant, the liver, is responsible for the first step in making medications that are ingested for pain relief ineffective once the work has been done.

**What is noted in connection with the treatment of pain?**
- Gastric and intestinal epithelial atrophy (the reduction in the cell surface for the absorption of medications) is an integral part of the aging process.
- The degeneration of the intestinal nerve tissues that already causes intestinal dysfunction will be increased by the use of opiate analgesics.

## THE AGING OF THE IMMUNE SYSTEM[7]

For several interactive reasons, the immune system ages and relative immune deficiency develops in the aging individual. As a result, the aging organism becomes more susceptible to microbial attacks and intrinsic attacks, including cancer and its pain. The immune activity is usually very intense between birth and sexual maturity. After the stage of sexual maturity, certain immune capacities decline in a linear manner up to the age of 85.

## THE AGING OF THE RENAL SYSTEM

**One important function, which must be kept intact when treating pain, is the renal function since it plays an unequivocally primordial role in gerialgia**. Most of the medications that we use to treat an illness, and pain is an illness, must be metabolized (transformed) by a hepatic enzyme system called "cytochromes" or by other different chemical reactions. At the best, the metabolites (transformed medications) must be eliminated, particularly if they are toxic as is the case of certain molecules used to treat pain. At the worst, they are eliminated, unchanged or almost unchanged, by the liver and the dosages must be adjusted.

**As a result of the aging of the renal system**, it is important for the physician treating an elderly person to know how the liver functions since he/she may occasionally have to adjust the dosage of the medication in keeping with the capacity of the liver to eliminate the chemical substance. Generally, the purification capacity of the liver varies according to gender and age as well as kidney function. "All people are not created equal when it comes to medications."

## 6. THE PERCEPTION OF PAIN AND AGING

With respect to the **perception of pain in geriatrics**, I have the impression that when we treat elderly people for acute or chronic pain, the clinicians that we are and the empirical and pragmatic conclusions we draw are ahead of the contradictory conclusions we find in basic research literature.

For example, in our clinical practice we have observed that:
- 45% of elderly adults suffering from acute appendicitis experience no pain in the right iliac fossa, compared to only 5% in the case of young people;
- The incidence of pain in the case of cancer patients varies according to age: 55% of young people experience pain, compared to 35% of adults and 26% of more elderly people;
- In the case of chest pain, it has been observed that 35% to 42% of adults over the age of 65 who have a heart attack do not experience the typical pain or simply feel no pain at all. In one study, people over the age of 70 took three times longer than younger adults to report ischemic myocardial pain, which means that it takes longer to detect an angina attack which could be quickly stopped by taking nitro-glycerine;
- Close to 40% of patients over the age of 65 will feel no pain to slight pain in the case of peritonitis, an intestinal obstruction or pneumonia.

If we compare these clinical examples with the results of laboratory research and interpret them in keeping with the literature on pain, it becomes clear that, during the last 50 years of life, we experience a modest and inconsistent reduction in mild pain in keeping with the increase in age. A recent meta-analysis[8] revealed that the pain threshold in the case of elderly people was higher than in the case of younger people. This might be considered an advantage for elderly people, but it is not, since the preventive aspect of pain must be taken into consideration (warning of potential danger). The more time it takes to sound the alarm and develop an awareness of the pain, the more serious the injury might be, compared to if the danger had been detected earlier.

In contrast to this higher pain threshold, both clinical and experimental studies seem to indicate that older people are more vulnerable to severe or persistent pain. Tolerance to these kinds of pain is reduced. Studies also seem to indicate that, in the case of humans and animals, the endogenous defence system against pain called "diffuse inhibitory controls" is less effective. Core studies seem to point the finger at a reduced plasticity of the nociceptive system and extended dysfunction following a tissue injury, an inflammation or a nerve injury. In all, it requires greater pain, of a shorter duration, before the situation becomes catastrophic.

## 7. THE PSYCHOLOGICAL FACTORS AND PAIN DURING AGING

The psychological parameters of the human being are generally fascinating and it is these particular attributes that result in an awareness of the originality of gerialgia.

The social context in which the nociceptive information (pain transmission) is handled, the cognitive beliefs of the individual and the meaning attributed to the painful symptoms will become important factors in the modelling of the perception of pain. Elderly people often think that pain is a phenomenon which they cannot expect to escape and a normal part of the aging process. A perverse normality is that is so. Elderly people feel less threatened by mild pain and are less inclined to seek out treatment or relief. However, when their pain is severe, the elderly have more of a tendency to think in terms of a serious illness and ask for help faster than their younger counterparts. It appears that the older patients have difficulty understanding that the pain leads to emotional problems. It has also been noted that younger patients experience less powerlessness, less guilt and a greater desire to find an adjunctive treatment.[9]

Younger people think that their conduct and their actions have a major impact on the intensity of their pain, whereas older people will opt for either destiny/fatality or good luck/bad luck. Often, in the case of younger people, the more active they are the more risk they run of increasing their pain. Older people, who do not think that their activities have a major impact on their pain, are less inclined to think like this; for them, **something that hurts is not necessarily bad**. However, this belief in destiny is associated with more depressive phenomena, more intense pain, a greater impact on functionality and a greater tendency to choose incorrect coping strategies. Older patients demonstrate more stoicism. The self-confidence perceived does not appear to differ from one age group to another when it comes time to find strategies for adapting to pain. In terms of the psychological strategies for dealing with chronic pain, studies have demonstrated that older patients use spirituality/religion and hope more.

**All in all, in an effort to reconcile all of these disparate and apparently contradictory results, we can summarize as follows:**
The more fleeting and mild the pain is, the more difference we will observe with respect to the coping mechanisms used by young adults and elderly patients. A greater propensity to catastrophize, pray and hope, without much personal initiative, is noted in the strategies adopted by older people. Nevertheless, in the case of severe pain, regardless of whether the patient is young or old, the search for coping strategies is at the same level.

In the case of the elderly person, when the pain is mild and short-lived, there is an unequivocal tendency to attribute the phenomenon to the inevitable and expected aging process, which gives rise to a certain sense of stoicism; acceptance is easier and is part of the unconscious coping strategy. This point of view tends to minimize the importance of the mildly painful system and, eventually, removes the meaning of this kind of pain, which is intended to be a warning signal to prevent a more important injury. These differences tend to disappear when the pain is intense and prolonged.

## 8. OTHER DISEASES (COMORBIDITIES) OF THE ELDERLY AND PAIN

Aging means accumulating the injuries of life. Twenty years ago, Gibson et al[9] demonstrated that the typical 70-year-old, living in his/her community had an average of 3.6 medical conditions and took an average of seven different medications. Let us imagine what the results would be today, a quarter of a century later, if we conducted the same research in the accumulation of life injuries and the taking of medication:

- The markers for biological normality have not stopped declining (ex.: blood sugar level, cholesterol level, blood pressure, etc.; as a result there are more diseases that are "artificially created");
- The "specialists'" list of guidelines for the pharmacological treatment has grown;
- The large pharmaceutical firms have invented new classes of medications that are usually added to the other medications without, however, replacing them (more medications, therefore more side effects, more drug interactions, more problems often created by medicine).

Cynically, it could be said that each physician treating one of the multiple problems of a single individual tells him/herself that the patient should not die from the disease that particular physician is treating the patient for. At what point should the limit for treating the comorbidities for a single individual be attained? This is always difficult to evaluate. There are associations of known pathologies for which the health professionals essentially have to choose which diseases to treat. As a result, it is important to have a physician who, much like the conductor of an orchestra, coordinates all of the treatments for all of the diseases and makes a list of priorities with respect to the diseases to be treated and the treatments to be given precedence as a result of the dangers involved in taking multiple medications. These cases have been documented by Guasti[10] and validated by D'Antono et al[11].

The following comorbidities will be considered as a result of their consequences on the pain experienced by elderly people: high blood pressure, diabetes mellitus, and dementia.

Silo medicine, medicine based on longevity and not quality of life... The longer an individual lives with a chronic disease, the more complications there will be, the more treatments will be used and the more problems will be created. **When do we enter the zone of therapeutic obstinacy or unreasonable treatment?** The answer to that is a matter of good medical practices and not exclusively good pharmacological practices or good surgical practices. It is a matter of ethics!

### REDUCING SENSITIVITY TO PAIN AND HIGH BLOOD PRESSURE IN THE ELDERLY

There is a directly proportional relationship between blood pressure and a reduction in sensitivity to pain. Thus, high systolic blood pressure is associated with a higher threshold for triggering pain.

As indicated earlier, a higher pain threshold may initially seem to be a good thing since the individual experiences less pain; however, there is the risk that the nervous system has lost its ability to warn the body about a potentially serious threat that could have serious consequences. **Lowering blood pressure is essential for preventing a dysfunction of the pain system.** But when the harm has been done and the pain has become chronic, these preventive means are no longer available.

Since 60% of the elderly have a systolic pressure higher than 140 mm Hg, **this single factor can account for the increase in the pain threshold of elderly people.**[12]

### DIABETES MELLITUS AND REDUCED SENSITIVITY

Let us consider another well-known example: diabetes mellitus. In 30% of the cases of diabetes of more or less long development, there is a peripheral neurological impact that can result in hypoesthesia (reduction in non-painful sensitivity) or neuropathic pain (dysfunctioning of the central nervous system with an increase in pain). In the presence of hypoesthesia that is responsible for a reduction in sensitivity, the pain threshold will be higher. Once again, with the loss of the alarm function of a normal pain threshold, there is a danger that elderly diabetic patients will injure their extremities. This is something we see on a regular basis in practice.

### DEMENTIA AND PAIN

Another problem that we see regularly in practice is the association of dementia and pain. For elderly patients with these comorbidities, the issues are different: the treatment for pain will almost certainly hamper their cognitive functions which have already been more or less reduced by the dementia since the medications use to treat pain have a great many negative side effects on concentration, judgment and memory. **The issue is to determine priorities with respect to the illnesses and symptoms to be treated**; treating pain with medications that affect the normal chemistry of cognition and will have a negative impact on a brain that is already affected or deciding to preserve the remaining function of the brain to the detriment of pain and suffering which will reduce the cognitive ability of the elderly in any case. The decision must be based on a process that involves analyzing ethical principles, legal principles, the code of ethics of those providing the care, and, above all, the wishes of the elderly patient, who is often forgotten in the medical-family decision-making chain.

The social issues are not limited to the perception of pain. Bradbeer et al[13] have demonstrated that "solitude and bereavement" are responsible for mood problems that in turn affect pain. By definition, pain is as much a sensation as an emotion. An emotion always results in a particular behaviour that promotes social interaction. Thus, it is possible that, as in the case of other age groups, pain leads to a behaviour of fragility and sadness that will cause the group to take care of the suffering member. However, in our urban and modern societies, what could be is not always the case. Families are often fragmented; the younger individuals have to cope with daily economic concerns; both spouses work to make ends meet. There is less space for the more elderly members within a family. Hospitals are overcrowded, home-care centres are too and natural caregivers are ill-prepared, and far too often overwhelmed and isolated and find themselves without medical or nursing support and without any relief team.

## 9. MAJOR PAIN SYNDROMES ENCOUNTERED IN GERIALGIA

In practice, we like to be able to identify the symptoms of a disease so that we can make a diagnosis that is as accurate as possible. Pain may be a symptom and it may be a disease. When is it which? The classification of pain is often based on various unrelated parameters. It is common to speak about acute pain and chronic pain. In these cases the reference factor is the speed at which the pain appears and the time it lasts.

### TYPES OF PAIN

#### Symptomatic pain

Any sudden and unexpected accident is considered acute. Examples are legion:
- the individual who falls and breaks a wrist;
- the individual who complains of abdominal pain that will result in a burst appendix and surgery; and
- the individual who experiences chest pain with radiation to the left arm, and will have a heart attack.

All of these kinds of pain are **symptoms** that warn the brain that a particular part of the body is injured, much like smoke detectors in our homes warn us about fire.

**This alarm has a precise function: to warn the brain so that it can decide which actions to take to allow the part of the body affected to rest and heal. This pain is important in terms of protection and is expected to end when the limb or organ in question heals.**

#### Chronic pain

Chronic pain is also defined in keeping with the time/duration parameter; for some, three months is the border between acute pain and chronic pain; others consider it to be six months. Finally, some would say that chronic pain is pain that lasts beyond the normal healing time. **This pain is no longer a reliable warning sign since it functions with no apparent reason**. It has lost its value for protection and healing. The sustained hope of seeing it disappear fades over time. Psychological problems are often the norm if coping is not possible or if the losses are too great to be overcome. In this case, the pain acts like a smoke detector, perpetually emitting its trident sound, when there is no smoke...

### Chronic pain as defined in terms of physiological or pathophysiological mechanisms

Other clinicians define chronic pain as a physiological mechanism or a pathophysiological mechanism. This means of classification is used by the doctor who wants to choose the treatment that is appropriate for the pain in keeping with the mechanisms involved in the various tissues and the central nervous system (from the spine to the brain) or the peripheral nervous system (from tissues to spine). **We generally use the term nociceptive pain to refer to a peripheral inflammation and neuropathic pain to refer to an injury of the nervous system or when there is a dysfunction of the nervous system.**

**Why is this terminology important?** Simply so that the pharmacological treatments can be directed at the defective mechanism, whether this is chemical or electrical. There is a large quantity of classes of analgesic medications because there are as many chemical mechanisms responsible for pain.

Finally, certain physicians speak of **cancerous pain** and **non-cancerous pain**. This classification is very vast and provides little enlightenment when it comes to selecting appropriate treatments. This is much like saying there are two types of road vehicles: cars and trucks! The label of cancerous pain and non-cancerous pain does not help and does not necessarily point to a particular treatment (although, occasionally, targeted radiotherapy can be the appropriate pain for some treatments much like chemotherapy that is focused on palliative care). There are animal models for bone cancer pain just as there are animal models for neuropathic pain or animal models for algodystrophic pain. It is true that chemical substances are encountered in cancers that modulate the rise in pain and the decline in the general state of patients. These particularities are added to the other electric and chemical mechanisms that are found in diseases with a non-cancerous etiology. **The pain of cancer has its own characteristics, but still obeys the other common characteristics of non-cancer pain.**

**In order to make an accurate diagnosis and clearly identify the patient's pain, it is important to know:**

· The duration (acute or chronic);
· The physiological mechanisms (nociceptive or neuropathic); and
· The etiology, which must be more specific than just cancerous or non-cancerous.

## SYNDROMES MORE SPECIFIC TO GERIATRICS

It would not be very appropriate to prepare a list of the various diseases to which an aging population is susceptible and then describe each one in detail. It is normal to think that the diseases of the bodily framework are preponderant since we are living older and older and the wear developed through repeated movements, the loss of the normal lubricants in the joints, the decalcification of bones and the new fragility means that we see diseases that develop over long periods of time and that have symptoms that result in a maximum loss of function, tissue destruction and pain. The osteo-articular diseases play a major role in the development of pain.[7]

Other types of pain are related to diseases, such as diabetes, shingles, strokes, etc.; a great many elderly individuals suffer from such diseases since they live longer, considering the fact that the primary disease is treated and postponed until the individual reaches a stage of multiple, major complications. Multi-system complications (involving several organs) are an integral part of the original diseases, to which chronic pain is added. Many types of chronic pain have exploded in number with the aging of our populations. Some diseases, present in limited numbers a few years ago since the individuals who have them die younger, now exist in large numbers as a result of the increase in life expectancy.

**Table 1** provides an overview of the diseases that a physician treating an elderly and continually aging population sees and treats. It is obvious that there are acute, chronic, cancerous, and non-cancerous diseases and that the explanation for such diseases is nociceptive or neuropathic.

All in all, elderly people have diseases that frequently start in the middle of their lives and will last much longer than they did one or two generations ago. Very often, these diseases do not cause death, but they do cause terrible suffering that lasts a long time.

TABLE 1 : Diseases and syndromes encountered more frequently in geriatrics

## DISEASES AND SYNDROMES ENCOUNTERED MORE FREQUENTLY IN GERIATRICS

| PAIN SITE | COMMON PAIN SYNDROMES |
|---|---|
| Head and neck | Facial neuralgia, vascular headache, temporal arthritis, osteoarthritis of the neck, strokes, Parkinson's, cancers |
| Joints | Osteoarthritis of the shoulder or hip, rheumatoid arthritis |
| Lower back | Lower back disc disease, spinal stenosis, osteoarthritis of the lower back, osteoporosis, crushed vertebra, widespread cancer, metastases |
| Limbs | Peripheral neuropathies, peripheral vascular diseases, complex regional pain syndromes, bone metastases |
| Heart - lungs - chest | Angina, cancers, nerve plexus invasion, invasion of the thoracic wall by cancer |
| Body | Post-shingles pain, diabetic radiculopathies, post-operative and post-radiation therapy intercostal neuralgia |
| Digestive system | Hiatus hernia, chronic constipation, irritable bowel syndrome, primary or metastasized cancer of the intra-abdominal organs, carcinomatosis |

# 10. CHRONIC PAIN AND ITS ASSESSMENT IN GERIATRICS

The assessment of pain must identify certain parameters with respect to the individual that are essential for developing a good treatment strategy.

## What is the definition of chronic pain in geriatrics?

Several definitions have appeared in the literature and caused confusion at one point or another. In the case of the elderly individual, the distinction between recurrent pain and chronic pain is blurry: talking about persistent acute pain or recurrent acute pain or benign chronic pain makes no sense.

Bonica[14] defined chronic pain as: **"Pain which persists a month beyond the usual course of an acute disease or a reasonable time for any injury to heal that is associated with chronic pathologic processes that causes a continuous pain or pain at intervals for months or years".**

**This definition provides a framework for the musculoskeletal-osteoarthritic diseases as well as certain degenerative diseases that accompany periodic pain in chronic pain in a categorical manner.** A very large number of our elderly patients suffer from these diseases.

Pain is a perception: This perception is particular in that it is both sensorial and emotional. Therefore, there is an intrinsic value of unpleasantness which is associated with the intensity of the nociceptive sensorial aspect of the pain. Pain, therefore, must be evaluated in a multi-dimensional manner with respect to both the intensity of the purely physical aspect of the pain and the psychological unpleasantness and the multiple functional problems it causes.

## The issues of the sensory and emotional components of the perception of the pain

These two simultaneous components of the pain perception (sensorial and emotional) lead to other issues that will dictate a behaviour that is both physical and psychological, ranging from an inability to cope to coping. The analysis of these two issues (inability to cope and coping) is of use with respect to the social interaction it creates within the immediate support group.

For example, an individual who is injured perceives an intensity of physical pain as well as a sense of anguish or fear or anger with respect to the lack of knowledge concerning the severity of the injury of the consequences of such an injury (a missed trip). If the intensity of the pain and the anguish result in crying and tears (a behaviour), a probable social interaction will be the consequence, mobilizing the community to come to the individual's assistance.

With chronic pain, the disease persists; the coping mechanisms or the inability to cope have often reached a plateau and the behaviours often reflect a certain despair with a negative impact on self esteem. When the pain first appears, the sympathy capital of loved ones and people close to the affected individual is high; over time, if the pain persists, this sympathy decreases as a result of their inability to help resolve the problem. It is at this point that the patient becomes depressive.

## PAIN ASSESSMENT TOOLS IN GERIALGIA

The first tools used to assess pain were described and used for patients dealing with the pain of cancer. Obviously, our elderly patients also suffer the pain caused by cancer, but a large number of other pathologies or diseases cause both acute and chronic pain. As a result, other types of assessment tools had to be developed.

## Pain assessment tool

We use the same pain assessment tools for our older patients as for our younger patients. **The first good tool for assessing geriatric pain is still a solid and disciplined medical examination**. We have to determine the cause of the pain, the location, the intensity, the characteristics of the pain (nociceptive, acute, chronic, neuropathic), the time of the pain, the actions or situations that exacerbate pain, as well as the actions and situations that relieve it and, finally, we must determine the repercussions of the pain on motor, psychological and social functioning. **Describing and quantifying the intensity of pain is a major challenge, especially in geriatrics**. Pain is, above all, a subjective perception that we try to rate quantitatively, so as to make it objective and comparable in order to offer a treatment that is appropriate for the type and intensity of the pain perceived. Afterwards, it will be easier to track the improvement (or lack of improvement) of this pain quantitatively and, as a result, the effectiveness or failure of our treatments. However, it is always difficult to quantify the quality of the pain experienced by an individual.

## Instruments

Since pain is both a sensation and an emotion, we also need instruments to recognize and evaluate the emotional issues as well as the behavioural and cognitive issues faced by individuals suffering from chronic pain. Certain instruments are subjective verbal measurements that examine the intensity and nature of the pain. Others measure the intensity, the quality, the history, the consequences and other variables of pain over time. Some questionnaires focus on measuring psychological functioning. Still other tools attempt to measure the coping strategies and certain cognitive variables as well as the social environment. And some tools focus on measuring the motor and behavioural components of pain and the multi-focus assessment.

Very recently, Davidson et all[17] reviewed the literature and proposed a pain assessment model that takes seven factors into consideration. They made an inventory of the multitude of measurement tools used to assess various interdependent dimensions such as: pain intensity scales, physical coping questionnaires, depression questionnaires, questionnaires to determine degrees of functionality, etc. Theses researchers concluded that **there are seven significant dimensions in the painful experience and that these dimensions are reliable and systematic.**

In order to assess pain adequately, we must, therefore, consider "pain-incapacity, the description of pain, emotional distress, support, the positive coping strategies, negative coping strategies and activity".

In the near future, it would be a good idea to develop a standardized and easy-to-use assessment kit, including a minimum number of scales and questionnaires that would serve to identify the dimensions of pain which are important but which vary from one person to the next.

## What instruments do we use in daily geriatric practice?

The first assessment scales that are still of use today are intended for elderly people who are sick but cognitively intact. It is easy to ask them: Do you hurt? It is more difficult to attribute a quantitative value to this pain and its intensity. The visual analog scale (VAS), the verbal scales, the digital scales and the face pain scales are used in practice to measure the intensity of pain.

### Examples of visual scales

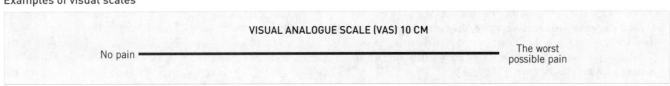

VISUAL ANALOGUE SCALE (VAS) 10 CM

No pain —————————————————————— The worst possible pain

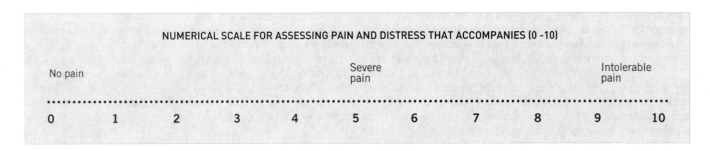

NUMERICAL SCALE FOR ASSESSING PAIN AND DISTRESS THAT ACCOMPANIES (0 -10)

No pain                          Severe pain                          Intolerable pain

0    1    2    3    4    5    6    7    8    9    10

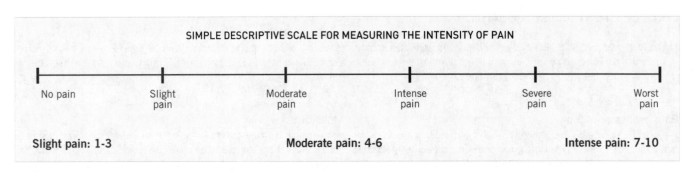

SIMPLE DESCRIPTIVE SCALE FOR MEASURING THE INTENSITY OF PAIN

No pain     Slight pain     Moderate pain     Intense pain     Severe pain     Worst pain

Slight pain: 1-3                    Moderate pain: 4-6                    Intense pain: 7-10

### Example of verbal and nominal scale

- [ ] 10 Unbearable
- [ ] 8 Severe
- [ ] 6 Strong
- [ ] 4 Uncomfortable
- [ ] 2 Slight
- [ ] 0 No pain

Visual scales can also be used to measure the unpleasant aspect of pain. The visual analog scales are reliable and they serve to make more accurate estimates of the pain sensations reported and the percentages of change in the intensity of pain. Unfortunately, some elderly people do not have the ability to use them adequately to describe their pain since their understanding of the process is often laborious, and they occasionally have difficulties with abstraction as well. Some scales use a range of colours that may be pointless in the cases of people with vision problems. Moreover, the meaning of the colours may differ according to the individuals' cultures. The verbal scales use adjectives to describe the level of the intensity of the pain (for example: no pain, slight pain, average pain, strong pain, unbearable pain). These scales are easy, but they do not work well and they provide little indication of the diversity of the pain the individual suffers.

EXAMPLE OF PAIN THERMOMETER WITH PAINFUL FACIAL EXPRESSIONS

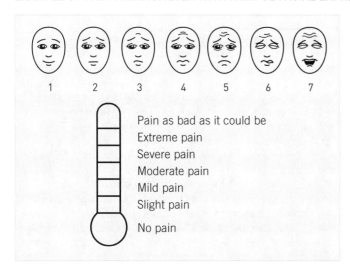

Pain as bad as it could be
Extreme pain
Severe pain
Moderate pain
Mild pain
Slight pain
No pain

## Elderly people with a reduced capacity to express pain

It is difficult to make a solid multi-dimensional assessment of the pain experienced by elderly people with dementia and have to deal with memory losses, personality changes, and a decrease or loss of judgement, the capacity for abstraction and language skills. Occasionally, the usual behaviours associated with pain are lacking in these individuals. However, symptoms that are attributed to dementia can be an indication of pain. For example, aggressive behaviour may be simply a defensive reflex. In this case, the main reason for analgesic under-treatment is under-detection. The self-evaluation of pain remains the best means but this self-evaluation may be deficient or lacking, even impossible in the case of clients with a loss of cognitive function, and this is not negligible. Therefore, other assessment tools were required. Vascular and degenerative dementia often complicates the diagnosis and assessment of pain as well.

### Assessment tools

The authors have concluded that none of the 12 tools they studied for assessing pain in the case of patients with cognitive losses stand out in any convincing manner and that, therefore, none of them is preferable over the others. Their conclusions, based on criteria of validity, reliability and homogeneity, do demonstrate, however, that PAINAD, PACSLAC, DOLOPLUS-2 and ECPA have the best psychometric qualities. Nevertheless, even if these four scales are the best known for their psychometric qualities, none would be rated better than average. Of these four scales, PACSLAC is the only one that identifies subtle changes in behaviour; moreover, it is also one of the few scales that focuses on painful items directed specifically at senile elderly people whereas several other scales were developed from previous scales used to assess pain in other categories of patients.

Of these four scales, DOLOPLUS-2 was the most completely tested (Link to DOLOPLUS-2: http://prc.coh.org/PainNOA/Doloplus%202_Tool. pdf). Holen et al[19] also examined the question of whether DOLOPLUS-2 was truly a good scale for assessing pain in the case of individuals with dementia. Their conclusions have led us to decide that, when used by experienced doctors and nurses, it is actually a good tool, but that in the case of users who are inexperienced and lack prior knowledge about the diseases, this scale was less reliable and sensitive. Moreover, the assessment of the psychosocial aspect of the test could easily be removed without any loss of reliability.

Zwakhalen[18] et al reviewed the existing literature and systematically analyzed 12 instruments and questionnaires (although there are at last [19] English questionnaires and 5 French questionnaires) for assessing pain in the case of elderly people with severe dementia. These assessment tools are based on behavioural changes that would be pain indicators and are usually revealed by facial expressions, verbalizations/vocalizations, body movements, changes in interpersonal interactions, changes in routine habits and changes in mental status.

**The current conclusion with respect to the tools used to evaluate pain in the case of elderly people with dementia: PACSLAC (Appendix 1) and DOLOPLUS-2 are the most appropriate scales for the time being since they examine the six fields (facial expressions, verbalization/vocalization, body movements, changes in interpersonal interaction, changes in routine activities, changes in mental condition) of the American Geriatrics Society[19] (AGS). The ABBEY scale deserves attention and will need to be validated, despite the fact that it only examines four of the AGS fields.**

## 11. PHARMACOLOGICAL TREATMENT IN GERIALGIA

Throughout this chapter, we have examined the characteristics of pain in geriatrics compared to pain experienced by younger patients. We are also interested in the physiological changes caused by aging and the emotional and cognitive components of pain, which make an adequate and professional evaluation more precise. Therefore, it is normal to have specific rules and stumbling blocks that must be taken into account when developing an analgesic treatment for elderly people.

The American Geriatrics society (AGS)[20], the British Pain Society (BPS) and the British Geriatrics Society (BGS)[21] have published – separately and at different times – guidelines for evaluating and treating elderly people. These three societies have essentially the same approach and many of the studies on which the AGS' 2002 rules were based were also used to develop the British rules of 2007. The six components of pain developed by the American Geriatrics Society to evaluate pain are found in their entirety in the guidelines issued by the British. The main difference between the two societies concerns the opinion given by the AGS concerning the pharmacological treatment of persistent pain in the case of the elderly; the British do not mention this and stick to major principles.

In addition to the general and universal rules of pharmacology to be applied to all patients, regardless of age, the AGS insists on stressing the fact that any pharmacological treatment has risks and benefits. It also stresses the fact that it is utopic, for both the doctor and the patient, to think that a pharmacological treatment can lead to complete relief when the pain is severe and chronic. The AGS also insists on the need to document the patient's physiological condition adequately in terms of liver and kidney function with respect to hydration and blood proteins before starting any medication treatment. It should be noted that older patients are more likely to experience drug reactions as a result of the large number of molecules they must ingest on a daily basis to treat their multiple comorbidities. It must be postulated and assumed that sensitivity to medications that act on the central nervous system (including opiate analgesics) increases with age.

> There is still one main clinical principle that must be reinforced: Start with a very low dosage (do not rely on the initial dosage indicated in the *Compendium of pharmaceuticals and specialties*), and increase this slowly, while applying the rules of drug half-life and the state of equilibrium of the medication used.

**The purpose of the analgesic treatment is to improve physical capacities and acquire or improve functionality. In this respect, the AGS stresses the importance of associating, in most cases, physical and even psychological treatments with the pharmacological treatment.** Since the analgesic pharmacopeia, which includes mild analgesics as well as very powerful opiates and a multitude of other co-analgesic agents or adjuvants is both enormous and developing exponentially, it is suggested that the results of analgesic treatment will be better with the use of more than one single medication acting on the various chemical and electrical mechanisms of pain. Health professionals must always remember to ask their elderly patients about the possibility of interactions with medications sold over the counter and medications based on herbal medicine.

A description of the various classes of analgesics and co-analgesics is provided in **chapter 30**. It should simply be noted that the galenic form is often as important as the molecule itself. Occasionally, the transdermal route, using medication patches applied to the skin, will be more appropriate than ingesting the medication by mouth. Some patients often prefer a topical application (by way of the mucous membrane or under the tongue), if the medication cannot be administered sub-cutaneously. For information about the dosages and possible drug combinations, the reader is encouraged to read all of the AGS' recommendations or refer to the recommendations of his/her attending physician. Finally, an important point has been raised with respect to the use of a placebo: in clinical practice, using a placebo is considered unethical for treating chronic pain.

For the elderly patient who manages his/her own medication, it is essential that the drug combination be as simple as possible in terms of both number of pills and number of times at which the pills are taken each day; **this also includes all medications other than analgesics**. Moreover, the physician may have to choose which diseases is more important to treat in order to reduce the medications that are considered less important and eliminate the very real risks of error.

### Recommended non-pharmacological therapies

We cannot conclude this chapter without mentioning the non-pharmacological therapies that are recommended and are an integral part of a readaptive treatment:

1. Physical activity programme for all so as to maintain flexibility, strength and endurance. For example, the programme included in *Pain Management for Older Adults, A self-help guide*[22];
2. Formal cognitive behavioural therapies will be indicated for certain individuals dealing with persistent pains;
3. Other means, such as massage, cold or heat, acupuncture, transcutaneous nerve stimulation, etc.

## 12. CONCLUSION

As we end this chapter, it would be easy to conclude that any kind of pain, whether it is chronic or not, is difficult to identify, diagnose and treat in the case of the elderly. This is only true in the event that you want to practice medicine focused on speed, superficiality and minimum involvement. When a human and attentive approach to medicine is applied, the pain suffered by elderly people becomes an unusual medical challenge that is of great value as a result of the help provided to people who are often fragile and have more difficulty obtaining aid. The painful syndromes are known and added to other cancerous, metabolic or organic syndromes that may co-exist in the same, suffering individual. This a global and general form of medicine, in which science mixes with ethics and research. It is by nature a form of medicine that is fascinating and constantly evolving.

Let us hope that the medical schools will take this into consideration and focus the teaching of the basic sciences on the understanding of painful phenomena in the case of the elderly so that a new generation of doctors will take an interest in it and conduct research specifically on this topic so as to develop balanced treatment strategies that minimize the negative results:

## "DOING GOOD
## WITHOUT CAUSING HARM."

## APPENDIX 1  PAIN ASSESSMENT CHECKLIST FOR SENIORS WITH LIMITED ABILITY TO COMMUNICATE - (PACSLAC)

| FACIAL EXPRESSION | PRESENT (√) |
|---|---|
| Grimacing | |
| Sad look | |
| Tighter face | |
| Dirty Look | |
| Change in eyes (e.g. squinting, dull, bright, increased eye movements) | |
| Frowning | |
| Pain expression | |
| Grim face | |
| Clenching teeth | |
| Wincing | |
| Open mouth | |
| Creasing forehead | |
| Screwing up nose | |

| ACTIVITY/BODY MOVEMENT | PRESENT (√) |
|---|---|
| Fidgeting | |
| Pulling away | |
| Flinching | |
| Restless | |
| Pacing | |
| Wandering | |
| Trying to leave | |
| Refusing to move | |
| Thrashing | |
| Decreased activity | |
| Refusing medications | |
| Moving slow | |
| Impulsive behaviours (repeat movements) | |
| Uncooperative/resistance to care | |
| Guarding sore area | |
| Touching/holding sore area | |
| Limping | |
| Clenching fist | |
| Going into fetal position | |
| Stiff/rigid | |

## APPENDIX 1 (CONT'D)  PAIN ASSESSMENT CHECKLIST FOR SENIORS WITH LIMITED ABILITY TO COMMUNICATE - (PACSLAC)

| SOCIAL/PERSONALITY/MOOD | PRESENT (√) |
| --- | --- |
| Physical aggression (e.g. pushing people and/or objects, scratching others, hitting others, striking, kicking) | |
| Verbal aggression | |
| Not wanting to be touched | |
| Not allowing people near | |
| Angry/mad | |
| Throwing things | |
| Increased confusion | |
| Anxious | |
| Upset | |
| Agitated | |
| Cranky/irritable | |
| Frustrated | |

| OTHER | PRESENT (√) |
| --- | --- |
| Pale Face | |
| Flushed, red face | |
| Teary eyed | |
| Sweating | |
| Shaking/trembling | |
| Cold clammy | |
| Changes in sleep routine **(please circle 1 or 2)** 1) Decreased sleep 2) Increased sleep during the day | |
| Changes in appetite **(please circle 1 or 2)** 1) Decreased appetite 2) Increased appetite | |
| Screaming/yelling | |
| Calling out (i.e. for help) | |
| Crying | |
| A specific sound of vocalization for pain (e.g. "ow," "ouch") | |
| Moaning and groaning | |
| Mumbling | |
| Grunting | |

# REFERENCES

1.  Stephen J. Gibson, PhD. Older People's Pain, Pain Clinical Updates, International Association for the Study of Pain, Seattle, U.S.A., volume XIV, No 3, June 2006.

2.  Kergoat, Marie-Jeanne, Paule Lebel. Aspects démographiques et épidémiologiques, Chapitre 1, pp. 19-27. Dans : Précis pratique de gériatrie de Arcand-Hébert, Edisem 1987 St-Hyacinthe, Québec, Canada.

3.  Hanschild. Pain Management in frail, community-living elderly patients. Archives of Internal Medecine, San Francisco, USA, 2001; 161:2721- 2724.

4.  Rose, Michael, Casandra Rauser, Laurence Mueller. Late Life: a new frontier for physiology, Physiological and Biochemical Zoology, Chicago, USA, 78(6): 869-878.

5.  Parmelle PA et al. Journal of American Geriatric Society, New-York, USA, 1993; 41:517-522

6.  Morrison, R. Sean, AL Siu. A Comparison of Pain and its Treatment in Advanced Dementia and Cognitively Intact Patients with Hip Fracture. Journal of Pain and Symptom Management, New-York, USA, vol. 19 No.4 April 2007.

7.  Laganière, Serge, Physiologie de la sénescence, chapitre 3, pp.41-55. Dans : Précis pratique de gériatrie de Arcand-Hébert, Edisem 1987 St-Hyacinthe, Québec, Canada.

8.  Cole, LJ, MJ Farrel, SJ Gibson, GF Egan. Age-related differences in pain sensitivity and regional brain activity evoked by noxious pressure. Neurobiol of Aging. 2008 May 29.

9.  Gibson, Stephen. The Pain Experience over the adult life span, Proceeding of the 10th World Congress on Pain. J Pain and Aging,Vol. 24, 2002; 767-791.

10. Guasti L., R. Cattaneo, O. Rinaldi et al. Twenty–four hours non-invasive blood pressure monitoring and pain perception. Hypertension 1995, 25: 1301-130

11. D'Antono, B., B. Ditto, N. Rios, DS Moskowitz. Risk for hypertension and diminished pain sensitivity in women: autonomic and daily correlates. International Journal of psychophysiology 1999; 31:175-187, New-York, USA.

12. Fagard, RH. Epidemiology of hypertension in the elderly. American Journal of Geriatric Cardiology 2002; 11: 23-28, Malden MA, USA.

13. Bradbeer, M., HH Hyong, HL Keng, RD Helme, SJ Gibson. Widowhood and other demographic associations of pain in independent older people. Clinical Journal of Pain, 2003.

14. Bonica, JJ. The Management of Pain (2e edition), Philadelphia, Lea & Febiger, 1990.

15. H. Flor, B. Knost Mesures standardisées pour évaluer la douleur - approche psychobiologique, chap 38; pp 389-408. Dans : L. Brasseur, M. Chauvin, G. Guilbaud. Douleurs, Bases fondamentales, Pharmacologie, Douleurs aigües, Douleurs chroniques, Thérapeutiques; Éditions Maloine,1997, Paris, France.

16. Harkins, SW, FM Bush, DD Price. La douleur chronique et son évaluation chez le sujet âgé, chap. 51 ; pp 547-566. Dans : Douleurs, Bases fondamentales, Pharmacologie, Douleurs aigües, Douleurs chroniques, Thérapeutiques; L. Brasseur, M. Chauvin, G. Guilbaud, Éditions Maloine 1997, Paris, France.

17. Davidson, Megan A., Dean A. Tripp, Léandre R. Fabrigar, Paul R. Davidson. Chronic Pain Assessment: A Seven-Factor. Pain Res Manage, Vol 13, No 4, July/August 2008.

18. Sandra MG, Zwakhalen, Jan PH Hamers, Huda HuijerAbu-Saad, Martin PF Berger. Pain in elderly people with severe dementia: A systematic review of behavioural pain assessment tools. BMC Geriatrics,2006, 6:3 doi: 10.1186/1471-2318-6-3.

19. Holen, Jacob C., Ingvild Saltvedt, Peter M. Fayers, Marianne J. Hjermstad, Jon H. Loge and Stein Kaasa. Doloplus-2, a valid tool for behavioural pain assessment? BMC Geriatr, 2007; 7: 29. PMCID: PMC2234400. Published online 2007 December 19. doi: 10.1186/1471-2318-7-29. Copyright © 2007 Holen et al; licensee BioMed Central Ltd.

20. The Management of Persistent Pain in Older Persons, Clinical Practice Guideline June 2002, vol.50, no 6, supplement, American Geriatrics Society, New-York, USA.

21. Assessment of pain in older people (2007), Royal College of Physicians, British Geriatrics Society and British Pain Society.

22. Hadjistavropoulos, Thomas & Heather D. Hadjistavropoulos, Editors. Pain Management for Older Adults. A self-help guide. IASP Press, Seattle. USA, 2008.

# ON AN APPROACH TO TREATMENT

**Gary Blank**, Dollard-des-Ormeaux, Quebec, Canada
Group leader, Montreal Chronic Pain Support Group (MCPSG),
Chronic Pain Association of Canada (CPAC), Montreal, Quebec, Canada

(See other testimonials, pages 124, 132 and 162. See Chapter 50, page 363.)

I'm happy to say that almost all of my experiences with doctors and specialists, clinics and hospitals, whether on the English or French side, have been good despite all the bad press and criticism our healthcare system receives. I've been treated with respect and compassion.

I believe strongly in taking a proactive approach to treatment, which includes taking medication responsibly, having an open mind, being informed and keeping informed, and communicating effectively with all your health professionals. That approach, together with hope, never giving up and a little luck, will keep you from falling through the cracks of the healthcare system. When asked for advice on living with chronic pain, I recommend what one of my physiotherapists at the Montreal General Hospital taught me (thank you, Denise!):

**The "P" words:**
**patience, posture, pace, plan, pride, persevere and prevail.**

# CHRONIC PAIN RESEARCH IN QUEBEC:
## UNCOVERING THE MYSTERIES OF PAIN

Luc Dupont, scientific journalist, Montreal, Quebec, Canada
for the journal *Recherche en Santé*, published by the Quebec Pain Research Network (QPRN)

The Quebec Pain Research Network (QPRN) was created in 2001. It focuses on understanding the mechanisms of chronic pain – from molecules to models, from psycho-physical measurement to clinical research and clinical testing – on a multidisciplinary and complementary basis in order to transfer new knowledge to clinical practice and other sectors of intervention. This research focuses on three main areas or strategic groups, each of which is designated by an action verb: Evaluate, Explain and See the pain.

With more than 50 regular members and 26 associate members affiliated with the four universities that form the basis for the *Réseaux universitaires intégrés de soins (RUIS)*, namely Laval, McGill, Sherbrooke and Montreal, the QPRN is now supported by mixed funding from the QPRN, the *Ministère de la Santé et des Services sociaux* (Quebec, Canada), and two pharmaceutical companies (Pfizer Canada and AstraZeneca).

Enjoy your reading!

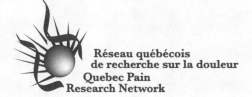

Réseau québécois
de recherche sur la douleur
Quebec Pain
Research Network

## FILE: THE QUEBEC PAIN RESEARCH NETWORK
UNCOVERING THE MYSTERIES OF PAIN

Pages 2 and 37 of Issue 42 of the journal *Recherche en santé*, published by the *Fonds de la recherche en santé du Québec (FRSQ)* are reproduced with the permission of the editor.

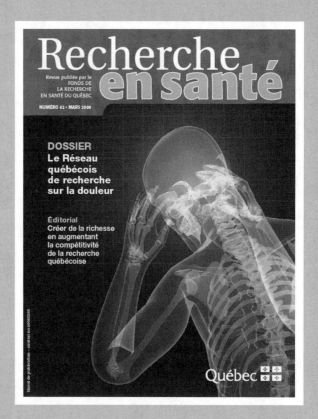

Complete file, in French only, available at:
http://www.frsq.gouv.qc.ca/fr/publications/recherche_en_sante/pdf/no42/dossier.pdf

"As I see it, the object (of medicine) is generally to relieve the suffering of patients and reduce the violence of disease"

– Hippocrates, On Ancient Medecine

"In many respects pain is a mystery[1]", according to a document produced by the Quebec Pain Research Network (QPRN). How can research unveil this mystery? How can it deal with such a varied set of human sensations?

Pain is what a young mother feels when giving birth; what the major burn victim feels throughout their body; what the amputee feels at the site of the missing limb; even what can be as common as a toothache. In any case, according to bioethicist Hubert Doucet, "Pain is what patients say their pain is. Palliative care services came to an understanding of this by establishing the most reliable evidence of pain through the description and the information the patient provides."

Specialized literature provides an initial definition of pain formulated by the International Association for the Study of Pain (IASP): "An unpleasant sensory and emotional experience associated with actual or potential tissue damage, or described in terms of such damage." As for chronic pain[2], it is "pain that extends beyond the expected period of healing, generally established as three months, or pain that is associated with a chronic disease, such as osteoarthritis."

The epidemiology of pain leaves no doubt as to its prevalence. According to statistics for Quebec taken from a Canadian study[3], 20% of adult males and 24% of adult women experienced chronic pain in 1996. Nevertheless, Quebecers do not suffer any more than others. A large European study (15 countries – 46,394 participants[4]) conducted in 2002 produced results similar to those for North America: 12% in Spain, 30% in Norway.

In response to what some already perceived as a serious health issue, the Quebec Pain Research Network (QPRN) was founded in 2001, as a result of an initial subsidy from *Valorisation-Recherche Québec*. Its members, which are affiliated with the four universities that provide the foundation for the *Réseaux universitaires intégrés de soins (RUIS)*, namely Laval, McGill, Sherbrooke and Montreal, grouped quite naturally around three main areas or strategic groups, each of which is designated by an action verb: ASSESS, EXPLAIN and SEE the pain. They share four major common resources – pan-Quebec research platforms that range from cellular and cerebral imaging to human and animal models.

With more than 50 regular members and 26 associate members, the QPRN is now supported by mixed funding from the FRSQ, the *Ministère de la Santé et des Services sociaux*, and two pharmaceutical companies (Pfizer Canada and AstraZeneca).

"Since pain is increasingly viewed not as a symptom but rather as a pathology on its own (and, in many cases, as a disease of the nervous system), the 1990s and the first decade of this century have been marked by an unprecedented acceleration in research," said Yves De Koninck, Professor, Psychiatry, *Université Laval*, Director of the cellular neurobiology unit of the *Centre de recherche Université Laval-Robert-Giffard*, Scientific Director, FRSQ national researcher.

Quebec, which is home to a major concentration of stakeholders in the field found itself in an excellent position. "There is a reason for this," continued the neurobiologist, "The presence in Montreal of a researcher with an international reputation, Ronald Melzack, who has moreover just been inducted into the Canadian Medical Hall of Fame. He is responsible for developing the first major theory of pain in the modern research era, a theory which is quite efficient and provides a foundation for even more leading-edge research throughout the world." (…)

But that is not the sole reason for the current galvanization in research at present. "Increasingly, the large pharmaceutical firms consider pain a target that can be medicated," he said. "And in this case, they are very interested in interfacing with a network such as ours which, in addition to including a wide variety of experts is also public and can rely on extremely powerful technology platforms (imaging, etc.)."

## NOTE TO READERS

We invite you to read pages 37 to 47 of the file on the Quebec Pain Research Network, **"CHRONIC PAIN RESEARCH IN QUEBEC: *PERCER LES MYSTÈRES DE LA DOULEUR*"**, written by Luc Dupont, scientific journalist, for the journal *Recherche en santé*, published by the Fonds de la recherche en santé du Québec *(FRSQ): "ÉVALUER la douleur, EXPLIQUER la douleur et VOIR la douleur"* at: www.frsq.gouv.qc.ca (available in French only).

---

1  *Sur la piste des douleurs neuropathiques*, RQRD-Coin recherche, March 2006.

2  Chronic pain can be classified in five categories: musculoskeletal pain, neuropathic pain, headaches and "other", each of which includes numbers sub-groups.

3  *Agence d'évaluation des technologies et des modes d'intervention en santé (AETMIS), Prise en charge de la douleur chronique (non cancéreuse)*, abstract, May 2006. www.aetmis.gouv.qc.ca (under « Publications » tab).

4  In this study, chronic pain is defined as pain that lasts for more than six months, was present in the month prior to the interview, is experienced at least two days per week, and is evaluated at greater than five on a intensity scale of 10.

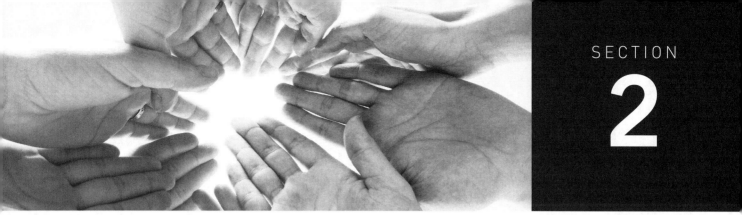

# PSYCHOLOGICAL AND SOCIAL
# ASPECTS OF CHRONIC PAIN

# PSYCHOLOGICAL AND **SOCIAL ASPECTS OF CHRONIC PAIN**

**Juliana Barcellos** de Souza Pht, PhD, Florianópolis, Brazil
Universidade Federal de Santa Catarina (UFSC)

http://lattes.cnpq.br/0009123389533752

## ABSTRACT

The traditional biomedical model cannot be used to explain chronic pain. This model associates the cause (injury) with the consequence (pain), using a rather linear approach. Yet, in the case of chronic pain, the tissue damage is frequently not identified, and does not necessarily account for the intensity and the severity of the problem. Understanding chronic pain requires a much more complex model that evaluates the symptoms on several levels (biological, psychological and social), and the interaction of these levels among one another. Using this biopsychosocial model, a few researchers will refer to an approach based on a circular cause.

Reading this chapter will help you develop a better understanding of the impact of psychological and social factors in the perception and expression of pain. We will also propose a few strategies for enhancing your management and control of chronic pain, such as positive thinking, which can have a major impact on your perception of your pain.

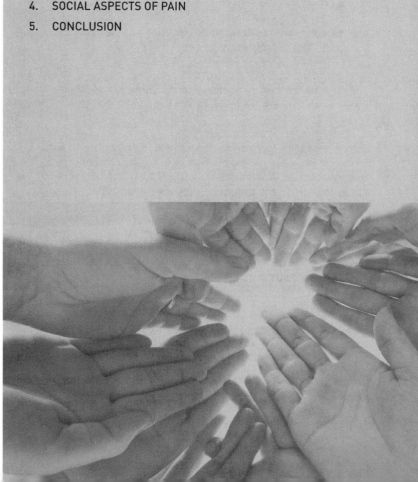

# 1. THE COMPLEXITY OF PAIN

Understanding chronic pain in all its complexity is one of the most important clinical challenges people suffering from chronic pain must face when learning to manage their pain better. Unlike chronic diseases such as diabetes and cardio-vascular disease, persistent chronic pain is not a disease that fits into the biomedical model (traditional), but rather a **biopsychosocial model** (complex). This change in paradigm from traditional to complex is the result of several limitations encountered by the biomedical approaches, such as the lack of tissue injury that could justify the persistence of pain.

> **How can pain occur when there is no injury?**
> **How can we justify persistent pain when we do not know what causes it?**

In order to answer these two questions, chronic pain must be viewed from the point of view of biopsychosocial models. These models consider chronic pain as a consequence of the interaction between biological predispositions, psychological characteristics, physiological changes, the perceptions of the individual suffering from pain, as well as their social and cultural status.

**In order to help you better understand the bio-psycho-social complexity of chronic pain, we will describe the interaction of the biological, psychological and social aspects of your condition.** Nevertheless, we will place more emphasis on the last two elements (psychological and social), since the biological aspect (the physical aspect of the pain) is discussed in detail in this work. The interaction among these three elements can, for example, explain how your mood influences your symptoms and how your symptoms affect your family activities. These three elements can be at the root of the problem, can be a consequence of it, or can even be one of the factors for maintaining your pain.

> The physical (biological), psychological and social elements interact among themselves as in a circular model, in which a **"consequence"** may affect its own **"cause"**.

# 2. PSYCHOLOGICAL ASPECTS OF PAIN

> The complexity of pain leads us to believe that several elements interact in the development and persistence of symptoms, such as learning responses to pain, the fear of experiencing pain and the dramatization of pain.

## CHRONIC PAIN AND MOOD DISORDERS

Both in clinical work and research, there seems to be a close link between chronic pain and mood disorders (which we call "conditions"), such as depression or anxiety. Although the co-occurrence of these conditions is frequent, they are not always present.

> **There is no linear reaction between chronic pain and mood disorders in which one of the two conditions depends on the other.**

Chronic pain and depression are two different problems, which may be associated or may not. Do not be surprised when observing those around you: **comorbidities** vary according to the individuals and their perceptions of life and pain; some people suffer and others do not necessarily do so. The advantage of mood disorders such as depression lies in the fact that they respond well to pharmacological treatment whereas finding the ideal pharmacological treatment for chronic pain takes much more time and is much more complex.

## THE FEAR OF PAIN

> The fear of pain is another characteristic that has a direct effect on perception and the persistence of pain as well as the inability to manage such pain.

On the one hand, fear increases the perception of pain since you become hypervigilant. On the other hand, fear can reduce your activities. For example, people suffering from lumbar pain (back pain) tend to stop taking part in any physical activity that may cause pain. This leads to a weakening of the muscles, which in turn serves to maintain the problem.

## ONE STRATEGY FOR MANAGING PAIN: DISTRACTION

One strategy for reducing **hypersensitivity** and **hypervigilance** to pain is distraction: going for a walk, listening to music, admiring the scenery, and a large variety of other activities.

> **Try to relax, take deep breaths and look somewhere else:**
> **It will be good for you.**

## THE DRAMATIZATION OF PAIN

> The dramatization of pain, once considered a factor in the predisposition to chronic pain, is now also considered a maintaining factor that plays an important role in the perception of pain and the patient's expectations.

## THE IMPORTANCE OF BEING BELIEVED

During research studies, we noted that women suffering from fibromyalgia wait an average of six years before obtaining a diagnosis. Living and suffering for all these years without knowing what the problem or disease may be is truly hellish. It is not surprising that these people become anxious! In cases of chronic pain syndrome, such as fibromyalgia, certain conditions present no objective signs (that a practitioner can observe clinically or detect by means of one or more tests) that can prove the existence of the problem. The fact of living with an invisible disease merely increases the importance of being believed for the patient.

> As in the case of the fear of pain, the dramatization of your condition can be relieved by changing the point of view from which you perceive it.

Your attitude to pain and even your perception of pain are influenced by your past experience and your emotions. The reactions of those around you to pain can also influence your response to painful sensations. This is a behaviour that the family and significant others transmit to children. The parents' attitude to their child's pain can also influence his/her future reactions to pain. It is important to note that the response to pain always depends on a context. For example, the parents' attitude toward a painful ritual that is culturally acceptable, such as ear piercing, is likely to relieve the pain, unlike a scenario involving an accident or illness.

## 3. FAMILY ASPECTS OF PAIN

### LEARNING TO MANAGE PAIN

Citizens are born within a family and it is there that they have their first experiences at communicating, where they learn to live in society, and where they learn to react to pain. The family, a social structure, can help a child build his/her strategies for managing pain, either by dramatizing this unpleasant sensation or not. Moreover, during this learning process, family, friends and loved ones play an important role in helping one of their own tolerate a painful sensation.

### PRESENCE MAKES A DIFFERENCE

The presence of a loved one at your side can enhance the management of pain. The expression on another's face can help – or not – a person who is experiencing pain to better tolerate this unpleasant sensation which is associated with an alarm signal for protecting the organism. For example, let us analyze various scenarios.

- A young child receives a vaccination (an injection), while accompanied by his/her mother. The mother's facial expression, transmitting a sense of protection, can attenuate her child's perception of pain and help him/her manage this unpleasant symptom, without dramatizing his/her pain. On the other hand, if the mother is anxious and if, moreover,

she is afraid of vaccinations, the child's response to the pain caused by the vaccination will be completely different.
- Likewise, the father's presence when the mother gives birth can reduce the analgesics taken by the mother.
- Patients suffering from fibromyalgia report experiencing less pain when a loved one accompanies them to a consultation or physical examination.

The presence of a loved one can either reduce pain or increase the perception of the pain syndrome, in keeping with:
- Personal beliefs and expectations;
- The interpersonal relationship between the two people.

Once again, let us consider the example of the child who receives a vaccination. The nurse giving the injection can have a friendly attitude without dramatizing the pain. However, the relationship is still new and the level of trust may not be great enough between the nurse and the child to attenuate the painful sensation. Trust in the health professional can also help the child tolerate painful stimuli, and even pain itself, better.

## 4. SOCIAL ASPECTS OF PAIN

The syndromes of chronic pain have a major socio-economic impact related to the functional incapacity of people who suffer from such pain. The work environment can facilitate the individual's return to work, depending on the flexibility available (such as working part-time, taking short breaks during the day, the availability of a break room or exercise room for employees to which the individual has access, etc.).

Moreover, another employment characteristic that can also facilitate a return to work is the willingness to adapt the employee's job to his/her physical and mental capacities. To promote the management of pain, we must also treat the depression, if any, that is associated with it.

## 5. CONCLUSION

Chronic pain is a complex phenomenon that depends on the interaction of several biological, psychological and socio-cultural factors. In short, we can say that chronic pain depends on each patient's memories, past experiences and perception of the future. Chronic pain can be related to predisposing factors from the past (genetics, for example) and past experiences (such as trauma, education, culture, beliefs and values). Also, the phenomena of the chronicity of pain can be triggered or maintained through the management of the patient's current experiences (for example, interpersonal relationships, trauma, difficulties at work) and his/her perceptions of the future (such as expectations and plans for resiliency).

# CHRONIC PAIN, FAMILY AND FRIENDS

**Gary Blank**, Dollard-des-Ormeaux, Quebec, Canada
Group leader, Montreal Chronic Pain Support Group (MCPSG), Chronic Pain Association of Canada (CPAC), Montreal, Quebec, Canada

(See other testimonials, pages 124 and 162. See Chapter 50, page 363.)

I remember some of my years with pain, but most I do not. The impact of my chronic pain not only affects me. While they don't suffer the physical aspects of my disease, my wife and daughter were forced to live with a different person whose mood varied according to the amount of pain, reactions to medication and lack of sleep. On one occasion, we travelled to New York City to take in a Broadway play and an NBA basketball game and do the tourist thing. Imagine how my daughter (who was 14 at the time) felt when I literally slept through the whole trip.

I am one of the lucky few whose family has stayed together. My family has supported me by accompanying me to doctor's appointments and counselling sessions. They have pitched in when I was too ill to shovel snow or cut the grass. Many times they said, "We understand," when I couldn't get out of bed to participate in family-oriented activities.

Over the last 10 years, we've learned who our real friends are: the ones who understood the many times my wife had to cancel plans at the last minute, not the ones that stopped calling.

# PERCEPTIONS AND
# EXPRESSIONS OF PAIN

**Juliana Barcellos** de Souza Pht, PhD, Florianópolis, Brazil
Universidade Federal de Santa Catarina (UFSC)

http://lattes.cnpq.br/0009123389533752

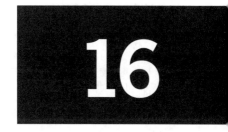

**16**

## ABSTRACT

Pain is a perception that is expressed in different manners by different individuals. Look at those around you. Look at how children react to pain: they react differently depending on those around them and even, depending on whether their parents are present or absent, their behaviour can change. Curiously, the expression of pain is not necessarily proportional to its intensity or its severity. Nevertheless, it must be taken into consideration in the development of a treatment plan. Several researchers have studied the variations in the expression of pain.

This chapter will present a brief summary of some of these studies. After reading it, you will be able to identify the important characteristics for taking charge of and controlling pain in children, adults, and elderly people.

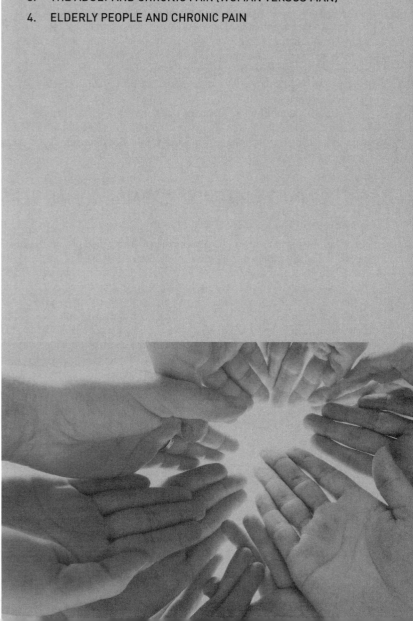

# 1. INTRODUCTION

Chronic pain is an unpleasant and subjective sensation associated with the values, beliefs and past experiences of the person who experiences it. The expression of pain will also be a result of the individual's experiences and the context in which he/she finds him/herself. For example, for a single individual, the perception and expression of pain will not necessarily be the same if he/she is at home with loved ones, or at the hospital with health professionals and care-giving personnel.

In the same context, living with chronic pain changes the colour of each phase of our life. Living with physical and mental disabilities caused by an invisible illness will change the life of children, adults and elderly people. The prejudices associated with chronic pain influence the development of the child and the social involvement of any patient regardless of whether they are male, female, young or old. In order to meet the needs of children, men, women and elderly people who are afflicted with chronic pain, we will describe a few of their specific needs briefly.

# 2. THE CHILD AND CHRONIC PAIN

The functional difficulties experienced by children or adolescents experiencing chronic pain are very different from those experienced by children with acute pain, such as following surgery. Even if the needs of children and adolescents and the attention they give to their pain have been stressed by several researchers and clinicians, we have observed that the pain experienced by children is often neglected and treated with means that are often inadequate since they rely on small dosages of analgesics. Living with chronic pain limits the ability of the child or adolescent to take part in daily activities such as walking and even being able to sit down for a long period time, as would be required, for example, to go to a movie. Moreover, persistent pain often prevents the child or adolescent from taking part in intense social activities or sports. Most children report problems sleeping. Some studies have associated sleeping difficulties with physical pain (muscular and joint pain) and mood disorders (depression and anxiety). (See **Chapter 12**.)

In order to manage and treat young patients with chronic pain, the following must be assessed and controlled:
a) The intensity of the pain;
b) The patient's physical capacity and participation in childhood activities;
c) The emotional response of the child to his/her pain and capacities;
d) The symptoms associated with pain (fatigue, stiffness, etc.);
e) The patient's satisfaction with the treatment;
f) Sleep;
g) The child's socio-economic situation; All without forgetting the impact that living with an invisible disease has on the child or adolescent.[1]

# 3. THE ADULT AND CHRONIC PAIN (WOMAN VERSUS MAN)

In the case of adults, frustration is one of the sensations most often associated with chronic pain since the functional, mental and physical disability limits, and makes most professional activities more difficult. Along with this frustration, the adults who suffer from chronic pain are often more likely to look for help than people with other problems, and women seem to be more likely to seek a consultation than men. Even more than children, adults often look for validation of their symptoms from their families and friends. While interviewing people suffering from fibromyalgia, we noted that men experience a loss of identity, which in turn places their virility in question, as a consequence of their hypersensitivity to pain and other sensations.

In order to manage and treat pain in the case of adults, the following must be assessed and controlled:
a) The intensity of the pain;
b) The patient's physical capacity, participation in family, leisure and professional activities;
c) The emotional response of the man or woman to his/her pain and capacities;
d) The symptoms associated with the pain (fatigue, stiffness, etc.);
e) The individual's satisfaction with and participation in the treatment;
f) The commitment to the treatment.[2]

## 4. ELDERLY PEOPLE AND CHRONIC PAIN

Elderly people and children make up a population for which the pharmacological treatment of pain is neglected and pain medication is under-used. It is estimated that one-third (1/3) of the elderly suffer chronic pain. Several studies have demonstrated that this population has a greater prevalence for a reduction in the quality of life, physical incapacity and severe depression, compared to adults. Despite severe disability, elderly people suffering with chronic pain desire independence, and want to control their pain; they fight, and ask for help to adapt their lives to chronic pain. Elderly people who successfully manage their pain have a better quality of life.[3]

In order to manage and treat pain in the case of elderly people, we recommend the same controls as for adults, namely:

a)  The intensity of the pain;

b)  The patient's physical capacity, participation in family, leisure and professional activities;

c)  The emotional response of the man or woman to his/her pain and capacities;

d)  The symptoms associated with pain (fatigue, stiffness, etc.);

e)  The patient's satisfaction with and participation in the treatment;

f)  The commitment to the treatment.[2]

## REFERENCES

1.  *PED IMMPACT: The Journal of Pain,* vol. 9, no 2, février 2008, p. 105-121.
2.  *The Journal of Pain*, vol. 9, No 9 septembre 2008, p. 771-783.
3.  *IMMPACT*: Pain, vol. 106, no 3, décembre 2003, p. 337-345.
4.  *Age and Ageing*, 34, 2005, p. 462–466.

# QUESTIONING

**Lucie Moisan,** St-Eustache, Quebec, Canada

(See pages 174 and 348 for other testimonials.)

Some days, I feel worse than others. This is one of them. So many questions run through my mind, so many uncertainties, and I don't know the answers. Unfortunately, I have no one at all to talk to about it.

I don't know where life wants to lead me. I do know that it is waiting for me to take a stand. Why is life hurting me like this? One thing is certain: I'm injured and disoriented, I no longer know what to think, I'm swimming in mystery, I'm walking towards the unknown – and I'm afraid. It's unsettling.

I'm well aware that many people are worse off than I am, but suffering is very difficult to deal with. A situation has been imposed on me, I've been forced to live with it, to keep quiet, and I have no choice. The physical and psychological suffering is one of the most painful periods in my life. My distress is so unbearable that I sometimes think about ending it all. I feel diminished, good for nothing. Others' joy in life and my inability to keep up with them have become intolerable. But, I always find the courage to get through this painful period, and to give it new meaning.

Everything will work out over time. It's always the word "time", and that hurts me. But what can I do? Nothing. I have to deal with it and let it guide me. But some days are so hard, and I have to fight against all the emotions that traumatize me, that upset me, injure me, and make me cry.

I'm growing stronger every day, but I just can't wait for the suffering to end!

If the shower could talk, it would have much to say since it is witness to my sadness, my distress and my tears. It is always there in moments of happiness or of sadness. Unfortunately, the shower can't do anything about my feelings, it cannot give advice, it can only listen, and sometimes make me feel better. It's probably the most intimate place, where my secrets and my reactions are the most explicit, but that's all.

This disease has covered me with a heavy cloak of anguish; it destroyed my life in record time. And now I have to live with all this while others are happy and moving ahead in joy. Why am I the one that has to suffer this pain? I will get over it, but what did I do to deserve this? Often, people ignore me and consider me like a shadow without feelings, without existence.

It's not easy since life goes on like a roller-coaster. With every passing day, I have to overcome my fear and my anguish, to move on, to take steps, and every time this takes an effort on my part. I have to find a new taste for living, and keep on going. I don't know what the future holds in store for me. I have to find a meaning for my life, and keep on moving towards my destiny, even if that frightens me. Yes, I'm heading into the unknown. Yes, my past and my memories hurt me. This is just another challenge of life, and I have to overcome it because I have a strength in me that tells me not to give up, and to stay strong.

I don't know what the outcome will be right away, but one day I'll know what purpose all my tears, my anguish, my efforts, my strength, my courage and my contradictory feelings have served.

I have to take charge of my life because no one else will do it for me. I have to move on, grow, and find fulfilment. Yes, I will still suffer, but time will help me get through it. People say that true wealth comes from giving. I give a lot of myself, of my time and that's my strength. I may not be a professional, but that doesn't prevent me from being an intelligent person and, above all, a responsible woman. Hierarchy means nothing in life; it's the soul that counts. Unfortunately, some people still haven't understood this. I will rediscover my personality, and I will get through life's difficulties. Little by little, my pain, my internal anger and my fears will dissipate. Joy will return to my heart, and I will move on with life. But I have to give myself time. I know that the disease still has its eye on me, and that it only needs one false step on my part to resurface. I will block it and fight it head on. Meanwhile, I ask for understanding and respect. I believe that life owes me that much.

# PAIN AND EMOTIONS:
# THE BENEFITS OF AFFECT REGULATION

**Stéphanie Cormier** PhD candidate (Psychology), Université de Montréal, Centre de recherche, IUGM, Montreal, Quebec, Canada,
Bachelor of Arts (Psychology), Université de Moncton, New-Brunswick, Canada, Recipient of a Vanier Canada Graduate Scholarship.
Read by Dr. Pierre Rainville, BSc., PhD, Montréal, Québec, Canada
Université du Québec, Biology, 1988; Major, Université de Montréal, Psychology, 1990; MPs, Université de Montréal, Clinical
Neuropsychology, 1992 ; PhD, Université de Montréal, Experimental Neuropsychology, 1998; Post-doctorate, University of Iowa,
USA, Cognitive Neurosciences, 2000.

## ABSTRACT

Although it is occasionally difficult to identify the source and causes of pain, pain is not "imaginary"; it is very real, and efforts should be made to relieve it. Health sciences are rigorously working to gain a better comprehension of pain, its treatments and the strategies for preventing it. For several of you, they cannot relieve your pain completely, but despite that, it is still possible to live a satisfying life.

The purpose of this chapter is to demonstrate the link between emotions and pain while presenting the benefits of appropriate emotion regulation. More specifically, it will help you understand the close relationship between your mood and your pain, while helping you understand the control you can have over your pain through the adequate management of your emotional state. This chapter will encourage you to regulate your emotional state while empowering you to effectively orchestrate and optimize the numerous treatments intended to manage your condition.

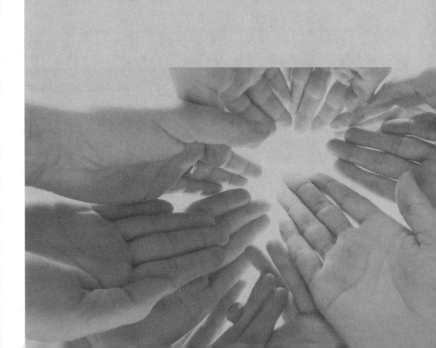

# 1. INTRODUCTION

It is not uncommon for people to consider pain as a strictly physical experience. In actual fact, the impact of pain is much wider, and includes social, mental and emotional components. Considering the numerous consequences that the necessity of living with pain on a daily basis may have, it would be absurd to believe that pain may be experienced without being accompanied by a wide range of thoughts, which in turn, make room for a variety of emotions that colour the individual's general mood. In addition to having a considerable impact on lifestyle, pain leads to significant losses and transformations on various levels (for example, a decrease in self-esteem, a deterioration in interpersonal relationships, loss of employment and financial difficulties, etc.). These life changes require a serious transition and adaptation period that is often accompanied by a wide range of negative emotions, including anger, fear, sadness, guilt and shame.

# 2. WHAT IS AN EMOTION?

Initially, this question appears to be rather simple. Most people are able to recognize and identify their own emotions, and those of others. Nevertheless, defining what we mean by "emotions" is rather complicated. For more than a century, several theorists have focused on this issue and have attempted to define and understand this phenomenon. This serious interest in the emotional experience gave rise to the formulation of a large number of theories.

## THE DIMENSIONS OF EMOTION

The theories formulated to explain emotions differ in significant ways. Nevertheless, most of them refer to the presence of certain important elements. Consequently, it is possible to define an emotion as an entity with three dimensions.

### a) A physical arousal

When we experience an emotion, we also experience certain physical changes, such as trembling, abundant perspiration, accelerated breathing and heartbeat, dryness of the mouth, etc. These changes are produced by the activation of the nervous system. More specifically, these responses are involuntary, and occur automatically through what we call the autonomic nervous system.

### b) A cognitive evaluation

An emotion is often accompanied by beliefs and thoughts. These are strongly influenced by the evaluation of the causes and the consequences of the emotion. This cognitive evaluation, which involves a complex mental information process, gives rise to various thoughts that automatically come to mind. For example, one morning you may have woken with unbearable pain. Several thoughts may have crossed your mind at that time, such as: "I won't be able to do what I had planned today" or "I'm fed up with this pain!"

### c) A reaction

It is not rare for an emotion to be accompanied by a facial expression. For example, anger is conveyed by frowning and clenching of the teeth, whereas surprise is accompanied by raising of the eyebrows and opening of the mouth. Emotion also leads us to adopt particular behaviours and react in a certain way. For example, anger can cause a person to be aggressive or violent, whereas joy can make a person laugh and move about.

All in all, an emotion can be defined as a state of the organism that occurs in response to an object or an event, and is accompanied by physical changes, thoughts and reactions. It is a brief period that is characterized by a negative valence (aversive emotion, ex.: anger) or a positive valence (attractive emotion, ex.: joy). In general, emotions are useful since they help us adapt to our environment, make decisions, communicate and develop relationships.

## EMOTIONS ET MOODS

The words "affect" and "emotion" are frequently used interchangeably, even if they don't represent exactly the same thing. Moreover, in common language, the word "mood" is used as a synonym for the word emotion. Nevertheless, moods and emotions differ in terms of time and intensity, and they should both be defined.

Mood is an extended affective state that, unlike an emotion, is not triggered directly by an identifiable stimulus, is less intense, develops gradually, and is maintained for a longer period of time. However, like an emotion, mood can have a negative or positive valence, and it can alter cognitive content and processes. As a result, emotion and mood can both influence the information processing mechanisms by modifying both the priority given to environmental elements and memories recalled. For example, someone dealing with a depressive mood will access sad memories and the related environmental aspects more easily whereas positive elements and memories will be much less accessible.

Although emotion and mood are two distinct concepts, they are related to one another. Mood may influence the threshold for triggering an emotion. For example, an individual who is irritable will be more prone to anger, whereas an individual in a neutral or positive mood will more likely be able to control his/her anger. Furthermore, mood interferes with the emotion regulation process. As a result, negative moods that persist on a long-term basis give rise to more negative emotions, which can lead to distress, and have a major negative impact on functioning.

# 3. WHAT IS PAIN?

The International Association for the Study of Pain (IASP) defines pain as "an unpleasant sensory and emotional experience associated with actual or potential tissue damage, or described in terms of such damage" (Merskey & Bogduk, 1994). This definition takes the subjective and multi-dimensional character of pain into consideration, and includes both the experience of a sensation and an emotion (Melzack & Casey, 1968). Each of these dimensions interacts with the cognitive processes of meaning attributed to pain, and the context in which it occurs. Moreover, the painful experience is characterized by responses of the autonomic nervous system and behaviours, both of which occur spontaneously.

## THE DIMENSIONS OF PAIN

It is generally acknowledged that pain has two major dimensions, namely the sensory-discriminative dimension and the affective-motivational dimension. The sensory-discriminative dimension concerns the intensity of the pain, the location, the type of pain and the factors that trigger it. These factors are directly related to the pain threshold, which varies from one individual to the next. This variation is one indication that pain is a multifaceted and highly individualized perception, and not just a simple sensation. The affective-motivational dimension translates the fundamentally aversive and unpleasant character of the painful experience, as well as the tendency to want to end it. This negative affective response that is generated by pain is strongly influenced by the individual's personal and socio-cultural background.

## THE AFFECTIVE DIMENSION OF PAIN

The emotional dimension of pain is complex and is characterized by a two-step experience (Price, 1999). The first stage refers to the immediate unpleasantness that is directly related to the sensory-discriminative dimension of pain. This first step constitutes the "primary pain affect" Subsequently, negative emotions arise and are generated by the understanding that an individual has of his/her own pain and the implications it may have. This secondary step in the treatment of pain constitutes the "secondary emotions".

### a) Primary pain affect

The primary affect or emotion is the unpleasantness caused by pain and is intimately related to its sense of threat. Therefore, this is the unpleasantness caused by pain. This component reflects the immediate experience that occurs in relation to the painful sensation. Moreover, the unpleasantness experienced in response to a painful stimulus is often closely related to the intensity of the painful stimulation, as well as the sensory characteristics attributed to it.

### b) Secondary affect

The unpleasantness caused by the pain frequently leads to emotions that are strongly influenced by our thoughts. These emotions, which are associated with the meaning we attribute to the pain and the evaluation of its potential consequences, correspond to the secondary emotions. Thus, pain-related emotions are often associated with suffering and distress, which is a result of the understanding an individual has of his/her own pain (i.e. its cause), and the implications that this pain may have (i.e. its consequences). As a result, the context in which the pain occurs, as well as the individual's attitude and expectations, contribute closely to the emotional dimension of the painful experience.

All in all, the emotional dimension of pain serves to explain why the painful experience may vary considerably from one individual to another. In fact, two people with the same injury may react quite differently as a result of the meaning they attribute to the physical problem, as well as the possible consequences of the pain. Each individual has beliefs, values, attitudes and memories that are his/her own and all of these determinants colour the painful experience, and the resulting emotions.

# 4. MODULATING PAIN THROUGH EMOTIONS

Research in the field of pain has demonstrated that the painful experience can be modulated by emotions. Whether it is a matter of pain-related emotions, namely secondary emotions, or emotions that can be attributed to sources independent of the pain, all of the research seems to agree that negative affect accentuates pain and positive affect generally reduces pain.

## PAIN-RELATED EMOTIONS

Rainville et al (2005) have used hypnotic suggestions to elucidate the impact of pain-related emotions in the painful experience. In this study, hypnotic suggestions were presented in order to provoke emotions associated with the pain experienced while immersing a hand in hot water. By comparing positive emotions (satisfaction and pride) to negative emotions (anxiety, sadness and frustration), and to the absence of emotions, it was possible to determine that the emotions related to pain influence the experience reported by the individuals, as well as their physiological responses.

The individuals who took part in this study evaluated the pain as less intense and less unpleasant when they experienced positive emotions, whereas the opposite was true in the presence of negative emotions. It was also noted that the negative emotions had a much greater influence on pain unpleasantness (affective component) than on pain intensity (sensory component). In a second experiment conducted by the same researchers, it was noted that the changes in the evaluation of the pain unpleasantness were related to significant increases in heartbeat. This relationship was only noted in the presence of negative emotions.

In summary, the results of these studies suggest that negative emotions with respect to pain have a greater impact on the unpleasantness than on the intensity of the pain. That said, even if the intensity of the pain remains the same, the experience is much worse for the individual who also experiences anxiety, frustration or depression with respect to his/her pain. It is all the more interesting to note that this impact is not limited to the subjective evaluation of pain, and that the modifications noted have repercussions on the body and the physiological systems.

Moreover, as explained above, the emotions related to pain are largely influenced by our interpretations of the experience. Other clinical studies conducted with patients suffering from chronic pain have also helped establish a connection between the emotions associated with pain and the painful experience. In recent years, pain catastrophizing has generated a lot of interest.

Pain catastrophizing involves a major negative focus on harmful stimuli and a tendency to overestimate the probability of the occurrence of negative consequences. It has been suggested that pain catastrophizing is characterized by three important elements, namely a) a tendency to amplify the gravity of the pain, b) an excessive focus on it, and c) a perception of being unable to cope with it (Sullivan et al, 2005). Catastrophizing about pain frequently leads to amplification ("I worry all the time about whether the pain will end."). Moreover, a tendency to ruminate and think continually about the pain ("I keep thinking about how much it hurts.") has been noted. Finally, it is common for people who catastrophize to experience a sense of helplessness with respect to their condition ("I feel I can't go on.").

Numerous studies have identified the harmful effects of this mode of thinking about pain. For example, it has been demonstrated that people who catastrophize tend to amplify and exaggerate the threat or the gravity of the painful sensation (Sullivan, Rodgers & Kirsch, 2001). Moreover, in a general manner, pain catastrophizing is associated with an amplified experience of pain, emotional distress and a variety of consequences related to pain, including the length of hospitalization, the use of analgesics and a reduced participation in daily activities and professional incapacity (Sullivan et al, 2002).

All in all, pain includes a considerable emotional dimension, which is translated into both the direct unpleasantness associated with the painful experience, as well as the meaning that is attributed to it (causes and consequences). Studies have demonstrated that the negative emotions associated with pain have a significant impact on the body and on the painful experience.

## EMOTIONS UNRELATED TO PAIN

It is possible to think of the impact of emotions on pain in another way. We can examine the influence that emotions unrelated to pain have on the painful experience. This influence has been covered in depth in studies conducted both in the laboratory and the clinical setting.

### Experimental studies

In the case of laboratory experiments, when individuals are asked to experience the emotions suggested by phrases with a positive connotation while their hand is immersed in painfully cold water, their tolerance to the pain is increased, whereas phrases with a negative connotation have the opposite effect (Zelman, Howland, Nichols, & Cleeland, 1991). In other cases, viewing humorous or erotic movies reduces sensitivity to the pain produced by applying painful pressure on the arm (Zillmann, de Wied, King-Jablonski, & Jenzowsky, 1996), or immersion of the hand in cold water (Weisenberg, Raz, & Hener, 1998).

Music has also been used to induce particular emotional states. Soothing music increases the tolerance to pain in women versus men whereas stimulating music tends to increase pain (Whipple & Glynn, 1992). Another study indicated that pleasant music reduces the pain caused by hot thermal stimulation applied to the forearm, without altering the non-painful thermal sensations (Roy, Peretz, & Rainville, 2008).

Moreover, pleasant odours relieve the pain produced by hot thermal stimulation (Villemure, Slotnick, & Bushnell, 2003). It has been demonstrated that sweet, pleasant odours inhaled while the subject's hand is immersed in icy water increases the tolerance to pain, whereas non-sweet odours do not cause any significant change (Prescott & Wilkie, 2007). Sweet tastes also reduce hot thermal pain in some individuals (Lewkowski et al, 2003).

The method most commonly used for inducing emotions is the presentation of images. Negative images that provoke fear (an animal baring its teeth) or disgust (mutilated limbs) result in a reduced tolerance to the pain caused by immersing the hand in icy water (de Wied & Verbaten, 2001), whereas positive images of an erotic nature generally increase the pain threshold in the case of men versus women (Meagher, Arnau, & Rhudy, 2001). Similar effects have been noted in studies using electric shock (Rhudy, Williams, McCabe, Nguyen, & Rambo, 2005). A recent study in cerebral neural imaging demonstrated that these changes are the consequence of an interaction between the regions of the brain involved in pain and those involved in emotions (Roy et al, 2009).

### Clinical studies

**Research studies involving individuals who suffer from chronic pain have also confirmed the existence of a significant connection between emotional state and pain.** These studies have mainly focused on specific problems, such as anxiety and depression. Among others, one large-scale study demonstrated that patients suffering from chronic pain had higher rates of mood and anxiety disorders (Gureje et al, 1998).

**Certain studies have managed to identify predisposing factors for the development of chronic pain.** It has been suggested that a negative mood is one of these factors. In other words, for an individual who is injured and maintains a positive mood, there is less risk that his/her acute pain will transform into chronic pain than for an individual whose mood is generally more negative. Moreover, there is a strong association between chronic pain and disability, or functional incapacity. Negative mood and emotions seem to mediate this relationship (Banks & Kerns, 1996; Holzberg et al, 1996). More specifically, the link between pain and disability can largely be attributed to a negative mood. Thus, an individual who manages to regulate his/her emotional state would be less inclined to develop a functional incapacity resulting from his/her pain.

All of these results have repercussions not only on pain and its consequences, but also on the treatments intended to relieve pain. It has been noted that the negative emotions commonly observed in the case of individuals who are suffering from chronic pain have a counter-productive impact on the effectiveness of the treatments used to reduce and manage their conditions. Furthermore, the different interventions focused on pain, including multidisciplinary treatments and traditional psychotherapy, do not attain their optimal effectiveness in the case of people who are negative, or have untreated depression or anxiety disorders. **All in all, such results illustrate the extent to which it is essential for you to regulate your emotional state in order to benefit fully from the treatments proposed to you.**

## 5. THE BENEFITS OF AFFECT REGULATION

Experimental and clinical research has demonstrated an association between emotions and pain, and several neurophysiological mechanisms have been proposed to explain their interactions. Therefore, we can no longer conceive the body and the mind as two completely distinct entities. You should now be able to understand how your psychological state can influence your body, and vice versa. Understanding this association is the first step in the process intended to help you develop a sense of self-efficacy with respect to the management of your pain.

Self-efficacy is the belief that it is possible to attain the desired objective, namely to reduce the pain experience, or at least to manage the pain effectively. In order to develop such a sense, it is essential that you adopt an active role regarding your condition, and that you develop the conviction that you can make the changes needed to achieve your objective. The very fact that you are reading this book means that you are on the right track.

### REGULATING AND MODIFYING EMOTIONS

Unsuitable emotions can be modified in three important steps (Greenberg, 2004):
a) Emotion awareness;
b) Emotion regulation; and
c) Emotion transformation.

### a) Emotion awareness
In order to have a certain amount of control over your emotional state, you must first live with and accept the emotions you are currently experiencing. Instead of avoiding or denying the negative emotions that are related to your pain, allow yourself to give them a place so that you can identify them and understand why they occur. Ask yourself what types of emotions are related to your pain. Which situations give rise to particularly intense and negative emotions? How often do you feel these emotions? What are the consequences of this emotional state on your thoughts, your behaviours, your activities? Getting into contact with these processes will help you identify the appropriate emotional states that will benefit you, and the inappropriate states that will hinder you and your ability to function on a daily basis.

### b) Emotion regulation
After identifying the emotions that you are currently experiencing, you must look into regulating them. A wide range of techniques are available to help you manage your mood and consequently your pain. Some of these strategies will be briefly presented in this chapter, and most of them will be discussed in greater depth elsewhere in this book. You do not need to practice and master each of these techniques. Instead, you are encouraged to identify the ones that are the most useful for you, and those that are effective to improve your mood. Moreover, remember that these techniques must be repeated and practiced a great deal before you can master them, and enjoy their full benefits.

### c) Emotion transformation
By regulating your negative emotions effectively, you will be able to access positive moods and emotions. Over time, you will be able to identify the situations that trigger negative emotions, and you will be able to use emotion regulation strategies as soon as they occur. In addition to slowing the rising of negative emotions, you will note that you are able to control your state of mind. In the long run, repeating this process will help you replace the negative emotions with more positive ones. Above all, do not get discouraged. **Learning to understand, identify and transform our emotions in order to develop a more appropriate and positive emotional state is hard work.**

## STRATEGIES TO REGULATE EMOTIONS

The following techniques have been proven to be effective with respect to managing emotions, and most of them are commonly used with individuals who are suffering pain. Although they are presented very briefly, you will find more details about each of these useful strategies elsewhere in this book. You are encouraged to practice all of these strategies at least a few times in order to identify those that will work best for you. It should also be noted that a large number of psychologists and psychiatrists are familiar with these techniques. Do not hesitate to consult these professionals to obtain the support you need to perfect your skills with these techniques. Once you realize that negative emotions can exacerbate your pain, and hamper the effectiveness of treatments intended to provide relief, it is to your advantage to learn and master the strategies that will help you control your emotional states

### a) Cognitive restructuring

Cognitive restructuring is based on the idea that it is not the events or situations that are the source of negative emotions, but rather our interpretation of them. Each individual interprets an event in keeping with his/her history and personal characteristics, and then reacts according to that interpretation. By simply modifying your inner speech, you can change your reactions and your behaviours, while reducing the intensity and frequency of negative emotions.

This technique leads you to verify if your thoughts and your interpretations are appropriate. Through cognitive restructuring, the thoughts that automatically come to mind in a situation that provokes strong emotions, are explored in order to identify the errors in thinking (cognitive distortions). It is these incorrect thoughts that give rise to negative emotions. In order to eliminate, or at least attenuate these negative moods, we focus on modifying inappropriate cognitions by considering alternative thoughts. All in all, integrating a new point of view into your daily life encourages the development of healthier emotions and reactions.

### b) Abdominal respiration and relaxation

Learning to breathe better serves to reduce stress, and prevent an escalation in emotions. Breathing with your abdomen allows better oxygenation, and reduces tension in the body. This type of breathing simply involves inhaling slowly by expanding the abdomen and exhaling by pulling it back in. Research has demonstrated that deep breathing increases tolerance to pain, enhances the action of analgesic medication, and reduces aggressivity and anxiety (Forbes & Pekala, 1993).

Once abdominal respiration has been mastered, it is possible to continue with relaxation. The most beneficial form of relaxation for individuals dealing with chronic pain is muscular relaxation. This involves relaxing the various limbs and muscles of the body one by one, without first contracting them (Schultz & Luthe, 1969). In addition to reducing muscular tension, this strategy also helps reduce stress and negative thinking, while having a beneficial effect on mood. You must, however, remember that relaxation is a skill that can only be developed through regular practice. The more you practice, the easier it will be for you to enter quickly into a relaxed state in various contexts.

### c) Behavioural activities and distraction

It is not uncommon for pain to be associated with a loss of interest in pleasant activities. In such cases, depression becomes a threat, which only accentuates the pain experienced. Therefore it is beneficial to introduce pleasant activities into daily life, to reduce negative emotions and thoughts, and to relieve pain (Keefe, 1996). It has been shown that increasing the frequency of pleasant activities facilitates social reintegration and a return to work (Turk & Flor, 2006). Therefore, you are strongly encouraged to identify the activities that will give you pleasure and practice them.

At the same time, as physical conditioning modulates pain, returning to a physical activity can be very beneficial. Individuals who are suffering from pain often wonder if it would not be better to rest, particularly when they note that certain actions accentuate their pain. This can lead to kinesiophobia (fear of movement), as people avoid all the physical activities that they believe will cause them pain (Picavet et al, 2002). In reality, you should remain active by selecting an activity adapted to your condition, which you can do with the assistance of your physician. You should also know that you have to avoid extremes, namely either overdoing activities, not doing enough activities, or avoiding them altogether. **Moreover, you should start gently and work at it progressively**.

Staying active is closely related to a very important principle: distraction. As our attention resources are limited, redirecting your attention to these activities serves to reduce the amount of attention given to painful sensations (Johnson & Petrie, 1997).

### d) Visualization and hypnosis

Through visualization, it is possible to project yourself into a comfortable and safe place of your choice, or to view yourself overcoming the difficulties of an upcoming event. This type of mental imaging uses the resources of the brain and the imagination in order to trigger a relaxed emotional and physiological state. Concentrating on the details of these visualizations while using all of the senses is distracting, and it encourages the appearance of positive emotions while improving well-being and reducing stress and anxiety (Gruzelier, 2002).

Hypnosis or hypnoanalgesia is a very useful technique for relieving pain. Although a good number of patients remain sceptical about this strategy, hypnotic analgesia is a phenomenon that is easy to induce and reproduce in most patients (Holroyd, 1996). In order to remain independent with respect to the management of your pain, you can learn self-hypnosis. You will be able to use the services of a professional who is certified in clinical hypnosis in order to help you develop this skill, or use audio recordings to attain this state, which is very similar to deep relaxation.

# 6. CONCLUSION

Emotions, whether they are triggered by your pain, or by something else in your life, have an impact on your pain experience. Living with pain on a daily basis is a serious challenge that provokes emotions that are sometimes very intense. Emotion regulation may become a strong complement to the other treatments you are already using, and this will help you reduce the distress you may experience and optimize your ability to function. Moreover, regaining control over your thoughts and your emotions can be extremely gratifying, and you will be satisfied to discover that you have a certain degree of control over your painful experience. Of course, for most readers, this will not be a cure for pain, but rather a means that will enable you to live a satisfying life despite the presence of pain.

# REFERENCES

- Banks, SM & RD Kerns (1996). Explaining high rates of depression in chronic pain: A diathesis-stress framework. Psychological Bulletin, 119(1), 95-110.
- Forbes, EJ & RJ Pekala (1993). Psychophysiological effects of several stress management techniques. Psychological Reports, 72, 19-27.
- Gureje, O., M. Von Korf, G. Simon & R. Gater (1998). Persistent pain and well-being: A World health organization study in primary care. Journal of the American Medical Association, 280, 147-151.
- Greenberg, LS (2004). Emotion-focused therapy. Clinical Psychology and Psychotherapy, 11, 3-16.
- Gruzelier, JH (2002). A review of the impact of hypnosis, relaxation, guided imagery and individual differences on aspects of immunity and health. Stress, 5(2), 147-163.
- Holroyd, J. (1996). Hypnosis treatment of clinical pain: Understanding why hypnosis is useful. International Journal of Clinical and Experimental Hypnosis, 44, 33-51.
- Holzberg, AD, ME Robinson, ME Geisser & HA Gremillion (1996). The effect of depression and chronic pain on psychosocial and physical functioning. Clinical Journal of Pain, 12,118–125.
- Johnson, MH & SM Petrie (1997). The effects of distraction on exercise and cold pressor tolerance for chronic low back pain sufferers. Pain, 69, 43-48.
- Keefe, FJ (1996). Cognitive behavioral therapy for managing pain. The Clinical Psychologist, 49, 4-5.
- Lewkowski, MD, RG Barr, A. Sherrard, J. Lessard, AR Harris & SN Young (2003). Effects of chewing gum on responses to routine painful procedures in children. Physiology & Behavior, 79, 257–265.
- Meagher, MW, RC Arnau & JL Rhudy (2001). Pain and emotion: effects of affective picture modulation. Psychosomatic Medicine, 63, 79–90.
- Merskey, H. & K. Bogduk (1994). Classification of chronic pain: Definitions of chronic pain syndromes and definition of pain terms. IASP press: Seattle.
- Melzack, R. & KL Casey (1968). Sensory, motivational, and central control determinants of pain. In: DR Kenshalo (Eds.), The Skin Senses (pp.423-435). Springfield, IL: Thomas.
- Picavet, S., J. Vlayen & J. Schouten (2002). Pain catastrophizing and kinesiophobia: Predictors of chronic low back pain. American Journal of Epidemiology, 156, 1028-1034.
- Prescott, J. & J. Wilkie (2007). Pain tolerance selectively increased by sweet-smelling odor. Psychological Science, 18, 308-311.
- Price, D. D. (1999). Psychological mechanisms of pain and analgesia. Seattle, WA: IASP press.
- Rainville, P., QV Huynh Bao & P. Chretien (2005). Pain-related emotions modulate experimental pain perception and autonomic responses. Pain, 118, 306–318.
- Rhudy, JL, AE Williams, KM McCabe, MA Nguyen & PA Rambo (2005). Affective modulation of nociception at spinal and supraspinal levels. Psychophysiology, 42, 579 – 587.
- Roy, M., I. Peretz & P. Rainville (2008). Emotional valence contributes to music-induced analgesia. Pain, 134, 140-147.
- Roy, M., M. Piché, J. Chen, I. Peretz & P. Rainville (2009). Cerebral and spinal modulation of pain by emotions. PNAS, 49, 1-6.
- Schultz, JH & V. Luthe (1969). Autogenic training. New York: Grune & Stratton.
- Sullivan, MJL, SR Bishop & J. Pivik (1995). The Pain Catastrophizing Scale: Development and Validation. Psychological Assessment, 7(4), 524-532.
- Sullivan, MJL, WM Rodgers & I. Kirsch (2001). Catastrophizing, depression and expectancies for pain and emotional distress. Pain, 91, 147-154.
- Sullivan, MJL, WM Rodgers, PM Wilson, GJ Bell, TC Murray, SN Fraser (2002). An experimental investigation of the relation between catastrophizing and activity intolerance. Pain, 100, 47-53.
- Turk, DC & H. Flor, (2006). The cognitive-behavioral approach to pain management. In Wall & Melzack's Texbook of Pain. McMahen, S. B., & Koitzenburg, M. (eds). 5th Ed. Philadelphia: Elsevier.
- Villemure, C., BM Slotnick, M. C. Bushnell (2003). Effects of odors on pain perception: deciphering the roles of emotion and attention. Pain, 106, 101–108.
- Zelman, DC, EW Howland, S. N. Nichols & C. S. Cleeland (1991). The effects of induced mood on laboratory pain. Pain, 46, 105–111.
- Zillmann, D., M. de Wied, C. King-Jablonski & M. A. Jenzowsky (1996). Drama-induced affect and pain sensitivity. Psychosomatic Medecine, 58, 333-341.
- Weisenberg, M., T. Raz & T. Hener (1998). The influence of film-induced mood on pain perception. Pain, 76, 365–375.
- Whipple, B. & NJ Glynn (1992). Quantification of the effects of listening to music as a non-invasive method of pain control. Scholarly Inquiry for Nursing Practice: An International Journal, 6, 43-62.
- de Wied, M. & MN Verbaten (2001). Affective pictures processing, attention, and pain tolerance. Pain, 90, 163–172.

# ON THE ROAD AGAIN...

**Mélanie R.**, Quebec, Canada

Thanks to my Mom, my family and my friends for your presence and your love.

When I woke up one winter morning, I had no idea just how much my life was going to change. I got ready, as I did every morning, to go to school, since I taught at primary school. I cleared the snow off my car and set out. That morning, there was a little snow on the road. As I drove in the right lane, my car started to skid toward the left lane and then the oncoming lanes. I was afraid! I pulled the steering wheel to the right, but I was driving along a curve. Then I felt that my car was no longer on the ground. I had time to think that I was only 30 years old and that was too young to die. I also had time to think about my Dad, who had died 13 years earlier. I asked him to take me in his arms to ease the shock of landing.

I landed in a rather deep ditch. Fortunately, there was a lot of snow at the bottom. That morning, my cell phone was in my pocket instead of at the bottom of my purse. Nervously, I called road assistance, then 911. Finally I called the principal at my school and asked her to find a replacement for the day. Two people came to my rescue before the ambulance arrived. I thought that was very generous of them. They could have continued on their way like most people did.

When the ambulance arrived, I told the medics that I had undergone surgery for herniated disks in 2002. There was no way I could get out of the car on my own two legs. I wanted to have an x-ray before moving. The medics were very nice. They called for reinforcements because the ditch was icy. They got me out and took me to the hospital.

The pain has never gone away since that day. It is located in my lower back and my left leg. In 2002, my sciatic nerve was caught between the herniated disks. I was hospitalized for one month before they operated on me and released my sciatic nerve. I suffered an enormous amount. After the operation, it took me five months to recover.

It was probably the shock of the accident that is largely responsible for my chronic pain. Following the accident, I had difficulty walking for a long time. I used a walker for several months. After that, I used Canadian crutches to get around. Finally, I used a cane for more than a year before I could walk on my own. In fact, I started to walk alone two and a half years after my accident.

I worked so hard to get to that point! I did physiotherapy, exercises, water fitness exercises and went swimming! I often think about all the effort I made when I walk. I feel a great sense of pride fill me when I think about my success. Yet, I still haven't reached the end of the road. My ultimate challenge is to go back to work. I've asked myself a thousand questions about work. I even consulted a guidance and vocational counsellor! And I came to the conclusion that going back to teaching would give me the most pleasure.

Meanwhile, I have to be able to wake up in order to go to work. I'm a real groundhog. I love to sleep. Unfortunately, my medication makes me sleep even deeper. I'm lucky that my mother calls me every morning to wake me up. Unfortunately, that doesn't always work. I also have to train regularly. I have to prepare my back and the rest of my body for this return to work. My legs have to be able to support me during my day. This is a challenge and I intend to face it.

Obviously, over the past five years, there have been good times and bad times. When they informed me that I was suffering from chronic pain, I was told that few couples survive chronic pain. Naturally, I thought that we would survive as a couple since we had been together for 10 years. Unfortunately, the man I loved decided to leave me. I thought that he was my friend and my lover. What a betrayal! My prince charming fell off his white horse... I had had such regard for this man and I believed that he was honourable. Unfortunately, I was wrong! In addition to losing the man I loved, I also lost some very good friends. Some failed to call me back or to answer my emails, whereas others were more direct and less delicate.

Fortunately, my mother, my family, my neighbours and some of my friends did not abandon me. They tried to help me by cheering me up, preparing my favourite dishes, accompanying me to appointments, taking out my garbage, cutting my grass or doing errands for me or with me, and so on. These people tried to put themselves in my place; they were sympathetic and they tried to make my life easier. I feel fortunate to have them close to me.

I was fortunate to be able to take part in meetings at the Montreal General Hospital pain clinic. I acquired some theoretical knowledge about chronic pain and that is very useful to me when the pain is unbearable. Also, I made a new friend during the meetings. It's been so good for me to have a friend who knows what pain is and what it's like to live with pain that never goes away. This friend is very important to me. We live far from one another, but the telephone helps us stay in contact. And then there was also one of the administrators of the Association québécoise de la douleur chronique who was of great help to me when my life was all topsy-turvy. Knowing that she was close to me, at the other end of the keyboard, was a great source of comfort.

Of course, the members of my family and my new partner are great sources of happiness and comfort. They watch over me. We have good times together. Since 2007, I've enjoyed the pleasure of being an aunt to Clémence. When I'm with her, it seems as if nothing else exists around us. She's a happy, funny little girl and simply quite marvellous. Her presence in my life is refreshing. In May, I'll have a nephew or maybe another niece. I really look forward to getting to know this new little baby.

The presence of Lélou in my life is another source of comfort. I didn't choose to have a dog. I met Lélou by accident one morning when she had been abandoned. I thought she was pretty and nice; she reminded me of Capitaine, a dog my family had when I was a child. Of course, now that I have a dog, I go for a lot more walks. But I don't always think about going for walks because that would be good for me. I do it for her because I know she needs exercise. In addition to being good for me physically, she's also beneficial psychologically. Yet, she does nothing special. She's just there. It's so simple yet at the same time so complex.

When I look over the past five years, I know full well that chronic pain has had some regrettable consequences. But, in everyday life, I don't think about what I don't have any more. I think about what I have. I try to think pleasant, positive thoughts. I want to see the glass half full instead of half empty. I still dream my dreams, plan projects and believe that the best is still to come...

# CHRONIC PAIN AND DISABILITY:
## THE BENEFITS OF PSYCHOLOGY

**Simon Laliberté,** PhD, psychologist, Montreal, Quebec, Canada
Clinique de gestion de la douleur de l'Hôpital Ste-Anne, Ste-Anne-de-Bellevue, Quebec, Canada.
Michael J. L. Sullivan. PhD, psychologist, Montreal, Quebec, Canada
Professor with the Department of Psychology at McGill University, Montreal, Quebec, Canada

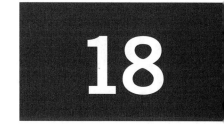

**18**

## ABSTRACT: PAIN AND PSYCHOLOGY

It has long been thought – and some people still believe this – that pain severity is proportional to the severity of a physical injury. It is now acknowledged that psychosocial factors play a major role in the perception of pain, and the level of disability associated with pain. These psychosocial factors need to be targeted by specific interventions that will attenuate their impact on the quality of life of people living with persistent pain. Although secondary and tertiary prevention programmes are available to effectively target these psychosocial factors, a certain amount of awareness raising is needed to facilitate access to such programmes. In this context, the psychologist can play the role of a 'coach' facilitating understanding of the chronic pain phenomenon and the return to significant activities.

ABSTRACT

1. PRESENTATION

2. PAIN AND DISABILITY

3. PSYCHOSOCIAL FACTORS

4. INTERVENTION

5. A REHABILITATION COACH

At the time of writing, Simon Laliberté was psychologist at the *Centre de réadaptation Lucie-Bruneau* and expert consultant at the *Société de l'assurance automobile du Québec*, Quebec, Canada. Michael J. L. Sullivan was professor in the department of psychology at the *Université de Montréal*, Quebec, Canada.

Reproduction rights granted by the *Ordre des psychologues du Québec*. This chapter has been revised to take into account developments made in the field since it was first published. The original chapter was published in the journal of the *Ordre des psychologues du Québec*, *Psychologie Québec*, Volume 21, No. 5, September 2004, pp. 23-26 and is available at: www.ordrepsy.qc.ca/pdf/Publ_PsyQc_Dossier_Douleur_Sept04.pdf

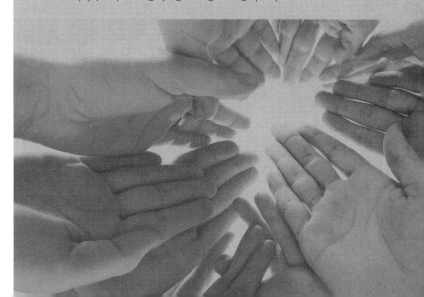

# 1. PRESENTATION

For a long time, it was believed that physical injuries were the sole cause of pain. Pain, one of the most unpleasant experiences, is an important signal that plays a major adaptive role in the physical protection and survival of living beings. Pain is the most common reason for consulting a physician (Turk and Melzack, 1992).

In most situations, pain helps an individual avoid actions that could be physically harmful. However, pain can also lead to a harmful degree of inactivity. In recent years, we have observed that physical inactivity following injury interferes with recovery. Moreover, pain can become a major stressor in an individual's life, particularly when it persists beyond the expected healing time.

For centuries, pain was treated as simply a symptom of a physical injury. In 1644, Descartes, who conceived of the body and the mind as being distinct and separate entities, suggested that pain was a direct signal of a physical injury (the greater the pain, the more serious the injury was). Gradually, we were able to observe that this linear explanation was not accurate. For example, it is common to see a child playing happily, hitting his/her head quite hard and, after taking a deep breath, returning to playing as if nothing has happened. Despite the fact that, objectively, the blow might be significant, the pain experienced is not proportional. Likewise a small scrape can become the "end of the world" for a child who is tired. Since Descartes could not explain these phenomena, others focused on this issue later.

**It can no longer be said that the more serious the injury is, the more significant the associated pain or disability will be.**

Over the past 40 years, theories have been developed that make more room for psychosocial aspects, which can provide a better understanding of phenomena that cannot be explained on a purely physical basis. Moreover, it is now acknowledged that pain is not a purely physical phenomenon. According to the International Association for the Study of Pain (International Association for the Study of Pain, Task Force on Taxonomy, Merskey and Bogduk, 1994), pain is defined as an "unpleasant sensory and emotional experience associated with actual or potential tissue damage, or described in terms of such damage". Therefore, it is increasingly recognized that pain is a phenomenon that is greatly influenced by physical, psychological, behavioural and social aspects, (Kerns and Payne, 1996; Turk, 1996; Waddell, 1998). The multidimensional nature of pain has been addressed in current biopsychosocial models of pain.

Following an injury, the general tendency is to undertake an intervention focused on the "bio" aspect of the problem (medicine, physiotherapy, etc.), frequently to the detriment of psychosocial factors. It is necessary to convince the treatment team of the importance of a psychosocial intervention. Moreover, even when we deal with difficulties for which it is obvious that psychosocial factors have been affected, as in the case of chronic pain, it is still difficult to convince the treatment team of the pertinence of a psychosocial intervention.

# 2. PAIN AND DISABILITY

It is now possible, using sophisticated robots, to observe the surface of the planet Mars and to determine if there was ever water and possibly even a form of life there. However, it is still impossible to measure an individual's pain objectively. There is no "pain meter". As in the case of many other experiences, pain must be evaluated subjectively.

Intuitively, we would expect the link between pain and disability to be linear. But clinical research has demonstrated that this link is much weaker than once believed (Waddell, 1998). For example, in the case of workers who have sustained musculoskeletal injuries, it has been observed that, with equivalent degrees of pain, a certain proportion of them report that their pain prevents them from working whereas others have already returned to work. In this respect, several studies (Jensen et al., 1999; Sullivan, Stanish, Waite, Sullivan and Tripp, 1998; Turk, 1990) indicate that pain severity accounts for only 10% of the variation in disability. How can we explain the fact that 90% of this variation cannot be attributed to pain?

Work and traffic injuries are still the most common causes of musculoskeletal pain. Despite progress made in terms of safety (both at work and on the road), the prevalence of disability caused by pain is increasing at an alarming rate. In 1970, 25 million days of work were lost in Great Britain as a result of pain whereas, in 2000, 125 million days of work were lost for the same reason, resulting in very significant social costs (Waddell, 1998). This increase occurred despite the fact that the number of injuries has remained stable. In other words, the number of injuries has not increased but, once they have been injured, individuals remain off work for longer periods of time.

Although pain contributes to disability, factors of an environmental, social, organization and psychological nature (Gatchel, Polatin and Mayer, 1995; Waddell, Burton and Main, 2003) also make major contributions to the development of disability. Several biopsychosocial models have been used to develop an understanding of pain-related disability (Turk, 2002; Waddell, 1998), which helps ensure a better explanation of the phenomenon and, above all, better treatment for it.

# 3. PSYCHOSOCIAL FACTORS

Psychosocial factors play a decisive role in the development of disability. They can be divided into two major categories: risk factors that cannot be modified and those that can (Linton, 2002; Sullivan and Stanish, 2003). Contrary to what people believed for a long time, the risk factors for chronicity or extended disability have very little to do with the medical condition or the severity of the injury, and much more to do with psychological, environmental and often behavioural aspects. Despite this reality, most interventions continue to focus almost exclusively on the physical injury.

> A multidimensional problem, a multidisciplinary response.

With respect to the risk factors that cannot be modified, it is very interesting to note that a woman in her forties who does not like her job is more likely to develop a chronic disability following an injury. This involves factors that cannot be modified such as age, gender and the fact that she dislikes her job. However, for a psychologist working with individuals who have sustained musculoskeletal injuries, it is essential to distinguish the risk factors that can be modified from those that cannot. In terms of factors that can be modified, we do know that, in the case of the woman mentioned above, regardless of the "objective" severity of her injury, she has more chances of developing a chronic disability if she reports a high degree of pain, expresses psychological distress, has catastrophic thoughts concerning her situation, is afraid of moving (kinesiophobia), is depressed, demonstrates pain behaviours and reports a great deal of disability. There are effective means for improving these aspects of her condition.

---

### TABLE 1 : PSYCHOSOCIAL RISK FACTORS THAT CAN BE MODIFIED (OR FACTORS MAINTAINING INVALIDITY)

| | |
|---|---|
| - Intensity of the pain | - Depression |
| - Psychological distress | - Acute behaviours (or pain) |
| - Catastrophic thoughts | - Perception of the disability |
| - Fear of movement | |

---

# 4. INTERVENTION

In recent years, research into intervention models has identified two major intervention priorities:
1) Reassuring the injured individual about the benign nature of his/her injury; and
2) Encouraging an early return to the activities of daily life (family, social and professional activities).

Reassuring the patient with respect to the prognosis for his/her injury and determining which physical activities he/she can maintain should be handled by professionals who are perceived as credible in matters of physical injuries (Waddell, 1998). As for the psychosocial factors that lead to inactivity, the psychologist can play a major role in this field by cooperating with the other members of the treatment team. Until very recently, no early rehabilitation programme included a psychosocial component, which was only dealt with once chronicity had occurred (Linton, 2002; Sullivan and Stanish, 2003). It is now acknowledged that, without an intervention specifically targeting the psychosocial factors, the success of the rehabilitation is compromised.

Recently, several intervention programmes have been implemented to target these modifiable risk factors at various points in the development of the problem. In these programmes, the participants are made aware of the psychosocial risk factors, among other things. The modifiable risk factors are above all covered through teaching in order to reduce the risk of developing a chronic condition. Programmes, referred to as secondary prevention programmes (Sullivan and Stanish, 2003) attempt to deal with the modifiable risk factors in the weeks following an accident. The Progressive Goal Attainment Program (PGAP) is an example of a programme which is available in the community of residence of accident victims and serves to target the risk factors in individuals with high levels of pain and pain-related disability. Using intervention strategies such as structured activity planning, goal setting, monitoring cognitive restructuring and problem-solving in the context of a gradual return to life activities, the PGAP focuses on reducing the psychosocial barriers that block progress and return to work (Sullivan and Stanish, 2003).

Tertiary prevention programmes are also useful for helping people whose pain problems have become chronic (Flor, Fydrich and Turk, 1992; Turk, 1996) and for whom the reduction or discontinuation of participation in certain activities has had major psychological repercussions (Boureau, 1991; Kerns and Payne, 1996). Such programmes (ex.: the musculoskeletal injury programme at the Centre de réadaptation Lucie-Bruneau, Montreal, Quebec, Canada) have often been implemented by professionals working in multidisciplinary teams, and focus on the social reintegration of individuals who have sustained debilitating injuries. At this stage, we do not refer to chronicity risk factors, but factors for maintaining the disability, since chronicity is already present.

These programmes all have their roles to play, depending on the stage at which people are referred to them. Unfortunately, even though the evidence seems to support early intervention in the case of individuals whose disability is at high risk of becoming chronic, many factors (bureaucracy, approach focused solely on the physical injury, prejudice against psychology) seem to delay referrals to the appropriate programs. The injured individuals may also be reticent to consult a psychologist soon after an injury: "The pain is in my back, not between my ears..." Thus, psychologists generally see injured people only after the vicious cycle of chronicity has developed. Psychosocial barriers to recovery and rehabilitation become more difficult ot treat effectively as the period of chronicity extends over time.

It is important to note that, regardless of when the intervention is initiated, particularly for the psychologist, the modifiable psychosocial risk factors (or factors that maintain disability; see **Table 1**) must remain the therapeutic targets for promoting a return to usual activities. Recent research has demonstrated that we must target these modifiable factors, regardless of how much time has passed since the accident (Vlaeyen et al, 2002). These interventions serve to reduce disability and therefore improve quality of life. The later the intervention occurs and the more numerous and complex the problems are, the less effective the intervention will be.

Psychologists are often consulted (often late in the process) at the request of a third-party payer (private insurers, CSST and SAAQ in Quebec, Canada) in order to help the accident victim return to the workplace. However, it is important, as a clinician, to review the importance of work from a clinical point of view. Work has direct effects on self esteem, daily structure, sense of autonomy, financial security, etc. It should not be forgotten that returning to work is an objective for third party payers, as well as a clinical objective for the well-being of accident victims.

## 5. A REHABILITATION COACH

In the context of post-accident rehabilitation, the role of the psychologist must be specified. It is essential that the psychologist working in this context adapt to the problems and the needs of this clientele. His/her role must be very targeted, of short duration and specific to the problem. His/her interventions must also be supported by evidence. When working on physical rehabilitation, the psychologist must play a role similar to that of a coach for an athlete. Therefore, it is important for the psychologist to accept and feel comfortable with this role of "coach". Obviously, this is outside the framework in which psychologists are often identified. Working with a major mental health issue is often quite different from working with chronicity risk factors.

With respect to preventing chronic disability, the role of the psychologist remains one of education, prevention through modifying behaviours and cognitive restructuring. In this short-term context, it would be advantageous to encourage the referral agents (insurers, attending physicians, other health professionals) to recognize the psychologist as a first-line resource for injuries that can result in chronic pain and disability. The psychologist can play a major role in the prevention of chronic disability. It is important to be familiar with this role and to support it better.

Traditionally, psychologists have been excluded from early interventions in rehabilitation but it is increasingly acknowledged that psychological interventions can have a significant impact on the reduction of disability related to pain. Psychologists must now make sure that they know how their intervention must be modified and adapted to the context of early rehabilitation. By adapting to these realities, the psychologist can become an essential part of early rehabilitation.

## REFERENCES

- Boureau, F. (1991). Contrôlez votre douleur. Paris, Petite Bibliothèque Payot.
- Flor, H., T. Fydrich, DC Turk (1992). Efficacy of multidisciplinary pain treatment centers: a meta-analytic review. Pain, 49 (2), 221-230.
- Frank, J. et al. (1998). Preventing disability from work-related low-back pain. New evidence gives new hope — if we can just get all the players onside. Cmaj, 158 (12), 1625-1631.
- Gatchel, R. J., PB Polatin, TG Mayer (1995). The dominant role of psychosocial risk factors in the development of chronic low back pain disability. Spine, 20 (24), 2702-2709.
- International Association for the Study of Pain. Task Force on Taxonomy, H. Merskey,
- N. Bogduk (1994). Classification of Chronic Pain: Descriptions of Chronic Pain Syndromes and Definitions of Pain Terms (2nd ed.). Seattle, IASP Press.
- Jensen, M. P. et al. (1999). Patient beliefs predict patient functioning: further support for a cognitive-behavioural model of chronic pain. Pain, 81 (1-2), 95-104.
- Kerns, R. A. Payne (1996). Treating families of chronic pain patients. In: Gatchel, R. J. & Turk, D. C. (ed.). Psychological Approaches to Pain Management: A Practitioner's Handbook. New York, Guilford Press.
- Linton, S. J. (2002). New Avenues for the Prevention of Chronic Musculoskeletal Pain and Disability (1st ed.). Amsterdam, Boston, London, Elsevier.
- Linton, S. J., M. Ryberg (2001). A cognitive-behavioral group intervention as prevention for persistent neck and back pain in a non-patient population: a randomized controlled trial. Pain, 90 (1-2), 83-90.
- Sullivan, M. J., W. Stanish, H. Waite, M. Sullivan, DA Tripp (1998). Catastrophizing, pain, and disability in patients with soft-tissue injuries. Pain, 77 (3), 253-260.
- Sullivan, M. J., WD Stanish (2003). Psychologically based occupational rehabilitation: the Pain-Disability Prevention Program. Clin J Pain, 19 (2), 97-104.
- Turk, DC (1990). Customizing treatment for chronic pain patients: Who, what, and why. The Clinical Journal of Pain, 6, 255-270.
- Turk, DC (1996). Biopsychosocial perspective on chronic pain. In: Gatchel, R. J., DC Turk (ed.), Psychological Approaches to Pain Management: A Practitioner's Handbook. Op. cit.
- Turk, D. C. (2002). A diathesis-stress model of chronic pain and disability following traumatic injury. Pain Res Manage, 7, p. 9-14.
- Turk, D. C., R. Melzack (1992). The measurement of pain and the assessment of people experiencing pain. In: Turk, D. C., R. Melzack (eds.), Handbook of Pain Assessment. London, The Guilford Press, p. 3-12.
- Vlaeyen, J. W. et al. (2002). Can pain-related fear be reduced? The application of cognitive-behavioural exposure in vivo». Pain Res Manag, 7 (3), p. 144-153.
- Waddell, G. (1998). The Back Pain Revolution. Edinburgh, New York, Churchill Livingstone.
- Waddell, G., K. Burton, CJ Main (2003). Screening to Identify People at Risk of Long-term Incapacity for Work: A Conceptual and Scientific Review. London, The Royal Society of Medicine.

# WORKING WITH CHRONIC PAIN SUFFERERS:
## A PSYCHOLOGIST'S REFLECTIONS

## 19

**Ann Gamsa,** PhD, psychologist, Montreal, Quebec, Canada
Associate Professor, McGill University, Department of Anaesthesia, Montreal, Quebec, Canada, Associate Director &
Director of Psychological Services, Alan Edwards Pain Management Unit, McGill University Health Centre (MUHC),
Montreal, Quebec, Canada; Director of Psychology Internship Training, McGill University, Montreal, Quebec, Canada

## ABSTRACT

By the time pain becomes chronic, it is often accompanied by emotional suffering. When people suffer from unremitting pain and can no longer work or participate in their usual activities, it is hardly surprising that they become depressed, anxious or angry. Unfortunately, the emotional distress resulting from pain may in turn exacerbate or even perpetuate the pain, sometimes rendering medical treatments ineffective. This does not in any way suggest that the pain is psychological in origin, but rather that emotional distress *caused* by chronic pain now also needs treatment for best overall results. There are some people with chronic pain who have suffered from psychological problems before the pain started. Such long-standing problems may contribute significantly to pain intensity and suffering, and may even maintain the condition.

The psychosocial assessment conducted by a pain psychologist in a multidisciplinary setting helps the treatment team understand how pain affects a person's life, and to what extent emotional distress plays a role in the pain or its response to treatment. This information, combined with that obtained by other team members, allows for an optimal treatment plan for each patient. Psychologists also provide short-term psychotherapy to help people cope with pain-related problems, and pain-management groups to improve quality of life, even with pain. This is a critical part of treatment because, sadly, we do not have the armamentarium to "cure" most types of chronic pain. While current treatments can often *reduce* pain — sometimes substantially — in most cases, the reduction will be insufficient to allow a person to return to many activities they did in the past.

Vignettes are offered throughout this chapter to illustrate ideas under discussion.

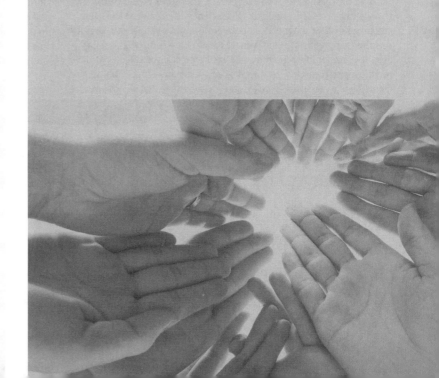

# 1. MY INTRODUCTION TO CHRONIC PAIN

I have been curious about the "mind-body" problem for as far back as I have posed philosophical questions to myself, long before I became a clinical psychologist. After hearing Ronald Melzack lecture at McGill University on the subject of pain, I realized that pain was the perfect example of the seamless connection between "body" and "mind." I wanted to learn more about the experience of people who suffered from constant pain, initially out of intellectual interest. I arranged to observe initial interviews conducted by a physician who treated patients with chronic pain.

This first encounter with a pain physician, Dr. L., was hardly what I expected, though perhaps more fortuitous than I knew at the time. Observing him conduct an initial assessment of a 67-year-old woman who had come in for treatment of unremitting trigeminal neuralgia pain, I was surprised to note his assessment was more psychological than medical. In response to his questions about her family, Mrs. G. told him that she lived with her husband and 32-year-old son on their farm. He asked, in a challenging tone, why her son wasn't married, to which she replied, "I guess he hasn't found the right girl yet." He suggested that maybe she liked it that way, keeping him single and to herself, and that the pain could be a means to keep him at home to help take care of her. To her protests, the doctor insisted that if she really wanted her son to marry, she would have found someone for him by now. After a few minutes of enduring his badgering, she looked helplessly in my direction, and asked, "Are you single dear?" (I was much younger then).

Dr. L. was an anaesthetist whose primary treatment was the administration of nerve blocks to help alleviate pain, but he also liked to use his form of psychotherapy — part psychoanalysis, part harassment. He asked many questions about her childhood. He seemed to be looking for a history of repressed psychological trauma expressing itself now in the body or evidence of early neglect or abuse to which he could ascribe the pain. According to his theory, pain in adulthood could supply the person with fulfilment of needs never met in childhood. From what I saw, Mrs. G. seemed a perfectly reasonable lady, whose considerable distress resulted from living with neuropathic pain. Dr. L. was no psychologist and certainly no healer.

It was as a result of observing this doctor humiliate his patients that I decided to pursue advanced studies in the field of chronic pain. Adding this speciality to my psychology training, I would be in a position to help people who live with such misery. I have Dr. L. to thank for launching me into my career, much of which I have spent happily working with McGill University Health Centre's Alan Edwards Pain Management Unit in Montreal, Quebec, Canada.

While the doctor I speak of was deplorably cruel, his belief that intractable pain could best be explained by psychological causes was not so remote from the view held by many doctors, psychiatrists and published researchers well into the 1990s. Having witnessed patients being "blamed" for their pain, I was determined to demonstrate in my doctoral research that psychological distress was not the *cause* but the *consequence* of pain. This is what I believed then. It turns out that I was only partly right.

# 2. IS THE PAIN IN YOUR HEAD?

Is the pain in your head? Short answer: Yes. All our sensations and perceptions, including pain, arise from signals registered in the brain, an organ that happens to reside in the head.

Earlier published literature characterized people with intractable pain as psychologically defective. It was widely assumed that if pain did not signal a known disease process or visible injury, and in addition failed to remit with treatments, it must be "in the head," "psychogenic," "imaginary," not "real," — whether or not there was evidence for psychological cause. The possibility that science might not be sufficiently advanced or that diagnostic tools were not yet available to identify the physical origins of some pain was given little consideration. Sadly, despite considerable research and some advances, we still do not have the means to pinpoint the specific cause of many chronic pains, nor do we have a cure. Nevertheless, the good news is that treatments are available to help attenuate the suffering of those who live with pain.

In the majority of cases, the *origin* of pain is not in the psyche. However, psychological difficulties, including anxiety or depression, do exacerbate pain experience, whether present before pain started or as a reaction to living with pain. Once pain becomes entrenched, it is not easy to separate out the relative contributions of organic and psychological factors to suffering. The pain may well have started with an injury or illness, but when it doesn't go away, it is "normal" for people to become depressed and anxious. Unable to work or do many of the things they used to do, there is little to focus on but pain. When there is no activity to create distraction, there is nothing but pain. Understandably, the person becomes depressed and, in turn, pain and suffering increase. This is what we call the "vicious cycle of pain."

---

1: There *are* rare cases of "conversion disorder," in which pain and disability may be wholly psychogenic (although, even then, brain circuitry is involved.)
2: There are many cases of disease previously believed to be "psychological" whose physical cause is now known.

## 3. DO PEOPLE WITH CHRONIC PAIN HAVE SIMILAR PERSONALITIES?

A common belief in the not-so-distant past was that people with chronic pain fit certain stable personality types. Because they often scored high on measures of anxiety, depression, "neuroticism," "hostility" and "hysteria" on tests never intended for people with pain, many authors concluded that psychopathology *caused* or, at the very least, perpetuated pain. More reasonable would be the conclusion that results on these tests revealed the distress experienced by people living with intractable pain. Tests administered after years of suffering tell us little about a person's psychological makeup *before* pain started. That intelligent researchers and clinicians could reach such obviously flawed conclusions is perhaps easier to understand in the context of earlier dominant beliefs.

Psychoanalytic views of psychosomatic disease carried considerable influence well into the 1980s. By extension, the belief that some kinds of pain were a somatic expression of repressed psychic conflict was much in fashion. As well, pain was dichotomized: it was *either* in the mind *or* in the body, but not both. From there, it's easy to see how pain, whose origins could not be found in a bodily mechanism, was relegated to the "mind" or "psyche." Gradually, as medical science developed better understanding of disease-causing pathogens, these ideas came to hold less sway. Interestingly, while the scientific community has largely discounted psychoanalytic notions of disease, the importance of the psyche looms larger than ever as a multitude of recent studies shows the influence of expectancy and other psychological factors on immune function and other neurophysiological processes.

After years of experience as a pain psychologist, I have come to acknowledge that there exists a subgroup of patients in whom psychological problems preceding pain onset have an important impact on pain intensity and intractability (however, in very few cases can psychological problems be said to have initiated the pain). These individuals have the greatest difficulty coping not only with pain but with life in general. Occasionally, there is even reason to believe that pain becomes a justification or rationale for a person's inability to succeed at life. Such individuals are likely to be overrepresented in tertiary hospital pain clinics to which they are referred by doctors who have exhausted their treatment options and, perhaps, their patience. They do not, however, represent the majority of people with chronic pain who, just like the rest of the general population, come from a variety of backgrounds and work situations and have unique personalities and ways of coping with adversity.

## 4. SUBGROUPS: ROLE OF PSYCHOLOGICAL FACTORS

The categories that follow classify patients according to the role played by psychological factors in generating, exacerbating and maintaining pain. This classification is based only on my clinical observation over the last two decades, and not on research. These are not airtight categories; nor should individuals within a subgroup be considered identical to each other. Each person comes with a unique personal "story" and pain problem. As long as this is understood, such groupings can help guide treatment.

We all develop strategies for coping with a variety of situations. Some people may find that pain prevents them from using strategies that were useful in the past. For example, people who used to be fiercely independent may find it difficult to ask for help, as will those who have always needed and managed to be "in control." Perfectionists may no longer be able to live up to their own standards. The inability to use earlier successful strategies can add significantly to a person's misery. Changes in coping style may be emotionally painful and are not easily attained but, over time and with the right kind of help, many people living with pain are able to adapt and enjoy life again.

---

3: It is important to note that such ideas have not gone completely out of circulation, and still exist in many forms.

## PSYCHOLOGICALLY HEALTHY AND FUNCTIONING WELL DESPITE PAIN

"Healthy copers" are rarely referred to a tertiary pain-treatment facility, and are seldom included in pain studies. They may well be the majority who suffer from chronic or ongoing intermittent pain. I assume they are adequately treated by their family doctor or manage to cope by using over-the-counter medication and/or self-taught pain management strategies and exercises. Those I have encountered outside the Pain Management Unit continue to work, having accepted and adapted to their limitations. Such adaptation is, of course, much easier for a professional person with a job over which they have control than, say, a construction worker with back pain.

People in both the following groups are emotionally distressed and function poorly.

## PSYCHOLOGICALLY HEALTHY BEFORE PAIN ONSET; PAIN CAUSES DISTRESS AND POOR FUNCTION

The larger subgroup of patients referred to the Pain Management Unit consists of people who functioned adequately before pain started, but who have become depressed, sleep deprived, anxious, low-functioning and sometimes angry because of the life changes resulting from pain (**figure 1**). In addition to treatments specifically targeting pain reduction, such patients usually require psychological intervention to help them cope better, manage their pain and readjust goals and expectations to fit their changed reality. Such learning and adjustments can vastly improve quality of life even with pain. Because most will be left with some residual pain and limitations even after treatment, this is a critical part of comprehensive pain management.

FIGURE 1: The chronic pain problem

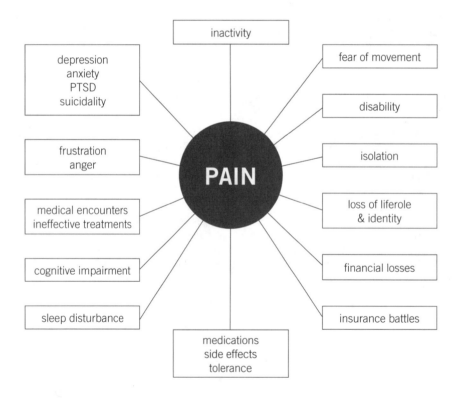

© Ann Gamsa

John, a CEO of a large corporation, was left with multiple pains and considerable disability after a car accident, necessitating two abdominal surgeries and another for a spine fracture. His life before had been happy and uneventful: a good marriage of 18 years, two healthy daughters in elementary school, a nice home and financial security. While the operations were successful, he was left with visceral pain in the abdomen, shooting pain in the scar area and intermittent "electric shock" pain in his back. Medications, injections, and an exercise program brought his pain from an average of 8–9/10 down to 5–6/10. Certainly this made a difference, but fell short of the improvement John had hoped for: to resume his life as it was before the accident. Sports, working as before, rough-and-tumble play with his daughters and sex with his wife were now out of the question. He became seriously depressed, withdrew from all social activity and barely talked to his wife or daughters. With appropriate psychological help, he gradually learned that despite pain and limitations, there were many things he still could do, including returning to work with reduced hours and a less central role, doing homework with his girls, helping with some household chores (which he had never done before) and a different but satisfying form of physical intimacy with his wife. Life was not the same as before, but he came to accept and even enjoy the slower pace. He had become more reflective, more sensitive to other people's needs, noticed and enjoyed springtime as never before and even liked himself better than he had in the past.

## PREVIOUSLY TROUBLED BUT USED EFFECTIVE COPING STRATEGIES; DISTRESSED AND FUNCTIONING POORLY BECAUSE PAIN LIMITS USE OF STRATEGIES

People in this group have suffered emotionally in the past but found strategies to maintain mental health and function well in their life. With the onset of pain, their previous problems (e.g. depression) tend to resurface while coping strategies, previously effective, are no longer available (e.g. a person who learned to control deep-seated depression by daily jogging may no longer be able to jog or even walk at a quick pace). When earlier problems resurface and are compounded by pain, the person's emotional suffering can be profound and difficult to treat. Psychotherapy can be helpful, but may need to be more intensive and prolonged than is usually offered in a multidisciplinary pain-treatment facility.

Mr. D. is a 31-year-old man born to alcoholic parents who abused him sexually and emotionally until he reached age 10 when his father was imprisoned, his mother disappeared and he was placed in foster care. He joined a violent gang when he was 16, abused and sold drugs, and served two years in prison at the age of 20, after which he was released on parole. During his time in jail and for some time after, Mr. D. was in rehabilitation, straightened himself out and eventually got a job as an orderly in a nursing home, turning patients in their beds, bathing them and sitting them up in chairs. He enjoyed the job, and the "old folks" loved him. He entertained them with rock music and made them laugh. They never judged him, and he got a smile every time he walked into a room. Home, a one-room basement apartment, was a lonely place, and he got depressed when he spent too much time there. So he got himself a second job of the same kind, working a total of 16 hours a day. That suited him fine; for the first time he felt loved and useful.

One morning on his way to work, a large truck struck his bicycle. He sustained severe injuries to one leg and his back. His leg was eventually amputated just below the knee and, despite surgery on his back, Mr. D. continued to suffer disabling pain. He could no longer do his job. He tried to go back on "light duties," but was not able to meet expectations. The automobile insurance company threatened to stop his salary replacement insurance, maintaining that the wounds had healed and he should be able to do some kind of work. Other than medical visits, he spent most of his time in his apartment. A couple of friends visited, but he became so depressed and enraged with his situation that their company, especially their attempts to cheer him up, only annoyed him, and he told them to stay away. He felt that all his best efforts to become a good citizen and a decent human being had only backfired. His landlord found him unconscious after his first suicide attempt. He took him to hospital, where Mr. D. was placed under psychiatric care. While the Pain Management Unit was able to offer some small relief for his pain, his mental health problems were too severe for us to treat with our resources. I feel sad whenever I think of Mr. D. In the face of many obstacles, he had worked so hard to make something of himself.

## LIFE-LONG INSTABILITY AND LOW FUNCTION

Significant psychological problems in this group explain much of the continued suffering with pain. Pain may start with an injury or illness, which then becomes the central focus of an already miserable, low-functioning life. Often, there has been early psychological, physical and/or sexual abuse, leaving irreparable emotional damage (and sometimes physical damage, too), which can later find its outlet in the form of chronic pain in or on the body. Such pain may serve to elicit care or fulfil some other emotional need and even — paradoxically — maintain the best psychological equilibrium available to such an unfortunate person. Despite the discomfort of pain, these individuals may feel better overall when care and attention are available. Alternately, persisting pain might provide a socially acceptable reason for a person with social anxiety or inability to function in the outside world to avoid emotionally threatening situations. The pain is not "faked" in such situations, but it looms much larger, enlists more treatment-seeking and is more intractable than it might be in a psychologically healthy individual or one without a troubled past.

When the medical system fails to recognize the important contribution of serious long-standing psychopathology, the patient may end up with side effects from medications, invasive pain treatments and even surgeries for pain — none of which help and may possibly cause harm. They can become increasingly "medicalized" and develop into a "career" patient who is deeply entrenched in the "sick role." The doctors are doing their best to help them, without realizing they are treating the wrong problem: such a person needs serious psychological help rather than treatment for pain.

A 38-year-old woman recently presented with chronic excruciating pain after 16 surgeries in the jaw area performed by six different oral surgeons (in different parts of the country). In the psychological assessment interview, I learned of her 20-year history of eating disorder for which she had been hospitalized and treated twice, without success. She has made four suicide attempts and has a diagnosis of factitious disorder (characterized by physical or psychological symptoms produced intentionally or feigned in order to assume the sick role). She was hoping for another operation, but this time her surgeon sent her to us for our opinion.

Another patient had had 11 pelvic and abdominal surgeries with pain increasing after each. She had been sexually abused by both parents, repeatedly raped by an uncle and had had three abortions before the age of 20. Unwittingly and with the best of intentions, the surgeons had betrayed the Hippocratic Oath: **to abstain from doing harm.**

## PSYCHOGENIC PAIN

An individual experiencing pain arising **entirely** from psychological causes is rarely seen in the Pain Management Unit —perhaps a couple of times a year. While we do not yet have a good understanding of "conversion disorder," we assume that symptoms such as a deficit or loss of function (e.g. inability to walk or incontinence) and pain appear to arise from severe psychological trauma. The problem is not produced intentionally by the patient, or with any conscious awareness. Multiple tests show no findings, and treatments for pain rarely provide much relief. Sometimes it lasts many years or, in severe cases, a lifetime, but it can also resolve on its own.

A woman who had been inexplicably wheelchair bound—in pain and unable to walk for seven years — suddenly stood up and walked with pain virtually gone after three weeks of hospitalization in psychiatry. To see such a dramatic recovery is rare.

Another patient, an acrobat, suffered from unremitting pain after falling from a height and severely injuring one leg. Previously, he had been well and very fit. In heroic attempts to restore his function and relieve pain, many medications and extreme forms of treatment had been tried in other pain treatment facilities. When we first saw him, he could barely speak or function at all, and was incontinent of urine. He had multiple side effects from taking large doses of many different medications, making it impossible for us to assess his true condition. We referred him to our detoxification unit, and by the time he completed the programme four weeks later, he was off all medications with pain neither better nor worse than before. His function was much improved; he spoke clearly, made good contact, and was no longer incontinent. Both he and our team were very happy. We now began to treat his pain, which, for a time, responded well to minimal medications. However, he was still unable to return to acrobatics, the only passion he had known in life. Sadly, over time, he became severely depressed and his condition seriously deteriorated. Soon, he was unable to use either of his legs, and later experienced paralysis in one arm, all in the absence of physical explanation. We never did learn much about his earlier history; we only knew that without acrobatics, his life had become meaningless and he didn't have the resilience to adapt.

4: This is not to suggest that all or even most people with such a history develop chronic pain, but for those who do, psychological factors may be major contributors.

## 5. "SECONDARY GAINS": TO TREAT OR NOT TO TREAT?

"Secondary gain" is a term usually used to describe how financial gain from insurance or disability payments impedes a person's motivation to get better. Malingering is sometimes implied.

The problem may be more pronounced when a patient's pain is being questioned or there is a court date to challenge the insurer's decision to stop payments. There are times when it is clear that compensation issues do hamper a patient's motivation to get better. However, the problem is usually more complex and nuanced, and an a priori assumption of malingering does patients a disservice.

> Often, the people we see with work injuries are labourers who are fearful of returning to a physical job where they risk re-injury, and return of pain intensity to pretreatment levels. I believe that if our treatments could completely eliminate pain, most people would gladly choose to return to work. Sadly, although pain intensity may substantially decrease with treatment, few are so fortunate as to have the pain completely relieved.

To best appreciate such a dilemma, consider the complexity of the problem from the patient's point of view. For example, a bricklayer with two years of back pain hovering around an intensity of 7–8 after surgery is unlikely to see a decrease of more than two to three points, even with the best combination of treatments. If a court case with the insurer is pending, he may fear (with good reason) that a pain reduction down to 5 on a scale of 0–10 may be considered sufficient to send him back to work, perhaps with modification of duties. While he may well have come in good faith for treatment, returning to a job while still in pain is frightening, especially if he believes compensation will be difficult to obtain the second time around should he again become injured, or if the pain increases. His apparent passivity does not reflect malevolent intent, but rather the difficult reality he faces. Most likely, he is not aware of these psychological processes.

The question remains: to treat or not to treat at a time when partial pain relief carries with it the risk of the patient losing compensation or being forced back to work prematurely. The literature on the subject is inconclusive with some studies showing that pain is more resistant to treatment when people receive or pursue compensation, while other studies show no such difference (Fishbain et al., 2004; Fishbain et al, 1995; Kwan, 2003).

Sometimes, when a patient is in the midst of a battle for disability payments, I openly suggest that they wait until the dispute is over before starting treatment. Only then are they likely to be "ready" to benefit. I have found that supportive but "straight" talk clarifies the situation for the patient and treatment provider alike. There is no virtue in investing energy, hope and resources at a time when a patient is more concerned with winning a court case or maintaining financial benefits than in participating actively in treatment. If there is reason to believe that treatment has minimal potential to help for any reason, it is hardly worth the risks of medication side effects, uncomfortable procedures or even the smallest possibility of causing harm. This does not mean that people receiving compensation should not be treated for pain, but that the situation deserves close scrutiny and honest, open communication between patient and clinician.

## 6. EFFECT OF CHRONIC PAIN ON FAMILIES

To watch a loved one suffer can be devastating. To see this person isolated, depressed and no longer involved in family activities can be painful for all. It feels worse for family members when the person with pain seems to push them away, especially when they are trying hard to help. For a couple, cessation of sexual activity, whether due to the sufferer's depression or pain, may be hard for both, especially when accompanied by withdrawal of all physical affection.

As difficult as it is for the person with pain to not know when and why pain is worse one day and better another, it can be even more trying for the partner who has no cues at all, and doesn't know how to react. Sometimes I hear family members say, "I can see it in his eyes; he doesn't have to tell me." Other times, the face of pain and depression remains blank and uncommunicative.

Financial problems caused by chronic pain also affect the entire household. Activities that a couple used to do together, including socializing, often cease. The lives of both people change, and silence can separate them further. Often they both feel guilty, one for disrupting family life by having pain, the other for not being able to help, and sometimes for getting fed up with their partner who does nothing but complain. The healthy person feels guilty going off and enjoying themselves alone, and the person with pain may feel guilty keeping their partner at home attending to their misery.

Pain makes a person irritable; often there are fights and arguments that were never there before. The person in pain no longer does their share of household chores, leaving the entire burden to the partner. Interactions with the children change. For example, Dad is lying on the couch when the kids get home. He can no longer throw a football around or wrestle with them. Or, Mom doesn't work or play anymore. This can become another source of guilty feelings and sadness for the parent with pain, who wants more than ever to be involved with their children.

Often the person in pain feels, not without justification, that others in the family don't understand or believe they are suffering. Indeed, pain, an internal, subjective, and invisible experience, is difficult for others to grasp. Sometimes, when people can't "see" the pain, they may believe the person is exaggerating. When this happens, pain becomes much more difficult to bear for the person living with it, and may engender hurt and anger in all.

When a family member asks for advice on how best to help, they are often surprised when I suggest they already help too much or are being overprotective. While the family's intent is to do everything possible to ease their loved one's pain, helping too much can increase the person's feelings of helplessness, uselessness and guilt, and even result in greater disability. People with chronic pain need to remain active to avoid becoming deconditioned, and to contribute as much as they are able in order to maintain their sense of worth and well-being.

## COMMUNICATION IN COUPLES

Improving communication is the first critical step to resolving family tension. Only then will misunderstandings — with their unfortunate consequences — abate. Avoidance of sexual activity is not rejection of the partner; rather, sexual activity may increase pain. The person in pain may shy away from any physical affection, fearing they will arouse their partner without being able to follow through. Or, the person with pain may stay alone in a room, door closed, not because of anger, but to avoid burdening others with their misery. A couple may have managed just fine in the past, even without the best communication skills. That was when life moved along trippingly, and everyone was busy and active.

Without clear communication, people make assumptions about what the other is thinking or feeling and then react as though these assumptions are true. This can initiate a pattern of successive misunderstandings with everyone feeling miserable.

## COMMUNICATING ABOUT PAIN

Patients often say they hate to be asked about their pain, especially because they believe the person who asks doesn't really want to hear the answer. They may be right. People sometimes feel obligated to ask, but only want good news. They may lose interest, feel uncomfortable or even express annoyance on hearing nothing has improved. Under such circumstances, I recommend a clear and courteous response such as: "Thank you for your concern, but I'd prefer you no longer ask me about my pain because I don't enjoy talking about it. I'll be happy to volunteer the good news when there's improvement." For those who don't abide by such a request, just reply with two words: "the same" (even if the pain is higher than usual).

On the other hand, family members may need a gauge of the person's pain level so they know what to expect. I have suggested some form of code or numerical system. For example, pain of 8-10 out of a maximum of 10, means "I'm feeling terrible; leave me alone;" 6-7, "you can talk to me, but I can't do much today;" 4-5, "it's a reasonably good day, maybe we can make some plans," and so on. Some families prefer to use a colour code, with "red" representing the worst days. Such clear, simple communications eliminate long complicated conversations around pain, and lighten the burden for all concerned.

# 7. PAIN SPECIALISTS: WHO ARE THEY?

Healthcare providers who treat patients with chronic pain come in all shapes, sizes and personalities, just like everyone else. Some are excellent at what they do while some are less so, just like other people in their jobs. However, people who are there to help those who suffer are more likely to be compassionate. Because pain has so great an impact on a person's mood, which in turn affects the pain and its response to treatment (the "vicious cycle" of pain), good pain specialists need to have a comprehensive awareness of the psychological problems arising from pain. By taking account of the "whole person" and not only the body part that hurts, they are more likely to take the time to "listen" (within reasonable time constraints).

Pain specialists represent many different disciplines, including anaesthesia, rheumatology, general medicine, neurology, neurosurgery, physiatry, dentistry, nursing, physiotherapy, occupational therapy, psychology and psychiatry. All are trained both in their own discipline and in its application to the treatment of pain. Practitioners of complementary and alternative medicine (e.g. acupuncture, chiropractic, osteopathy, massage therapy) also treat pain, but rarely work as part of a medical team in a pain clinic.

Interdisciplinary teamwork creates a special environment, with pain specialists from different disciplines learning from each other and understanding the complexity of pain from many points of view. Such collaboration fosters motivation, enthusiasm and learning, all of which promote better treatment for patients.

While most pain specialists I have known are compassionate, the task can be difficult and sometimes frustrating. Despite the many scientific and technological advances, there is still, unfortunately, no "magic bullet" to treat chronic pain. Furthermore, because of large individual differences in genetic makeup, constitution and psychosocial factors, we cannot always predict which treatment will work best for which patient. The endeavour is as much an art as it is a science. Despite our best efforts, many continue to suffer, even when pain improves with treatment. The goal then becomes optimal management of pain rather than cure. Many patients are pleased with whatever pain reduction and improvement in well-being our treatment offers. They accept that they themselves must participate actively in their treatment, as well as learn how best to cope with whatever pain remains. Other patients feel differently, believing, unrealistically that medicine should be able to take all the pain away so they can return to life as it was before. It can be hard to have unsatisfied patients, and sometimes even the most understanding clinician becomes frustrated. On the other hand, we feel a sense of triumph when a patient returns for a follow-up visit with a smile, feeling better, more active, involved again in life and happier than before.

## 8. **ROLE OF PSYCHOLOGY IN PAIN TREATMENT**

Since Drs. Ronald Melzack and Patrick Wall published their "gate control" theory of pain in 1965, we have understood that the perception of pain is affected not only by severity of an injury or wound, but also by a complex array of neurophysiological and psychological processes. Before you feel pain, neurochemical messages travel from the wound site to multiple areas in the brain that register pain sensations (intensity and quality of pain) as well as emotions ("this pain feels horrible"). Sometimes there is no wound as such to trigger pain messages that originate from within the nervous system or even the brain itself (e.g. phantom limb pain). At the same time as pain signals travel toward the brain, the brain is already occupied with other activities and thoughts that also contribute to the intensity and unpleasantness of the pain a person feels. Such brain activities are associated with processes such as attention, distraction, memory, beliefs, thoughts, feelings, fears and expectations. Clinical psychologists concern themselves with this latter group of factors that play an important role in exacerbating, as well as reducing, pain and suffering.

Psychologists who work as part of a multidisciplinary pain team conduct psychological assessments, offer brief psychotherapy (including relaxation training or hypnosis) and conduct pain-management groups. The primary objective of the psychological assessment is to clarify the role played by psychological and social factors in the person's suffering. The information obtained allows the team to tailor a multidisciplinary treatment plan to individual needs. For example, if a nerve block or other injection is recommended for a patient who is afraid of needles,

a psychologist may provide a few sessions to help the person overcome their fear. If exercise is part of the plan, but the patient is too depressed or sleep-deprived to comply, antidepressant medication together with short-term psychotherapy may be offered. Depression in the patients we see is so common that it is considered almost "normal." Without treating both depression and pain, chances for improvement are small—even when pain is the initiating cause of depression.

While patients tend to think, "If they only take my pain away, my mood will improve and I'll be fine," the problem, unfortunately, is not so easily solved. As previously mentioned, most people referred for treatment of chronic pain won't leave cured. A reduction of pain is likely, but few can expect to resume their lifestyle as it was before the pain. Strategies taught by psychologists can help people better *manage* pain and live a happier, more fulfilling life. Such strategies include adapting to limitations (not the same as "resigning" oneself), learning new skills, creating new goals in line with new limitations, coping with residual pain and short-term exacerbations and finding new or different ways to live an enjoyable, productive life. Pain most certainly changes a person's life options, but identifying new — or reviving old — interests, and becoming involved in meaningful activities can go a long way to diminishing the focus on pain and alleviating suffering.

When pain brings life to a halt, the only image that occupies the "mental screen" is **pain**. With only pain to focus on, suffering increases. When other, more interesting activities occupy the "screen," there is less room for pain and suffering.

---

A man with a passion for the piano had not played for several years because of back pain. I suggested he start by playing for five minutes. He did so, but instead of five minutes, he became so absorbed that he played for an hour without any awareness of pain. Not surprisingly, soon after he stopped, the pain returned, at a more intense level than before he had started This example points out an important principle of pain management: the need to pace activities; to start slowly and gradually increase[5]. However, while he was completely involved in a pleasurable activity, pain remained outside his conscious awareness. Essentially, it ceased to exist.

---

Lest the reader think this effect is "only psychological," there is substantial evidence showing that brain activity changes when a person is involved in an endeavour that distracts from pain.

**This does not mean that pain has been cured or decreased for all time, but for the time of engagement a person feels better. The more such times, the more enjoyment and the less overall suffering.**

---

5 : This example points out an important principle of pain management: the need to pace activities; to start slowly and gradually increase.

A patient who suffers from severe "electric shock"-like sensations in the face has worked hard to resume activities even through times of unbearable pain. She has gone back to school, carrying a heavy graduate programme, and continues with her full range of activities. When I asked her how she manages to do it, she thought for a while before saying, "Distraction, immersing myself in my studies and learning. It's hard, but that's what enables me to tolerate the pain, sometimes to even forget about it." She is also helped by medications that decrease her pain, although not reliably.

**On their own, chronic pain patients spend so much time thinking about all the things they _can't_ do anymore that they forget the many things they still know or _can_ do.**

A psychologist can explore with the patient the knowledge, abilities and interests they still possess, and from there look at new possible directions for work, learning or recreation. When such help is effective, well-being increases and pain stops being the dominant force in life. While the pain is still present, suffering is decreased. Getting there is hard; it requires persistence, hard work, hope and an environment that makes it possible.

### COGNITIVE-BEHAVIOUR THERAPY

Cognitive-behaviour therapy (CBT) is the most commonly used psychological intervention for patients with chronic pain. It is efficient, goal-oriented, concrete and pragmatic, and lends itself well to research. The techniques are easy for therapists to learn, the methods can be standardized and the results can be observed and measured. According to cognitive-behaviour theory, how we think shapes how we feel and what we do. If a person thinks, "I can't do anything, I'm useless," they will become depressed, sit around doing nothing and then become even more depressed. The thought "I'm useless" is termed "distorted" or "irrational" thinking, because it is not strictly true, and it makes the person feel worse. Persisting in such a belief, and continuing to do nothing, leads to a self-fulfilling prophecy: the person does indeed become useless. If, on the other hand, the thought can change to: "Maybe I can't do what I used to, but there are still useful things I can do," action will replace inaction, self-esteem will improve and depression will lift. A major objective of CBT is to help a person shift from "distorted," self-undermining thinking to more "realistic," helpful and productive thoughts and beliefs.

**Too often, CBT is used in only a formulaic way, without attention to the _particular_ suffering of a specific individual or what they need in order to recover a sense of meaning and purpose in life.** CBT as a theory fails to address the existential losses of meaning, identity and other aspects of a person's spiritual[7] needs so crucial for a sense of well-being. CBT on its own is but a useful **technique**; it is not the whole of therapy. If we know **only** technique, we can't have true understanding of the suffering individual who has lost the capacity to experience beauty, joy, hope and sometimes the feeling of connection to loved ones. The work of the psychologist is care of the human psyche, a mysterious, complex, capricious entity, demanding thoughtful attention and sensitivity to the unique needs and meanings of the individual. With this in mind, CBT can be a useful tool within a broader multifaceted approach.

## 9. LIMITS OF PSYCHOLOGICAL SERVICES

Unfortunately, we are unable to offer long-term psychotherapy or therapy for psychosocial problems not directly related to pain. When patients come in with needs that are beyond the scope of our services, we make efforts to recommend alternate facilities with appropriate psychological and psychiatric services. Unfortunately, suitable services within the medical system are very limited, and wait times may be long. Most cannot afford to pay the fees of psychologists in private practice. This is a difficult situation, without clear solution and with which the patient and our staff continue to struggle.

6 : Trying to find an image to help me understand a pain I have never experienced, I imagine my face perpetually attacked by insects, or of climbing endlessly up a hill in a ferocious blizzard, with snow pellets whipping my burning face.

7 : "Spiritual" here refers to the deepest part of a person, the part connected to how a person makes meaning of their world. It is integral to one's identity, purpose and place in the world, providing the nourishment for strength and hope.

## TWO STORIES

The personal stories I hear from patients are many, colourful and diverse. There are stories of courage, abandonment, hope, loss, despair, pride, shame, ingenuity, love, adventure and triumph. The stories come from the rich and famous, the poor and abandoned and those from every situation in between.[8] Regardless of social or economic status, pain is a great leveller. Suffering does not discriminate.

The following stories belong to two of the many extraordinary people I have had the privilege to treat.

### Elisabeth

Elisabeth is an artist and art instructor. She first came in the winter for treatment of a painful shoulder and neck, the result of years of painting finely detailed watercolours. Anti-inflammatory medications were not an option because she has ulcerative colitis. She could no longer paint or lift or carry very much, and she had stopped teaching because that required her to do all three. She was approaching 50, had insufficient income and felt alone and bereft of her identity as an artist. That she was depressed was no surprise. Still, throughout the interview I could sense a warm, passionate, dynamic woman with enormous capacity to enjoy life's small pleasures and quirks. But not at the moment. Now, with pain and depression, she seemed to have lost her moorings.

Not surprisingly, Elisabeth has good friends who were sticking by her and offering help. She and I talked about what she might be able to enjoy and do without increasing her pain. Was there something she had done in the past, perhaps as far back as childhood, some hobby or pleasure she had since forgotten that she might pick up again? I encouraged her to ask for help with lifting and carrying, and to think about how she might modify her teaching so she could return to a job she loved.

She was also receiving treatments from our physiotherapist who showed her exercises and recommended she walk as much as possible in order to keep fit and maintain energy. Elisabeth is one of those rare people who, despite pain and depression, latch on to any helpful suggestions, putting one foot in front of the other as best she can.

At an appointment a few weeks later, she told me she had gone home after the last meeting and asked herself, "What do I already know that I could use now to help me?" She remembered her love of poetry, a pleasure she had abandoned many years ago because life had become so busy. She found a notebook of poems she had copied by hand years ago, and read them again. From there, she gathered some poetry-loving friends to meet once a month in her home to read and discuss their favourite poems. She had also rediscovered photography, an art form less physically demanding than painting.

She was taking long daily walks. When friends drove anywhere in the city, she went with them to wherever they were going, and from there she explored the local area on foot before walking home. This became an adventure she looked forward to each day. A friend bought her a treadmill to use on days of inclement weather. Another friend was teaching her T'ai Chi.

By the following autumn, Elisabeth was teaching again, having learned how to accommodate to her physical limitations. She resumed painting only after a difficult period of adjustment, feeling limited at the beginning, and unable to carry out her usual intensive projects. Later, she found a freer, more immediate way of painting, a less technical and more spontaneous style. She was painting outdoors, fortuitously with shorter sessions than she was used to due to changes of light and weather. As well, she was pleased that the whole endeavour involved more physical exercise.

Whereas her previous work had been detailed and labour-intensive, she now paints more spontaneously and with broad dynamic strokes and colour washes, mostly nature scenes. Every summer she and an artist friend, with their faithful dogs in tow, spend days outdoors in the country, painting. Elisabeth has devised contrivances that allow her to carry her brushes, tools and easel around her waist, so as not to aggravate the shoulder pain. She still has pain, sometimes intense, sometimes moderate, but usually she manages it well enough to live her life again with energy and pleasure. As I walked around the gallery looking at the exhibit of watercolours she had painted last summer, I couldn't stop smiling.

---

8: I have seen people from a vast array of occupations and preoccupations at the Pain Management Unit, including labourers, office workers, teachers, nurses, company presidents, pilots, sex workers, doctors, homeless people, judges, soldiers, victims of torture, dancers, politicians, cleaners, students, parents, designers, mechanics, artists, political refugees, lawyers and university professors.

## Mr. T.

Mr. T., born in 1931 in Hungary, is a Holocaust survivor. A charming man, always ready with a joke and a smile, he suffers from intolerable pain in his abdomen, a pain so severe that it makes him want to "jump out of [his] skin." This pain has been his constant, unwelcome companion since age 12 or 13, soon after he got out of the concentration camp. His parents had died or been killed, and he was left to find his own way. He tells a story of "running non-stop" from one country to another, seeking a home, safety and peace. Coming to Canada in early adulthood, he finally found home and safety, but not yet peace of mind. In one way or another, he still keeps running, in search of calm, away from pain. Whether his pain is emotional or physiological in origin was difficult to discern[9] He believes "experiments" done on him in the concentration camp are the cause of his pain, but has no actual memory of them.

Mr. T. married in Montreal, worked hard as a dressmaker until his retirement, created a life for himself and his family and now has grandchildren who adore him and see him often. At one of his sessions he proudly showed my psychology intern Jodie and me a calendar one of his grandsons had made for him, each page a photograph of family members. His wife ("the love of my life") had died a decade earlier.

Every day for many years, Mr. T. (who also suffers from lung problems) walks about 10 kilometres, no matter the weather. On waking, his pain is always severe. He takes his pills, drinks his coffee and perhaps has a little breakfast, then heads out for his walk across town, always following the same route. He greets people, spreading good cheer as he goes. People along his route have come to know him. He stops at the same restaurant for lunch every day, then walks back, reaching home at around 4:00 p.m. While out and walking, he feels no pain. The pain reappears as soon as he gets home, and is most intense between 4:00 and 8:00 p.m., at which time he takes his next set of antianxiety and analgesic pills. He is adamant that he cannot do without the pills, and afraid they might be taken away.

He has found many creative ways to remain busy, and to distract himself from pain. He reads, listens to music and is a formidable dancer (he showed us a tap dance routine). Nevertheless, he told us, "The pain never goes away." By this he means that even when medication takes effect, or when he is fully distracted and not bothered by pain, he knows it is there, waiting to resurface.

Mr. T. is currently trying to piece together things that have happened to him that he can't quite grasp, hoping to make sense of his life since the start of the Holocaust. He believes such understanding will bring peace and maybe relief from pain. His quest to unravel this mystery has become relentless.

After the first interview, Jodie and I were concerned about the amount of antianxiety medication he was taking. The doctor agreed to reduce these pills, while at the same time increasing the dose of analgesic medications. Interestingly, both seemed equally effective in decreasing pain. In psychotherapy sessions, Jodie made every attempt to decrease Mr. T's anxiety, hoping this would lessen the pain and reduce his need for medication. He was eager to come to every session and very much enjoyed talking to her. Unfortunately, the sessions failed in their objective. Mr. T. was too restless to learn relaxation techniques and not much interested in other therapeutic strategies we tried. He was fidgety, needing always to be "on the move." Walking, as he had figured out on his own, was probably his best form of relaxation.

### Mr. T.'s case presented us with a couple of dilemmas:

1) Was the problem we were treating one of anxiety or of pain?
2) Should medications continue to be prescribed at the high doses he was using?

We discussed the matter with the entire team, weighing the risks and benefits. Benefits: The medications seemed to decrease Mr. T.'s pain and certainly made him feel better. He suffered no ill effects, and these medications were not dangerous to his health. Risk: There was every indication that he would continue to require escalated doses. This raised some concern, but in the end we decided that with appropriate medical monitoring, the problem could be managed. I believe the real problem resided in us, the treatment professionals: we are not used to such doses in our clinic, and we also felt uncomfortable using pain medication for what seemed to be mostly an anxiety problem. After some judicious thought, we concluded that there was no good reason to deprive Mr. T. of a treatment with demonstrable effectiveness for him and, in his case, without any harmful effects. For other patients this might be an unwise choice, but not for Mr. T.

There are no tried and true formulas in this business; the pain of each individual must be assessed, understood and treated as a unique problem. At the same time, we must use our training, knowledge base, clinical experience and best judgement to provide patients with treatments demonstrated to be effective for a given type of pain.

In Mr. T.'s case we decided to stray a little from the norm. He is living his life the best way he can: he remains functional and fully active, and brings love and happiness to others. Why would we risk changing this in a man who has suffered so much, a man who says of himself, "I'm a clown on the outside, crying on the inside"?

I believe Mr. T. suffers from "life pain;" a pain that can decrease with medications or go into the background with distraction but, as he says, "It never really goes away." Such life pain is deeply embedded in the core of a person. I have seen it in Holocaust survivors as well as in others who have endured torture or serious psychological trauma. Whether its origin is in the psyche or in the body is an irrelevant question, and probably has no answer. As healthcare providers in the face of such indomitable pain, we must do whatever is in our power to diminish suffering (while being cautious to cause no harm).

---

9: This question is not easily answered because psychological stress produces physiological changes.

## 10. CONCLUSION

Doing the best we can to alleviate pain and suffering, we are still unable to help everyone. Some we help a lot, others a moderate amount, and a few not at all. Most patients find the Alan Edwards Pain Management Unit to be a comforting and supportive place with doctors, nurses, physiotherapists and psychologists who can be counted on to care. Even when pain is not improved, patients regard our unit as a safe haven.

The hard part comes when it's time for discharge — after we have tried all appropriate treatments and medications, and have nothing more to offer. Because many people are on the wait-list to be treated, we cannot continue seeing the same patients indefinitely, especially when there's nothing more we can do. For some, discharge from our unit feels like expulsion from the one place that gives them succour and hope. We try to say "goodbye" gently and make suggestions for how they might continue to help themselves, but sadly, some feel that, without our continued support, they are being thrown to the wolves.

Before discharge, medications are stabilized. Patients are taught coping skills to manage their pain, and many are given an exercise program. We send a letter with our recommendations for continued care to the referring doctor and/or family physician, whom we welcome to contact us in the future for any further advice.

When patients come to a pain treatment facility, they want their pain taken away so they can return to the life they lived before pain intruded. Pain treatment specialists share these goals, but with the available treatment armamentarium, it is rarely possible to completely eradicate entrenched chronic pain. While we explain this early on, patients coming to a world-class university pain-management unit find it hard to believe and accept. Science and technology can send people to outer space and can clone animals; medicine can work miracles, keeping people alive when their organs fail, transplanting hearts and livers. It seems impossible to believe that a cure for pain has not been found.

Unfortunately, despite extensive research, we do not yet understand pain very well. In the past four decades, basic researchers have been trying to solve the mystery of pain by looking for the molecule or molecules that will lead to new medications, without having made any spectacular discoveries so far. It is possible — even likely — that some day molecules will be found to completely alleviate some types of chronic pain, but other types are likely to remain impervious to a "magic bullet." As long as medicine has no cure for chronic pain, psychological factors such as mood, coping, distraction, social supports, acceptance and finding meaning will remain essential ingredients of treatment, both for managing pain and improving quality of life.

## REFERENCES

- Alghalyini, B. & M. Oldfield. That sinking feeling. Can Fam Physician, Vol. 54, No. 11, Nov 2008, 1576-1577.
- Fishbain DA, HL Rosomoff, RB Cutler & RS Rosomoff. Is there a relationship between nonorganic physical findings (Waddell signs) and secondary gain/malingering? Clin J Pain, 2004, Nov-Dec, 20(6): 399-408.
- Fishbain DA, RB Cutler, HLRosomoff & RS Rosomoff. Secondary gain concepts: a review of the scientific evidence. Clin J Pain, 1995, March: 11(1), 6-21.
- Freud, S. Studies in Hysteria. In: J. Strachey. ed. «Complete psychological works», 1955, v. 2, 1893-1895.
- Kwan, O. & J. Friel. A review and methodological critique of the literature supporting 'chronic whiplash injury': part 1 – research articles. Med Sci Monit 2003, Aug: 9(8): RA 2003-15.
- Melzack, R. & P. Wall. Pain mechanisms: a new theory. Science, 1965, 150, 971-979.

# WHERE DO I GO FROM HERE?

Gary Blank, Dollard-des-Ormeaux, Quebec, Canada
Group leader, Montreal Chronic Pain Support Group (MCPSG), Chronic Pain Association of Canada (CPAC), Montreal, Quebec, Canada

(See other testimonials, pages 124 and 132. See Chapter 50, page 363.)

Ten years ago, I received good news and bad news. The bad news was that I had a brain tumour. The good news was that 99% of acoustic neuromas[1] are benign. The tumour was growing from my inner ear, wrapping around the facial and auditory nerves, and eventually pressed on my brain stem. Although these tumours are not cancerous, they can continue to grow with deadly consequences if not removed.

I underwent an 11-hour craniotomy in July of 1999, the infamous day of the nurses' strike. I received excellent care. The following morning, my surgeon told me that my operation had been routine except for my hearing. Though they tried to preserve my auditory nerve, part of the tumour was adhered to it. I was now deaf in my right ear, had a hearing loss in my other ear, and developed tinnitus (ringing in the ear/head) for which there is no cure. Otherwise, the surgery was considered a complete success. After 5 to 6 weeks of convalescence, I could resume my life and return to work. Unfortunately that never happened. One in 200,000 people develop this kind of brain tumour. Less than 1% of those who have the tumour surgically removed end up with chronic head and neck pain. I hit the jackpot.

I had excruciating headaches and neck pain that totally immobilized me. I rarely could get out of bed; any movement would increase my pain score. For the next nine months, I lived on Advil and Tylenol cocktails. I kept going back to see my surgeon and he kept telling me I'd get better; he never uttered the words "chronic pain." He once told me I had benign fibromyalgia. On another occasion, he told me to rub cayenne pepper paste into my scar. What a burn! One day, I gave up. I went to see my general practitioner who explained the difference between acute and chronic pain. He then referred me a neurologist, and then finally to a pain clinic.

After my first visit to the pain clinic, I was told that that what I was feeling was not all in my head. Finally, I received an answer to my question: "What's wrong with me?" The diagnosis was neuropathic pain, possibly caused by disturbing my sub-occipital nerve during my surgery.

Since then, I have tried a vast array of medications and a myriad of treatments in my search for relief: osteopathy, acupuncture, cranial massage, myofascial physiotherapy, head and neck physiotherapy, a tens machine, different types of nerve blocks, steroid injections, masso-therapy, reiki, different forms of psychological counselling, as well as a few visits to a psychiatric pharmacologist because of the complex drug interactions and different forms of depression I experienced at various stages of my disease. Living with chronic pain and treatments has been a series of trade-offs and cycles. Medications sometimes trigger side effects that are worse than my pain.

Getting into my pain clinic was like reaching an oasis in the desert. I was taken seriously and, more importantly, believed! In addition to seeing a pain specialist, I was one of the lucky few who were invited to participate in a pain management course at my pain clinic. I say lucky because only a very small percentage of patients are accepted into this course. Once a week for 6 weeks, I spent 5 hours with about 10 other pain sufferers. The course included a pain nurse specialist, psychologist and physiotherapist. For me it was a Pain 101 course for dummies, which I was. Nobody knows beforehand that they're going to end up with chronic pain. We were all newly diagnosed, and for the first time I was spending time with other people damaged by pain. The experience was good but, once it ended, I became isolated again. All my friends were continuing their lives in the workforce while I remained at home in pain. Few were interested in hearing about my suffering; many probably didn't believe it could be that bad. I had no one to share or commiserate with about my new life sentence. I didn't want to burden my family every day, nor could they really understand what I was going through.

At a follow-up pain clinic visit, I noticed a sign on a bulletin board. It was from the Chronic Pain Association of Canada (CPAC) looking for volunteers to start a pain support group. I had never belonged to a support group of any kind, but this caught my interest because these groups are patient-run. At the meeting I met Terry Bremner, CPAC's support group co-ordinator. (See Terry Bremner's testimonial, page 10.) When no one volunteered to become a volunteer, I decided to step up. To me, this was the answer to "Where do I go from here?" once the pain management course ended. After all, I had nothing but time in my "new" life.

That was six years ago. The Montreal Chronic Pain Support Group (MCPSG) was founded. It hasn't been easy given the very nature of what brings us together: chronic pain. For a long time, I was barely able to care for myself, let alone organize and attend our monthly meetings. But I persevered. Our members come from all cultures, ages and lifestyles. Pain does not discriminate. I've met and made wonderful friends that I would have otherwise never met if I had been in good health. When people who have recently been diagnosed contact me for information on our group, I tell them from the heart that attending our meeting is like meeting good family you didn't know you had.

---

1: An acoustic neuroma is a benign tumor on the sheath surrounding the eighth cranial nerve, affecting the functions of the inner ear. http://www.anac.ca/index.html

# WHY YOU SHOULD YOU SEE
# A PAIN MANAGEMENT PSYCHIATRIST

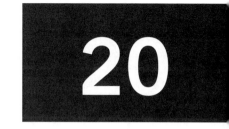

**Sarah Whitman** MD, psychiatrist, Philadelphia, Pennsylvania, United States

Parts of this chapter were previously published on the How to Cope with Pain
Web site at http://www.howtocopewithpain.org/
©: Sarah Whitman, MD Rights to reproduce granted by Sarah Whitman, MD

## ABSTRACT

For many people, when their doctor recommends seeing a pain-management psychiatrist or psychologist, it's not clear to them exactly why this might be helpful. They may have thoughts such as, "Does my doctor think my pain is all in my head?" and "Will I have to lie on a couch and recount my dreams?"

The answer is no. No, it's not all in your head. And no, you'll do other things instead of psychoanalysis. There are many ways that visits to a pain-management psychiatrist might be helpful.

This chapter presents what a psychiatric evaluation covers for patients with chronic pain, the treatment of psychiatric symptoms and the benefits of supportive therapy and pain support groups. A pain-management psychiatrist will also teach techniques from which the patients can benefit, as well as new psychological skills to manage daily life that includes a pain condition. New brain-based treatments will be explained as well as the importance of physical activity, both of which will ask the patient to play an active role.

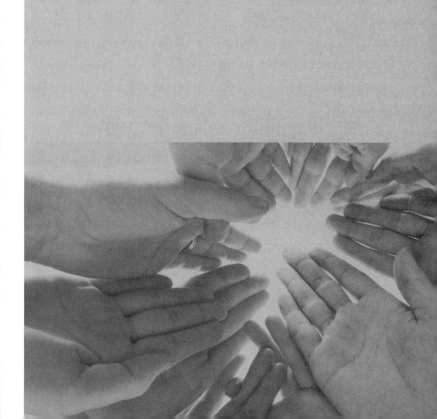

# 1. INTRODUCTION

We now know that comprehensive pain management works best. That is, having a group of specialists helping you get better gives better results than just approaching pain treatment from one angle. The pain-management team often includes a pain-management doctor, physical therapist, psychologist or psychiatrist and perhaps other healthcare professionals and therapists providing acupuncture, occupational therapy or massage treatments, etc.

**The benefits of having a pain management psychiatrist include:**

- receiving a psychiatric evaluation
- recognizing and treating any psychiatric symptoms, such as anxiety, depression, post-traumatic stress disorder (PTSD) and sleep problems
- using psychiatric medications for pain; many medications that are considered psychiatric can be helpful for the pain alone, even if you don't have psychiatric symptoms
- learning psychological skills

- making positive behavioural changes
- making positive psychological changes
- benefiting from supportive therapy
- benefiting from a pain support group
- considering new brain-based treatments such as mirror therapy and graded motor imagery, which can re-train your brain away from pain in some conditions

# 2. WHAT YOU GET OUT OF A PSYCHIATRIC EVALUATION

Link: http://www.howtocopewithpain.org/blog/830/psychiatric-evaluation-for-pain/

When I see someone for psychiatric pain management, I initially perform a psychiatric evaluation comprising the following areas:

### Prior psychiatric functioning and psychiatric diagnoses
Prior psychiatric functioning and psychiatric diagnoses enable the psychiatrist to understand if someone has had difficulty with anxiety, depression, sleep, etc., even before confronting a pain disorder. They may be at higher risk for these symptoms to recur.

### Current psychiatric symptoms
Unfortunately, pain is often buddies with psychiatric disorders, such as depression, anxiety and sleep problems. We know that if multiple disorders are present, it's crucial to treat them all.

### Psychiatric interactions with medications
Many drugs used for pain cause psychiatric symptoms, including sedation, depression or more serious side effects. It's important for someone on your treatment team to figure out what's causing what and make recommendations to minimize side effects.

### Treatment of psychiatric disorders
If psychiatric symptoms or disorders are found, treatment is crucial. Having an expert in this area is important. Treatment might include therapy, medication or both.

It's also helpful to know that a good pain-management psychiatrist will know how to treat issues related to pain. Your treatment shouldn't be just talking about how bad things are or treating a medical pain disorder as if it was psychiatric.

# 3. TREATING PSYCHIATRIC SYMPTOMS

Link : http://www.howtocopewithpain.org/blog/870/treating-psychiatric-symptoms/

Psychiatric symptoms, such as depression, anxiety, etc., often accompany chronic pain. A psychiatrist can identify these symptoms, take them seriously and treat them appropriately with therapy, medication or both.

## 4. BENEFITS OF SUPPORTIVE THERAPY

Link: http://www.howtocopewithpain.org/blog/998/supportive-therapy-benefit/

**How can supportive therapy be useful to you?**
Supportive therapy consists of helping people living with pain cope with a difficult situation through listening and support, problem -solving, and instilling hope.

Supportive therapy helps people living with pain by:
· Providing an opportunity to tell their story and make sense of their experience
· Providing an opportunity to work on adjusting to their changed situation
· Receiving family support

A good resource for families is *SURVIVING A LOVED ONE'S CHRONIC PAIN*. (See **Chapter 21.**)
• Link: http://www.ppmjournal.com/Handout.pdf

## 5. BENEFITS OF A PAIN SUPPORT GROUP

Link: http://www.howtocopewithpain.org/blog/1023/pain-support-group-benefits/

Why might you join a pain support group? Benefits of participating in a group can include:
· decreased isolation
· solving problems with others on ways to cope with pain
· helping others, instead of always receiving help
· expanding your support network
· sharing resources

One important challenge of any group is to keep it focused on coping with pain. Groups should not settle into complaining, focusing on pain, or focusing on whose pain is worse.

## 6. MAKING POSITIVE PSYCHOLOGICAL CHANGES

Link: http://www.howtocopewithpain.org/blog/978/pain-management-positive-psychological-changes/

In the psychiatric pain-management process, it is an essential step to make positive psychological changes in how you see your pain condition and the disability it causes. Although you may go through feelings of grief in response to the losses associated with pain, it is important to continue to work on moving forward.

One goal is increasing acceptance of both pain and the changes in your life. To be clear, acceptance is not liking pain or giving up. It's no longer struggling with pain, taking a realistic approach to pain and engaging in positive everyday activities. **How can one move towards acceptance? First, recognize that the process is often slow. You must grieve for what you've lost, then have a goal of living a full life despite pain.**

## 7. LEARNING NEW PSYCHOLOGICAL SKILLS

Link: http://www.howtocopewithpain.org/blog/924/psychological-skills-for-pain-relief/

Psychological skills can help to decrease pain and cope with it. There are many types of relaxation exercises you can learn, including breathing, basic relaxation exercises and visualization. The benefits of theses exercises are many:
· Help with relaxation and decreased anxiety
· Decreased stress response associated with pain
· Help getting better sleep
· Help decreasing pain.

Visit the How to Cope with Pain Web site for breathing, relaxation and guided imagery exercises.
Link: http://www.howtocopewithpain.org
   Guided imagery and hypnosis, where suggestions of decreasing pain are paired with imagery, help in the same way that relaxation exercises do. In addition, these exercises can directly decrease pain through these suggestions.
   You can learn all of these skills and then practise them regularly on your own. Regular practice is key!

## 8. NEW BRAIN-BASED TREATMENTS FOR PAIN

Link: http://www.howtocopewithpain.org/blog/1044/new-brain-based-treatments-for-pain/

There are more recent advances in brain-based treatments for certain pain conditions. These treatments are based on the theory that, in chronic pain, pain signals get "stuck" in pain-mode and no longer provide helpful information to you. Chronic pain creates actual changes in your brain that perpetuate a repetitive pain cycle.

How can you break this cycle? These newer treatments retrain your brain to reverse the pain cycle and the changes in your brain. Mirror therapy uses your visual system to retrain your brain into thinking that movement is safe. Motor imagery programs break up movement into components, allowing your brain to slowly resume normal movement without producing pain.

## 9. STAYING ACTIVE

Links: http://www.howtocopewithpain.org/blog/941/staying-active-despite-pain/
http://www.howtocopewithpain.org/blog/13/use-100-to-help-you-measure-how-much-to-do/

### What kind of behaviour changes can help you live better and get better?

It is important that you keep up activities when you have chronic pain. A pain-management psychiatrist will help you with pacing so that you can avoid doing too much or too little. They will also work with you to figure out what activities you can do, what you should avoid and, if you need to, how to replace or *alter* favourite activities so you can still do them. Let's say you love gardening but you can't do as much as you once did. It's important not to drop this activity that you really enjoy. So figure out what aspect of gardening you love. If it's seeing green by your front door, try container gardening instead of doing the whole yard. If it's being outside, garden for 15 minutes instead of 5 hours, then sit in or walk through a garden to enjoy the outdoors. You get the idea — alter what you need to so you can continue to enjoy your favourites.

## 10. CONCLUSION

A pain-management psychiatrist knows that comprehensive pain management works best. They are an important member of the group of specialists who help people living with chronic pain get better and get better results for their overall treatment, and not just approach pain treatment from one angle.

# SURVIVING A LOVED ONE'S CHRONIC PAIN -
## A GUIDE FOR FAMILY AND FRIENDS OF PAIN PATIENTS

**David Kannerstein** PhD, psychologist, Philadelphia, Pennsylvania, United States
**Sarah Whitman** MD, psychiatrist, Philadelphia, Pennsylvania, United States

Practical PAIN MANAGEMENT, January/February 2007

## NOTE

Editor's note from *Practical Pain Management*: The following article is suggested as a handout to your patients' families or loved ones to help them understand what patients are going through and encourage them to communicate with them and provide support. This article is available online (at www.PPMjournal.com/Handout.pdf) as a printer-ready PDF to allow free unlimited printing of handouts.

## PRESENTATION

1. WHAT IS CHRONIC PAIN?
2. HOW IS IT DIFFERENT FROM ACUTE PAIN?
3. HOW AM I AFFECTED BY THEIR PAIN?
4. WHAT DO I DO TO TAKE CARE OF MYSELF?
5. IS IT ALL IN THEIR HEADS?
6. COULD THEY BE FAKING IT, SAY, TO GET OUT OF WORK?
7. HOW SHOULD I RESPOND TO MY LOVED ONE WHEN (S)HE'S IN PAIN? HOW MUCH SHOULD I DO TO BE HELPFUL?
8. HOW CAN I TELL HOW HE OR SHE IS DOING?
9. WHAT TREATMENTS ARE THERE FOR CHRONIC PAIN?
10. WILL MY LOVED ONE GET ADDICTED TO HIS OR HER MEDICATIONS?
11. WHAT QUESTIONS DO I NEED TO ASK THE DOCTOR?
12. WHAT ELSE HELPS BESIDES MEDICATION?
13. HOW DO I COMMUNICATE WITH MY FAMILY MEMBER?
14. CONCLUSION

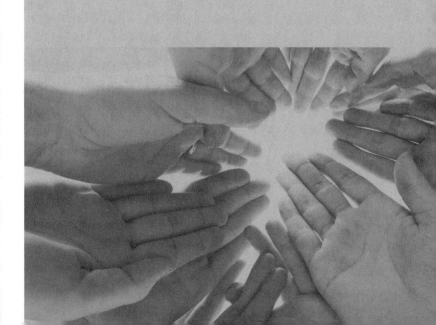

## PRESENTATION

This handout was inspired by a patient of mine who came into my office and inquired what resources were available for the family members of patients with pain to help them understand what their loved ones were going through. He discussed how his wife was frequently angry at him for not doing more physically at home while she was at work and how she often yelled at him. He felt guilty about it, but felt he did as much as he could tolerate. I was embarrassed to admit that I did not know of any handouts explicitly directed at spouses, family members, and other loved ones. After doing some research on the Internet, I discovered several very helpful publications, specifically Julie Silver's 2004 book, *Chronic Pain and the Family: A New Guide* (Harvard University Press) and the American Chronic Pain Association family manual, *ACPA Family Manual: A Manual for Families of Persons with Pain*, written by Penny Cowen (ACPA, 1998). I also found some helpful articles by Mark Grant, a psychologist in Australia, especially his "Ten Tips for Communicating With a Person Suffering From Chronic Pain," which is available on his website, www.overcomingpain.com. Mark was kind enough to allow us to summarize his suggestions here. As well, one of us (Whitman) has a website to help patients cope with chronic pain, and occasionally discusses family issues on it (www.howtocopewithpain.org). Much of what is in this handout is taken from these sources. What was striking, however, is how little material there was oriented toward the family compared to the massive amount of self-help material oriented to the patient with pain. In view of the profound effect the patient's pain has on the family and the equally profound effect the family's (and friends') responses have on the patient with pain, I found this troubling. I also felt that while Silver's book and the ACPA manual were very helpful, few family members would get them and fewer read through them. What was needed, I felt, was something brief and to the point. This is the result of that determination.

*- David Kannerstein*

## 1. WHAT IS CHRONIC PAIN?

Chronic pain is pain which persists beyond the time usually required for the healing of an injury or illness. Some definitions set a specific time period; for example, pain which lasts longer than three months or longer than six months.

## 2. HOW IS IT DIFFERENT FROM ACUTE PAIN?

Acute pain is what most of us are familiar with. It's what happens when you twist your ankle or burn your fingers on the stove. It's a signal that tissue damage is happening. While it may be severe, it is time limited and responds to appropriate treatment. Chronic pain is different. It may occur without ongoing tissue damage. This is what happens when nerves get injured (known as neuropathic pain). Examples include shingles (postherpetic neuralgia), diabetic neuropathy, and Reflex Sympathetic Dystrophy (RSD, also known as Complex Regional Pain Syndrome). It is difficult (or impossible) to imagine someone can be in severe pain continually if one has not experienced it. It's normal for you not to understand it if you haven't lived through it. It may also be hard to stand by and accept that your loved one's pain cannot be fixed or cured (although it may be eased and the suffering associated with it may be reduced). It may also be hard to accept that you cannot make it better.

## 3. HOW AM I AFFECTED BY THEIR PAIN?

If you are in a close relationship (spouse, significant other, parent, child, sibling or even close friend) with someone with chronic pain, you are likely to develop a variety of negative feelings as a result. For example, you may feel guilty at times for not being able to help them more. You may feel angry at them if they are irritable or withdrawn. You may resent having to take over tasks they previously performed. You may feel depressed as a result of a withdrawal of affection or a decline in your sex life. You may get anxious about financial problems which result from your loved one's disability. You may feel stressed by the reactions of others. For example, relatives or neighbors may say "He (she) doesn't look that disabled to me" or "Should he (she) be taking that addictive pain medication?" In fact, both you and the family member in pain are victims of the pain problem, as are those others who are part of the family (and this applies to close friends too). You may experience significant lifestyle changes. You may have to live on a reduced income or have to work harder to stay afloat financially. You may have to spend time getting your family member to medical or other appointments if they can't drive. You may end up doing most or all household chores and child-rearing activities. You may have less time for friends and experience reduced social support. You may experience intrusions into your life from outside agencies. For example, some insurance companies (primarily worker's compensation) may follow or film your family member. You may also be stressed by lawsuits, disability evaluations, or independent medical examinations (IME's). You may also experience some positive outcomes, although this is less common. For example, if your spouse was controlling, you may actually have more freedom. If you have very strong needs to help others, you may feel good about helping your loved one. If you were experiencing intimacy with your loved one (including sex) as unwanted, a decrease in intimacy may feel positive. You may get additional support or sympathy from other family members. These positive outcomes can lead one (not always intentionally) to try to maintain the situation. These have been referred to as "tertiary gains." Being aware of these can help you identify more effective ways of dealing with problems in your relationship. If you are the spouse of a patient with pain and you have children, you may worry about the effect of the pain on them. Children may blame themselves for their parent's pain. It is important to let the children know it is not their fault. They may also get depressed about the loss of attention and affection from the parent in pain or from the loss of activities due to financial limitations.

## 4. WHAT DO I DO TO TAKE CARE OF MYSELF?

If any of the above applies to you, you are not alone! In addition to discussing things with your loved one's doctor, you may also benefit from talking things over with a therapist or counsellor to help you cope better. In addition, consider the suggestions below.

- Try to maintain a healthy life style. Keep exercising (or start), socialize as much as possible, and eat right.
- Try to find others to help with the care of your loved one. This may be other family members or friends. This will allow you to take a break at times. (Your loved one may also feel less guilty if the burden does not all fall on you!)
- Try not to personalize your loved one's behaviour. If they are grouchy or depressed, don't see it as an attack on you but as a reflection of their pain.

- Try to avoid being either too babying or too harsh toward your loved one. Remember they are not doing this on purpose and are suffering just as you are. Gently encourage them to function in spite of the pain and to do as much as possible for themselves.
- Look for support wherever you can find it. If there is a support group for loved ones of patients with pain, join it (or start one if there isn't already one). Don't isolate yourself from friends and family. Participate in your church, synagogue, mosque, or other religious or spiritual organization. If prayer (or chanting or meditation) is helpful, keep doing it.

Learn as much as you can about your family member's condition and the available medical and other treatment options, and discuss them with your loved one when he or she is ready to talk about them.

Remember, this is a family problem, not just an individual one. Try to see it as one that you face all together , "we" — not "he" or "she" — will fight this together.

The following sections (5 to 13) present some questions you may have about your loved one's pain.

## 5. IS IT ALL IN THEIR HEADS?

Chronic pain is rarely imaginary (psychogenic) or simply a way for your loved one's psychological problems to come out. However, negative emotions such as depressed mood, anger, or anxiety can play an important role in making pain worse. For example, anxiety or anger can cause an increase in muscle tension leading to more pain. Post-Traumatic Stress Disorder (PTSD) causes one's nervous system to become very sensitive and can make it harder to recover from a physical injury. Certain types of personalities may find it more difficult to cope with pain and/or the losses and disabilities it brings. For example, many people get their self-esteem from working and cannot tolerate being disabled. This can make it difficult to treat their pain.

## 6. COULD THEY BE FAKING IT, SAY, TO GET OUT OF WORK?

Consciously faking pain to get out of something or to get a reward is known as malingering. While it does occur, it is rare. Most patients will feel very guilty about not being able to do the things they used to do, whether working at a job or doing chores around the house. Very few patients with pain get rewarded financially for their pain. Most suffer severe financial losses. Unconsciously producing symptoms to get rewards or get out of unpleasant things is called "secondary gain." It is rarely the cause of someone's pain, although it sometimes may reinforce a negative situation. For example, someone on disability may fear vocational training because they are afraid to lose the income, in case it doesn't work out if they go back to work at a new job. For some, there may be positive outcomes that make it easier to accept one's situation. However, for most pain patients, the losses far outweigh the gains.

## 7. HOW SHOULD I RESPOND TO MY LOVED ONE WHEN (S)HE'S IN PAIN?

### HOW MUCH SHOULD I DO TO BE HELPFUL?

People in chronic pain seem most helped when those closest express concern for their suffering and offer help that is genuinely needed, along with encouragement for them to be as active as possible. Don't overdo sympathy or try to remove all obstacles and challenges from someone in pain. On the other hand, don't punish the pain sufferer by blame and hostility. If you are not sure how best to be helpful, you might ask the person in pain what kind of attention (s)he feels is most helpful and respectful. There are a number of signs that you can look for. The following are some important ones.

## 8. HOW CAN I TELL HOW HE OR SHE IS DOING?

Are they able to communicate? Can they speak clearly and audibly and does what they say make sense? Are they aware of where they are, who they are, and what day it is? Are they able to stay focused and to remember things? Problems with memory and concentration may indicate depressed mood or medication side effects. Not knowing where or who they are, and what day it is, is known as disorientation. It is a serious symptom and should be discussed immediately with the patient's physician. Are they sleeping at night for the right number of hours? Sleeping too much or too little may indicate depression or anxiety. Insomnia can also result from being in a lot of pain. Has their appetite increased or decreased, or have they gained or lost weight? This can also be a sign of depression.

Weight gain may also result from taking certain medications and/or a reduction in activity. Do they appear depressed? Do they look sad or do they seem "slowed down"? Are they frequently grimacing, crying, groaning, or otherwise indicating extreme distress? Do they appear anxious or irritable? Have they maintained their relationships with family and friends or have they become withdrawn? Have they increased use of tobacco or alcohol? Are they overusing prescription drugs? Do they appear 'out of it' or intoxicated? Are they using street drugs of any kind, including marijuana, cocaine, or amphetamines (speed)? If the answer to any of the above is "yes," these concerns should be discussed with the patient's physician and, if he or she is seeing one, their therapist.

## 9. WHAT TREATMENTS ARE THERE FOR CHRONIC PAIN?

There are numerous medical and other treatments which can help patients with pain live happier and more productive lives. Sometimes complete pain relief can't be reached, but reducing suffering and increasing a patient's functioning can almost always be accomplished. As a loved one of a patient with pain, you need to be aware of these to help your loved one get the appropriate treatment. As every patient is different, this information is not meant as medical advice, but to give you a sense of the range of treatments.

Let's start with medications. There are many medications which can be helpful in making your loved one's pain more tolerable. You and your loved one should be aware of both common and serious side effects from any medication being taken.

**NSAIDs:** For mild to moderate pain and inflammation, a non-steroidal anti-inflammatory Drug (NSAID) may be recommended. This includes over-the-counter medicines like aspirin, Advil and Motrin (forms of ibuprofen) and prescription drugs like Rufen (ibuprofen), Toradol (ketorolac), Naprosyn (naproxen), and Inderol (indomethacin) as well as many others. Tylenol (acetaminophen) operates on pain like a non-steroidal anti-inflammatory, but does not reduce inflammation.

**Narcotics:** For more severe pain, narcotics (opioids) are often prescribed. These include drugs such as hydrocodone (Vicodin), morphine, hydromorphone (Dilaudid), and oxycodone (as in oxycontin). Narcotics may be short acting (taken every 4-6 hours) or longer acting (12-24 hours). They may be in the form of a patch put on the skin, such as Fentanyl in the Duragesic patch. A non-opiate which works much like narcotics is tramadol (Ultram) which is also available combined with acetaminophen (Ultracet).

**Antidepressants:** Some medications used to treat depression are useful to help with pain, and 2 types of antidepressants are most effective. These are the tricyclic antidepressants, including Elavil (amitriptyline) and Pamelor (nortriptyline); and the dual-action antidepressants, including Effexor (venlaxafine) and Cymbalta (duloxetine). Another class of commonly prescribed antidepressants, the SSRI's (Selective Serotonin Reuptake Inhibitors) are generally less effective in treating pain, but they may work for some people. Examples include Prozac, Zoloft, Paxil, Celexa, and Lexapro. Antidepressants are helpful in treating the depression that patients with pain may develop, but they treat pain even without accompanying depression.

**Anticonvulsants:** Medications used to treat seizure disorders may be used in treating pain, especially nerve pain. They include Neurontin (gabapentin), Tegretol (carbamazepine), and Topamax (topirimate).

**Others:** Other drugs used to treat pain include muscle relaxants like Soma (carisoprodol) and Flexeril (cyclobenzaprine). Medication to help improve sleep is often used, as patients with pain often have difficulty sleeping. These include Ambien and Lunesta. In addition to oral medication, patients may use creams on the skin.

Procedural interventions can also be useful to decrease pain. For example, patients may receive injections, including trigger point injections or spinal injections such as nerve root blocks and facet blocks. Anesthetic and/or steroidal medication may be used in injections. Radiofrequency procedures can sometimes provide longer-term benefits than steroid injections.

## 10. WILL MY LOVED ONE GET ADDICTED TO HIS OR HER MEDICATIONS?

Many patients with pain and their families worry about addiction to medication. Much, although not all, of this concern is the result of confusion about the meaning of terms like "addiction," "dependency," and "tolerance." The American Pain Society's definitions are paraphrased below.

**Addiction:** Addiction is a disease with genetic, psychological, social, and environmental factors influencing its development and symptoms. It consists of behaviors such as poor control over drug use, compulsive use, continued use despite harm, and craving.

**Physical Dependence:** Physical dependence is when the body is used to a certain medication or drug, and withdrawal symptoms occur when the drug is stopped or decreased in dose.

**Tolerance:** Tolerance means that the body gets less effect from a certain dose of a medication or drug, or needs a higher dosage to get the same effect.

In other words, addiction always involves abuse of a substance. Physical dependence and tolerance do not. If your loved one uses narcotics or benzodiazepines (e.g. Ativan or Klonopin) regularly, they may become dependent and may develop tolerance for them. By themselves, these are not signs of addiction. If your loved one is not abusing the medication, notice whether or not the medication is improving his or her functioning. Can they do more? Are they more cheerful? These are signs of appropriate use of medication. Patients who are not getting adequate relief may complain and demand more medication — this may look like the behaviour of an addict. This is sometimes called "pseudo-addiction." So how can you tell real addiction? If your loved one repeatedly says (s)he has lost prescriptions, gets the same medication prescribed by different doctors, gets prescriptions filled in different pharmacies, or gets medication off the streets — all to get more medication than is prescribed — then this may be addiction and needs to be discussed with the doctor.

## 11. WHAT QUESTIONS DO I NEED TO ASK THE DOCTOR?

You should go with your family member to the doctor at times and understand what the overall treatment plan is. Ask the doctor what medications are prescribed, in what dosages, and how often. You should also ask what the medication does (for example relieve pain, combat depression, help with sleep, etc.), what the possible side effects are, and how you will know if your loved one is taking too much or too little? A doctor (or physical therapist) can also help you understand what the appropriate level of activity is for your loved one, given his or her physical limitations.

## 12. WHAT ELSE HELPS BESIDES MEDICATION?

Many other techniques have been found helpful with pain. Physical therapy includes exercise and other treatments. Exercises can focus on strengthening, flexibility, and aerobic or cardiovascular functioning and must be tailored to the individual to be effective. Other treatments include heat, cold, Transcutaneous Electrical Nerve Stimulation (TENS), ultrasound, and massage.

Assistive devices like braces, canes, telephone headsets, and orthotics can help reduce pain. So can making adjustments in seating arrangements at home or work. Adjusting the placement of computer keyboards, for example, can help reduce repetitive strain injuries.

Surgery is an option when it can address a specific cause of the pain. For example, some individuals with herniated discs or spinal instability may need spinal fusions (fusing vertebrae together) or discectomies (removal of the disc). Less invasive surgical options are now available to help stabilize the spine without undergoing a formal fusion. Surgery may also be used to implant pain-relieving devices such as dorsal column stimulators or spinal medication pumps. Patients' and families' coping strategies are important determinants of successful outcomes in these surgeries, and psychological evaluation is generally important to maximize non-medical coping strategies and chances for the success of the proposed implants. In addition to spinal surgery, other surgery may be indicated to relieve nerve compression (in the wrist or elbow, for example).

Alternative medicine includes a wide variety of approaches which can be helpful to many patients including chiropractic, acupuncture, the use of herbal and other nutritional supplements, traditional techniques including yoga, Tai Chi, qigong and many more. These should be seen as working with — and not as opposed to — medical treatments, and their use should be discussed with the physician. (Many herbs, for example, can interact with medications.)

Psychological interventions can also be very helpful for many patients with pain. Therapists help individuals change negative thinking styles and behaviours. This is especially crucial if the patient with pain has developed significant emotional disturbances. These interventions may also help with decreasing pain or increasing the patient's tolerance for pain through "mind-body" techniques including hypnosis, meditation, biofeedback, guided imagery, progressive muscle relaxation, breathing techniques, and other relaxation approaches. Additionally, they may help the patient identify and stick to an appropriate activity schedule.

## 13. HOW DO I COMMUNICATE WITH MY FAMILY MEMBER?

(Adapted from Mark Grant, "10 Tips for Communicating with a Person Suffering from Chronic Pain" at www.overcomingpain.com.)

**Listen.** Pay attention not only to what your loved one is saying, but to their nonverbal communication and how they're saying it. They may be reluctant to talk about how they feel but give indications in their behaviour.

**Be genuine.** Don't pretend to be interested in their feelings if you're not.

**Believe.** Accept that their pain is whatever they say it is. Don't tell them it can't be that bad.

**Accentuate the positive.** Repeat and summarize what they say and ask questions that show you're interested. Avoid hurtful comments like "You'll just have to live with it." Ask questions which help patients get in touch with their strengths, like "What helps you get through this?"

Remember the idea of positive reinforcement; when your loved one acts in a more positive manner, reinforce this with praise and attention. When they act more aggressively, don't pay too much attention. Acknowledge they feel bad and wait for an opportunity to reinforce the positive.

**Be aware of your nonverbal communication.** Remember that you can also communicate rejection, not only through the words you choose but also by how you say them — your tone of voice and volume, for example. You also communicate by facial expression (frowns, sneers, gestures, putting hands up to indicate "enough!"), and by eye contact (looking away).

## 14. CONCLUSION

We hope the information in this handout will be useful. Remember, dealing with severe pain can be overwhelming for both patients and those who care for them. This handout is not intended to substitute for the expertise of a professional when needed. Before the burden becomes too great, speak with a professional therapist — psychologist, clinical social worker, or psychiatrist — with experience in the field of pain management. The more involved you get, the less helpless you will feel!

**David Kannerstein,** PhD is a psychologist in private practice with Margolis Berman Byrne Health Psychology in Philadelphia and SRI Psychological Services in Jenkintown, Pa. He specializes in helping individuals and their families manage chronic pain as well as people with mood disorders, anxiety, and trauma-related conditions. He also is a coach whose focus is helping people identify their career goals, manage stress and conflict, achieve greater satisfaction, and reach their full potential in their personal and professional lives. He can be reached at dkanner@comcast.net

Sarah Whitman, MD is a psychiatrist in private practice in Philadelphia, specializing in chronic pain. She is a Clinical Assistant Professor in Psychiatry at Drexel University College of Medicine in Philadelphia. She can be reached at Sarah.Whitman@drexelmed.edu

# LETTER TO MY CHILD

Lucie Moisan, St-Eustache, Quebec, Canada

(See pages 136 and 348 for other testimonials.)

Ever since the moment you were conceived, you have been a ray of sunshine in my life, an endless source of happiness. You were, you are and you will always be a part of my life and nothing, and no one can change the bond that ties us.

Even if the days are getting more and more difficult, I want you to know that I love you. A mother's love, the love I offer you, is unconditional love. Don't be afraid of me; take the time to discover and appreciate what I can give you. I know that sometimes it's not easy, and that there are days when you need me. Unfortunately, my physical and psychological pain prevents me from being as attentive to your needs as I would like to be. There are days when I feel bad because I'm not strong enough to deal with my suffering. But I'm there. I know that my distress and my anger against this disease upset you and affects you at the same time, since you often suffer its consequences. But, believe me, it has nothing to do with you, and I often regret my attitude towards pain. All I ask is that you give me the chance to prove that you can trust me. I will always be there, concerned for you, and I want to be with you through all the moments of your life. I want to help you during the difficult times, and watch you grow up. Sometimes, life is filled with stumbling blocks. However, I will always be there to support you, to listen to you, or just to be there. The important thing is that I will always give you my time since there is nothing more valuable. Let me offer you the warmth of my arms, the tenderness of my caresses, and the love of my heart. Please, I beg you, never turn your back on me. Accept my love, let me watch over you and share your life. My shoulders are broad enough and strong enough to support your sorrow, my ears are attentive enough to respect your silence, and my mouth is respectful enough to abstain from making any noise.

But you must give me a little time because I have to fight. I will need your love as well. Don't be angry at me. Please understand me, instead. I humbly ask you to help me make my way through this tunnel of trials while hoping that, together, we will be able to see the light at the end of it.

I love you with all my heart.

Mom

# MOOD DISORDERS AND CHRONIC PAIN:
## WHEN PAIN IS SYNONYMOUS WITH UNHAPPINESS...

## 22

Guylène Cloutier MD, psychiatrist, Rouyn-Noranda, Quebec, Canada

## ABSTRACT

The psychiatrist plays an important role within the inter-disciplinary team that treats pain. The phenomenon of chronic pain is associated with several central and peripheral neurotransmission systems that are also involved in psychiatric disorders. Naturally, psychiatrists are interested in pain, and have contributed to evaluating and treating it. They have also been called on by their colleagues, both general practitioners and specialists, to reflect on certain ethical and moral dilemmas faced by individuals suffering from chronic pain.

**Depression strikes randomly:
it's a disease, not a mood.**
  Tahar Ben Jelloun

Translation of an extract from
*L'auberge des pauvres*

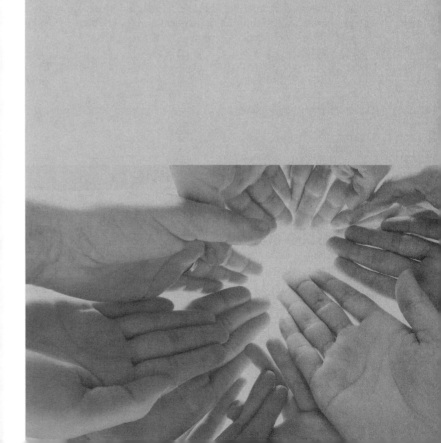

## 1. THE ROLE OF THE PSYCHIATRIST WITHIN A PAIN CLINIC

The psychiatrist plays an important role within the interdisciplinary team that treats pain. He uses a rigorous medical approach so as to make a diagnosis and propose treatment. He is the expert that confirms the existence of a mood disorder, an anxiety disorder, a somatoform disorder or any other psychiatric illness.

## 2. CHRONIC PAIN AND DEPRESSION: THE CHICKEN OR THE EGG?

Pain is a sensation that plays a role in survival when it is acute. When this sensation extends over a long period of time, regardless of whether the cause can be identified and treated, it becomes chronic pain. This condition is a predisposing factor for depression. Approximately 40%-60% of individuals with chronic pain will suffer a major depression. Depression itself also brings with it pain, pain that is not only moral but also physical.

For several years now, although the symptom of pain is not a diagnostic criterion for major depression, researchers have agreed that pain symptoms (headaches, back pain, musculoskeletal pain, muscular tension, heartburn, etc.) can be part of a mood disorder in about 60% to 85% of cases. Some people have criticized the diagnostic criteria of the *Diagnostic and Statistical Manual of Mental Disorders* (DSM-IV-Tr) for giving psychological criteria priority over somatic criteria. Not only are these types of pain part of the clinical table, but the treatment of this disease can occasionally lead to the complete resolution, or at least the alleviation of this category of symptoms.

Depression and pain have a complex and reciprocal relationship. Each of these conditions aggravates the severity of the other. Pain is an obstacle to the achievement of remission in the patient who suffers from a depressive episode. Depression accentuates an individual's pain. This overlapping of pain and depression demonstrates the need for combined and simultaneous treatment of both medical conditions.

## 3. DEPRESSION: A CHARACTER WEAKNESS?

Depression is a disease that is still too often tainted with shame. In Canada, in 2002, 4.8% of the population suffered from a major depressive disorder. One person out of five will suffer from depression during the course of their life. Depression does not strike randomly: clearly identified risk factors can predispose us to develop this medical condition.

**The presence of chronic pain increases the risk of developing a major depression. A major depression can be qualified as mild, but it will still require pharmacological treatment or psychotherapy. Left untreated, it modifies the neurobiological structure of the brain and causes emotional, physical and/or cognitive symptoms that are occasionally irreversible if they persist for several years.**

Fortunately, major depression, which is treated early and effectively, can occasionally be healed completely. This is one of the reasons why we must continue to demand better access to first-, second-, and third-line care. People suffering from depression and those around them tend to find a multitude of reasons to account for the presence of depressive symptoms: "You have to understand, she's just lost her job." – "Her daughter is very ill." – "He's suffering so much; I'd be depressed too if I were in his shoes." – "He just has to push a little." – "She likes to wallow in her unhappiness."

Depression must be treated as early as possible to prevent it from becoming chronic.

## 4. TREATING MAJOR DEPRESSION

Several chronic painful conditions are being treated more and more effectively. Certain types of chronic pain, combined with a mood disorder or a functional somatic syndrome, have not been characterized as well and are occasionally attributed, at least partially, to faking or exaggeration on the part of the patient. If the treatment is to succeed, the health professional and the patient must have the same understanding of the clinical picture.

Therapeutic partnership is an essential condition and is based on the quality of the dialogue between the care-giver and the patient.

Several therapeutic models can be chosen for treating a mild or moderate depression. Commonsense is always appropriate and good personal health practices will possibly lead to a prompt recovery. It is often necessary and essential to add other therapeutic means, such as a pharmacological treatment or psychotherapy, or a combination of these means of treatment.

Medication includes antidepressants of various classes. Several of these antidepressants are also used to treat painful conditions that are not necessarily associated with depression. As mentioned earlier, these various conditions probably share common psychopathological mechanisms.

Along the same lines, psychotherapy also plays an essential role. Psychotherapy must focus on change and not only on giving meaning to an individual's difficulties. Cognitive and behavioural interventions have been studied most often.

## 5. CRITICAL CONCLUSION

Some people have wanted to believe that major depression was a lack of courage, or that depression was a failure, a reflection of your inability to adapt to a painful condition. This is not so. Depression is not a synonym of weakness. Depression is a disease that can have lasting effects, and can also recur if it is not treated in time. Depression is contagious: the spouses and children of those who suffer from depression are more at risk of becoming depressed themselves. Depression can result in death, either your own or that of your loved ones (15% risk of successful suicide). Depression must be treated, whatever its cause.

### ISABELLE'S STORY

Isabelle's life was complicated. Since she hurt everywhere for several months, her family physician diagnosed a possible fibromyalgia. She was referred to us by her neurologist, who was no longer able to treat her migraines. When we met her for the first time, she had just lost her job, her spouse had been diagnosed with cancer and she had two demanding teenagers. She no longer thought she could find a new job at the age of 42. The unpaid bills were piling up. She suffered from horrific migraines that did not respond to migraine medication. She had to go to the ER at least three to four times every month to receive intravenous medication to relieve her migraines. She had been irritable and difficult to live with for several months, and had had a conflict at work, which resulted in her dismissal. She could no longer sleep, was constantly lacking energy, and was openly thinking about ending it all whenever she found herself behind the wheel of her car and saw a truck coming in the opposite direction.

We diagnosed a major depression. She had already had depression twice in the past, one during a post-partum period, from which she had never really recovered, since no one had considered that diagnosis. By starting on antidepressants and recovering her ability to sleep, she was able to eliminate all of these symptoms and continue her university training in accounting. Her spouse went into remission from his cancer. Isabelle found a new job. Her migraines disappeared almost completely, and she now treats them at home. She will have to continue taking an antidepressant for several years if she wants to avoid a relapse.

### MICHAEL'S STORY

Michael is 48 years old. He had a work accident in 2000 which left him with lower back pain that became increasingly serious and chronic. He had to stop work for several years. His work was essentially physical. He valued his ability to support for his family. Feeling useless and finding it difficult to put up with his pain despite treatment with powerful pharmaceuticals, he soon developed suicidal ideas. He did not want to live with his reduced capacities, unable to empty his dishwasher, at the mercy of the weather and snowstorms, barely able to take long trips to visit his grandchildren.

He went to the ER to seek help for his depressive condition (a courageous exploit for a man). He was sad and had felt powerless for several weeks. He felt tired, did not feel like doing anything, and did not feel like laughing. He found it hard to concentrate when watching a TV show or having a conversation. His sleep was disturbed, by both the pain and an inability to sleep in, waking up in the early hours of the morning. His wife was no longer able to encourage him, and make him see that the future would be better.

Michael was convinced that the pain would kill him.

Michael suffered from a persistent psychiatric and painful condition. After seven years of treatment, he still suffered a great deal. Nevertheless, he recently realized that after he stopped taking antidepressants, he was much less able to tolerate his condition. As a result, he started taking the antidepressants again, and was able to continue working. Michael is a very courageous man.

# REFERENCES

· CME Institute. Academic Highlights, Depression and Pain. J Clin Psychiatry, 69: Décembre 2008: 1970-1978.

· Fava, M. Somatic symptoms, depression, and antidepressant treatment. J Clin Psychiatry, 2002; 63: 305-307.

· Gameroff, MJ & M. Olfson. Major depressive disorder, somatic pain, and health care costs in an urban primary care practice. J Clin Psychiatry, 2006; 67: 1232-1239.

· Graziono, O. & R. Bernabei. Association between pain and depression among older adults in Europe: Results from the aged in home care (AdHOC) project: a cross-sectional study. J Clin Psychiatry, 2005; 66: 982-988.

· Lee, P. & M. Dossenbach. Frequency of painful physical symptoms with major depressive disorder in Asia: Relationship with disease severity and quality of life. J Clin Psychiatry 2009; 70: 83-91.

· Ohayon, MM. Specific characteristics of the pain/depression association in the general population. J Clin Psychiatry, 2004; 65 (suppl 12): 5-9.

· Stahl, SM. Stahls'essential psychopharmacology, Neuroscientific basis and practical applications. Cambridge University Press, Third Edition, 2008.

· Workman, EA, JR Hubbard & BL Felker. Comorbid psychiatric disorders and predictors of pain management success in patients with chronic pain. Primary Care Companion, J Clin Psychiatry, 2002; 4: 137-140.

· Zimmerman, M., JB McGlischey, MA Posternack, M. Friedman., D. Boerescu & M. Attiullah. Differences between minimally depressed patients who do and do not consider themselves to be in remission. J Clin Psychiatry, 2005; 66: 1134-1138.

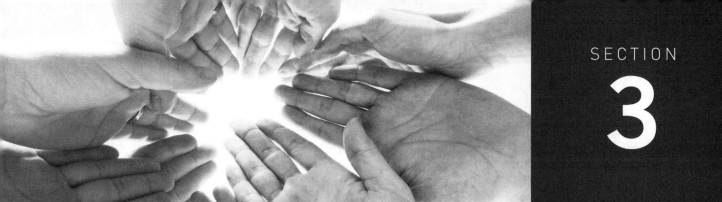

# TREATMENT OPTIONS
# AND PAIN MANAGEMENT

# SMART MANAGEMENT
## OF YOUR CAPACITIES

**Jacques Charest** PhD, psychologist, Rouyn-Noranda, Quebec, Canada
**Dat-Nhut Nguyen** MD, anaesthesiologist, Rouyn-Noranda, Quebec, Canada

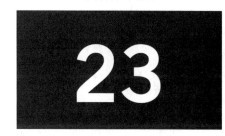

**23**

## ABSTRACT

Continuing to manage your capacities in the same manner as before will merely increase your pain and fatigue. In order to improve your painful condition, you must act differently: modify certain habits and change the way in which you perform certain movements or accomplish tasks.

To help you do this, this chapter proposes several means, organized around five strategies. These strategies are based on the two following premises: your pain is real and elastic; and you are the sole expert when it comes to evaluating your pain. By practising on a regular basis these strategies to manage your capacities, you will discover your own way in which to act differently.

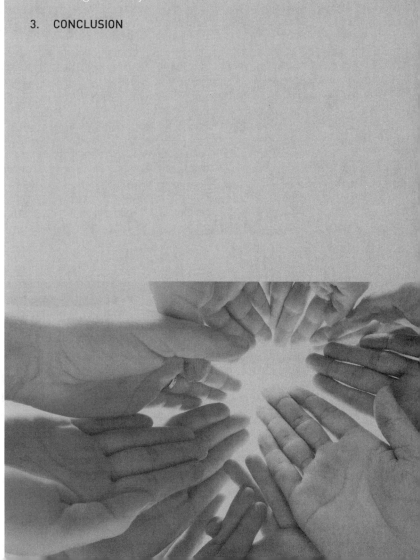

A chronic health problem often creates an imbalance between what we want to do and what we can do. What we want to do is ruled by our will. What we can do is ruled by our real physical capacity. For a person without loss of capacity, «will» and «capacity» balance out in a natural way. For example, we don't run up the steps all the way from the ground floor to the 5th floor. Rather, we will progress up the stairs, slowing our cadence as needed, thus maintaining balance between our will to go to the 5th floor and our capacity to do so. When a loss of capacity occurs, the adjustment between will and capacity is not automatic. We often continue to want to act like before, even if our body cannot do so any longer.

Unfortunately, the more we persist in acting the same way as before the loss of capacity, the more the pain and fatigue will increase and reduce the capacity that we still have. It is as if we are caught up in a vicious circle: as soon as there is finally a day with little or no pain, we try to make up for lost time by doubling our efforts, continuing into the evening. This one day of intense activity is inevitably followed by several days of exhaustion. Sometimes, our capacity is diminished to the point that we must go to bed. Then, after a few days of forced bed rest, the discomfort decreases until another day without much pain appears then, the cycle, starting with intense activity, begins again. Continuing this pattern of managing our capacities increases fatigue and pain, leading invariably to a total halt. Going from relapse to relapse has dramatic repercussions for us, our loved ones, and our colleagues. The joy of living and physical capacity are greatly affected by chronic pain[2, 22].

Fortunately, we can gradually increase our capacities, even the most diminished ones, by their smart management. In the pages that follow, five strategies for the smart management of our capacities, as well as the two important underlying premises, are presented.

## 1. BASIC PREMISES

The smart management of your capacities has a single goal: learning to self-manage chronic pain, or to put it more simply, learning to **act differently** in the face of chronic pain. This new way of acting is accomplished by applying the five strategies described in this chapter. Underlying this smart management of your capacities are two basic premises.

**Basic Premises**
1. Your chronic pain is at the same time real and elastic.
2. You are the sole expert of the evaluation of your pain.

### First Premise: Your chronic pain is at the same time real and elastic.

Healthcare professionals receive little training regarding the difference between acute and chronic pain.[1] Moreover, not so very long ago, for your acute or chronic pain to be considered believable, it had to be directly proportional to the nature and the extent of tissue damage. Thus, some healthcare professionals could explain to you that they believe that your chronic pain is imaginary or «caused either by unresolved tissue damage or by psychological disorder».[20] Such explanations can lead to mutual misunderstanding or to your conviction of their incompetence. However, new technologies, like magnetic resonance, show without a shadow of a doubt that chronic pain is indeed real.[23] In other words, your chronic pain is not imaginary.

In addition, your pain is elastic in the sense that the perception of pain varies. Indeed, science now supports the fact that the brain plays a major role in the perception of pain. Your brain can, for example, ward off painful impulses by releasing endorphins. These natural sedatives temporarily block pain transmission by a mechanism called «diffuse inhibiting control».

Research also shows that the perception of pain is influenced by such factors as your expectations[11], stress[9], perception of pain as threatening[17], emotions[4], attention[13], social exclusion[19], sex hormones[10], satisfaction with the information provided by your doctor[12], and the context[21].

As we will see in the next section, the smart management of your capacities act upon several of the above factors influencing the elasticity of your pain.

### Second Premise: You are the sole expert of the evaluation of your pain.

The second premise at the base of the smart management of your capacities is that **you are the only one able to evaluate your own pain**. Pain is defined as a subjective experience or «an unpleasant emotional and sensory experience associated with a real or potential tissue lesion or described according to such a lesion».[16] This means that you remain the sole expert able to find the movements and postures which do not trigger your pain. However, to be the only expert is not enough. You also need to be sure of the reliability of your pain evaluation.

For example, the level of improvement or relief is often evaluated by comparing current pain with pain experienced before any treatment. However, research studies confirm that **the memory of pain is not reliable**. On one hand, it is difficult to remember the precise level of symptoms beyond a few days and, on the other hand, pain experiences tend to become exaggerated in our memory.[3] To counteract this situation, you should always evaluate your current pain, without comparing it to past pain. You can use a numerical scale from 0 (no pain) to 10 (the worst possible pain imaginable).

However, the most reliable pain evaluation tool proves to be the Visual Analogue Scale or VAS. Placing a simple mark on the line of the scale indicates your level of pain at any specific times.

At each extremity of the scale, two descriptors guide the evaluation of pain: left, no pain and right, worst possible pain imaginable. Evaluate your pain's intensity first, then the unpleasant aspect of that pain. The evaluation of each aspect of pain is not necessarily the same. For example, for labour pains, the intensity clearly exceeds the unpleasant aspect; for a slap, the unpleasant aspect overrides the intensity of the pain; and for a crushed finger, evaluation of both aspects is similar.[5] In addition, both aspects of pain vary from one day to the next or over time on a given day.[27] It is preferable to evaluate pain at home, every two hours during three days (consecutive or not), at the beginning and the end of any treatment for which you want to evaluate the impact on pain. An example of a daily sheet of VAS is shown in **Figure 1**. Make copies of this one, to measure your pain over time.

**FIGURE 1** : Visual Analogue Scale or VAS

Examples of visual scales

**NUMERICAL SCALE FOR ASSESSING PAIN AND DISTRESS THAT ACCOMPANIES (0 -10)**

| No pain | | | | | Severe pain | | | | Intolerable pain |
|---|---|---|---|---|---|---|---|---|---|
| 0 | 1 | 2 | 3 | 4 | 5 | 6 | 7 | 8 | 9 | 10 |

**VISUAL ANALOGUE SCALE (VAS) 10 CM**

No pain ——————————————————————————— The worst possible pain

| INTENSITY OF PAIN | | UNPLEASANTNESS OF PAIN | |
|---|---|---|---|
| No pain | Worst possible pain | Not unpleasant | Most unpleasant pain imaginable |
| 10 p.m. | ................................................ | 10 p.m. | ................................................ |
| 8 p.m. | ................................................ | 8 p.m. | ................................................ |
| 6 p.m. | ................................................ | 6 p.m. | ................................................ |
| 4 p.m. | ................................................ | 4 p.m. | ................................................ |
| 2 p.m. | ................................................ | 2 p.m. | ................................................ |
| Noon | ................................................ | Noon | ................................................ |
| 10 a.m. | ................................................ | 10 a.m. | ................................................ |
| 8 a.m. | ................................................ | 8 a.m. | ................................................ |
| 6 a.m. | ................................................ | 6 a.m. | ................................................ |
| 4 a.m. | ................................................ | 4 a.m. | ................................................ |
| 2 a.m. | ................................................ | 2 a.m. | ................................................ |
| Midnight | ................................................ | Midnight | ................................................ |

Name : ————————————————————— Date : —————————————————————

These two basic premises also underlie our group interventions for chronic pain (called Interactional Schools). The results obtained up to now with various types of chronic pain are very encouraging. For example, the Interactional School of Low Back Pain (ISLBP) has proven to be an effective group treatment for severe chronic low back pain.[6] The detailed description of the steps, as well as the educational materials required, for applying the ISLBP are described in detail in a book written specifically on the subject.[5] Moreover, all the program information is available for free on the low back pain clinic web site at http://ecoledudos.uqat.ca (in French and Chinese). A similar group intervention was developed for fibromyalgia. The Interactional School of Fibromyalgia (ISF) produced major short-term and long-term (one year follow-up) clinical improvements with fibromyalgia patients.[25,26] In addition, the preliminary results of our Interactional School of Neck Pain and in our Interactional School of Chronic Abdominal Pain are equally promising. These schools have demonstrated the efficacy of strategies for managing capacities in the context of chronic pain, of which five are described in **Table 2**.

## 2. STRATEGIES FOR THE SMART MANAGEMENT OF YOUR CAPACITIES:
Find your own way of acting differently

TABLE 2: Strategies for managing your capacities

| | |
|---|---|
| **1. REFUSE, ACCEPT, OR DELEGATE A TASK** | A. "Saying no, is saying yes to me!"<br>B. Prioritizing and planning<br>C. Delegating tasks and accepting the consequences |
| **2. AIM FOR A MINIMAL GOAL** | Looking for the first signs of improvement |
| **3. CHANGE THE MEANING OF YOUR PAIN** | Giving a non threatening meaning to pain |
| **4. BREATHE PEACEFULY** | Mastering abdominal breathing (in 6 steps) |
| **5. MOVE DIFFERENTLY** | A. Find your Neutral Zone<br>B. «Going around» your pain |

### STRATEGY 1: REFUSE, ACCEPT, OR DELEGATE A TASK

#### A. "Saying no, is saying yes to me!"
A smart strategy for managing your capacities is to exercise control by **refusing, accepting or delegating tasks**. Most of the time, we refuse a task by simply saying "no". However, it can be very difficult to say "no" because we feel guilty. One of the participants of an intervention group shared a great trick. When faced with a request, she simply repeats the following sentence to herself: «**Saying no, is saying yes to me!**» Using this sentence will perhaps help alleviate any guilt feelings and, thus, help you refuse the task. You may word your refusal in various ways, for example: "Sorry, I've done my share of work." "Sorry, I don't have time to do it.» You can also give yourself time to "sleep on it" by simply saying «I will think about it and give you my answer tomorrow.» Finally, it may be easier to say "no", if you give yourself the right to reassess your decision and change your mind if need be.

#### B. Prioritizing and planning
If you accept a task, remember the followings two points:
- **Prioritize**. If you could accomplish only one task today, which one would you choose? Begin with the task you like the least or the one you prefer. If you have energy for more, vary the number and type of tasks. Remain flexible in your choices by always granting yourself the right to change the order of your priorities.
- **Plan breaks**. Sometimes, we can invest ourselves so much in a task that we even forget to eat. One patient shared her solution with us: before beginning a task that is likely to monopolize all her attention, she sets a timer to make sure she takes a break from time to time.

#### C. Delegating tasks and accepting the consequences
Another way of dealing with a task is to **delegate it to another person**. First of all, this involves previously identifying your available alternative resources. Next, you must accept that the task may be done differently. This sounds easy but it may be very difficult for some. For example, if you decide with your spouse that he will now have the task of emptying the dishwasher, you must accept the fact that dishes and cutlery may be arranged in a different way in the cupboards. If you don't accept that things will be done differently, conflicts will likely come up and the task will be even more tiresome. In sum, either you delegate without supervising or you do it yourself.

## STRATEGY 2: AIM FOR A MINIMAL GOAL

### Looking for the first signs of improvement

Aiming for a minimal goal consists primarily of looking for the first signs of an improvement that justifies, in your eyes, the efforts required to incorporate into your daily life these strategies or any other treatment, for that matter. In other words, you have reached the minimal goal if your condition starts to improve. By definition, the minimal goal is still a far cry from the total relief of symptoms. This particular way of setting a goal can raise a question: **"Why aim for a minimal goal if I am looking for total relief of my pain?"**

Several facts justify the advantages of aiming for a minimal goal. On the one hand, from a clinical point of view, to achieve (or exceed) a goal is always gratifying, no matter how small it may be. On the other hand, not achieving a goal (because it was set too high) always remains disappointing even though a minimal improvement was achieved. In addition, from a scientific point of view, it has been proven that a strong will to relieve pain actually increases a person's distress and vigilance to pain.[8] In fact, a simple increase in the desire for pain relief (induced by using hypnotic suggestions) significantly increases the unpleasant aspect of the pain.[24] Thus, by decreasing the desire for pain relief, aiming for a minimal change eliminates the pain increase associated with intense efforts to reduce it. Well before the establishment of these facts, Paul Watzlawick, internationally known as one of the founders of strategic interactional therapy, had already advocated the same point: «one should never aim at the complete, total solution of a problem, but only at its improvement or lessening; for instance, that [we] feel *less* pain, or that [we] will sleep a *little* longer, or that this discomfort [...], will be tolerable.»[28]

Here are some examples of the minimal goals set by group intervention participants. A patient, currently experiencing continuous back pain, set this minimal goal for the end of the treatment: «to go for half a day per week with little or no back pain».

Another patient, who had stopped playing with his young children for fear of increasing his pain, wants to play with them again. His minimal goal: "not to be afraid to play with my children two evenings a week". Another patient with back pain is currently unable to travel 100 km in his car without having to stop three to five times to relieve his back pain. His minimal goal is: "to be able to travel by car to a city located at approximately 100 km in having to stop not more than once because of back pain".

Here are other examples of minimal goals chosen by patients with fibromyalgia. At the beginning of treatment, a patient considers her energy level to be very low. On a scale of 1 (the lowest energy level you can imagine) to 10 (the highest energy level you can imagine), she evaluates her energy level at 1. She chooses a goal of 2.5 on this scale by the end of the treatment. Another patient with fibromyalgia wishes to improve the quality of her sleep without using any medications. She evaluates her current quality of sleep at 4 on a scale from 1 (the lowest quality of sleep you can imagine) to 10 (the highest quality of sleep you can imagine). She aims for a sleep quality level of 6 by the end of the treatment.

In sum, to aim for a minimal goal makes it possible to avoid the increase in distress which invariably happens when we seek total relief of our pain. More importantly, this strategy ensures success which, in turn, builds your confidence in your ability to self-manage your pain.

## STRATEGY 3: CHANGE THE MEANING OF YOUR PAIN

### Giving a non-threatening meaning to pain

**Can the meaning you give to pain affect your tolerance to pain?**

An interesting experimental study showed for the first time that the meaning you give to pain affects not only your tolerance to this pain but also affects your loved ones' attempts to encourage you.[17] The experiment was done in a laboratory environment. The tolerance to pain was measured by a cold-water-immersion test. This test consists of immersing one's arm in a basin filled with very cold water (2° C) for the longest possible time. During the test, each individual is accompanied by a trusted person who verbally encourages the individual to maintain his or her arm in the cold water for as long as possible by using the following coping strategies.

**Diverting attention**: The accompanying person tries to distract the partner by inviting him or her to speak about a past pleasant experience or to hum a song in his or her head.
**Reinterpreting**: The accompanying person suggests to the partner to think of the sensations as a dull warm feeling rather than pain.
**Ignoring**: The accompanying person suggests that the partner ignore the pain.

### The experiment

At the beginning, the partners and the accompanying persons read an instruction describing the uses and security of the cold-water-immersion test that gives either a reassuring or threatening meaning to the pain resulting from the immersion. The instructions are the same except in the threatening condition a passage describing the symptoms of frostbite have been added: feelings of tingling, numbness, reduced mobility and, in serious cases, the skin turning blue, gangrene and amputation. This instruction thus gives a threatening meaning to the pain resulting from the immersion. The partners and the accompanying persons do not necessarily have the same instructions.

Three aspects of the results are pertinent here. First, giving a reassuring meaning to pain makes it much easier to tolerate. The partners tested under the reassuring condition maintained their arm in cold water a little more than three minutes, on average, whereas those under the threatening condition barely exceeded two minutes. Secondly, the support of the accompanying person is modified according to the meaning he or she gives to the pain. Under the reassuring condition, the accompanying person spontaneously uses coping strategies to help the partner increase tolerance to pain, which is not the case in the threatening condition. Third, the conversation between the accompanying person and the partner is focused on pain if, and only if, it is perceived as threatening by both the accompanying person and the partner.

This study leads to an important practical implication: giving a reassuring meaning to pain increases both your pain tolerance and the support from your entourage. In turn, higher pain tolerance makes maintaining healthy activities possible. For example, imagine that each painful sensation means to you that muscular or tissue damage is occurring (threatening meaning). You will rapidly and drastically reduce your movement to avoid worsening the damage or interrupting the healing process. However, this reaction – logical in light of your meaning of the pain – in fact maintains the problem because restricting movement inevitably worsens the initial pain.

To avoid such counterproductive actions, you and your entourage need to give a reassuring meaning to your pain, like "this pain is due to body dysfunction not affected by movement".[7] This could raise your pain tolerance sufficiently to continue moderate physical activity.

## STRATEGY 4: BREATHE PEACEFULLY

Pain can prevent us from living in the present moment. When we are in pain, we tend to project ourselves into the future (for example, when hoping for relief dominates all our thoughts) or into the past (for example, when we continually think of the past causes - real or hypothetical - of our pain). The smart management of your capacities requires centring on the present moment in order to modulate your pain and stress. Peaceful (abdominal) breathing is a powerful tool for this.

Breathing is part of every second of our lives. It changes according to our needs, moods and social interactions. For example, watching a sleeping child calms our own breathing, while facing an angry "pumped up" person accelerates our breathing. In addition, pain and breathing are closely interrelated. When an individual is injured, he takes a deep breath, blocks his breathing and grimaces. His breathing then becomes short and shallow, muscle tension is at a maximum. Once the danger or the shock has passed, the individual calms down and his breathing becomes more peaceful, the muscles relax and pain decreases. This story has a good ending. However, in another situation, if an individual continues to feel his health or physical integrity in danger, the muscles remain tense, short and shallow breathing persists, and pain is maintained. In this kind of situation, learning to relax your muscles and return to peaceful breathing helps to modulate pain.

Three types of breathing are most frequent: stressed, effort, and abdominal (peaceful).

- *Stressed breathing* (**Figure 2**, third image) communicates our state of stress to our entourage and prepares us for confrontation or escape. It occurs primarily in the upper part of the chest and in the shoulders, characterized by a shallow inhalation, exhalation, followed by a shallow inhalation, exhalation, and so on. If this type of breathing persists over a long time, it can provoke hyperventilation, with dizzy spells, numbness and heart palpitations, feeling a lack of air, as well as pain in the neck and shoulders.
- *Effort breathing* (**Figure 2**, second image) occurs during physical effort where simultaneously, the heart rate accelerates, the muscles warm up, and the skin perspires. It takes place in both the belly and chest, characterized by a deep inhalation, exhalation, followed directly by another deep inhalation, exhalation, and so on.
- *Abdominal breathing* is associated with peaceful rest. It takes place primarily in the abdomen (belly) area; this is why it's called "abdominal breathing". As illustrated in **Figure 2** (first image), your diaphragm descends downward into your abdomen – swelling your abdomen slightly – when you fill your lungs with an inhalation while relaxing your abdominal muscles. Abdominal breathing includes a brief pause after exhalation and before inhalation, thus characterized by a cycle of inhalation, exhalation, pause, then inhalation, exhalation, pause, and so on. Rediscovering natural and peaceful breathing is an important tool to modulate your pain and stress, so important that the next few pages are devoted to a description of the six steps to mastering abdominal breathing.

FIGURE 2 : Three types of breathing: abdominal breathing, effort breathing, stressed breathing

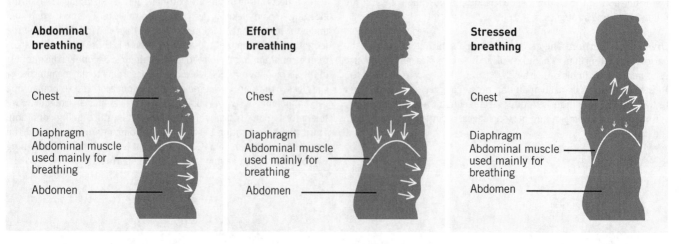

## Mastering abdominal breathing (in 6 steps)

It is important to take the time to master each step presented here before going to the next, even if this means practising more days than indicated. However, notwithstanding the number of days you take to learn each exercise, be sure to take one day per week "vacation" from practising.

### 1st Step: Observing Yourself

Lie down comfortably. Put one hand on your abdomen below the navel and the other hand on your chest at the breast level. Relax for a few minutes, and then observe how your hands move in rhythm with your breathing. Observe that during inhalation (breathing in), the belly (or the chest) inflates and the respectively placed hand rises. During exhalation (breathing out), the abdomen (or the chest) empties and the respectively placed hand lowers. Pause a brief moment after exhalation, before you take the next inhalation. Observe now the cycle inhalation-exhalation-pause, inhalation-exhalation-pause, and so on.

**Practice: 5 minutes, once a day, 3 days consecutive if possible.**

### 2nd Step: Directing the air toward your abdomen

Lie down comfortably. Place one hand on your abdomen below the navel and the other hand on your chest at the breast level. Relax for a few minutes, and then at each inhalation, direct the air towards the abdomen as if it were a balloon, filling up with air every time you breathe in. This image of a balloon filling with air will help you relax your abdominal muscles sufficiently to allow your diaphragm to descend into your abdomen so that it swells slightly "like a balloon" (see **Figure 2**, first image). Note that you may have to go through a period of trial and error before discovering how to relax certain abdominal muscles in order to allow abdominal breathing. The hand placed on your abdomen will perceive more inflation than the other hand. Then, simply let the air out of your lungs. Pause for a second before inhaling, starting thereby another cycle of inhalation, exhalation, pause. Observe the movement of your body (your hands on your chest and abdomen) while you continue to repeat this type of breathing.

**Practice: for 5 minutes, once a day, for 6 days.**

### 3rd Step: Restoring abdominal breathing

The purpose of this third step is to restore natural, spontaneous abdominal breathing, what your body easily does when relaxed. This step is similar to the previous one, but this time you do not deliberately inhale after the pause. Instead, you wait until your body starts the inhalation. This step may seem difficult at first if you have the impression that you will lack air. Rest assured, however, that your body will inhale spontaneously when it lacks oxygen. Lie down comfortably. Relax a few minutes, observing your breathing: inhalation-exhalation-pause, inhalation-exhalation-pause, and so on. When you feel ready, do not intentionally start the next inhalation. **Wait until your body inhales spontaneously**, and then go back to your usual inhalation-exhalation-pause cycle for several breaths.

Start by doing this exercise with one breath. Then, when you feel ready, let your body inhale by itself for 2 breaths and then for 3 breaths – until you can observe that your body is naturally breathing abdominally, without effort.

Note: This is a good exercise when you are stressed or in pain in order to restore abdominal breathing.

**Practice: for 5 minutes, once a day, for 6 days.**

### 4th Step: Integrating abdominal breathing in a sitting position

This step is similar to the preceding steps 2nd and 3rd, only this time you are in a sitting position. Sit comfortably, place one hand on your abdomen below the navel and the other hand on your chest at the breast level. Relax for a few minutes. Then, at each inhalation, direct air towards the belly, relaxing your abdominal muscles sufficiently to allow your diaphragm to descend into your abdomen so that it swells slightly "like a balloon". Note that you may have to go through a period of trial and error before discovering how to relax certain abdominal muscles in a sitting position to allow abdominal breathing.

Observe your breathing for one minute: inhalation-exhalation-pause, inhalation-exhalation-pause, and so on. When you feel ready, do not intentionally start the next inhalation (like in the 3rd step). Wait until your body inhales spontaneously.

Start by doing this exercise with one breath, then 2 breaths, then 3 – until you can observe that your body is naturally breathing abdominally in a sitting position.

**Practice: for 5 minutes, once a day, for 6 days.**

## 5th Step: Integrating abdominal breathing in a standing position

This step is similar to the preceding steps, only this time you are standing upright. Place one hand on your abdomen below the navel and the other hand on your chest at the breast level. Relax for a few minutes. Then, at each inhalation, direct air towards the abdomen, relaxing your abdominal muscles sufficiently to allow your diaphragm to descend into your abdomen so that it swells slightly "like a balloon". Note that you may have to go through a period of trial and error before discovering how to relax certain abdominal muscles while standing upright to allow abdominal breathing.

Observe your breathing for one minute: inhalation-exhalation-pause, inhalation-exhalation-pause, and so on. When you feel ready, do not intentionally start the next inhalation (like in the 3rd step). Wait until your body inhales spontaneously.

Start by doing this exercise with one breath, then 2 breaths, then 3 – until you can observe that your body is naturally breathing abdominally while standing upright.

**Practice: for 5 minutes, once a day, for 6 days.**

## 6th Step: Integrating abdominal breathing when walking

This step is to practice when walking, the abdominal breathing you have learned in the prior steps. First, relax while standing in an upright position, until you are using abdominal breathing. Then, start walking as you usually do. After two minutes, observe how you are breathing.

Gradually incorporate your abdominal breathing as you walk. Combining walking and abdominal breathing is a very challenging feat. Keep at it!

**Practice:  Once a day for one minute.**

## STRATEGY 5: MOVING DIFFERENTLY

People living with chronic pain move (direct their body through space) with less precision; their movements are jerkier; they experience creaks, blockages and balance problems. This is related to subtle losses of tactile sensitivity and of motor skills produced by chronic pain.[18] Over time, these losses lead to the following pernicious effects.

· People with chronic pain take painful and stationary positions, often and for long periods of time.[14] In addition, they injure themselves repeatedly because they make certain mistakes in their muscle contraction sequence and their stabilization sequence.[15] Unfortunately, they don't know this, and thus, they keep on moving in the same way, again and again, even though it is more and more painful.

· There is only one possible way to avoid repetitive injuries due to the subtle losses of sensitivity and of motor skills: **moving differently**. Acquiring the following two skills will change your way of moving: finding your neutral zone and «going around» your pain.

### A. Finding your neutral zone

The neutral zone is that position of your body in which you feel the most comfort, the least pain, the best alignment and balance. Being able to find your neutral zone will help you avoid the pernicious effects of

your chronic pain, mentioned above. The exercise described in **Figure 3** takes you through the steps required to discover your neutral zone, to feel your body moving slowly and to precisely perceive the sensations of tension, pain, comfort and alignment. **Figure 3** describes specifically the neutral zone of the pelvis. However, even if your chronic pain is in your neck, it is still important that you are able to find the neutral zone of your pelvis, as it will balance your whole body. You can then apply the same steps to your neck or other part of your body that is in pain. Once you know how to subtly move your body to find your neutral zone, practice finding it when sitting, standing, and walking.

The goal is to integrate into your daily life the neutral zone. So that **finding the neutral zone** becomes automatic, here is a good trick. Put a round red sticker on 20 different objects in your environment that you see or use every day. For example: place a red sticker on the refrigerator, the mirror of your room or bathroom, the front door, the filing cabinet, the remote control of the TV, etc. These stickers act as "exercise alarms". As soon as you see a red sticker, find your neutral zone once. These sticker "alarms" ensure the 50 daily repetitions of this new skill which, once automatic, will help you move differently.

FIGURE 3: Steps to finding your neutral zone

1. **Lie down** on your back, on a firm surface, with your knees bent and your feet flat on the floor. Take several abdominal breaths.

   **Note:** During the entire exercise, use the least muscular force possible and keep your abdominal muscles relaxed. The objective of this exercise is the mastery of subtle movements and sensations. If it is done correctly, the exercise should be comfortable from the beginning to the end.

   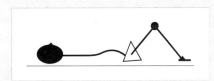

2. **Rock your pelvis up**, gently and slowly, while slightly pressing your feet on the floor. This subtle movement will flatten the curve of your lower back against the floor (second image). Then, push the curve of your lower back into the floor by slightly contracting your abdominal muscles (third image).

   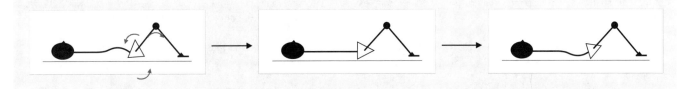

3. **Rock your pelvis down**, gently and slowly, while releasing any contraction of your abdominal muscles which will flatten the curve of your lower back against the floor (second image). Then, put less weight on your feet without taking them off the floor and curve your lower back away from the floor (third image).

   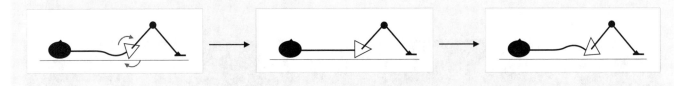

4. **Find the neutral zone.** Your neutral zone is that position of your pelvis which is the most comfortable or the least painful. In your neutral zone, you will feel your lower back and pelvis in alignment, well balanced, at ease. You are the only expert able to find your neutral zone.

5. **Repeat slowly** the entire exercise, 10 times, while keeping your attention on your pelvis as it rocks up, and then as it rocks down, passing through the neutral zone. Identify each time, as precisely as you can, your neutral zone. Remain in your neutral zone as long as necessary for you to perfectly memorize the comfortable sensation.

## B. «Going around» your pain

To avoid the pernicious effects of your chronic pain, described above, you must make subtle movements continually like, for example, moving every 10 or 20 minutes and frequently changing positions. Here are a few tricks: set a timer to ring every 15 minutes, placed so that you have to get up to turn it off and reset it; sit on an exercise ball or on the end of your chair so you must move subtly and frequently to keep your balance.

You must also look for ways to move without pain, without any blockage, jerking or cracking. This implies looking for ways to "go around your pain" in your daily movements. It is like, when walking in the forest you find an enormous tree fallen across your path and instead of labouring to cut and move it or instead of abandoning your walk, you simply go around it and continue on your way.

Here are several exercises that show you how to "go around" shoulder pain, back pain and elbow pain (epicondylitis).

---

**Exercise 1:** Going around your shoulder pain

This exercise explains how to bring your hand to your head by going around your shoulder pain (refer to **Figure 4**).

- Lie on your back and, with subtle movements, find the neutral zone for your shoulder pain (a position where your shoulder is in less pain, is more comfortable).

- Slowly seek the sequence of movements that allow you a pain-free way of bringing your hand to your head, with no blocking, jerking or cracking.

- If your movement causes any pain or blocking, stop and go back to your neutral zone and try a different movement. For example, move your arm more to the left or more to the right; keep your arm closer to your body or further away from your body, etc.

- Looking for ways of "going around» pain involves much trial and error and many dead ends; but if you keep trying, you will find ways of moving with no pain, no blocking, jerking or cracking.

- Once you have found your way of going around your shoulder pain, practice the movements often to remember them well.

- Next, practice your movements for going around your pain while in a different position, such as sitting, standing, lying at a 30° or 45° angle.

FIGURE 4: Finding how to move without pain (arm movement)

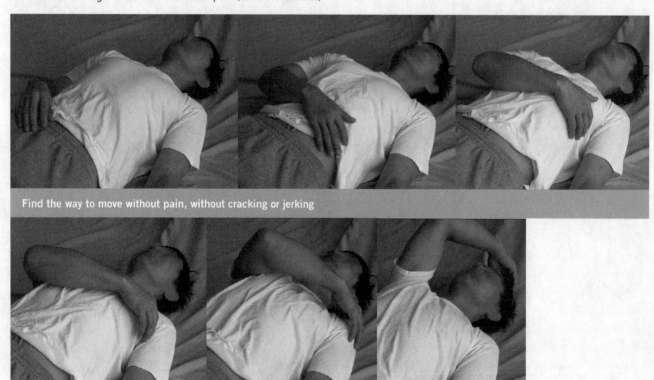

Find the way to move without pain, without cracking or jerking

## Exercice 2: Going around your back pain

This exercise explains how to turn over in bed by going around your back pain (refer to **Figure 5**).

- Lie down on your back and, with subtle movements, find the neutral zone for your back pain (as in **Figure 3**).

- Slowly seek the sequence of movements that allow you a pain-free way of turning over in your bed with no blocking, jerking or cracking.

- If your movement causes any pain or blocking, stop and go back to your neutral zone and try a different movement. For example: move your pelvis more to the left or more to the right, accentuate the curve in your lower back, reduce the curve in your lower back, etc.

- Looking for ways of "going around» pain involves much trial and error and many dead ends; but if you keep trying, you will find ways of moving with no pain, no blocking, jerking or cracking.

- Once you have found your way of going around your back pain, practice the movements often to remember them well.

- Next, practice the movements for going around your back pain as you go from a lying position to sitting, then from a sitting to a standing position, and then while taking some steps.

FIGURE 5: Turning around without pain

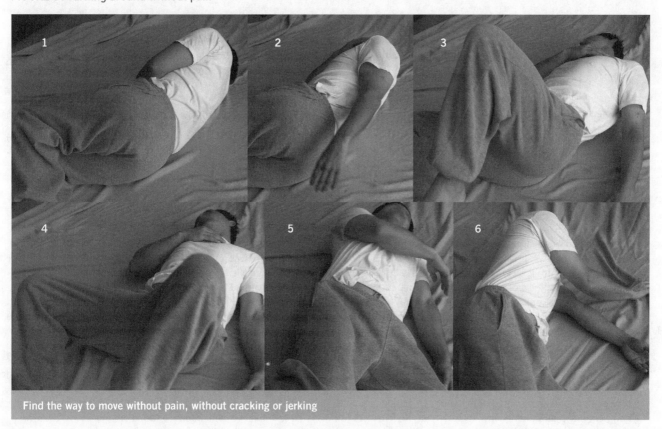

Find the way to move without pain, without cracking or jerking

**Exercice 3:** Going around your elbow pain (epicondylitis)

This exercise, in three steps, explains how to achieve everyday movements by going around your elbow pain.

- Hold a small apple in the hand on the side of your elbow pain. Try different ways of holding the apple, for example: palm upwards, downwards or at an angle; elbow close to the body or far away from the body, etc. Check which position is the most comfortable and painless (neutral zone). Learn how to pick up or to put down the apple on a table in a flexible, comfortable and painless way.

  **Practise: 5 minutes a day for 3 days.**

- Do the same exercise with objects a little heavier or a bit more cumbersome (cup of coffee, small tool, etc). Always look for a better way to making the movement.

  **Practise: 5 minutes a day for 3 days.**

- Slowly try going around your pain in order to do everyday movements such as opening a gate, taking a bag, turning the ignition key of a car. Always pay careful attention to your movement as if it was the most important movement of the day.

## 3. CONCLUSION

- **Your pain is real and elastic.**

- **You are the sole expert of the evaluation of your pain.**

To continue managing your chronic pain in the same old way only increases your pain and fatigue. You must act differently by applying the strategies described in this chapter: refuse, accept or delegate tasks, aim for a minimal goal, change the meaning of your pain, breath peacefully, and move differently. Remember also that you are the sole expert able to find the ways of going around your pain. Through the regular practice of these strategies, you will discover your own way of doing things differently; you will attain the smart management of your capacities.

## REFERENCES

1. Ali, N. & Thomson, D. (2008). A comparison of the knowledge of chronic pain and its management between final year physiotherapy and medical students. European Journal of Pain, 13, p. 38-50

2. Baune, B. T., Caniato, R. N., Garcia-Alcaraz, M. A., & Berger, K. (2008). Combined effects of major depression, pain and somatic disorders on general functioning in the general adult population. Pain, 138, p. 310-317.

3. Broderick, J. E., Schwartz, J. E., Vikingstad, G., Pribbernow, M., Grossman, S., & Stone, A. A. (2008). The accuracy of pain and fatigue items across different reporting periods. Pain, 139, p. 146-157.

4. Bruehl, S., Burns, J. W., Chung, O. Y., & Quartana, P. (2008). Anger management style and emotional reactivity to noxious stimuli among chronic pain patients and healthy controls: The role of endogenous opioids. Health Psychology, 27, p. 204-214.

5. Charest, J., Chenard, J. R., Lavignolle, B., & Marchand, S. (1996). Lombalgie: École interactionnelle du dos. Paris: Masson.

6. Charest, J., Lavignolle, B., Chenard, J. R., Provencher, M., & Marchand, S. (1994). École interactionnelle du dos. Rhumatologie, 46, p. 221-237.

7. Daniel, H. C., Narewska, J., Serpell, M., Hoggart, B., Johnson, R., & Rice, A. S. (2008). Comparison of psychological and physical function in neuropathic pain and nociceptive pain: implications for cognitive behavioral pain management programs. European Journal of Pain, 12, p. 731-741.

8. Eccleston, C. & Crombez, G. (2007). Worry and chronic pain: a misdirected problem solving model. Pain, 132, p. 233-236.

9. Finestone, H. M., Alfeeli, A., & Fisher, W. A. (2008). Stress-induced physiologic changes as a basis for the biopsychosocial model of chronic musculoskeletal pain: a new theory? Clinical Journal of Pain, 24, p. 767-775.

10. Gaumond, I. & Marchand, S. (2006). La douleur est-elle sexiste? Mécanismes endogènes et hormones sexuelles. Médecine/Sciences, 22, p .901-903.

11. Goffaux, P., Redmond, W. J., Rainville, P., & Marchand, S. (2007). Descending analgesia-when the spine echoes what the brain expects. Pain, 130, p. 137-143.

12. Hadjistavropoulos, H. & Shymkiw, J. (2007). Predicting readiness to self-manage pain. Clinical Journal of Pain, 23, p. 259-266.

13. Hasenbring, M. (2000). Attentional control of pain and the process of chronification. Progress in Brain Research, 129, p. 525-534.

14. Haugstad, G. K., Haugstad, T. S., Kirste, U. M., Leganger, S., Wojniusz, S., Klemmetsen, I., & Malt, U. F. (2006). Posture, movement patterns, and body awareness in women with chronic pelvic pain. Journal of Psychosomatic Research, 61, p. 637-644.

15. Hodges, P. W. & Moseley, G. L. (2003). Pain and motor control of the lumbopelvic region: effect and possible mechanisms. Journal of Electromyography and Kinesiology, 13, p. 361-370.

16. International Association for the Study of Pain (1979). Pain terms: A list definitions and notes on usage. Pain, 6, p. 249-252.

17. Jackson, T., Huang, X., Chen, H., & Phillips, H. (2008). Effects of threatening information on interpersonal responses to pain. Eur.J.Pain, doi:10.1016/j.ejpain.2008.05.012, European Journal of Pain, 13, p. 431-438

18. Johnston, V., Jimmieson, N. L., Jull, G., & Souvlis, T. (2008). Quantitative sensory measures distinguish office workers with varying levels of neck pain and disability. Pain, 137, p. 257-265.

19. Macdonald, G. & Leary, M. R. (2005). Why does social exclusion hurt? The relationship between social and physical pain. Psychological Bulletin, 131, p. 202-223.

20. Moseley, G. L. (2003). Unraveling the barriers to reconceptualization of the problem in chronic pain: The actual and perceived ability of patients and health professionals to understand the neurophysiology. The Journal of Pain, 4, p. 184-189.

21. Moseley, G. L. & Arntz, A. (2007). The context of a noxious stimulus affects the pain it evokes. Pain, 133, p. 64-71.

22. Murphy, S. L., Smith, D. M., Clauw, D. J., & Alexander, N. B. (2008). The impact of momentary pain and fatigue on physical activity in women with osteoarthritis. Arthritis & Rheumatism, 59, p. 849-856.

23. Owen, D. G., Bureau, Y., Thomas, A. W., Prato, F. S., & St Lawrence, K. S. (2008). Quantification of pain-induced changes in cerebral blood flow by perfusion MRI. Pain, 136, p. 85-96.

24. Rainville, P., Bao, Q. V., & Chrétien, P. (2005). Pain-related emotions modulate experimental pain perception and autonomic responses. Pain, 118, p. 306-318.

25. Barcellos de Souza, J., Bourgault, P., Charest, J., & Marchand, S. (2008). Escola Inter-relacional de Fibromialgia: Aprendendo a lidar com a dor - Estudo clinico randomizado [Interactional School of Fibromyalgia: Learning to cope with pain - a randomized controlled study]. Revista Brasileira de Reumatologia, 48, p. 218-225.

26. Barcellos de Souza, J., Charest, J., & Marchand, S. (2007). École interactionnelle de fibromyalgie: description et évaluation. Douleur et analgésie, 20, p. 213-218.

27. Straub, R. H. & Cutolo, M. (2007). Circadian rhythms in rheumatoid arthritis: implications for pathophysiology and therapeutic management. Arthritis & Rheumatism, 56, p. 399-408.

28. Watzlawick, P. (1980). Le langage du changement. Paris: Seuil.

# ON COPING

Janice Sumpton, RPh, BSc Phm, London, Ontario, Canada

(See other testimonials, pages 222 and 358. See chapter 31 page 247.)

As a result of the frustrations linked to fibromyalgia, and with time, I have learned different coping skills, which help me to do the best I can. I rely on my family and friends to be understanding, especially when I need reminding to look after myself and take a rest. My family is very good at reading my irritability barometer, and they tell me to sit down when I continue to do more than my body allows. I am only a patient when I am at a medical appointment.

Accepting assistance, while very hard to do, can be very beneficial. Learning to ask people for help is very difficult too, especially because I am an independent person. I am still struggling to learn this skill even though I know the benefits. Asking people to help with chores will save me energy to do an activity that is a pleasure to me.

I have coped by reading and attending conferences to learn everything I can about fibromyalgia and chronic pain. Knowledge is power. I have written articles in peer-reviewed journals and web-based modules, and given lectures to physicians and healthcare professionals on chronic pain. This helps me by using my skills as a pharmacist to advocate, increase acceptance and expand the knowledge of healthcare professionals.

I became a support group leader to persons with fibromyalgia. This allows me to pass along knowledge to them and provide a network where we can support each other. I recently was appointed to the Board of Directors of the Canadian Pain Coalition (See Chapter 43), which gives me another way to help fellow Canadians suffering with chronic pain.

Letting others know that I have chronic pain and fibromyalgia is a difficult and huge step. How much information I share depends on my comfort level. Becoming more public with my chronic pain, fatigue and thinking challenges helped me to cope. It was a load off my shoulders. An article about my experience with pain along with my picture appeared in the city newspaper. As a result of the article many people in pain contacted me with their questions. It helped me knowing that I could help them.

I reduced my workweek from five to four days to give me rest time and ability to do activities I wanted to do. Not working every Wednesday gives me breathing space between two workdays. It comes with decreased income and missing things that happen that day at work. But what I gain in physical, mental, and emotional rest is well worth it.

I have learned to pace my activities. It is the best coping tool in my arsenal, but it is the hardest one to do. Pacing allows for rest periods in the day. It requires thinking differently. Everything does not need to be finished in one go. Listening to what my body is telling me (sometimes screaming) is learning how to live differently. Rest more on "bad pain days." On "good pain days" I try not to overextend myself because I pay for it on the following days.

Relaxation techniques help decrease stress and pain. Finding an activity that works for you is most effective. I have found deep breathing to be helpful and it can be done anywhere. Where possible, I remove myself from the situation if the environment is increasing my pain and worsening my cognition.

So that I can accomplish what I need to do in a day, I make a list and refer to it often. There is great satisfaction in crossing something off the list. I always start the list with "make a list" as the first task. Then I can cross something off right away! I have lists at work and at home to keep me focused. I accept that some items on the list may be there for some time.

The therapeutic benefits of my dog help decrease pain and stress! I have had golden retriever dogs for many years and their faithful devotion has helped me cope. The endless love and comfort they give me is tremendous, no matter how much I hurt and how little I have been able to do in a day.

While I had to give up skiing I still have hobbies that relax me and help with the pain. The accomplishment of knitting and the gentle rhythm of the needles and stitches is relaxing. The serenity of my garden, whether I am glancing at its beauty, or working in it on "good days," is rejuvenating. Going for a walk, even a short distance to get fresh air and some exercise, is very helpful. Listening to soothing music is restful and helps me to gear down at the end of the day and have a better sleep. I try to sit down with a cup of tea as soon as I get home from work so I can de-stress. Even 20 minutes helps give me energy for the evening with my family.

I have found some pain medications and sleep medication helpful to decrease my pain and reduce the number of "bad pain days"

After repeated suggestions from family members I got a handicapped parking permit. This has been one of the most helpful aids. I conserve energy and decrease pain by parking closer to the door. After much procrastination I began using a cane to improve my balance and increase my endurance in walking. This has helped my balance and I am not as tired when I get home. I have a few different canes, all of them pretty and in different colour combinations, to match whatever outfit I am wearing.

My coping mantra is: Try to live in the present, think positively and be thankful for those "good pain days." Be kind to yourself.

# CHRONIC PAIN
# **PREVENTION**

**Dat-Nhut Nguyen** MD, anaesthesiologist, Rouyn-Noranda, Quebec, Canada
**Jacques Charest** PhD, psychologist, Rouyn-Noranda, Quebec, Canada

## 24

## ABSTRACT

The purpose of pain is to motivate us to protect the injured part, to indicate the right pace for returning to our activities following an injury, to show us that certain postures, and ways of working injure our body. As a result, striving to constantly improve the work environment, work tools and work procedures is a good strategy for preventing injuries and chronic pain. Proprioception and stabilization are necessary for good musculo-skeletal health. These functions are altered following an injury. Rehabilitating them early stops pain from becoming chronic. Finally, interpersonal relations, work overloads and stress are also serious risk factors for chronic pain. All in all, this chapter presents several means of preventive maintenance for our body, that formidable machine.

Page 200:
**The Workstyle Short Form** was reproduced with the permission of the editor **Oxford University Press**: Michael Feuerstein and Rena A. Nicholas. Development of a short form of the Workstyle measure. Occupational Medicine 2006; 56: 97-98, Published online 15 December 2005 doi: 10.1093/occmed/kqi 197

ABSTRACT
1. INTRODUCTION
2. MECHANISMS OF INJURIES AND HEALING
3. PROPRIOCEPTION AND STABILIZATION DEFICITS
4. PREVENTING THE CHRONICIZATION OF PAIN
5. CONCLUSION

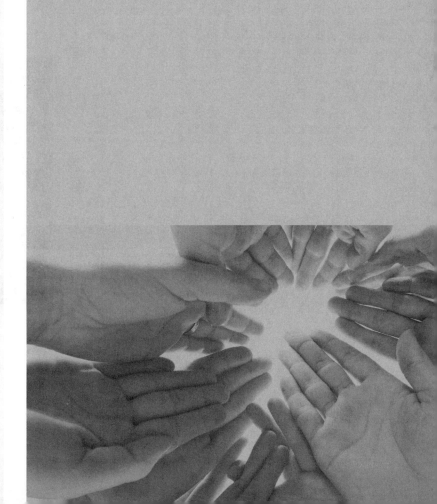

# 1. INTRODUCTION

Walking, moving or picking up an object are simple, ordinary actions for people in good health. Yet, each of these actions involves dozens of muscles that work in a complex activation sequence. It is so complex that current technology still cannot build a robot that is capable of taking a bowl out of a cupboard and serving soup! In addition to my eyes that guide me and my nervous system, which controls all action, I need healthy bones, muscles, joints, tendons and ligaments to perform each of these simple actions. I also need proprioception to feel the movements of each segment of my body and stabilization to position the joint properly during the movement.

Unfortunately, the functioning of this formidable machinery is compromised when an injury occurs, whether it is minor (secondary to small repeated traumas) or major (following a serious trauma). Moreover, actions taken in good faith after that to facilitate healing can, on the contrary, perpetuate the injury and contribute to the development of chronic pain. Such a possibility raises an important question: what can we do to improve our chances of living actively without chronic pain while continuing to do the things we like to do? In the following pages, we will describe several means for preventing the chronicization of pain. These means have grown out of three processes that have been studied in the science of musculo-skeletal injuries, namely **the mechanisms of injuries and healing, proprioception and stabilization deficits, and risk factors at work.**

## KEY CONCEPTS

Proprioception: ability to feel the position and the movements of each segment of the body (position of one hand with respect to the other, for example), accurately and at any moment.

Stabilization: ability to use the small "stabilizing" muscles to position and keep the joints aligned properly during movement.

# 2. MECHANISMS OF INJURIES AND HEALING

All the tissues in our body (muscles, tendons, ligaments, bones) have a certain resistance that enables them to support the **load** imposed by each of our movements. This resistance, however, has a limit called the **breaking point**. An injury occurs when the load is greater than the breaking point.

**Figure 1** illustrates active people who are using their muscles and their tendons regularly and without injury. **Figure 2** represents an individual who is too sedentary and whose inactivity has progressively caused the tendons, muscles and ligaments to deteriorate.

FIGURE 1: Active life without injury

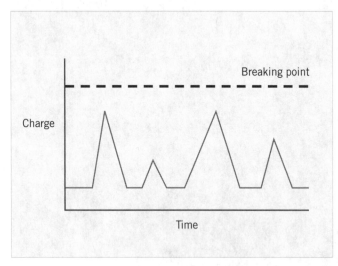

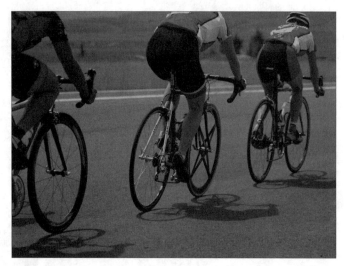

FIGURE 2: Inactive life without injury

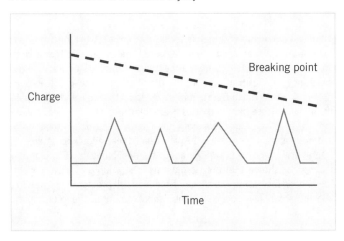

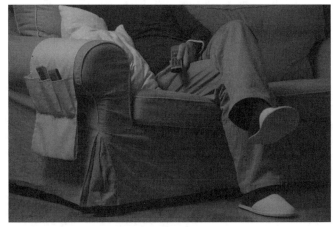

As **Figures 3** and **4** show, an injury occurs as soon as the load exceeds the breaking point. In the case of an individual who leads an inactive life, the breaking point is so low that simply bending over to pick up a box of tissues can cause an injury.

FIGURE 3: An injury occurs when the load exceeds the breaking point in the case of an active individual

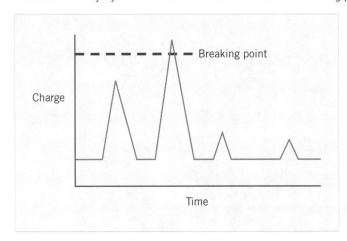

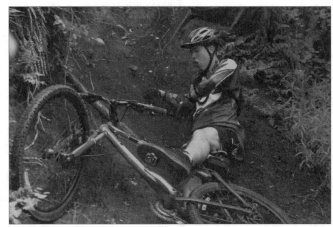

FIGURE 4: An injury occurs when the load (picking up a box of tissues in this case) exceeds the breaking point, which has become very low in the case of an individual who is inactive and out of shape

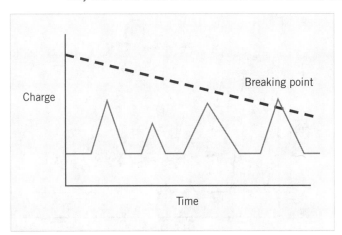

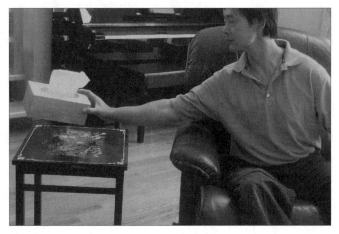

After the injury, the tissues are more fragile and the breaking point decreases significantly. The usual reaction is to slow down and move cautiously so as to protect the injured part. This slowing gives the tissues time to heal as long as the individual returns to normal activities progressively and does not exceed the breaking point (see **Figure 5**).

Sometimes people react differently following an injury, unknowingly contributing to the chronicization of their pain. The most common reactions that interfere with tissue healing result from the two following opposing strategies.[9]

**Endurance coping.** Despite the injury, you feel obliged to continue using your muscles, tendons and ligaments to a significant degree, causing other injuries (**Figure 6**). In this situation, the tissue healing process never catches up with repetitive injuries. The tissues deteriorate more and more. Pain becomes chronic.

**Pain-related fear-avoidance.** Once injured, you take refuge in complete inactivity out of fear of inflicting more pain on yourself. But tissues need movement and action in order to heal. With inactivity, your tissues will deteriorate more and more. You move less and less. The pain becomes chronic.

It is not uncommon for people to use both strategies in the same day. For example, research[10] has demonstrated that people suffering from chronic back pain work *as much* as people without back pain (using the endurance coping strategy). But the distribution of the activities over the course of the day differs significantly. In fact, people with back pain often concentrate their activities in the morning and then, exhausted and suffering, they lie down motionless for long periods of time in the afternoon and evening (using the pain-related fear-avoidance strategy).

In short, current knowledge about the mechanisms of injury and healing has shown that people must use the injured part cautiously. This means increasing the range of movements progressively, finding a pace that will lead to a continuous improvement of the injured part.

FIGURE 5: Following the injury, tissues heal naturally if the individual slows down and returns to his/her usual activities without exceeding the breaking point

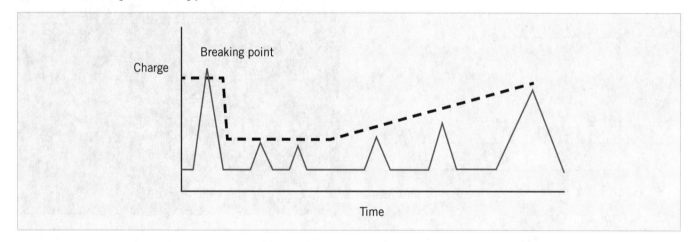

FIGURE 6: Endurance coping

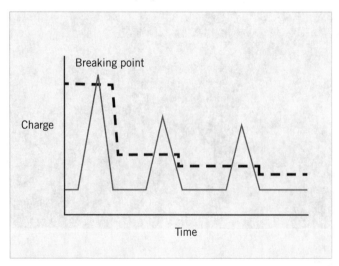

FIGURE 7: Pain-related fear-avoidance

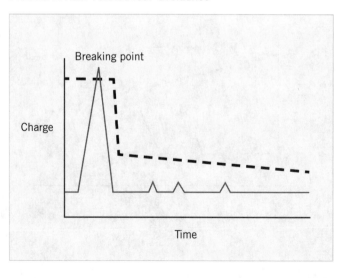

# 3. PROPRIOCEPTION AND STABILIZATION DEFICITS

Following a serious injury such as a herniated disk, people improve slowly with a short-term rest programme, followed by progressive mobilization. After three months, 80% return to their usual activities, with good pain control. For many years, however, these people will continue to experience proprioception and stabilization deficits.[3]

These deficits are evident through small instabilities when moving, cracking and clicking sounds during joint movements, a leg that gives out from time to time, a lack of balance, movements that are less precise and perception of the body in space that is not as adequate (they will brush up against door frames, bump into furniture). As a result of these deficits, these people are more at risk of getting injured again, in the same place or somewhere else in their body. This risk increases even more in the presence of the five following external factors.

1. **Vibrations.** Vibrations interfere with proprioception signals and make stabilization more difficult. Vibrating plates, cars, trucks and airplanes are risks for musculo-skeletal injuries.
2. **Fatigue.** Think about when you are tired, your actions are not as precise, your balance is precarious and you make more mistakes. Many accidents occur when people are tired.
3. **Strong negative emotions (anxiety, anger, a sense of injustice).** In one of his studies, Dr. Moseley asked healthy volunteers to perform simple actions with neutral emotions or strong negative emotions (he criticized them harshly). The strong negative emotions prevented stabilization even for movements as simple as lifting an arm.[7]

4. **Doing several things at the same time.** You know that talking on your cell phone while driving increases the risk of accident. Paying attention to several activities at the same time reduces the quality and the speed of your reflexes. In a similar manner, working "with your mind elsewhere" increases the risk of injury since coordination and stabilization are less precise. You may have already heard stories about people who are able to lift heavy loads but then injure themselves when moving a wastepaper basket. Check with these people. Their minds were probably elsewhere or they were in a rush when the injury occurred.
5. **Medications.** Certain medications have side effects such as drowsiness or reduced attention. They slow your reflexes and reduce your coordination and the precision of your movements. They may cause accidents.

All of the patients we have met in our clinical practice present several of the risk factors listed above: using endurance coping and pain-related fear-avoidance strategies, proprioception and stabilization deficits, and the use of medications that affect their attention and reflexes. Moreover, for most of them, the way in which they work also leads to the chronicization of pain.

## RISK FACTORS AT WORK

A report on musculo-skeletal injuries at work showed that 73% of the workers reported that they suffered from musculo-skeletal pain to varying degrees.[4] This means that most of us have to or will have to deal with a minor injury such as a sprain, a tendinitis, a bursitis and so on. Following this, we usually try to identify the cause: a bad movement or an effort that was too strong or too repetitive. Then, depending on the cause identified, we decide what action to take to improve it and avoid getting injured again. If the first solution does not work, we try another… and then another if the problem persists, including asking for help. Unfortunately, for some people, the injury lasts or is repeated over and over. This report on injuries at work identifies several risk factors that lead to chronic musculo-skeletal pain.

In fact, workers are at risk in each of the following situations.

1. They are dissatisfied with the company's internal communications;
2. They do not play a sufficient role in decisions concerning their own work;
3. They feel that the work load is too heavy;
4. They feel that their salaries are unjust and inequitable;
5. They have personal, family or social problems;
6. They are too conscientious and they want things to be perfect at all times;
7. The speed of their movements at work is rapid or jerky;
8. There are no micro pauses in their movements;
9. Their work is very repetitive;
10. The ergonomics of their workstations are insufficient.

In other words, the way in which you work may contribute to the chronicization of the pain.[6] In this respect, researchers have developed a questionnaire to evaluate your risk of developing or maintaining chronic pain as a result of your work environment.[1] In order to identify your own reactions to the various difficulties encountered at work and determine if changes are necessary, we suggest you take 10 minutes to answer the questionnaire the following pages.

## WORKSTYLE SHORT FORM

The Workstyle Short Form was reproduced with the permission of the editor: Oxford University Press: Michael Feuerstein and Rena A. Nicholas. Development of a short form of the Workstyle measure. Occupational Medicine 2006; 56: 97-98, Published online 15 December 2005 doi: 10.1093/occmed/kqi 197

Please complete the following survey by checking the boxes that describe your experience at work.

PART 1: Rate the degree to which each of the following items describes you at WORK by selecting the appropriate option.

| | ALMOST NEVER | RARELY | SOMETIMES | FREQUENTLY | ALMOST ALWAYS |
|---|---|---|---|---|---|
| **ITEMS TO SUM** | 0 pt | 1 pt | 2 pts | 3 pts | 4 pts |

1. I continue to work with pain and discomfort so that the quality of my work won't suffer.

2. My hands and arms feel tired during the workday.

3. I feel achy when I work at my workstation.

4. Since there is really nothing that I can do about my pain in my hands/arms/shoulders/neck, I just have to work through the pain.

5. There really isn't much I can do to help myself in terms of eliminating or reducing my symptoms in my hands/arms/shoulders/neck.

6. My fingers/wrists/hands/arms (any one or combination) make jerky, quick, sudden movements.

7. I can't take off from work because other people at work will think less of me.

8. I can't take off from work because I'd be letting down or burdening my boss.

9. I can't take off from work because I'd be letting down or burdening my co-workers.

10. I can't take off from work because it will negatively affect myevaluations, promotions and/or job security.

11. If I take time off to take care of my health or to exercise, my co-workers/boss will think less of me.

12. I don't really know where I stand despite all the effort I put into my work.

Rate the degree to which each of the following items describes you at WORK by selecting the appropriate option.

13. The boss doesn't let you forget it if you don't get your work finished.

14. If I bring up problem(s) to my supervisor, like a coworker not pulling his/her weight, it won't make any difference anyway, so I just go ahead and do the work myself.

15. It is frustrating to work for those who don't have the same sense of quality that I do.

16. I have too many deadlines and will never be able to get all my work done.

17. Even if I organize my work so that I can meet deadlines, things change and then I have to work even harder to get my work done on time.

18. My schedule at work is very uncontrollable.

19. I feel pressured when I'm working at my workstation.

20. I push myself and have higher expectations than my supervisor and others that I have to deal with at work.

21. My co-workers don't pull their weight and I have to take up the slack.

22. Others tell me I should slow down and not work so hard.

**SUM FOR QUESTIONS 1 TO 22**

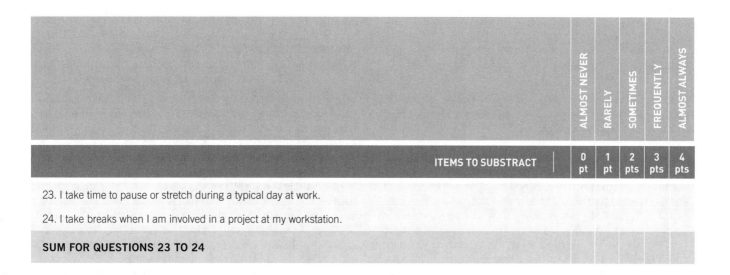

| | | ALMOST NEVER | RARELY | SOMETIMES | FREQUENTLY | ALMOST ALWAYS |
|---|---|---|---|---|---|---|
| **ITEMS TO SUBSTRACT** | | 0 pt | 1 pt | 2 pts | 3 pts | 4 pts |
| 23. I take time to pause or stretch during a typical day at work. | | | | | | |
| 24. I take breaks when I am involved in a project at my workstation. | | | | | | |
| **SUM FOR QUESTIONS 23 TO 24** | | | | | | |

**PART 2: Check all the behaviours/emotions/symptoms that you experience only during periods of high work demands/workload.**

| | PRESENT | ABSENT |
|---|---|---|
| **ITEMS TO SUM** | 1 pt | 0 pt |
| 25. Anger | | |
| 26. Out of control | | |
| 27. Have trouble concentrating/focusing on work | | |
| 28. Depleted/worn-out | | |
| 29. Overwhelmed | | |
| 30. Short fuse/irritable | | |
| 31. Cold feet | | |
| 32. Cold hands | | |
| **SUM FOR QUESTIONS 25 TO 32** | | |

## INTERPRETING THE RESULTS

- Calculate the sum by subtracting the points obtained for Questions 23 and 24.
- A result higher than 28 is of concern. It means that you have a high risk of developing and maintaining chronic pain. Changes may be required in your approach, and the way in which you communicate with colleagues at work, your boss or bosses or your clients. You may need to step back and examine the place that work occupies in your life, and study the possible alternatives.

- Questions 1 to 6 measure your propensity to continue working despite pain. If this is your case, we suggest that you take the time to re-read **Chapter 23**. The information provided later will serve to answer the other elements of this questionnaire: stress at work (Questions 7 to 15); work under pressure (Questions 16 to 19); work pace (Questions 20 to 22); breaks at work (Questions 23 to 24); and too much stress during periods of work overload (Questions 25 to 32).

# 4. PREVENTING THE CHRONICIZATION OF PAIN

We are proposing several steps you can already take on your own. Take the time to examine them and identify those which apply to your situation; they will provide possible solutions for your problem. Four principal categories of means can be used to prevent the chronicization of pain: **stop rules, stress management, ergonomics and biomechanics, and rehabilitation of proprioception and stabilization.**

## STOP RULES

We all have rules for stopping and starting an activity; sometimes we choose them and other times we apply them unknowingly. For example, let us imagine the following situation.

> Ben-I-stop-when-the job-is-done is a good worker. His rule is clear: if he starts something, he stops when the work is finished, namely when he is satisfied with the result. And that works well for Ben. He's proud of being a hard worker, of his performance, of earning a good salary… But recently, Ben got a new boss. The work climate has become difficult, stressful. Too much work, always rushing about, and it's never enough, never good enough. But, remember, Ben stops when he is satisfied with the result. When Ben is frustrated, he is never satisfied with the result and so he doesn't know how to stop. Ben works until he's exhausted every day and then he gets injured. But Ben has never stopped working because of an injury. So, he continues to work, despite his injury… and injures himself more.

This story is intended to illustrate that we are sometimes trapped by our "rule". The rule of "doing as much as I am capable of" or "I stop when the work is finished" works very well when you're in a good mood and everything is going well. However, frustration or a bad mood could lead to overwork, exhaustion and injury. In this respect, according to one of the models of chronic pain, being in a bad mood motivates people to stop or to continue, depending on the stopping rule in effect at a particular time.[11] For example, if "I work as much as I can" (or until I'm

satisfied with the work done), the fact that I am in a bad mood indicates to me that I have not made enough progress and motivates me to work even more. On the other hand, with the rule "I work until I feel like stopping" (or until I'm no longer enjoying the work), the fact that I'm in a bad mood indicates that it is no longer appropriate for me to continue working and motivates me to stop.

Another rule that we often see in the clinic is "I stop when my pain reaches 8 on a scale of 10". This rule is simple, but it has two major inconveniences. First, you only stop when the pain reaches 8 on a scale of 10, which means that you regularly suffer until your pain reaches 7 on a scale of 10. Then, from time to time, you exceed 8 on a scale of 10 and you run the risk of injuring yourself seriously.

The key to protecting yourself involves **remaining flexible** as you pursue your goals. We suggest that you try other rules for stopping that are safer and more comfortable, such as those indicated in the following list.

1. Taking a break every 90 minutes.
2. Changing your position every 15 minutes.
3. Making sure that you are comfortable on a regular basis.
4. Dividing the work to be done into realistic phases.
5. Stopping when you feel tired.
6. Stopping when your movements start to be less precise.
7. Stopping when you start making small "stupid" mistakes.

## STRESS MANAGEMENT

Stress is omnipresent in daily life: criticism from colleagues, too much work, unexpected events, financial problems… When it is managed well, our stress sharpens our reflexes, keeps us alert and vigilant, temporarily increases our energy and our capacities and temporarily reduces the perception of fatigue and pain. But when stress goes on for too long, or becomes too significant, it becomes harmful. It will become obvious through the following signs.

We all already have techniques for managing stress. We would like to explore four means of stress management with you that may possibly help you.

### SIGNS OF SERIOUS STRESS

- Cold hands and feet
- Shaking
- Muscular tension and pain
- Difficulty concentrating
- Sleep disorders
- Tightness in the chest, impression that you can't catch your breath

### a) Reducing the effect of stress on the body

**Physical exercises.** We are all familiar with the benefits of taking a good walk in order to take in some fresh air and admire nature. In fact, all of the activities that make our muscles work, that increase our circulation, our respiration, our heart beat and make us feel hot and sweat for at least 30 minutes reduce the effect of stress on our body: our muscles become more supple, our hands and feet warm up, we sleep better, we breathe better. Practising physical activity regularly and moderately prevents chronic pain. In fact, as shown in **Figure 8**, either too few or too many physical activities increase the risk of chronic back pain.[2]

**Relaxation.** Visualization, meditation, relaxation techniques, relaxation cassettes, Tai Chi, yoga... All of these techniques are intended to regulate respiration, focus the mind, turn your attention inwards, towards the signals of our body. With regular practice, 20 minutes, 3 times per week, the effects are impressive: better control of your heart beat, blood pressure, anger, pain and sleep.

The important thing is to identify the technique that you enjoy, to practice it regularly for one month and then to note the effect it has on your life. Following this, you will be able to decide if long-term practice of the technique is part of your life choice.

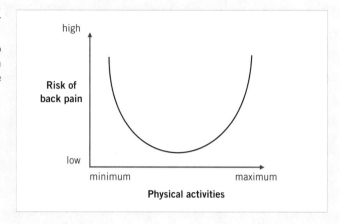

FIGURE 8: There is a U-shaped relationship between chronic back pain and physical activities: only the moderate practice of U-shaped activities reduces the risk of back pain

## b) Acting to resolve the stressful situation

Dealing with criticism from your boss, refusing to do certain jobs that people try to impose on you, re-establishing communication after a family quarrel, negotiating with an organization that does not want to pay you, etc. are all sources of stress. Learning to communicate without making the conflict even more bitter is an effective means for resolving a dispute and stopping the stress at the source. There are many good books on this topic. We suggest the following strategy, which is effective.

• Choose to communicate with the right person, at an opportune time. This may be the person with whom you have the conflict, an individual who can mediate or someone interested in resolving the same conflict. First, prepare your initial communication carefully in writing.

• Start with a positive point. In order to place the person with whom you are communicating in the best possible position, highlight a recent action or accomplishment that you appreciate. A positive point that works is one that is concrete and recent. The positive point must be sincere. It is intended to provoke agreement or a smile on the part of that individual.

• Agree on the event that is causing the problem. Take the time to describe what you saw or heard about the event that is behind the conflict. Check to see if the person with whom you are communicating understood the same thing. As needed, adjust your understanding before proceeding to the next step.

• Express how you feel. At this stage it is important to use the following wording: "I felt ......" and you must make a particular effort not to make accusations. For example, "I felt rejected by you" may be interpreted as an accusation, whereas "I felt as if I were isolated, without any power to act" probably sounds less like an accusation.

• Then, work with the other person to find a solution to the problem together. If you want to read more about this, we suggest you read a short and simple book by Marshal Rosenberg.[8]

## c) Take a step back

Taking a step back from the difficult situation can give you an opportunity to see it from a broader perspective and find other alternatives. To illustrate this, let us take a look at Patrick's story.

Patrick has been growing frustrated over the past few weeks: work is piling up, and his days end later and later. Patrick is exhausted at the end of the day. His neck hurts after he spends long periods immobile. Moreover, his boss keeps bringing him other tasks that can't wait. He has tried to reason with his boss several times, but the answer is always "We have no choice". The tension is rising... In order to have a broader perspective, Patrick looks into the company's situation. He learns that the company is seriously in debt, but sales and orders are good. The boss' attitude is a little easier to understand.

The tension decreases. Working with other employees, Patrick suggests a reorganization of the work to the boss. The employees agree to take on a heavier work load on a temporary basis and to help train new recruits. For his part, the boss agrees to more flexible schedules and the principle of taking back time. Harmony and mutual trust return to the company. Patrick is still working long hours but he is motivated and he is pleased to know that after this difficult period his family and he will lead a pleasant life exempt from financial need.

Taking a step back means you have to set aside your anger and your resentment and try to look at the situation through the eyes of the other (i.e., the target of your anger). To do this, you need to choose to believe that the other individual is a person like you, with work, a family, friends, colleagues, concerns, self-esteem, trying to live comfortably and develop good relationships with others. You can then try to understand why an individual acts in a given way. By proceeding in this manner, you see that the other is no longer an "evil person" who is trying to poison your life. He/she becomes a worker, a parent, a human being with whom you do not agree upon the way in which to resolve the current difficulties. And the tension decreases. And other solutions become obvious.

### d) Letting go

Here is another story.

Marie-Ève is seriously fed up. She had worked so hard on this project. She had given up her weekends and evenings for it. Then, at the last minute, someone else took the credit for this wonderful project and earned a great promotion. Marie-Ève received no sign of acknowledgement. She tries to make people see her point of view; she loses her temper. She cries out against injustice. No one dares to support her in her fight. And every day, every night, she goes over and over the injustice and feeds her desire for vengeance. Moreover, she has financial problems. She's seriously in debt. She bought things recently, thinking she would be promoted soon. She is always tired. She hurts all over and finds it difficult to concentrate. And to top it all off, her boss has criticized her for her bad mood and her recent drop in productivity. One morning, after a night spent crying, Marie-Ève makes a decision. She decides to let go. The past is the past. She can't change anything. She bravely decides to set this episode behind her and return to her life as it was before. Getting up early in the morning, starting the day with a healthy walk, eating a good breakfast, going to work with a smile, taking on each project enthusiastically, talking with her colleagues on a regular basis. Moreover, she now makes sure that her boss is informed about her efforts and her good ideas. Later, she finally gets her promotion.

Sometimes the evil is done and we can no longer go back. Maybe, you have been the victim of injustice. And maybe the injustice has not been repaired, despite all your efforts. The anger and rage were useful in giving you the energy to fight, to make an effort to obtain justice. But if, today, that rage and anger are merely eating you up inside, a possible choice would be to let go, to turn the page and use the experience acquired to build the future. To decide to rebuild as if it were the first time. Like the victims of hurricanes or tsunamis: they have lost everything, they have wept, and they have rolled up their sleeves and rebuilt.

Choosing the right moment to rebuild is difficult. Letting ago is very difficult. But once you have set aside your burden you will feel as if a great weight has been taken from your shoulders. You will feel light. Then you can start to rebuild something else.

## ERGONOMICS AND BIOMECHANICS

Another way to prevent the chronicization of pain, involves either adapting the work environment to your body and your abilities (ergonomics), or using your body in a safe manner in the work environment (biomechanics).

**ERGONOMICS**
Science that studies the optimal and safe way in which to adapt tasks, work environments and machines to the human body. Adapting the tools to the worker and not the worker to the tools

FIGURE 9: Examples of bad and good ergonomics

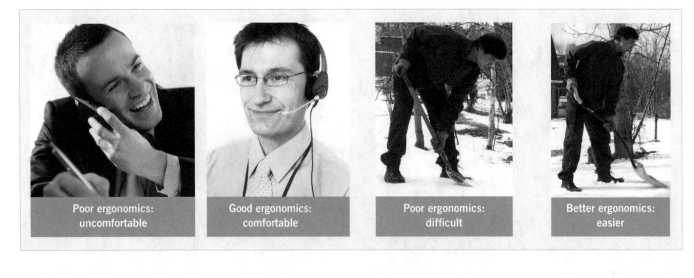

Poor ergonomics: uncomfortable

Good ergonomics: comfortable

Poor ergonomics: difficult

Better ergonomics: easier

Is the activity that caused your injury adapted to your situation? For example, if several people working at the same workstation are injured, perhaps the ergonomics of the workstation should be improved (**Figure 9**). It should be noted that the most effective ergonomic changes are those designed by experienced employees for their own workstation.[5] Here are five steps for introducing an ergonomic change.

**Step 1 – Identify.** Discover the activity, the movement or the action that injures you. Take time to observe in which circumstances that action is painful. What is its purpose?

**Step 2 – Analyze.** Take time to analyze everything surrounding that action. Can you modify the way you do it? Can you change the posture in which you do this action, or the height of the work table, or the position of the tool? Can you add or modify a tool, can you use a lever or a handle in order to make the action more effective, easier and less likely to cause an injury? Can you take small breaks (a few seconds) when you perform the action? Can you make frequent posture changes during your work?

**Step 3 – Plan.** Plan ahead the changes you want to make in your workstation. Discuss it with the other people who are involved in the work or who also perform this action. Their ideas can be useful for improving the workstation.

**Step 4 – Change.** Start to make changes at an opportune time. Select a moment when you can take your time and pay attention when performing the action to be changed so that you can verify if there are other improvements to be made.

**Step 5 – Persevere.** Maintaining the change is a challenge. Find simple and practical ways to remind yourself to perform the action in the improved manner. This might involve placing a sticker on the workstation, or agreeing with your colleagues to watch one another while performing the dangerous action or other related movements.

## BIOMECHANICS

Science that uses physics and mechanics to study the movements of the human body. One of the purposes is to discover optimal and safe ways in which to do movements, in keeping with individual physiognomy. The optimal and safe movement is the one that enables to perform the desired task easily, effectively, without jerkiness and without catching.

Are you suited for the activity that injured you? For example, loggers who have trained for years can carry armloads of wood all day long. But if you are someone who is not used to this type of work, the only way you can keep from injuring yourself is to learn professional techniques, start slowly and increase the loads and the duration progressively. In this manner, you will give yourself time to build up the muscles, the coordination and the techniques needed to work in a safe manner.

Does the movement that hurts or injures respect biomechanical principles? Can your technique be improved? Injuries resulting from repetitive movements are often caused by a deficient technique, or a technique that is poorly adapted to your body. For example, in the case of golfer's tendinitis, a small correction in the starting position can correct the movement that caused a small injury with each swing. In other situations, such as musician's dystonia, the musician must spend long months re-learning the action performed by each finger.

FIGURE 10: Back muscles in a position of strength
This lift respects the biomechanics of the back

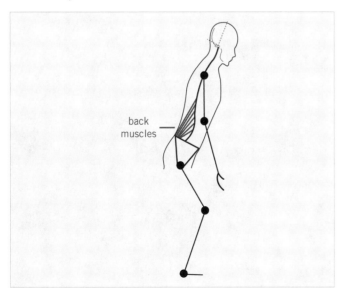

FIGURE 11: Back muscles in a position of weakness
This lift does not respect the biomechanics of the back

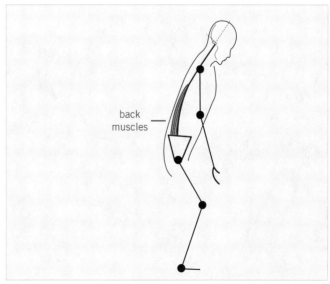

## REHABILITATION OF PROPRIOCEPTION AND STABILIZATION

Have you ever watched a one-year-old child learning to walk? After several attempts, the child manages to stand while holding on to a piece of furniture. Proudly, he/she smiles and tries to remain standing for longer and longer periods of time. Children learning to walk try to find their balance, try different positions for their feet, knees, and pelvis. They concentrate. The most important thing is their search for balance. Certain positions are good and keep them standing; others are not so good and they fall onto their bottoms. And they keep starting all over again. Then, one day, they cautiously let go of the furniture and fall on their bottoms. Then they keep starting over and over again. How happy they look when, one day, they manage to stand alone, without any support! Eventually, they learn to take a step, another immense joy… then a second and so on.

That's how we learned proprioception and stabilization. After an injury, proprioception and stabilization are altered. The good news is that they can be recovered with exercises. Most physiotherapists and sports professionals offer many programmes. Some are done with balls and proprioceptive planks. Others look more like mediation standing up (Tai-chi, Qi-gong). All of these exercises share four basic principles:

1. The most important part involves focusing all your attention on the sensations and functioning of your muscles, tendons, balance and joint control.
2. Precision, balance and gentleness are essential. Strength, speed and movement amplitude will come later.
3. The feet support the weight of the body (swimming and cycling are not stabilization exercises).
4. Start on a solid floor, then slowly progress to other, more demanding surfaces. Start with a basic activity, then progress slowly to more demanding activities.

FIGURE 12: Examples of progression in a rehabilitation programme

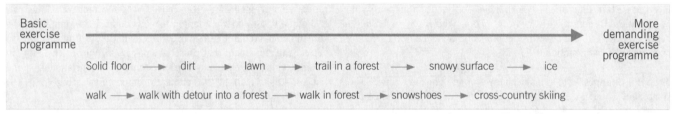

After an injury, the first steps are decisive. For these first steps, we have chosen a few **basic, simple exercises** that do not require specialized equipment, that you can do anywhere, and that you can do often. First, the **pelvic tilt**. Look for the neutral zone (**Figure 11**).

## PROPRIOCEPTION EXERCISE PROGRAMME FOR THE LUMBAR SACRAL SPINE

### Pelvic tilt STANDING

1. Start the pelvic tilt exercise lying down so as to be able to memorize the comfortable sensation of the neutral zone. Then stand up, with your back about 2 inches from the wall.
2. Tilt your pelvis backward to the neutral zone, then forward. Picture shifting your buttocks toward the ground and your genital organs forward. Or imagine contracting the muscles at the back of your thighs (hamstrings) and letting your knees bend passively as the pelvis is tilted forward.
3. Then slowly release the muscles at the back of your thighs and move your pelvis forward to the neutral zone, and then back.
4. Do the pelvis tilt exercise slowly, while standing, ten times. Identify the neutral zone as accurately as possible and stay in that zone as long as you need to memorize the comfortable sensation of the neutral zone perfectly.

5. **Congratulations!** Now you have discovered how to find the neutral zone easily while standing. Keep your spinal column in the neutral zone and take a few steps. Try to find the neutral zone accurately once again and take a few more steps. Repeat the exercise as often as needed so that the spinal column is always perfectly aligned and comfortable in the neutral zone in the various postures, and during various activities. You can perhaps practice as often as children who have just learned to write their name. They are so happy that they write it everywhere, on sheets of paper, blackboards or posters. They are proud of being able to write their names and they write them as often as possible, without realizing that one day they will no longer remember the time when writing did not come easily and naturally.

FIGURE 11: Pelvic tilt STANDING

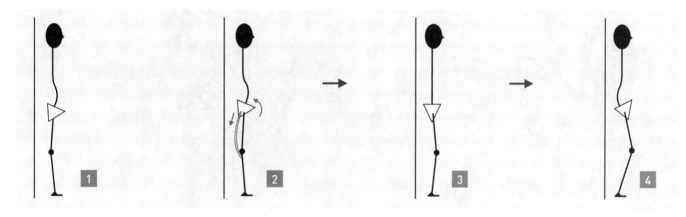

## Balance exercises

1. Stand, with your eyes closed, for a few moments. Observe (from within) the movements of your body, from your feet, which are continuously re-establishing the balance. Feel your centre of gravity as it shifts and the pressure that moves from one place to another in your feet (**Figure 12**).
2. As you get more comfortable, the goal is to keep the pressure point in the safe zone well within the feet (**Figure 13**). Progressively, increase the time during which you can maintain your balance with your eyes closed. Later, you can position your feet closer together to increase the challenge.
3. Walk with the pressure point in the safe zone within each foot (**Figure 14**). First, walk ten steps, paying particular attention to each action. Later, when walking has become easier, take 10 very stable steps to each door your pass through.

4. Walk while picturing your pelvis stable. You can imagine that your pelvis is a container that is filled to the top with water and your goal is to walk without spilling water (**Figure 15**). First, take 10 steps, paying particular attention to each movement. Later, when walking has become easier, take 10 very stable steps to each door you pass through.
5. Have some fun standing on one leg. For a few seconds at first. As you improve, change the position of your knees (knees locked or unlocked), pelvis, body, head (look ahead or look at your feet) to extend your time. Later, when you are an expert, stand on one leg with your eyes closed.

### FIGURES 12,13, 14, 15: Balance exercises

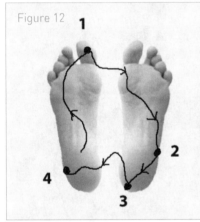

Figure 12

In this case, the person is standing, eyes closed. The pressure point moves about. At Point 1, the pressure point is very far forward (big toe); the individual feels very off-balance, to the front, then regains his/her balance. At Point 2, the pressure point is far to the left and the back, and the individual is off-balance to the rear left. At Point 3, off-balance to the back. At Point 4, off-balance to the rear right.

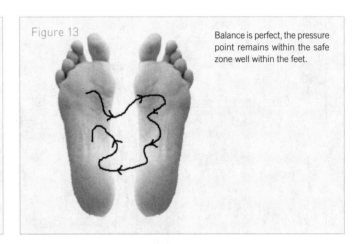

Figure 13

Balance is perfect, the pressure point remains within the safe zone well within the feet.

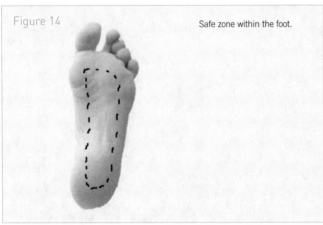

Figure 14

Safe zone within the foot.

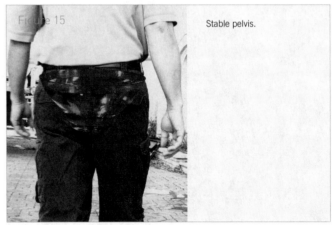

Figure 15

Stable pelvis.

Once you have mastered these exercises, you can move on to more demanding activities. We have learned from experience that patients who achieve and maintain musculo-skeletal health have developed the following winning strategies.

- Integrate exercises in brief periods throughout the day;
- Schedule a walk or sport at particular times reserved just for that;
- Progress slowly to activities that please them or fulfil their aspirations (preferred sport or new sport, with friends or alone, outdoors or at a gym);
- Dare to try new activities and make the necessary adjustments; and
- Choose to take part in a regular exercise programme outside work, even if they walk a lot at work or do physical work.

# 5. CONCLUSION

In order to prevent chronic pain, people must listen to the signals from their bodies. Here is an illustration.

Joe-on-the-go is an enterprising guy. He repairs everything; he can build anything, he makes things work. One day, the yellow engine light lit up on his dashboard. Joe-on-the-go checked the oil, the battery, the engine was running... "It can't be that serious" and Joe didn't give it another thought. One month later, the red engine light lit up. Joe checked everything out and it was all working. Nothing to worry about. Joe didn't give it another thought. A while later, the brake light lit up. Joe checked the brake fluid, looked at the brake pads... everything was fine. Joe felt reassured. The important thing was that the car worked. A week later, in addition to the lights, an alarm started sounding, all the time. Joe inspected the engine and the car, saw nothing abnormal and decided to dismantle the dashboard. He found a way to disconnect the lights and also cut the wire to the speaker and the alarm. And that was that! The car still worked, with no light signals or alarm. The important thing was that it worked without a fuss. A week later, the car made a strange noise when Joe braked: "Crrrr...". Joe inspected the brake fluid and the pads again. Everything was fine. "I won't brake as much," Joe said to himself. And that worked; the car made less noise. But, a few days later, the motor started making a "click, click, click" sound all the time. Joe inspected the oil, the belts and the battery. Everything was fine, so it couldn't be anything serious. Joe decided to turn the radio on full blast. No more "click, click, click", until one day, as Joe was driving home from work, the engine blew, with a lot of noise and smoke. When Joe tried to stop the car by the side of the road, he had no brakes! Fortunately, Joe was not injured; but he left the car smoking at the bottom of a ditch.

This grotesque tale illustrates the fact that ignoring alarm signals all the time can have serious long-term consequences. Hunger, thirst, pain, a need for sleep and fatigue are all important alarm signals that ensure the well-being of our bodies. Pain motivates us to protect the injured part, indicates the right pace for returning to activities after an injury, and reveals that certain postures and certain ways we work injure our bodies. As a result, continuously trying to improve the work environment, work tools and the way we work is a good strategy for preventing injuries and chronic pain.

Two other functions are also necessary for good musculo-skeletal health: proprioception and stabilization. These functions are altered following an injury. Rehabilitating them quickly serves to prevent the chronicization of pain. (In the same way that it is important to watch what you eat and rebuild your intestinal flora following a gastroenteritis.)

We have discussed means for managing the interpersonal relationships, work overloads and stress that are other major risk factors for the development of chronic pain. They can be summed up as follows.

- Remain flexible when pursuing your goals by trying other stop rules, which are more comfortable and safer.
- Practice a relaxation, meditation or visualization technique on a regular basis, three times per week.
- Walk or take part in other physical activities three times per week.
- Improve your interpersonal relationships by learning to communicate without making the situation worse.
- Take a step back from conflict situations.
- Let go, when necessary.

We have all learned to perform preventive maintenance on our cars. And we do so regularly so that our vehicles don't break down on the road. Today, we have the scientific knowledge we need to perform preventive maintenance on these formidable machines: our bodies. Learning to do so regularly and carefully is a major challenge in daily life.

# BIBLIOGRAPHY

- Feuerstein, M. & Nicholas, R. A. (2006). Development of a short form of the Workstyle measure. Occupational Medicine, 56, 94-99.
- Heneweer, H., Vanhees, L., & Picavet, H. S. (2009). Physical activity and low back pain: a U-shaped relation? Pain, 143, p. 21-25.
- Macdonald, D., Moseley, G. L., & Hodges, P. W. (2009). Why do some patients keep hurting their back? Evidence of ongoing back muscle dysfunction during remission from recurrent back pain. Pain, 142, p. 183-188.
- Malchaire, J., Cock, N., Indesteege, B., Piette, A., & Vergracht, S. (1999). Influence des facteurs psychosociaux sur les troubles musculosquelettiques. Bruxelles: INRCT : Institut national de la recherche sur les conditions de travail (Belgique).
- McGill, S. (2007). Reducing the risk of low back pain. In Low back disorders: Evidence-based prevention and rehabilitation (p. 133-158). Champaign, IL, USA: Human Kinetics,Inc.
- Meijer, E. M., Sluiter, J. K., & Frings-Dresen, M. H. (2008). Is workstyle a mediating factor for pain in the upper extremity over time? Journal of Occupational Rehabilitation, 18, p. 262-266.
- Moseley, G. L., Nicholas, M. K., & Hodges, P. W. (2004). Pain differs from non-painful attention-demanding or stressful tasks in its effect on postural control patterns of trunk muscles. Experimental Brain Research, 156, p. 64-71.
- Rosenberg, M. B. (2003). La communication non violente au quotidien. St Julien-en-Genevois: Éditions Jouvence.
- Rusu, A. C. & Hasenbring, M. (2008). Multidimensional Pain Inventory derived classifications of chronic pain: evidence for maladaptive pain-related coping within the dysfunctional group. Pain, 134, p. 80-90.
- van Weering, M. G., Vollenbroek-Hutten, M. M., Tonis, T. M., & Hermens, H. J. (2009). Daily physical activities in chronic lower back pain patients assessed with accelerometry. Eur.J.Pain.
- Vlaeyen, J. W. & Morley, S. (2004). Active despite pain: the putative role of stop-rules and current mood. Pain, 110, p. 512-516.

# THE PATIENT'S
# ROLE

**Juliana Barcellos** de Souza Pht, PhD, Florianópolis, Brazil
Universidade Federal de Santa Catarina (UFSC)

http://lattes.cnpq.br/0009123389533752

## ABSTRACT

In all life's situations, we have a role to play and an attitude to adopt. Whether we are active or passive with respect to life, we take part and we communicate. This also applies to the treatment for chronic pain, in which **the active participation of the patient is essential if the treatment is to succeed.** Immersed in pain, your role as an active patient may occasionally appear somewhat abstract. During the course of this chapter, we will describe several strategies to help you with this process, which focuses on you and in which you should play an active role. This process starts with a search for help. This means that you must first identify the pain issue. Don't forget that pain is a subjective symptom, and you are the **only one** that is able to evaluate it. The treatment team (the experts) can do nothing without your comments. In order to develop an action plan for the treatment of pain, first your symptoms must be identified (and you are the expert in this field) and next, adjustments must be made to respond to your needs (to reduce undesirable side effects and adapt the activities to your capacities and your objectives).

In clinical practice, the treatment of pain is a dynamic process. The prescriptions (medication, exercises, etc.) you will be given will not help you if you do not take action. Taking action means: taking the medications, doing the exercises, etc., in short, trying the strategies discussed with the treatment team. This dynamic process evolves through your communication with the treatment team: inform them about your perceptions since this will lead to adjustments in the strategies proposed and tested.

This chapter also proposes strategies for improving communication with the treatment team. The end of this chapter deals with group interventions. These interventions, which are generally multidisciplinary in nature, are enriched as the patients share their experiences. This can serve to encourage you as well as show you other ways of managing your pain and even stressful situations, such as developing an attitude to "let go" rather than "dramatizing the situation". After reading this chapter, you will have a small box of "tools" you can use to help you become a participatory patient and improve your condition and your health. Enjoy your reading, and don't forget to take action! Trying the strategies is the starting point for the participatory patient!

# 1. INTRODUCTION

More and more, patients want to be kept informed about their condition to be able to make decisions, and understand the benefits and side effects of the interventions proposed to them. Patients do not want to be a passive part of the treatment; they want to take part. Such a change in patient behaviour enables them to take control of their pain. Patients play an active role in improving their health; they learn to manage their symptoms better, and they adopt lifestyle habits that lead to sustainable change. **This participatory behaviour is a key part in the success of any treatment.**

In the following pages, we will help you better understand your role as a participatory patient, the attitude to be adopted with respect to health professionals and your responsibilities and duties toward yourself. The role of the active patient is often learned through observing those around you: how your friends and family behave during your treatment. This is not a role that requires academic training, but rather one that is built over the course of a life. At the end of this section, we will present multidisciplinary treatment programmes as a group (interactive schools), since patients can help one another manage their symptoms better through working together.

Your participation is important at all stages of the treatment, starting from the search for assistance up until improvements are experienced. Make decisions! Stay active throughout the process!

# 2. LOOKING FOR HELP AND CONSULTATION

Consulting a health professional is an action that depends directly on the patient and those around him/her. This desire to consult and look for help is often motivated by one of the three following wishes:
- To identify the cause of the problem;
- To obtain a precise diagnosis;
- To identify the strategies that can relieve or heal the problem (Hamilton et al. 2005).

Regardless of the initial goal, any treatment starts with the patient making the following decision – "I want to consult" – and this desire must persist throughout the treatment. The patient must be A PARTICIPATORY PATIENT.

At the time of the consultation, the role of health professionals is relatively clear: their expertise should help us resolve our problem. Their years of training should enable them to identify the solutions to their patients' health issues. For example, a doctor and a pharmacist should be skilled at identifying the medications that can relieve the patient's pain. Unlike the health professionals, patients have received no formal training in their role. This role has to be learned day by day, starting in early childhood.

Let us continue with our example about medication. The participatory patient asks: "How can these medications help me? Is this the right prescription? Will going to the drug store for pills help me?"

Even without knowing the biochemistry of the pharmacological substance that is prescribed, we are fully aware of our role as a patient. From early childhood, we have learned that, in order to benefit from the beneficial effects of medications, we must follow the prescription and take the medications.

If we consider the role of the patient from the point of view of the **participatory patient**, the patient is positioned at the heart of his/her treatment. If the patient does not follow the prescription for medication or physical activity (for example, going for walks), the treatment will not have the desired effect.

The patient is the "active principle" in any treatment. As a patient, the health professionals must **guide** you through the process and your change in attitude so as to **trigger an improvement** in your health condition. **The success of any treatment depends on the efforts of the patient.**

# 3. AT THE HEART OF THE TREATMENT TEAM AND THE TREATMENT PLAN: THE PATIENT

The treatment for chronic pain must be multidisciplinary and adapted to the physical, psychological and social needs of each patient. Since several factors must be taken into consideration in order to bypass the complexity of the painful phenomenon, several health professionals must be committed to the patient throughout the treatment. It is important to note that, for this treatment team, which includes doctors, physiotherapists, psychologists, occupational therapists and pharmacists, the patient is at the heart of the treatment plan. All of the therapeutic strategies and techniques are prescribed in keeping with his/her individual needs.

## The patient at the heart of a dynamic process

This focus on the patient should not be viewed in a static context. The healing process is far from static, and the prescriptions are not the only element in the solution for the painful condition. **You experience this, as a patient, when the pills prescribed have no beneficial effect if you do not take them.** Since the patient is at the heart of the treatment plan, let us make an analogy that compares the patient with that very important organ: the heart.

| THE HEART | | |
|---|---|---|
| The movements of the heart are essential for keeping the body alive: it receives blood and moves it along, by distributing it to all the cells in our body. | *If the patient doesn't collaborate any longer...* | If the heart stops, **there is no need for new blood** since there is no body to be kept alive. |

| THE PATIENT | | |
|---|---|---|
| For the patient, the "blood" translates into the strategies and the prescriptions for medication or physical activities. | *If the patient doesn't collaborate any longer...* | If the patient does not cooperate with his/her treatment plan, new prescriptions will be useless. The "blood" translates into new prescriptions. Therefore, there is no need for new strategies, medications and therapy if we do not take action. |

**A static attitude is contrary to progress, whether that is progress in life or progress in our treatment. Healing is the end result of a dynamic process that involves the cooperation of the entire treatment team: the patient and the health professionals.**

# 4. MOTIVATION UNDER CONTROL

In order for the treatment to be a success, **action must be taken.** A static attitude will not help us advance. Since early childhood, we have developed our motor skills by observing the world and through a good many trial and error activities. So, taking action is not something new. However, if you are aware of the importance of the various prescriptions your care team gives you, why is it so difficult to follow them?

"Am I the problem? Is it a lack of motivation on my part? Yet, I truly do want to improve my health."

In order to answer these questions, let us look at the problem from three points of view:
• The person who gives the prescriptions;
• The prescription for physical activities;
• The person who takes action.

### The person who gives the prescriptions (generally, the health professional or the practitioner)

In order to be able to give the correct prescription, the practitioner must have adequate information about the patient's health. He/she must also know the patient's objectives (since the patient is at the heart of the treatment plan), namely personal objectives that are realistic and can be measured in keeping with his/her medical condition. Equipped with all this information, the practitioner will be able to better choose the physical activity to prescribe for the patient. He/she can help the patient directly to improve his/her quality of life on a short- or medium-term basis, while promoting the attainment of the initial objectives.

Moreover, the practitioner may encourage the patient to get motivated by choosing physical activities that are in keeping with his/her tastes and values, and that help to achieve his/her personal objectives, which are realistic and measurable (established at the outset).

### The prescription for physical activities

As we have seen, the prescription for physical activities must be adapted to the tastes and values of each patient. It must respect the patient's physical and mental capacities, as well as his/her leisure activities and needs. For example, dozens of scientific research studies have demonstrated the beneficial effects of physical exercise in water (hydrogymnastics or hydrotherapy) for people suffering from chronic pain. Despite these results, we must, however, acknowledge that in real life there are patients who appreciate physical exercise in water whereas some do not appreciate the routine of getting into and out of the pool once or twice a week. This is a personal choice. The decision to take part in hydrogymnastics (exercises in the water) is solely up to the patient. But be careful! This does not mean making a choice between **doing exercise and not doing exercise**, but between the place where the exercise is to be done (namely in the water, at home, in a fitness centre or elsewhere).

As a participatory patient, you must discuss this with your physician and any other practitioner treating you so as to identify the activities that you enjoy and that are suitable for you.

### The person who takes action (you!)

The person who takes action is you, the patient. **You are the only one that can guarantee the success of your treatment.**

Before taking action, you must understand the following elements: your prescription for physical activities, the way in which the activities function, their benefits, the possible side effects and, finally, overdoses of activities that could be potentially harmful or dangerous for you.

Here are a few questions and answers that could help you have a better understanding of your role as a patient who participates in the prescription for physical activities that you are given.

### THE EFFECT OF THE PRESCRIPTION FOR PHYSICAL ACTIVITIES AND HOW TO MOTIVATE YOURSELF

| | |
|---|---|
| How can this strategy help me? | Sometimes, understanding "why" can help you get motivated. |
| How can I organize myself so as to take action? | Make an action plan, choose the best time for following the prescriptions for physical activity and including them in your routine. |
| When will I take walks? After a meal? When will I do my stretching exercises? When I get up or when I come home from work? When will I listen to music in order to relax, and where will I relax? In the living room? In my bedroom? In the basement? | Your action plan should answer each of these questions. |

Motivation is the decisive element that will enable you to take action, but there is a risk. Excessive motivation can cause us to do too much, and too much is as bad as not enough! Physical exercise is a classic example of this. When we make a decision to start practising the physical activities prescribed, we want to make up for lost time and we want to attain our goal quickly. This inevitably leads to too much exercise, intense pain and a lack of motivation for continuing.

Here is some advice that will help you get motivated without getting overly zealous.

**First:** You will never make up for lost time.

**Second:** If you do too much, you simply encourage pain and giving up on the prescribed activity. For example, if you walk for 60 minutes, four times a week, whereas before, you never went for walks. Making a decision to follow the prescription for physical activity also means making a decision to start slowly: **you have to control your motivation!** If the prescription for physical activity says walk for 20 minutes, three times a week, you should not walk for 40 minutes or four times a week. The goal is not to exceed the prescription and do more. Your long-term goal: you want to persevere and include the physical activity in your routine. Your period of physical activity must be easy and pleasant!

**Third:** Make the easiest choice: do only what has been prescribed, and progress slowly without jumping a step.

## 5. ALWAYS TAKE PART! YES, BUT HOW DO I DO THAT?

Living with chronic pain is not easy. Progress and looking for help is often lengthy for patients who have to deal with chronic pain. They must schedule and attend numerous medical consultations, try dozens of medications, undergo several treatments and deal with the costs in time, money and energy, alone or with their loved ones, in order to glimpse the possibility of relieving their symptoms and their pain. These patients undergo several treatments, some of which are lengthy, merely to obtain results that are often discrete. The costs are not always proportional to the benefits.

### Taking part means communicating!
**Taking part also means looking for help!** In order to obtain a service that is appropriate and satisfactory, it is important to communicate well with your treatment team, and take action!

The communication between you and your health professional or your treatment team is, without a doubt, the best strategy for avoiding both multiple treatments and disappointing benefits. For example, the best indicator for measuring the effectiveness of a medication is your perception of the relief of your symptoms.

Without your participation, the physician, the psychologist and the physiotherapist will not be able to evaluate the reduction of your pain. Pain is a subjective perception that you are the only one to experience, and to be in a position to measure.

## Taking part means sharing your experiences

Always taking part means sharing your experiences. In order to be able to communicate well with your treatment team, you must take the following recommendations into consideration.

Always remember to report on the extent of your pain clearly and objectively. You are the one in the best position to do so. You must learn how to **describe** your pain and your symptoms as well as your relief clearly. Although researchers have developed indirect means for measuring pain, such as through perspiration or pulse, these measurements are indirect. The direct measurement is the one you take.

- Keep your doctor or any health professional in your treatment team informed about the difficulties you have following the prescription for physical activities or medication. In this way, they will be able to help you.
- Have you already thought about it? Why don't you take your walks? Why don't you take the pills prescribed?
- Identify your limits and go to your treatment team for specific help. For example, the psychologist can help you get motivated.
- Share ideas with your loved ones and friends: they can help you remember to take long breaths during the day, to relax or take a short walk. In pairs it's often more motivating and pleasant! But take care with respect to your pace! Those who accompany you have to go at your pace, slowly and progressively. Change partners if you have to and always progress slowly.

## Taking part, means taking action!

In order to progress in a symptom management process and take action, you have to change your lifestyle habits.

- Report the intensity of your symptoms to the health professionals.
- Follow the prescriptions for physical activities or medications.
- Adapt your routine: take walks, take deep breaths, observe what you do in daily life.
- Develop new habits.
- Recount your experiences and discuss them.
- Practice your techniques.
- Choose the right time of the day and the right place to practice your new habits.

It is not easy to make changes in lifestyle habits. This requires your commitment and discipline. Even if some tasks seem simple, do not hesitate to talk about them with your loved ones. For example, breathing and relaxing seem to be easy tasks, but they are far from simple. **It's a learning process.** Talk with those around you who are practising relaxation or meditation. The benefits will come as you practice each new technique. Moreover, you have to choose the right time of the day so that you are not disturbed and choose a small pleasant nook in the house where you are comfortable. Consider turning off your computer or letting voice mail pick up your calls. Develop your own ritual; you have to practice it and adapt it to your needs.

## 6. HOW CAN I IMPROVE MY CONDITION?

Learning to manage your pain and your symptoms requires a disciplined commitment on your part. The treatment team can serve as guides, proposing strategies that are adapted to each patient. **The common goal is to increase the capacity to manage symptoms.**

How can I play an active role in the process to manage my pain and my symptoms? What can I do? Is my attitude really important to my recovery?

Some patients recount the progress they make towards managing their own chronic pain and they help us better understand the role of the participatory patient. We've noted that these patients tell us that they have to be realistic with respect to their capacities and their limits, without fearing change. Participatory patients have the courage to take action and get involved in a lengthy change process, one small step at a time. Regardless of how long you have been suffering, you can learn to manage your symptoms and relieve your pain. You will adapt your activities and your hobbies along the way, without having to give them up.

"When I had painful crises, I was no longer able to walk straight. I was ashamed. People would point at me and would think I was drunk. I've learned balance exercises that have enabled me to increase my endurance and now I can go for walks. I've learned to manage my capacities and my limits in order to reduce the intensity of my crises."
*47-year-old patient, suffering from chronic pain for 5 years*

"Now that I listen to my body more, I'm more positive and more motivated. I feel like taking charge of myself. Since I've been taking regular walks, my husband is more sensitive to the disease and encourages me more. I feel a lot more assured and I'm less afraid to agree to an outing. I enjoy myself more. I plan my outings and I rest the next day."
*45-year-old patient, suffering from chronic pain for 15 years*

"By listening to my body, the signs of fatigue, pain and sleep, I have learned to demystify fibromyalgia. Now I have a better understanding of the disease. This has helped me regain a certain amount of confidence in myself. I learned various tricks for dealing with my pain [eating well, having positive ideas, having fun, listening to music, laughing, going for walks in nature, taking deep breaths …]. My quality of life is better now than a few months ago. This has enabled me to take better care of myself. I've been able to explain the symptoms better to my family and make them understand that I don't have the same amount of energy as before. I've started to go out a little more, but at my pace and in keeping with the amount of energy I have. My patience has increased because I've managed to control my pain and I respect my limitations a little more as well as those of others. I'm less tired after a day of work."

*40-year-old patient, suffering from chronic pain for 5 years*

### The first step : considering realistic objectives

Agreeing on an objective that is both realistic and measurable gives the practitioner and the patient a unique opportunity to modulate the patient's expectations with respect to the treatments. A few realistic and measurable objectives are presented in **Table 1**.

For example, let's consider the objective of taking walks. A patient with fibromyalgia, who has been suffering from chronic pain for more than six years, presents her objective to us: **to take walks lasting two to three hours, once a week.**

Is this realistic? She also told us that she used to take walks like this ten years ago! At this point in time, she can barely manage to walk for 15 consecutive minutes. She may not be able to achieve her goal during the course of the treatment (three or four months). After discussion, the patient and the practitioner agree on an attainable objective (and one that the patient can exceed if she wants), namely: **training progressively so as to be able to take 30-minute walks, three times per week.**

The patient is also reminded that taking walks lasting two to three hours is a goal that is possible to attain in the future, if she continues her training.

TABLE 1: Realistic and measurable objectives

| REALISTIC AND MEASURABLE OBJECTIVES | |
|---|---|
| **TYPE OF OBJECTIVE** | **PERSONAL OBJECTIVES** |
| **Physical** | • Walking for 30 minutes, three times per week.<br>• Being able to play with my grandchildren for 30 minutes (bent over)<br>• Walking for an hour, once per month.<br>• Driving a car for an hour, without having to stop because of the pain.<br>• Being able to go out once per month (dinner, visiting friends).<br>• Having friends or family over once per semester. |
| **Mental / cognitive** | • Reading an eight-line paragraph without having to go back over it in order to understand.<br>• Recounting a brief event (ex.: sharing news heard on the TV).<br>• Planning a trip. |

### Second step: follow your prescriptions!

Is taking action a choice that you agree with? You have sought assistance. Are you prepared to make a commitment to the process now? Just going to see your practitioner will not relieve your pain **if you do not take action.** Take things seriously, try the new prescriptions, and change the details of your routine: **you are the active element in the treatment. Without your participation, the results will be minor and short-lived.**

Nutrition prescription

If you are given nutritional advice to help increase your energy throughout the day, what will you do? There are two easy options: try it or not. It's your choice.

The prescription is as follows: eat protein three times per day (approximately 15g/meal: morning noon and night).

Is this simple? Realistic? Of course. Particularly when you have to eat everything and add protein to your meal. Why? Neurotransmitters, enzymes, muscles, among other things, are proteins! Therefore, we need

protein, and in good quantities! Moreover it takes longer to digest protein than carbohydrates (ex.: rice, potatoes, bread, etc.), which releases energy over a longer period of time and will help you maintain an optimal level of energy all day long.

So? Are you ready to take action? Try it!

### Third step: observe yourself!

Every day, you're working on improving your condition. You are the person in the best position to evaluate the effect of a treatment and to assess the intensity of the activities during the course of a day. **Observing yourself and evaluating your day is a profitable strategy!** Have you noticed that participatory patients often speak of "listening to their body"? If you want to evaluate your capacities and your limitations, you have to observe yourself, you have to observe your environment and you have to always try to arrange your day accordingly. **Don't ask too much of yourself!** It's better to have three days of moderate activities than one day of excessive activity followed by two days of exhaustion. What do you think?

# 7. WHY PERSIST?

Three aspects are most important when it comes to improving your condition and in your involvement in doing that: the prescription for physical activity, breathing and relaxation, and nutrition.

## Prescription for exercise

Physical activity is an essential component in the treatment of chronic pain. This is justified by the effects physical activity has on the patients' physical functionality (Valim 2003), mood, particularly with respect to reducing depression and anxiety (North, 1990), as well as in neurophysiological terms through the phenomenon of analgesia that is induced by exercise (Koltyn, 2002). In order for the patient to enjoy these benefits, the exercise must be of moderate intensity (Souza et al. 2007) and it must be in keeping with his/her pain level and limitations so as to encourage compliance (Jones et al. 2002).

## Respiration and relaxation

Managing chronic pain is enhanced through the practice of mental techniques such as relaxation and meditation. There are several techniques for respiration and relaxation and their beneficial effects vary according to the instructions given, the pleasure experienced and the patient's experience with the various techniques. In this respect, practising breathing techniques, with slow, deep breaths, also serve to reduce anxiety, depression, stress and pain (Meuret 2005). Moreover, as noticed in clinics, the patients perceive an improvement in their state of health after taking slow deep breaths (Villien et al. 2005) and this can also enhance mental activity and pulmonary capacity (Fluge et al. 1994).

## Nutrition

The nutritional component is rarely described in the treatment and management of chronic pain. In fact, chronic pain seems to inhibit the patient's appetite, thereby reducing the ingestion of nutriments and the energy they produce. Also, there are two messages that are important to communicate to patients with respect to increasing their energy levels during the treatment: first, the importance of eating protein regularly (15 g/meal) and, second, the importance of ingesting iron every day, both to carry oxygen through the blood and to reduce the iron deficiency that is so widespread among women.

# 8. INTERVENTION GROUPS (FIBROMYALGIA, CHRONIC PAIN)

**Therefore, the patient's participation is the principal element in the intervention! Without the patient's commitment, he/she will see no change in his/her condition.**

The treatment of chronic pain requires a multifactorial approach in which the patient is evaluated and treated in various respects in order to satisfy his/her biopsychosocial needs. Multifactorial approaches are characterized by the association of at least two therapeutic treatments. Physical exercises are the most popular, since they are frequently associated with relaxation, stress management strategies (education) and psychotherapy. These programmes are often offered in groups (from 6 to 25 participants), with several facilitators (from 3 to 20 participants). These programmes are costly in terms of time and money, since they require several contributors and several hours of meetings. Moreover, despite proven satisfactory results, patient participation is low, specifically as a result of the time required for the meetings and the activities to be undertaken at home. A few years ago, in order to resolve this problem and guarantee the interdisciplinarity of the programmes, group treatment was proposed in which, in addition to discussions between the patients and the health professionals, each patient can also share ideas and experiences with other patients in the group. Patient participation in these programmes tends to be higher, particularly when the programmes are adapted to the patients' objectives as is done at the interactive schools.

**Links:**
**Back pain**: http://ecoledudos.uqat.ca/    http://web2.uqat.ca/lombalgie/examens/ecoledosliste.htm
**Fibromyalgia**: http://www.springerlink.com/content/627r0jl65677w022/fulltext.pdf?page=1

Several types of chronic pain are treated in Quebec using the model of the interactive schools: lower back pain, fibromyalgia, neck pain, abdominal pain and breast cancer. The goal of these schools is to teach patients strategies for managing their symptoms. They offer weekly meetings for groups of eight patients assisted by two facilitators. Each meeting lasts two hours and takes place as follows:
- Greeting, practice of a motor routine adapted for each patient (15 to 20 minutes), review of the activity prescribed the week before, presentation of a new theme and group discussion, broken up by a break. The meeting ends with a relaxation exercise, a summary of the meeting and a prescription of a new activity to be integrated for the following week.
- The meetings are organized around certain themes. In the case of fibromyalgia, the themes are as follows:

- To sign a therapeutic contract (patient and care givers) to establish realistic and measurable objectives;
- To identify the strategies used by the participants to relieve pain, fatigue, stress and sleep;
- To discuss the importance of physical activity and prescribe walks and the motor routine adapted to the needs of each individual;
- To discuss and prescribe relaxation or mediation techniques;
- To discuss strategies for managing capacities and limitations;
- To discuss the importance of nutrition in fighting fatigue and pain;
- To discuss the impact of chronic pain in life (sexuality and undesirable effects of the "healing");
- To discuss the effects of medication;
- To discuss the progress made by the members of the groups.

**What should you do to return to your initial condition, before you started interaction school?**

The results of the interactive schools demonstrate that the therapeutic strategies used there as intervention tools are effective for teaching patients how to treat themselves. Significant improvements are obtained in terms of pain at sensitive points, clinical pain, quality of life and the perception of the ability to manage the symptoms and they are maintained on a short- and long-term basis.

## 9. CONCLUSION

Your role as a patient in the treatment of chronic pain is simple, yet very demanding. The treatment is a long, dynamic process that depends directly on your participation. The entire process is influenced by your motivation. In order to be able to take action and persist, you must be motivated. Having realistic short-term objectives may be an excellent strategy that will help you to persevere. A few examples of objectives have been proposed and you will find others. Just don't forget to modulate your expectations; don't be in a hurry to attain major objectives. Move ahead slowly and you will come out a winner!

# SLEEP AND
# CHRONIC PAIN

**Sarah Whitman** MD, psychiatrist, Philadelphia, Pennsylvania, United States

## 26

## ABSTRACT

Unfortunately, sleep difficulties often go along with chronic pain. Even in people without pain, occasional sleep problems are common – 75% of people report occasional sleep problems. But for people with chronic pain, sleep problems can be worse. Some basic changes can help you sleep better.

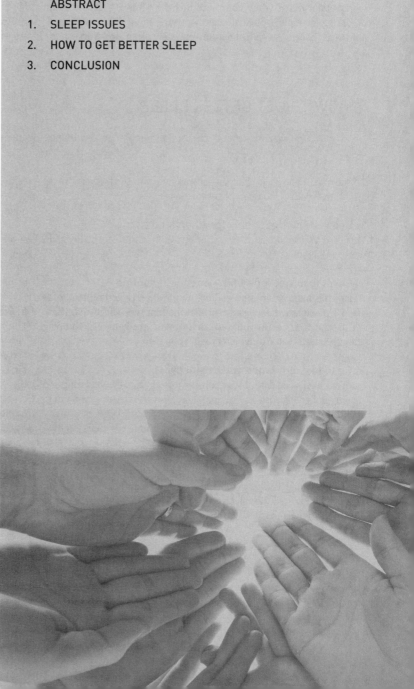

# 1. SLEEP ISSUES

Link: http://www.howtocopewithpain.org/resources/sleep-issues.html

For people with chronic pain, sleep problems can be worse, for reasons which include the following.

## Pain
Falling asleep can be difficult because pain keeps you awake, or pain can wake you up in the middle of the night.

## Decreased activity
If you aren't able to do very much during the day, you might not be tired at night.

## Anxiety and worry
These two notorious culprits can make falling asleep difficult if you worry about things when your head hits the pillow. Or, if you wake up during the night, you might start worrying about things and not be able to get back to sleep. Things unfortunately often look worse in the wee hours of the morning. You might wake up earlier than you'd like to and not be able to fall back to sleep.

## Depression
This often accompanies anxiety and worry. And actually, one of the symptoms we look for to diagnose depression is sleep problems, especially waking up earlier than you'd like. We call this "early morning awakening."

## Sleep problems as part of your medical disorder
For example, difficulty sleeping or sleep that doesn't refresh you ("non-restorative sleep") is part of the disease of fibromyalgia.

## Medication
Although most of the medications that are used to treat chronic pain are sedating, a few can cause sleep problems.

# 2. HOW TO GET BETTER SLEEP

Link : http://www.howtocopewithpain.org/resources/how-to-get-better-sleep.html

To start, try some basic changes that can help you sleep better. These are often called "sleep hygiene techniques."

## 1. Use your bedroom only for sleep (and sex)
This is so your mind associates your bedroom with sleep, rather than work, TV, reading, etc.

## 2. Develop a "getting-ready-for-sleep" routine
Again, this helps your mind and body know you're getting ready for sleep. Do relaxing, calming activities the hour or two before bed. Then, brush your teeth, wash your face, and turn off the lights. Even doing activities in the same order every night can help.

## 3. Go to bed only when you're sleepy
It's more likely you'll be able to fall asleep, and you'll avoid tossing and turning in bed because you're not sleepy. But remember, you have to spend the hour or two before your bedtime slowing down your body and mind, so you naturally become sleepy. It's unlikely you'll begin to feel sleepy if you're engrossed in a book, doing an online search, etc.

## 4. If you can't fall asleep, get out of bed
The average time it takes to fall asleep is 5 to 30 minutes. To keep your bedroom associated with sleep, you don't want to lie in bed unable to sleep, which can also make you start worrying about when you're going to fall asleep. So if you're unable to fall asleep after 20 minutes or so, get out of bed and do a quiet activity – perhaps a relaxation exercise or quiet reading – and then return to bed when you begin to get sleepy. You may then fall asleep, but if not, get out of bed again, and do this as many times as you're unable to fall asleep. Again, the first few nights you do this, you may not sleep very much at all, but keep at it. You're working on establishing good sleep habits! And the next night, you'll be more likely to fall asleep sooner.

## 5. Get up at the same time every morning
This helps to establish a sleeping routine. You might be tired, or even very tired, the first few days you do this, but you'll then be ready for bed at night. On weekends and vacations, you can change this a little bit, but get up no more than one hour later than your usual getting-up time, and don't do this until you're sleeping well.

## 6. No naps
Naps go against the sleep routine you're trying to establish of sleeping at night, and confuse your body. If you find yourself tired, try exercise, getting fresh air, or some other alerting activity. Again, after you're sleeping well, if you still find you get tired, a brief – _ hour – nap in the early afternoon may be acceptable, especially for older adults.

**7. No alcohol before bed**
  **No caffeine within 8 hours of your bedtime**
  **No tobacco within 3 hours of your bedtime**
No, this isn't to take away things you might enjoy – it's because all of these disrupt your sleep! Caffeine and nicotine are stimulants – what you don't need at bedtime. Alcohol disrupts your sleep cycles, especially deep sleep. While it may help you get to sleep, you'll wake up more often.

**8. Exercise regularly, but not right before bedtime**
Exercise tires your body and decreases anxiety, in addition to all the other good reasons to exercise. Just don't do it right before bedtime, when it can wake you up.

**9. Make your bedroom a good place to sleep**
Be sure your bedroom is not too hot or cold. Make sure it's dark enough, even as the sun starts to come up. And make sure sounds don't disturb your sleep – you can try a fan or white noise machine.

## 3. CONCLUSION

Remember, everyone experiences occasional sleep problems. But if you regularly have sleep problems, try these techniques all together. If after trying them, you're still unable to sleep better, talk to your doctor about other options. Good sleep is very important – for your mood, for healing, and to reduce your pain.

## Shot down by pain and getting up again

Janice Sumpton, RPh, BSc Phm, London, Ontario, Canada

(See other testimonials, pages 194 and 358. See chapter 31 page 247.)

I want to share with you the frustrations of living with pain, my constant companion, how it affects me every day, its impact on my family, and ways I have found to cope with the intrusiveness of persistent pain.

I am currently 50 years old and my pain began at age 38. I was given the diagnosis of fibromyalgia 7 years later. I am happily married with two children, now 19 and 17 years old. I have practised as a hospital pharmacist for over 27 years.

**The frustrations of chronic pain are many**. Pain is always present and I cannot escape it. The most frustrating aspect of pain is that it is invisible to others.

**There is the frustration of waiting years for a diagnosis**. Why do I have this pain? Am I going "crazy"? The pain and overwhelming fatigue are real. As a healthcare professional I know there aren't always answers, but as a patient I need an answer. I felt relief when given a diagnosis, despite the news that pain would be with me for the rest of my life. I could now put on my pharmacist hat, and find out everything that I could about fibromyalgia so I could live with this condition the best way possible.

**Constant pain is frustrating**. It is very difficult to explain precisely what the pain feels like. Pain is what the patient says it is. My muscles feel like I'm going through the worst flu ever. The pain is throbbing, twisting, burning, aching, tingling or like a knife turning inside muscle. Sometimes it feels like a bug or snake crawling under my skin and I feel it moving.

**There is frustration with the stigma of fibromyalgia**. Despite great strides in understanding the causes of fibromyalgia, and official label indications for two or three drugs in Canada and the United States, respectively, many don't believe fibromyalgia exists. This disbelief is prevalent among many in the medical community. There is a lack of education about fibromyalgia. It mostly affects women, and many people feel patients are "a bunch of whining women." That hurts.

**There is frustration with how chronic pain affects the relationships and activities I share with my family**. My family bears the brunt of my pain and exhaustion at the end of a work day, especially when I need to crash on the couch. I am irritable and that isn't fair to them. My poor memory is frustrating for me and my children who have to say things over and over again. My husband is very patient. I can't walk as quickly as I used to. A heart-wrenching comment from my child as we were walking in a shopping mall was, "I liked it much better when you could walk fast like you used to." I liked that, too.

**The unpredictability of the pain is frustrating**. Is it going to be a "good day" or "bad day"? I cannot plan ahead. A bad day can come out of the blue and I am sidelined.

**Poor sleep is frustrating**. I don't feel rested or restored, and poor sleep worsens the pain. It can be difficult to find a comfortable sleeping position.

**Work restrictions are frustrating**. I became a pharmacist to help people. Now, because of pain and non-restorative sleep, there are duties that I am unable to perform. I feel guilty that I am not pulling my weight, even though I am doing the best I can. The more stressful the environment is, the greater the impact on pain, thinking and fatigue. The pain is heightened in a work environment that is noisy and busy with multiple demands. Fibromyalgia increases my sensitivity to noise, smells and temperature changes, which are common in a hospital environment.

**The inability to multitask is frustrating**. I can no longer juggle many things at once, which I was easily able to do in the past. Fibromyalgia has robbed me of that skill. As a person who likes to be busy, it is frustrating when my body fails me and I have to lie on the couch and do absolutely nothing. I cannot accomplish what I want to do because I hurt too much. I feel that I have let down my family, my friends and my co-workers. I do not like myself when I am irritable because of the pain.

**As a result of these frustrations I have learned different coping skills, which help me to do the best I can.** (See page 194.)

# BREATHING, RELAXATION AND
## VISUALIZATION EXERCISES

**Sarah Whitman** MD, psychiatrist, Philadelphia, Pennsylvania, United States

**27**

## ABSTRACT

People who live with chronic pain can learn many psychological skills to decrease and cope with pain. Among those skills, many types of relaxation exercises can be beneficial. Breathing, basic relaxation and visualization may help people to relax and decrease anxiety, lower the stress response associated with pain, get better sleep and indirectly decrease pain.

This chapter presents basic breathing, basic relaxation and visualization exercises, and links to such exercises on the How to Cope with Pain Web site at http://www.howtocopewithpain.org/

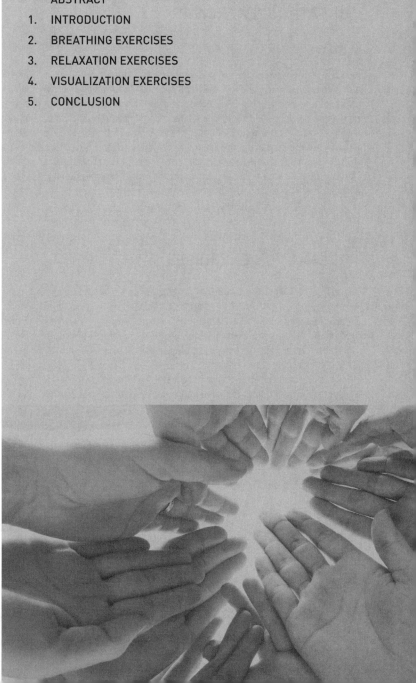

# 1. INTRODUCTION

What psychological skills can you learn to decrease and cope with pain? There are many types of relaxation exercises you can learn.

Breathing, basic relaxation and visualization may help you to:
· Relax and decrease anxiety;
· Decrease the stress response associated with pain;
· Get better sleep; and
· Indirectly decrease pain.

Breathing and relaxation exercises are meant to help you relax. You may very well feel more comfortable physically as anxiety and tension decrease. Pain management skills and exercises are most helpful when used regularly. Regular practice brings the best results!

There are several ways to use these exercises:
· Read through the exercise and then do it from memory — you can do it your way!;
· Record the exercise and play it back for yourself to do;
· Have someone read the exercise to you.

If you record a relaxation exercise or have someone read it to you, eventually try to be able to do it on your own. This lets you do it anytime and anywhere — a great skill to have in your back pocket!

Each exercise will take about 20 minutes and will help relax both your body and mind.

# 2. BREATHING EXERCISES

Link: http://www.howtocopewithpain.org/resources/breathing-exercises-2.html

Several breathing exercises are presented on the How to Cope with Pain Web site (see link above), which all focus on breathing patterns, and imagining that healing is occurring with breathing. These can be practised at any time, with your eyes open or shut, for a short or long amount of time. You can do just one, or let one flow into the next. By focusing on your breathing you can help your body relax, which often results in less pain. These exercises can also decrease the anxiety that often accompanies pain. When you're instructed to breathe deeply, moderately deeply is fine so that you don't hyperventilate.

**Pointers**

Do any of the breathing exercises only for as long as you're comfortable. If you begin to feel light-headed or tingly, simply return your breathing to normal, and shorten the number of deep breaths you take the next time you do the exercise.

Adding gentle, pleasant, natural smells to your environment while doing these breathing exercises is great. Fresh flowers, citrus or other enjoyable smells can be used. Using any and all of your senses—sight, taste, hearing, touch and smell — can add to your relaxation experience. There are many avenues to your relaxation destination.

# 3. RELAXATION EXERCISES

Link: http://www.howtocopewithpain.org/resources/relaxation-exercises.html

Use any imagery you'd like to imagine your discomfort or worries decreasing, such as a grassy field in the morning, the sun slowly evaporating in the mist or a sandcastle being slowly washed away by gentle waves.

At bedtime, omit the ending countdown and the phrase "with energy to resume your day," and instead simply continue to focus on your breathing.

**Pointers**

Hold your muscles tense for at least seven seconds, for a better contrast between tension and relaxation. If you are prone to muscle spasms, or feel a spasm coming on, you can shorten this time.

If you practise the exercise often, your body will learn to relax more quickly when you use the exercise. Soon you may find that you become very relaxed just by starting the exercise. After you learn the exercise, you may also find that just doing parts of the exercise relaxes you. For example, during a meeting where you can't close your eyes, just focusing on your breathing for a few moments brings calm and relaxation.

# 4. VISUALIZATION EXERCISES

Link: http://www.howtocopewithpain.org/resources/relaxation-visualization-exercise.html

This exercise will take about 20 minutes, and will help relax both your body and mind. Many people find that imagining a special, relaxing place helps them relax more easily. For this exercise, I've used the imagery of the beach. You can use whatever is your favourite place.

1. To get started, sit up straight in a comfortable chair, with your feet on the floor. If there is a more comfortable position for you, certainly use it. Unless you want to fall asleep, do the exercise sitting up. At bedtime, you can lie in bed and simply fall asleep with this exercise. If any step in the exercise isn't comfortable, either physically or emotionally, just focus on your breathing during that step instead.

2. Slowly close your eyes, or focus on one spot on the floor or wall if that is more comfortable for you. Invite your body and mind to begin to relax. If worries or concerns come to you, now or during this exercise, imagine placing them on clouds slowing drifting across the sky. You might notice these clouds as they drift by, but you don't have to get involved with these thoughts. Slowly your mind will settle down and begin to feel more relaxed and comfortable.

3. Begin to focus on your breathing. Take two slow, relaxed deep breaths, watching your breathing come in, and then go out. Then return your breathing to a normal rate and depth, and continue to watch your breath. Imagine that with each breath in you're breathing in comfort and relaxation, and with each breath out you're breathing out any discomfort or worry.

4. Next I'll have you turn your focus to a couple of different areas of your body, first tightening the muscles, and then letting them relax.

5. To start, I'll have you focus on your hands. Tighten those muscles into tight, tense fists and on the count of three relax. One, two, three. Let any tension or discomfort flow out through your fingertips.

6. Next, focus on the muscles of your face. Tighten those muscles by tightly shutting your eyes and clenching your jaw, and on the count of three relax. One, two, three. Let your forehead become smooth, and your jaw droop slightly.

7. Now I'll have you focus on your feet. Tighten those muscles by pushing your feet into the floor and on the count of three relax. One, two, three. Let any tension or discomfort flow out through the tips of your toes.

8. Imagine a wave of relaxation starting at the top of your head, flowing down over your face and the back of your head … flowing down the front and back of your neck … down your shoulders … down your chest and stomach … down your back … and down your legs to the tips of your toes.

9. Now take two more deep breaths in through your nose, blowing the air out through your mouth. Then return your breathing to normal. Next I'll describe a scene in which you can imagine yourself. Imagine walking over the sand, heading toward the beach. You can imagine slipping off your shoes, and feeling the warm, comfortable temperature of the sand. Notice how smooth the sand feels between your toes. As you walk toward the ocean, imagine looking out over the water, looking out toward the horizon. Notice the different colours of the water, the light and dark blues of the ocean. You might even see a cloud reflected on the water. You might see some whitecaps on the waves away from the shore. Then watch the water come into shore, and go back out again. You can also look up into the sky, noticing how many clouds there are, and if they're fluffy.

10. As you approach the water, imagine laying out a blanket on the sand and sitting down. Notice the comfortable warmth of the sun on your face and shoulders. Imagine picking up some sand in your hands, and letting it drift through your fingers, noticing how smooth it is. You can again look out over the water and watch the waves come in, and go out … come in, and go out.

11. Now imagine lying down on your blanket and closing your eyes. Notice what sounds you hear … perhaps some seagulls calling … perhaps some children playing off in the distance. Listen to the water as the waves come in, and go out. And take a deep breath, noticing what smells come to you … the clean, fresh smell of the ocean air … perhaps the coconut smell of suntan lotion. Enjoy resting on the beach for several minutes, noticing what each of your senses is experiencing. **(Pause for several minutes.)**

12. Then imagine sitting up again, looking out over the ocean, and then standing up and walking back away from the shore. You can brush off your feet with your blanket, and put your shoes back on. Even as we get ready to end this exercise, you know that you can return here at any time. Invite your body and mind to continue to feel comfortable and relaxed, even as your attention turns elsewhere.

13. Now to bring this exercise to a close, I'll count down from 10 to 0, and when I reach 0, you can slowly open your eyes.

14. 10 … 9 … 8 … 7 … 6 … 5 …

15. Continuing to feel comfortable and relaxed, and with energy to resume your day.

16. 4 … 3 … 2 … 1 … 0.

17. Slowly open your eyes, take a deep breath in and out, and gently wiggle your fingers and toes. You are ready to continue your day.

**Alternatives**

When you use your own favourite places for this imagery exercise, imagine what each of your senses is noticing. The more senses you involve in your imagery, the more real it will be for you. Real or imaginary places are fine.

As with the basic relaxation exercise, at bedtime, omit the ending countdown and the phrase "with energy to resume your day", and instead simply continue to imagine the beach scene, or whatever imagery you're using.

## 5. CONCLUSION

Many psychological skills can be learned to decrease and cope with pain. Breathing, basic relaxation and visualization exercises are effective strategies through which you can become more active in the healing process, and in taking charge of your pain. Active personal involvement in such beneficial exercises can help you to relax and decrease anxiety, decrease the stress response associated with pain, get better sleep, and indirectly decrease pain.

Helpful writings and new exercises are frequently added to the *v* Web site to support people who live with pain in coping better and living fuller lives.

# PHYSICAL ACTIVITY:
## A TOOL AND
# A NECESSITY FOR THE PATIENT

Pierre Beaulieu MD, PhD, FRCAD, Associate Professor, Department of Anaesthesiology,
Centre hospitalier universitaire de Montréal (CHUM) - Pavillon Hôtel-Dieu, Montreal, Quebec, Canada

## ABSTRACT

Regular physical activity is not a universal practice. For example, 25% of adults in the United States are sedentary, compared to 22% in Canada and 29% in Montreal (Quebec, Canada). Moreover, 40% of people over 65 years old are also sedentary. At the same time, the link between being sedentary and pain is an interesting one, since **most studies indicate that people with chronic pain are sedentary or not very active**. Intuitively, people with chronic pain think that physical activity will make their pain worse, and they tend to reduce their activities. While this attitude is justified following an acute trauma (such as a fracture or a sprain), treating pain involves a **progressive return to activities** in which people will experience the benefits in terms of both their pain and their quality of life. For example, their morale will be better, they will feel more sociable, and they will sleep better.

The physical condition of those who suffer from chronic pain can be improved by means of a training programme that includes various types of exercises, including endurance exercises, development of muscular strength, stretching, etc. With a programme such as this, people can generally return to work more quickly even though it is true that their perception (self-evaluation) of pain has not generally changed.

In this chapter, we will start by presenting the model for understanding chronic pain on which the chapter is based: the global approach to pain. **Following this, we will set aside certain prejudices concerning physical activity, while pointing out the problems of a sedentary lifestyle**. We will show how physical activity can be a tool for preventing and relieving chronic pain, in the case of various pathologies. At the end of the chapter, we will suggest physical activity programmes adapted to these pathologies.

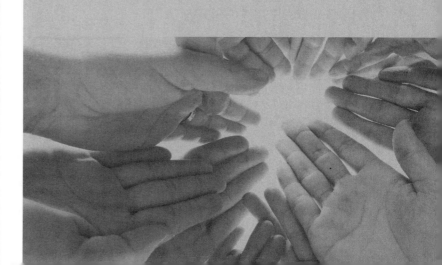

# 1. RISK FACTORS RELATED TO REDUCED PHYSICAL ACTIVITY

The development and maintenance of chronic pain following an injury or an accident is a complex process involving numerous factors. These factors interact on several levels and can cause the individual suffering from a chronic pain syndrome to develop a form of physical and moral handicap. **In fact, there is the risk that the individual will find him/herself in a vicious circle that results in a reduction of physical activity, that is frequently and rapidly reinforced by a fear of moving**. In such a case, in addition to his/her condition, the individual will experience frustration and anger, emotions that are caused by various factors, such as socio-economic situation, a work stoppage and family concern. All of these conditions can cause the individual to withdraw from his/her daily activities, go into a depression, get out of "training" or experience physical deconditioning and/or fixate on the painful symptoms. **Figure 1** (modified, based on Main et al 2000) shows the many factors that can intervene in physical deconditioning (immobilization and physical inactivity) and depression in the case of an individual with a chronic pain syndrome, and that can also help **maintain this syndrome**.

FIGURE 1 : Factors involved in the development of physical deconditioning and depression following a painful event

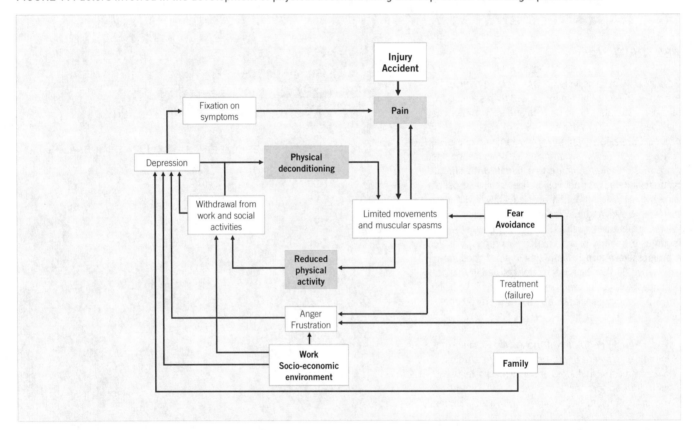

# 2. THE DAMAGES OF SEDENTARITY

Since the last century, people living in the so-called developed countries have grown progressively less physically active. This situation is a result of deep changes that have occurred with respect to the nature of the work they do, and the use of machinery to replace manpower. This sedentarity or physical inactivity is associated with a higher incidence of chronic diseases, such as obesity, type II diabetes, osteoporosis and cardiovascular diseases.

Physical inactivity is more specific to the mechanisms of pain, and is accompanied, on a musculo-skeletal level, by a reduction in bone density (and an increased risk of fractures), a deterioration of certain structures (connective tissues and joint cartilage), a reduction in joint function, strength and muscular endurance (muscle fatigue) and, finally, an overall decline in physical capacity, as indicated in **Table 1** on next page (modified according to Gifford et al 2006).

**TABLE 1: Principal harmful effects of immobility and physical inactivity with respect to maintaining pain**

- Muscle loss, weakness and loss of endurance
- Musculo-skeletal degeneration and atrophy with loss of muscle strength and elasticity
- Altered proprioception, loss of balance
- Joint stiffness and slowing of movements
- Reduced capacity to use energy substitutes
- Modifications to the automatic nervous system (sweating, oedema, skin changes, etc.)

- Pain and increased sensitivity (allodynia)
- Memory and concentration problems
- Loss of vitality and energy
- Problems with the circadian rhythm (wake/sleep rhythm)
- Increased risk of work accidents
- Increased incidence of back pain
- Cardiovascular deconditioning

## 3. PHYSICAL ACTIVITY AND THE PREVENTION OF CHRONIC PAIN

Unlike sedentary, physical activity has beneficial effects for both the nervous system (for example, mood and anxiety), and the immune system, which is involved in the fight against external attacks, and the body's defence mechanisms (for example, reduced incidence of certain cancers). **Figure 2** indicates the benefits of physical activity.

In the case of individuals suffering from chronic pain, a large portion of the benefits of physical activity are all the more interesting since they can also help to prevent the painful phenomena. Thus, in concrete terms, physical activity improves mood and sleep, and reduces anxiety, depression and stress. In musculo-skeletal terms, large muscle groups are mobilized by physical activity, facilitating the nutritional supply to tissues. Moreover, the proprioception function of the joint ligaments and capsules is optimized.

Overall, these positive effects of physical activity help reduce the number of injuries (such as at work) and, more globally, the health costs associated with treating them.

Thus, it is strongly recommended that people integrate simple physical training, which is motivating and stimulating, in their daily routine, and do this outdoors, if possible. Walking, jogging, cross-country skiing, swimming and dancing are all ideal physical activities for preventing chronic pain. Physical activity, which has long been forgotten, is to a certain extent a type of very relevant intervention when it comes to preventing a handicap and occasionally excessive medicalization (medical consultation and medications), particularly in the treatment of chronic pain. (See **Chapter 24**.)

Contrary to popular beliefs, the progressive increase in physical activity is not associated with an increase in pain, but rather, in most cases, in a reduction in pain.

**FIGURE 2: Benefits of physical activity**

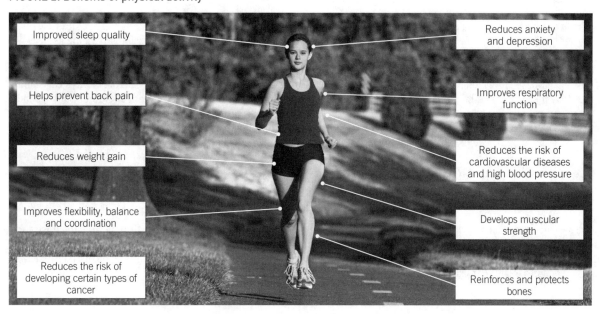

- Improved sleep quality
- Helps prevent back pain
- Reduces weight gain
- Improves flexibility, balance and coordination
- Reduces the risk of developing certain types of cancer
- Reduces anxiety and depression
- Improves respiratory function
- Reduces the risk of cardiovascular diseases and high blood pressure
- Develops muscular strength
- Reinforces and protects bones

## 4. PHYSICAL RE-EDUCATION AND RELIEF OF CHRONIC PAIN

Pain can cause individuals to reduce their mobility and lead to stiffness, which is in turn a source of pain.

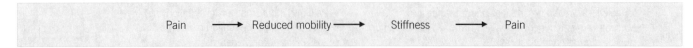

**FIGURE 3: Hypothetical connection between physical activity, pain and tissue integrity over time**
(based on Ljunggren & Bjordal, 2003.)

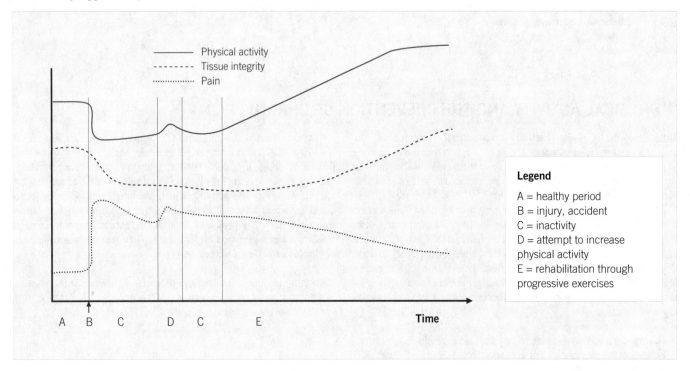

Musculo-skeletal diseases, such as osteoarthritis, are most often the result of a progressive attack on soft tissues, such as collagen. Thus, following an injury or an accident, the soft tissues may become more vulnerable. Moreover, physical inactivity or hyperactivity may be related to the appearance of chronic pain and other symptoms.

Numerous studies suggest that, in addition to contributing to the relief of pain, physical activity improves functional recovery. In this respect, there are many means that can be used by an individual suffering from chronic pain, either on their own or in combination: antalgic physiotherapy, massages, passive and active joint mobilizations, recovery of muscle strength, balneotherapy (bath therapy) and occupational therapy. Passive treatments such as the application of heat and cold, TENS, biofeedback or self-massage are also possible in the case of exacerbated chronic pain.

In order to relieve chronic pain, we focus on stretching exercises, a selection of physical exercises to increase muscle strength (isometric or isotonic), an endurance activity (aerobics) or aquatic exercise (swimming, aquafitness). Nevertheless, the role of physical training (or physical re-education) in the treatment of chronic pain depends, in the case of an injury or accident, on the extent to which the injury has consolidated or healed and, in the case of a disease, on the evolution of the condition.

### PHYSICAL ACTIVITY FOR RELIEVING ACUTE PAIN

Physical activity is also recommended for relieving acute pain. Generally, early functional re-education, such as after surgery, helps patients recover their natural functions (joint movements and intestinal movements), which makes it easier and more certain for them to return to their daily activities. In addition to relieving pain through the administration of medication and the use of local/regional anaesthetics (blocking nerves), optimal treatment involves the implementation of a physiotherapy programme as often as possible.

In more specific cases of osteoarticular and musculo-skeletal pain, treatment will involve physical interventions (for example, the application of heat and cold to the painful site and electrostimulation) and adapted mobilization exercises (for example, active or passive mobilization exercises, see page 233). On a short-term basis, the development of musculo-tendon adherences (adherences are fibrous strips that connect tissue surfaces that are normally isolated: in this case, we are discussing adherences of muscle and ligament tissues) is limited and muscle loss (amyotrophy or reduced muscle volume) is less important; on a medium-term basis, the secondary recovery of the function of the muscle or joint affected is improved.

Nevertheless, functional recovery depends, as we have seen, on many other factors affecting the individuals in question, such as their relationships, the cessation of all physical activity (rest), which in turn may lead to physical deconditioning, and become a source of a more definitive handicap.

Finally, it should be noted that inadequate or insufficient treatment of acute pain can lead to chronic pain.

**It is absolutely essential that any acute pain be treated adequately so as to prevent the secondary development of chronic pain.**

## RELIEVING CHRONIC PAIN THROUGH PHYSICAL ACTIVITY

Relieving chronic pain through physical activity is based on certain principles that are presented below. But, be careful! First, you must make sure that the application of physical activity in functional re-education is supported by clinical practice based on evidence. **In other words, it is essential that you make sure, <u>before starting a physical activity programme</u>, that research studies have demonstrated that the intervention methods considered for people suffering from chronic pain are effective and risk-free for them.** Nevertheless, since the ultimate objective it to improve the quality of care offered to these people, this criteria concerning providing care based on evidence would be incomplete without calling on the expertise of the clinician (case by case intervention), and the values of the individuals to be treated. Namely, a scientific culture must be created by prioritizing the objectives in cooperation with the other professionals involved, and through communication with people suffering from chronic pain.

**Before undertaking the planned physical activity programme:**

1. Prioritize the individual's objectives with the health care team;
2. Make sure that studies indicate that it is effective and safe;
3. Have the practitioner validate the programme;
4. Tailor the programme to the values of the individual to be treated.

| Principle 1 | Principle 2 | Principle 3 |
| --- | --- | --- |
| As a general rule, any functional improvement in an osteoarticular or musculo-skeletal context requires an ergonomic evaluation of the patient's environment (home, work), the implementation of a physical conditioning programme, and efforts to return to a normal level of physical activity. Moreover, it is important to define the individual's base performance in various activities, such as the number of times an exercise can be repeated, while taking into account limitations, such as pain, weaknesses and fatigue. **Following this, it is possible to prescribe a programme of daily exercises and physical activities based on the base performance with regular progression.** | In order for this type of approach to succeed, objectives must be established in cooperation with the individual to be treated (for example, a return to work). The time required to attain the objectives must be determined, and the individual's current disabilities and any eventual physical, social and work disabilities must be identified. | Educating the individual to be treated is also a key to success. He/she must be able to differentiate between acute pain and chronic pain, clarify the connection between the nature of the diagnosis and the possibility of a treatment and, finally, recognize the multi-dimensional nature of pain. Moreover, he/she must have recourse to systematic training, be aware of the risks of deconditioning, and the importance of physical activity. Finally, he/she must be open with respect to his/her expectations with respect to the pain. |

To sum up, the elements of an **active approach** include the following for each individual to be treated:

1. Functional movement selected in keeping with his/her needs;
2. Concentration on the disabilities that limit normal functioning;
3. Normalization of joint movement, muscular strength and endurance (aerobic work) as well of the capacity for physical work (aerobic shape);
4. Gradual progression with the exercises prescribed.

To complement this, cognitive-behavioural therapy could serve to modify the individual's beliefs and behaviours with respect to physical activity in particular, using the following strategies:
· Playing down (fear of movement, catastrophization); and
· Reinforcing the conviction of success in the rehabilitation process.
Other strategies can be added (operant conditioning) that will reduce the focus on pain.

In order to illustrate these comments, the major lines of the treatment of chronic pain specific to certain pathologies will now be discussed.

## MANAGEMENT OF CHRONIC PAIN CONDITION: EXAMPLES OF THE REHABILITATION PROCESS

### Chronic back pain

Approximately 70% of the Canadian population will suffer from back pain and 30% of these people will develop chronic back pain. In this manner, back pain, one of the most common forms of chronic pain, will be prevented by the practice of regular physical activity, through exercises to reinforce muscle groups, and by a certain amount of basic practical advice (bending one's knees when picking up an object, avoiding long car rides or planning regular breaks).

The objective of reconditioning programmes for effort (or rehabilitation, functional restoration) in the treatment of chronic back pain is based on an overall approach to the individual, and is intended to correct physical, functional, mental and social components in seriously handicapped people suffering from chronic pain. The originality of these functional rehabilitation programmes lies in not focusing on the pain, but rather on the patient's physical performances.

In a similar manner, a relatively recent study on a back to fitness programme for patients with back pain demonstrated the persistent, long-term positive effects with two major discoveries:

1. An exercise programme directed by a community physiotherapist helped people manage their pain and their performances better;
2. The people in the group who received this help used fewer health resources and were absent from work less often than other members in the group who did not benefit from this programme.

In clinical practice, the recommended approaches vary, depending on whether we are dealing with acute or sub-acute and chronic back pain.
· **During the acute stage of the pathology**, certain medications (for example, non-steroidal anti-inflammatory drugs, muscle relaxants) are as effective as staying physically active and practising stretching exercises, whereas specific exercises would not be effective. Numerous stabilization exercises have been proposed, and will be presented in this chapter.
· During the **sub-acute and chronic stages of the pathology**, we recommend a multidisciplinary approach with specific therapeutic exercises associated with behavioural therapy.

TABLE 2 : Guidelines for the treatment of back pain lasting less than three months

**For treating back pain lasting less than three months, it is recommended that you:**

- Reassure the patients (give a good prognosis);
- Advise against bed rest;
- Advise the patients to remain active;
- Prescribe general exercises;
- Do not prescribe passive treatments;
- Prescribe an anti-inflammatory medication or acetaminophen;
- Do not prescribe x-rays, laboratory tests or a specialized consultation.

### Arthritis of the knee

Chronic knee pain is very common and arthritis of the knee is the main cause of such pain. The few clinical studies based on evidence, and published in scientific journals, have noted a clinical advantage to exercises and the use of TENS with people with this problem, but there is a lack of proof concerning massages, the application of heat, ultrasounds or electrical stimulations.

**The purpose, for the person with this condition, is to improve or maintain his/her functional independence through better education (instruction)**, by controlling the pain (antalgic medication), modifying activities so as to reduce mechanical stress (tension), improving the biomechanical function of the knee (injections into the joint), and using technical aids (cane, orthotics).

TABLE 3: Example of treatment for arthritis of the knee

---

**For treating arthritis of the knee, the recommendations are as follows:**

- Continue using a cane;
- Acetaminophen and ice for the pain;
- Physiotherapy to improve the stabilization capacity of the particular muscles of the knee;
- Viscosupplementation (injection of a gel in the joint);
- Orthosis to decompress the medial compartment of the knee;
- Start an aquafitness programme;
- Stable shoes for walking.

---

## Neck pain

Neck pain is the second most important reason for absenteeism at work. Neck pain is most often the result of an injury or accident (whiplash). When neck pain becomes chronic it is the object of recommendations that encourage the use of proprioceptive exercises, as well as therapeutic stretching and strengthening exercises.

There is little evidence to support or eliminate the use of heat therapy, therapeutic massages, mechanical traction, therapeutic ultrasounds, TENS or electrical stimulation.

## Fibromyalgia

The treatment for fibromyalgia involves an interdisciplinary approach. It will be based on education (coping with pain and stress), aerobic exercises, cognitive-behavioural therapy and medication. Thus, in the data based on evidence concerning the use of physical activity to treat fibromyalgia, aerobic exercise holds a very important place. This type of exercise improves the aerobic capacity of the individual with fibromyalgia, increases the pain threshold at tender points, and reduces pain in general. It should be noted that this effectiveness is not maintained if the exercise programme is stopped.

The literature provides only weak or moderate support for the use of anerobic exercises, hydrotherapy, manual therapeutics, massages, electrotherapy or ultrasounds.

## 5. PHYSICAL ACTIVITY PROGRAMME

There are two major kinds of exercises: anaerobic and aerobic. **Anaerobic exercises** involve short-term, high-intensity activities that use the individual's reserves of energy and carbohydrates (sugars). Examples include a quick race lasting a few seconds, jumping and lifting weights. **Aerobic exercises** on the other hand are medium- and long-term activities that use carbohydrates, as well as lipids and proteins. Examples include a race or a swim lasting longer than three to five minutes.

The data in the literature has indicated that stretching and activities to increase muscular endurance and strength are associated with a decrease in chronic pain, although the exact mechanisms behind these effects are not completely known.

### Stretching exercises

Stretching (flexibility) exercises are the first step in an exercise programme. Flexibility makes a joint movement more fluid in all respects. It can be limited by problems with the muscles or tendons or the joint capsule, as well as by an underlying neurological condition (muscular hypertonia) and excess weight. Regular and appropriate stretching can prevent injuries of a muscular or tendinous origin.

**Thus, two stretching techniques must be used:**

- **Passive stretching:** progressive stretching of a muscle group until a certain amount of discomfort is obtained (for example, creating tension of 4 on a scale of 10), and holding the position for 30 seconds, then repeating this exercise ideally three times with 30 seconds of rest between each series;
- **Contract-relax per neuromuscular facilitation:** maximum contraction of a muscle or a muscle group for 10 seconds followed by relaxation and progressive stretching combined with a contraction of the opposite muscles. Take note: although this exercise is good for improving movement amplitude and flexibility, it requires a good warm-up.

Slow and progressive stretching for a few minutes is better than stretching repeatedly and briefly.

## Development of muscular strength

With stretching exercises, the **development of muscular strength** or muscular reinforcement is also crucial. Muscular strength can be developed by lifting weights (lower or upper limbs) to the point of fatigue. Generally, 10 to 15 repetitions are recommended, and make a good compromise between the development of muscular strength and endurance. The frequency of these sessions is ideally three times a week. It has been demonstrated that training to develop leg muscles (thighs) five times per week has been associated with a 40% increase in muscular strength after 10 weeks. When a weight can be lifted 15 to 20 times in a row, it is recommended that the weight be increased by 10%.

## Endurance exersices

Endurance exercises, namely aerobic exercises, involve the rapid and alternate contraction of a large muscle group with little resistance for a sustained period of time. These exercises include walking, jogging, cycling, swimming, cross-country skiing, etc. Certain notions concerning the use of aerobic exercises for the treatment of chronic pain should be noted.

**Aerobic exercises are:**

1. Dynamic exercises, free movements, based on respiration;

2. Of moderate intensity, under the threshold of respiratory fatigue or breathlessness;

3. Ideally last at least than 30 minutes, with breaks as needed (for example, 3 sessions lasting a minimum of 10 minutes);

4. Performed at a frequency of 3 to 5 times per week; although if they last less than 30 minutes, it is recommended that they be done at least once per day. Ideally, the intensity of the exercise must be enough to achieve a heart beat between 60% and 85% of the maximum rate for the patient's age, easily calculated using the following formula: 220 – age. Thus, for a 50-year-old, the maximum theoretical heart rate is 170 beats per minute; physical exercise at 70% of that rate should be approximately 120 beats per minute.

## EXAMPLES OF PROGRAMMES

### A. Exercise programmes for lower back pain

A progressive rehabilitation programme including walking and cycling for six weeks is associated with an improvement in the performance of a person suffering from chronic lower back pain. Moreover, the therapist signs a contract with the patient, and the exercises programmed for two to three times a week must be completed despite the pain. Throughout the programme, the physical activity is increased progressively, based on the patient's physical performances and not the pain. The exercises involve stretching of the back muscles and the quadratus lumborum muscle along with flexibility exercises for the lower limbs including the tensor of the fascia lata, and the hamstring and buttock muscles. (See **Photo 1**.)

Muscles can be strengthened through specific exercises for the pelvis (seesaw movement), and the back muscles ("crushing" and extension). (See **Photo 2**.)

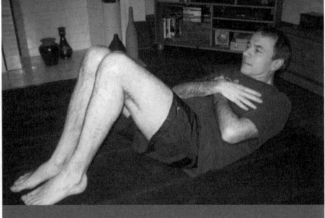

**Photo 1:** Standing up with knees and hips bent, heel flat on the ground; the arms are crossed over the chest, and only the head and the shoulders are raised.

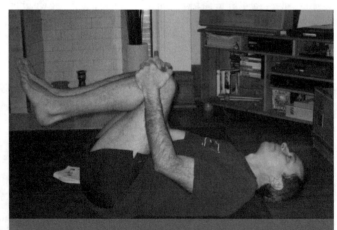

**Photo 2:** Knees against chest, and stretching of buttock muscles. May be done one leg at a time, with the other extended.

## B. Exercise programme for arthritis of the knee

Sustained stretching of the hamstring muscles is recommended first. (See **Photo 3**.) Muscular reinforcement will focus first on the isometric work of the quadriceps (thigh) muscle. (See **Photo 4**.)

Following this, proprioceptive muscles for movement around the knee will be done with assistance at the beginning, and then alone. Low impact endurance exercises for the knee will be done; this may involve, for example, walking while immersed to the waist in a swimming pool. Ideally, the water in the pool should be approximately 32-36 °C. In addition to the aerobic walking activity, stretching, muscle reinforcement and joint movement exercises may also be done in the pool. Out of the pool, physical activities should be done with a physiotherapist three times a week, with work to be done twice a day, three days per week.

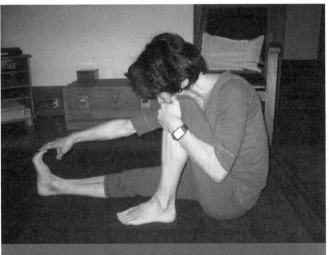

**Photo 3:** Stretching of the hamstring muscles: one knee is bent and the other extended while the individual tries to touch his/her toes.

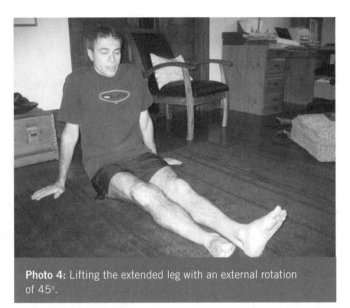

**Photo 4:** Lifting the extended leg with an external rotation of 45°.

## C. Exercise programme for fibromyalgia

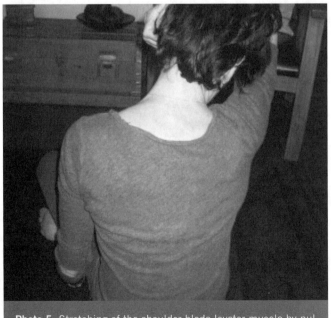

**Photo 5:** Stretching of the shoulder blade levator muscle by pulling the head forward and to the side.

The importance of physical activity for the treatment of fibromyalgia has been clearly demonstrated. This physical activity includes stretching exercises, joint mobilizations, walking, swimming or cycling.

Stretching exercise for the shoulder blade levator muscles (see **Photo 5**), the pectoral muscles and the posterior capsule of the shoulder. These exercises will be combined with flexibility exercises for the lower limbs. A regular endurance activity (2 or 3 three times a week) that lasts 30 to 60 minutes and causes an increase in heart beat above 70% is also beneficial.

# 6. CONCLUSION

Patients must set goals that can be attained, are relevant, interesting and measurable, and affect three different spheres: physical (exercise programme), functional (tasks associated with everyday activities) and social (enjoyment in taking part in social activities). Thus, we will conclude this discussion on the importance of physical activity in the treatment of pain with a quote from Watson (2000):

« Physical activity is perhaps the most powerful component in pain management programmes. Increasing fitness is important not only in reversing the disuse syndrome, but in giving a powerful signal to patients that they are beginning to regain a degree of control over their musculoskeletal system. It is therefore extremely important from both the physical and the psychological point of view. »

# REFERENCES

- Bartels EM, Lund H, Hagen KB, Dagfinrud H, Christensen R, Danneskiold-Samsøe N. Aquatic exercise for the treatment of knee and hip osteoarthritis. Cochrane Database of Systematic Reviews, 2007, Issue 4. Art. No.: CD005523.
- Bonnin-Koang HY, Richard D, Luigi A, Villy J, Alméras N, Pélissier J. Mobilisation des raideurs articulaires et gestion de la douleur induite. In: Pélissier J, Viel E (eds) Douleur et Soins en médecine physique et de réadaptation. Sauramps Médical, Montpellier, 2006, p. 66-74.
- Busch AJ, Barber KA, Overend TJ, Peloso PMJ, Schachter CL. Exercise for treating fibromyalgia syndrome. Cochrane Database of Systematic Reviews 2007, Issue 4. Art. No.: CD003786.
- Chapman EC. Pathophysiologie de l'intolérance à l'activité physique. Réadaptation de la douleur: approches physiothérapiques. Dans le cadre du cours PHT-2321 — Physiothérapie de la douleur. Hiver 2008. Université de Montréal.
- Feldman D. Pratique centrée sur les preuves et normes de pratiques cliniques en réadaptation des douleurs musculo-squelettiques. Dans le cadre du cours PHT-2321 — Physiothérapie de la douleur. Hiver 2008. Université de Montréal.
- Klaber Moffett JA, Frost H. Back to fitness programme: 'the manual for physiotherapists to set up the classes'. Physiotherapy 2000; 86: 295-305.
- Liddle SD, Gracey JH, Baxter GD. Advice for the management of low back pain: a systematic review of randomized controlled trials. Man Ther 2007; 12: 310-327.
- Ljunggren AE, Bjordal JM. Physiotherapy. In: Breivik H, Campbell W, Eccleston C (eds) Clinical Pain Management – Practical applications and procedures. Arnold, London, 2003, p. 179-193.
- Main CJ, Spanswick CC, Watson P. The nature of disability. In: Main CJ, Spanswick CC (eds) Pain management: an interdisciplinary approach. Churchill Livingstone, Edinburgh, 2000, p. 89-106.
- Pedersen BK, Saltin B. Evidence for prescribing exercise as therapy in chronic disease. Scand J Med Sci Sports 2006; 1: p. 3-63.
- Rannou F, Macé Y, Poiraudeau S, Revel M. Douleur et réentrainement à l'effort du lombalgique. In: Pélissier J, Viel E (eds) Douleur et Soins en médecine physique et de réadaptation. Sauramps Médical, Montpellier, 2006, p. 81-83.
- Schramm-Bloodworth D, Grabois M. Physical medicine and rehabilitation. In: Warfield CA, Bajwa SH (eds) Principles and practice of pain medicine. McGraw-Hill, New York, 2004, p. 792-810.
- Watson P. Physical activities programme content. In: Main CJ, Spanswick CC (eds) Pain management: an interdisciplinary approach. Churchill Livingstone, Edinburgh, 2000. p. 285-301.
- Wittink H, Cohen LJ, Michel TH. Pain rehabilitation: Physical therapy treatment. In: Wittink H, Michel TH (eds) Chronic management for physical therapists. Butterworth Heinemann, Boston, 2002. p 127-59.

# CHRONIC PAIN
# AND CLINICAL HYPNOSIS

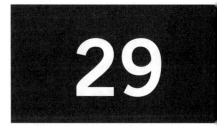

## 29

**Gaston Brosseau,** Psychologist, Saint-Lambert, Quebec, Canada

## ABSTRACT

Chronic pain and clinical hypnosis provide succinct answers for the questions people ask with respect to a therapeutic approach that still has an aura of mystery. In just a few brief years, clinical hypnosis has gone from the world of beliefs to the world of science as a result of work done in experimental research, as well as functional cerebral imaging. The hypnotic effect requires a combination of letting go and abandoning resistance on the part of the individual. How can this be managed?

The characteristics and the coaching approach specific to hypnotherapy are covered in the process for learning to deal with pain, giving subjects an opportunity to speak and "name" their pain, and make the most of their own resources.

ABSTRACT

1. DOES HYPNOSIS REALLY EXIST AND HOW IS IT DIFFERENT FROM THE PLACEBO EFFECT?

2. MY DEFINITION OF CLINICAL HYPNOSIS

3. IS HYPNOSIS AN ALTERED STATE OF CONSCIOUSNESS OR RATHER AN EFFECTIVE STATE OF CONSCIOUSNESS?

4. THE COACHING APPROACH SPECIFIC TO HYPNOTHERAPY

5. PARTICULAR CHARACTERISTICS OF HYPNOTHERAPY

6. THE PATIENT IS OFTEN SURPRISED THAT THEY DO NOT HAVE TO PROVIDE THEIR ENTIRE HISTORY

7. BYPASSING THE SUBJECT'S RESISTANCE ZONES

8. BEING ABLE TO OFFER SUBJECTS A PLACE FOR SPEECH WHERE THEY CAN «NAME» THEIR PAIN

9. KNOWING HOW TO USE THE HEALTHY PART OF THE SUBJECT

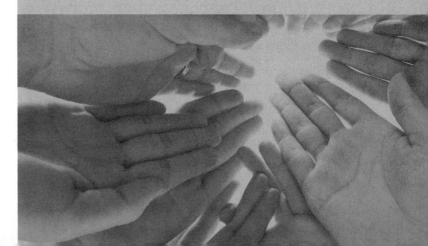

## 1. DOES HYPNOSIS REALLY EXIST AND HOW IS IT DIFFERENT FROM THE PLACEBO EFFECT?

At the risk of confusing certain hypnosis specialists, I have adopted the definition developed by Dr. Jean-Roch Laurence, PhD., and Dr. Campbell Perry, PhD, two psychologists at Concordia University (Montreal, Quebec, Canada) who have distinguished themselves for their experimental research in hypnosis. They have concluded, like Hippolyte Bernheim[1], that **"Hypnosis does not exist. What does exist in fact is the interaction between a specific context and the subject's ability to respond to that context."** Moreover, I admit that I use the hypnotic effect without fully understanding the very essence of that phenomenon. Personally, this type of semantic question does not really bother me and I have continued to teach hypnosis for more than 25 years. To my credit, I quote the informed pedagogue who stated, "If you don't know something, teach it," something I have been doing for more than two decades.

## 2. MY DEFINITION OF CLINICAL HYPNOSIS

At most, I dare to propose a personal definition of clinical hypnosis as the "re-initialization of the five senses in order to improve well-being". Above all, hypnosis requires a combination of letting go and abandoning resistance on the part of the individual. In this sense, hypnosis would act as a mediator or a connection between the conscious and the unconscious. Experimental research work done by Dr. Pierre Rainville, PhD, neuropsychologist at the *Université de Montréal* (Montreal, Quebec, Canada), in functional cerebral imaging to provide an understanding of hypnosis has served to position hypnosis, for the first time, on the scientific chessboard, demonstrating the specific activity of certain regions of the right hemisphere of the brain during hypnotic inductions. Thus, hypnosis has moved from the world of beliefs to the world of knowledge. This distinction is essential and sets hypnosis apart from the placebo effect. We speak of the placebo effect when we observe something in fact that should not exist. It is logical to think that when the cause is removed, the effect should be eliminated, with the exception of the placebo effect when we observe that an effect occurs without a cause. Recent publications on the placebo effect highlight a significantly higher response in the case of children. Saying that "mommy" has an excellent placebo effect is, in my opinion, obvious. She is worth more than many remedies and her effectiveness is proverbial.

I will let you reflect on this conclusion drawn by François Roustang[2], and taken from his book, *La fin de la plainte*:

> "The conclusion is obvious: it is the placebo and its irritating effect that circumscribe the purely scientific field. The placebo is not part of medical science and yet medical science is the sole field capable of validating it. Both beyond and within this science, it is science that defines its limits. If pharmacological science were to reject the placebo on moral grounds, it would destroy itself because it would no longer be able to establish its own scientificalness. In short, the unscientific placebo provides the foundation for the scientificalness of any medication."

## 3. IS HYPNOSIS AN ALTERED STATE OF CONSCIOUSNESS OR RATHER AN EFFECTIVE STATE OF CONSCIOUSNESS?

The people who consult me argue: What exactly are you leading us to do? Visualization, meditation, concentration or what else? It doesn't bother me how you interpret it. Above all, I make sure that you will be able to "re-initialize your life through clinical hypnosis" exactly as you want to. Instead of conceiving of hypnosis as an altered state of conscience, I think that it would be more accurate to speak of mobilizing the subject's effective conscience (an element I will define later) in real time. Thus, I will attribute all credit for the healing to the subject's ability to use their own resources.

## 4. THE COACHING APPROACH SPECIFIC TO HYPNOTHERAPY

The quality of the therapeutic alliance is acknowledged as the decisive element in the success of any therapy. The therapeutic alliance must remain the foundation of any psychological consultation. In order to manage this, the hypnotic relationship (based on letting go and abandoning resistance) provides an excellent tool for galvanizing the helping relationship. By using one of the characteristics of hypnosis, namely the sudden creation of motherhood contact (people often tell us that they have the impression that they have known us a long time after only one or two meetings, I first invite the person to "DO NOTHING" sparing them the anxious or fastidious task of spilling out their personal history (patient history). The form of clinical hypnosis that I practice means that I have to lead the subject to experience a success at each of the sessions so as to counterbalance the failures accumulated in the past with their specialists. In this case, the impasse will be undone. To do this, as of the very first consultation, I like to introduce, among other things, an exercise that is exempt from any form of failure. For seven years, I have been using a very simple exercise that involves DOING NOTHING, as I mentioned previously. This exercise liberates the subject from any constraints, eliminating their fear of being unable to attain their personal objective. This paradoxical induction is discussed in the book *L'hypnose aujourd'hui*, produced under the direction of Dr. Jean-Marc Benhaiem (2005)[3].

Then, I use the subject's ability to help them obtain an instantaneous induction in keeping with their degree of creativity so that they can use it in real time and access the sensory universe of their effective conscious (refers to a cause that produces an effect on its own). This sensory re-initialization initialisation gives the subject the feeling that he/she is re-appropriating his/her body and "naming" him/herself in the here and now, saving a spectacular amount of time and energy, compared to hypnotherapy as used in the analytical approach. These last lines may give rise to many questions and deserve some clarification. In order to lead the patient to a knowledge of how to manage his/her pain through hypnosis, I invite him/her to find a simple induction based on identifying a sensory element that will come spontaneously to mind: what the subject hears, sees, feels, tastes or touches, with the focus constantly on the here and now. In my specific vocabulary, I refer to this as being the ability to return to "zero". Based on numerous clinical observations, I am of the opinion that, when the patient manages to experience this moment, he/she no longer experiences pain and suffering. The patient is no longer anticipating the future or ruminating over the past; he/she has returned to "zero" and is living completely in the here and now. And it is the patient who does all the work. The patient observes this on their own, thereby regaining their self confidence and motivation to find a way out of their chronic pain and chronic fatigue. Moreover, this process has worked very well with people suffering from fibromyalgia.

## 5. PARTICULAR CHARACTERISTICS OF HYPNOTHERAPY

In passing, I would like to clarify the fact that the practice of hypnotherapy is also characterized, with respect to other forms of treatment, by the fact that the patient adopts an active role as of the first visit. There is something tangible, something physical, that is characteristic of the hypnotic experience, setting it apart from most other psychological approaches. This dimension is essential and it is often passed over in silence. Hypnosis serves to unify the somatic and psychic components that are often dissociated in the human being and can cause discomfort.

## 6. THE SUBJECT IS OFTEN SURPRISED THAT THEY DO NOT HAVE TO PROVIDE THEIR ENTIRE HISTORY

In my practice, I invite the subject to use all five senses, to move about physically and take action. Moreover, the individual does not have to recount their history and, in this respect, I like to unsettle the patient by telling them that I don't really listen to what they "say" but rather to what they "are". I like to tell myself that I am not seeing a back ache, a migraine headache, an irritable colon or insomnia in my office, but above all a "person". The subject feels this and notes it quickly. This procedure quickly reduces the subject's anxiety about recounting everything in detail and ensures that they no longer feel as if they have forgotten an element that we should know about. Consequently, the subject's sense of guilt is reduced. As a result, we have to lead the patient to shed their sense of guilt for their condition. This element is often observed as an aggravating factor in the experience of pain. Another characteristic to be noted is the effectiveness and rapidity of the method used to obtain tangible results. Since the subject deals with sensory experiences as of the first session, he/she is able to evaluate his/her level of functioning without assistance and determine the expected results.

## 7. BYPASSING THE SUBJECT'S RESISTANCE ZONES

It should be noted that, as a result of the fact that the subject uses their own vocabulary based on their own culture, there is ordinarily no form of resistance and the subject lets go naturally. It is crucial for the subject to identify their zones of resistance so as to be able to hope to regain mobility and flexibility. The support provided is destined to failure if we bypass the subject's messages of resistance. This is what we refer to as the "therapist's art", distancing ourselves from the recipes established by too many practitioners of hypnosis who focus on using traditional induction techniques that do not really take the patient's personality into consideration. Subjects must be able to step back from their problems if they want to access their own resources.

## 8. BEING ABLE TO OFFER SUBJECTS A PLACE FOR SPEECH WHERE THEY CAN NAME THEIR PAIN

Yes, it is possible to succeed when using hypnotherapy to treat chronic pain if we know how to listen to the subject's pain and suffering since: "Knowing how to listen involves possessing the brain of others as well as your own." (Leonardo da Vinci). First, we agree on the very concept of pain, which is a subjective experience, namely one that is modulated by the subject's experience. Everyone interprets pain in their own way. Everyone has their own personal code for registering pain. We must offer subjects a place where they can speak and express their distress. Listening quality is a decisive factor when coaching subjects with respect to the way in which they "name" the pain. The common understanding that results has a direct impact on the progress of the treatment. The fact of agreeing on a common vocabulary pulls the subject from his/her torpor with respect to his/her pain and personal distress. The subject no longer feels alone; he/she has found support in us. As needed, I use the McGill-Melzack (1975)[4] questionnaire, which has been translated into a dozen languages and is now used throughout the world. This questionnaire makes it easier for the subject to "name" his/her pain. We must take the time needed for the subject to be able to explain his/her benchmarks, beliefs and personal convictions. We are in slippery ground when we deal with people's convictions. This is a conscious and unconscious source of resistance that must not be neglected. When reflecting on the search for truth, Nietzche said that convictions are more dangerous enemies of truth than lies. For just a moment, let us consider the religious convictions, all religions taken together, that have justified, for centuries, and continue to justify the worst humanitarian atrocities. I suggest that you read a book that strips down our popular beliefs, written by Gérard Zwang (1975), entitled *Lettre ouverte aux mals baisants*, and published by Albin Michel[5].

## 9. KNOWING HOW TO USE THE HEALTHY PART OF THE SUBJECT

This sentence must be banished from our language, "Sorry, but there is nothing science can do for you." In that case, what use is all of our knowledge if we lack the creativity and imagination needed to relieve the individual's chronic pain or suffering? I believe that this is precisely where our support as therapists starts. We have to be able to use the subject's potential in order to improve their quality of life. The difference between the medical world and the psychological world lies in the patient's approach. The doctor or the psychiatrist will take care of the patient's physical or psychological problem. These specialists will focus on the pathological part of the patient using, as needed, the appropriate pharmacological treatment or surgery, whereas psychologists will focus on the subject's potential since they have no tools other than the patient's resources. The psychologist focuses on updating the healthy part of the subject. Albert Einstein said: "Imagination is more important than knowledge." Contrary to popular thinking, I claim that every individual can make use of hypnosis if we take the time to show them how they can access their personal resources. The success of our intervention depends on our ability to listen and understand when the individual is at. Therefore, the quality of our coaching is essential to the treatment of chronic pain.

## REFERENCES

1. Godin, J. La nouvelle hypnose, 1992 Albin Michel, Paris.
2. Roustang, F. La fin de la plainte, 2001, Odile Jacob.
3. Benhaiem, JM. L'hypnose aujourd'hui, 2005, IN PRESS. (Ne rien faire : l'induction paradoxale).
4. Melzack, R. & P. Wall. Le Défi de la douleur, Chenelière & Stanké.
5. Zwang, G. Lettre ouverte aux mals baisants, 1975, Albin Michel.

# MEDICATIONS

**Aline Boulanger** MD, FRCPC, MPH, anaesthesiologist, Director, Pain Clinic, Centre hospitalier universitaire de Montréal (CHUM) - Pavillon Hôtel-Dieu, Hôpital du Sacré-Cœur, Montreal, Quebec, Canada

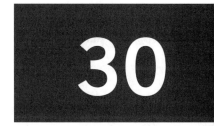

**30**

## ABSTRACT

**Treating chronic pain with medication is useful when it is accompanied by an overall treatment of the individual, involving physical rehabilitation, psychological support and the cooperation of the treatment team.**

Analgesics belong to various families of medications. They alleviate pain while reducing transduction (the forwarding of information from the site of the injury to the posterior horn of the spinal cord) and transmission (the forwarding of information from the spinal cord to the brain), or changing the modulation (mechanisms by which the painful message can be intensified or decreased), and the perception of pain (integration of the information in the brain). They can be used alone or in combination, depending on the individual's basic problem and his/her medical history and current medication.

In the following pages, you will find a summary of the most commonly prescribed analgesics. Nevertheless, it is important to note that the treatment of chronic pain is not limited solely to taking tablets or pills and that medication is only a part of the solution. For several people, medication is contra-indicated.

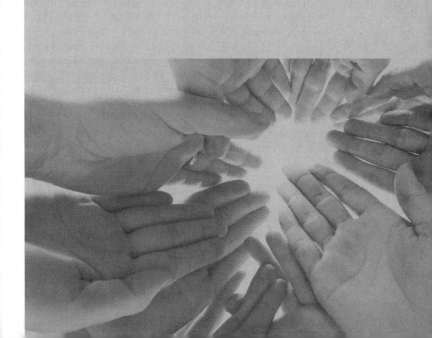

# 1. NON-OPIOID ANALGESICS

## ACETAMINOPHEN

Acetaminophen is a medication that is used to reduce fever, relieve headaches and treat pain. It was first prescribed by a German physician, Dr. Josef Von Mering, in 1893. More than a century has passed and yet the manner in which acetaminophen acts is still uncertain. Acetaminophen is the product that is most used throughout the world to treat mild to moderate pain. As a result of the low risk of complications associated with the use of acetaminophen, it is almost systematically prescribed as a basic analgesic treatment. Nevertheless, the dosages recommended by the physician or the manufacturer must be respected. When larger dosages are used, acetaminophen may cause irreparable damage to the liver.

## NONSTEROIDAL ANTI-INFLAMMATORIES (NSAIDs)

Nonsteroidal anti-inflammatories (NSAIDs) inhibit the cyclooxygenase enzyme. This enzyme is involved in the production of prostaglandins. Prostaglandins play a major role in the appearance of fever and inflammation. By preventing the cyclooxygenase enzyme from producing prostaglandins, NSAIDs alleviate pain, lower fever and reduce inflammation.

NSAIDs are a large family of medications that include various agents belonging to different chemical classes. For example: salicylates (aspirin), indole derivatives (indomethacin: Indocid), oxicams (piroxicam: Feldene; meloxicam: Mobicox)), arylacetates (diclofenac: Voltaren and Arthrotec), and derivatives of propionic acid (ibuprofen: Advil; ketoprofen: Orudis; naproxen: Naprosyn).

NSAIDs are used in the treatment of rheumatic and inflammatory diseases with mild to moderate pains (dysmenorrhoea, trauma, dental pain, post-operatory pain), alone or in combinaison with other analgesics. The maximum dosages indicated for NSAIDs should not be exceeded since the analgesic effect does not increase and the side effects are serious. **NSAIDs have many side effects.** When taken regularly, they can cause stomach ulcers, digestive track bleeding, coagulation disorders and kidney failure. Cyclooxygenase-2 inhibitors (rofecoxib: Vioxx; celecoxib: Celebrex; valdecoxib: Bextra; lumiracoxib: Prexige) were marketed in order to reduce the risk of undesirable effects caused by NSAIDs. Selective COX-2 inhibitors do, in fact, cause less damage to the stomach and do not interfere with blood coagulation. Nevertheless, they have the same negative effects on kidneys as the traditional NSAIDs and studies have indicated that they can cause heart attacks, strokes and high blood pressure. Since the publication of these studies, rofecoxib and valdecoxib have been withdrawn from the market as a result of the negative impact on cardio-vascular function and lumiracoxib has been taken off the market since there is a risk of liver failure when it is taken in high dosages. Only celecoxib is still available at drug stores.

# 2. OPIOID ANALGESICS

Opium, which comes from the *Papaver somniferum* plant, contains numerous natural alkaloids, including morphine and codeine. The organism produces molecules, namely endorphins, which resemble opium alkaloids. The endorphins, the opium alkaloids and the related synthetic products alleviate pain by reducing neuron excitability in various manners.

Opioids are used to treat pain following surgery, cancer pain and certain types of chronic pain. Commonly used opioid medications include morphine (Statex, MS-Contin, M-Eslon, Kadian, etc.), codeine (Codeine Contin), hydromorphone (Dilaudid, Hydromorph Contin), oxycodone (Supeudol, Oxycontin), and fentanyl (Duragesic). Codeine is also available in combination with acetaminophen (Empracet), and the same applies to oxycodone (Percocet). The choice of opioid is often arbitrary. No opioid has been proven superior to the others with respect to analgesic effectiveness, side effects or patient satisfaction. Nevertheless, for various pharmacological reasons, certain opioids seem more beneficial than others for certain people.

Two opioids have particular properties: methadone and tramadol. Methadone has been prescribed for several years for the maintenance or withdrawal of drug addicts. It has been discovered that it is able to block the receptors involved in the maintenance of neuropathic pain. This benefit accounts for its recent popularity in the treatment of chronic pain. Tramadol is considered an atypical central analgesic. This molecule is both an opioid and an antidepressant. It is particularly useful in the case of people with pain of neuropathic origin. Tramadol is available in a slow release formula (Zytram XL, Ralivia, and Tridural) or in combination with acetaminophen (Tramacet).

## SIDE EFFECTS OF OPIOIDS

As in the case of any other medication, opioids have side effects. For several of these side effects (nausea, vomiting, pruritis and urinary retention), tolerance develops over time, and the side effects can decrease, and even disappear. As for constipation, the symptoms persist despite extended usage of opioids. It must be expected and treated. Drowsiness is also a side effect of concern with respect to opioids. Single doses of opioids administered to individuals who have never taken them before have significant effects on reaction time, muscular coordination, attention and short-term memory. When these agents are taken on a regular basis, most people develop a tolerance with respect to this sedative effect. Nevertheless, a small proportion of the population continues to experience drowsiness that can interfere with their ability to perform their professional activities adequately or to drive their car, despite their long-term usage of such medications. People who experience such effects on a long-term basis should not drive vehicles or handle dangerous objects. It was recently demonstrated that the extended use of opioids can modify the hormone balance. The concentration of cortisol, testosterone and estrogens may decrease, where the concentration of prolactin may increase. This can cause a decline in libido and amenorrhea (cessation of menstruation). Finally, opioids both inhibit and stimulate the central nervous system. Although they can provide significant relief at low or moderate dosages, at high dosages they can increase the pain experienced by an individual. It is not possible to determine the maximum dosage to be administered to an individual in advance without incurring the risk of increasing their pain. **In this respect, it is important that each individual for whom an opioid is prescribed respect the dosage prescribed, and make no attempt to self-manage the medication.**

## RISKS OF DEPENDENCY

One of the major concerns associated with the use of opioids is the risk of dependency. It is, nevertheless, important to define some terms that are frequently confused:

### Tolerance

Tolerance is a normal bodily process in which the effect of a medication decreases following long-term use. In practice, this translates into a need to increase the dosage in order to maintain the same therapeutic effect. Tolerance does not affect everyone and it does not mean that there is a psychological dependency (addiction).

### Physical dependency

Physical dependency is a normal physiological response, resulting from the continuous administration of an opioid. It is characterized by a syndrome of withdrawal (sensation of general malaise, rhinorrhea, shaking, sweating, shivering, abdominal cramps, myalgia, etc.) if the patient suddenly stops taking an opioid or if an opioid antagonist is administered. Physical dependency occurs in almost all patients who must take opiates on a regular basis. The withdrawal reaction can be avoided by gradually reducing the medication dosage. Physical dependency does not mean that there is a psychological dependency (addiction).

### Psychological dependency (addiction)

Psychological dependency is a biopsychosocial disorder characterized by an inappropriate use of opioids. One or more of the following will be observed in the individual:
· Loss of control with respect to the use of the opioid;
· Compulsive use;
· An irrepressible desire to use the medication (craving); and
· Continuous use despite the negative physical, emotional, social or economic consequences.

Genetic, psychosocial and environmental factors affect the development of psychological dependency. The risk of psychological dependency associated with the medical use of opioids is not known. This risk is probably low. Nevertheless, a patient who already has problems with substance abuse (dependency on alcohol or illicit drugs) is more likely to develop a dependency than one who has no such history.

## 3. CO-ANALGESIC MEDICATIONS OF ADJUVANTS

**Co-analgesics or adjuvants** are medications that have been developed to treat other pathologies, but were discovered to have analgesic properties. Co-analgesics can modulate the intensity of pain of muscular-skeletal and visceral origin although they were primarily intended to treat chronic neuropathic pain. **The principal co-analgesics used in practice are antidepressants and anticonvulsants.**

## ANTIDEPRESSANTS

Almost all antidepressants can modulate pain. They alleviate pain by improving the modulation capacity by means of two neurotransmitters: serotonin and noradrenaline. The oldest such medications, tricyclic antidepressants (TCAs), are the most effective, but cause many side effects. Tricyclic antidepressants include amitriptyline (Elavil), desipramine (Norpramin), doxepine (Sinequan), and nortriptyline (Aventyl). When a patient cannot take a tricyclic antidepressant for medical reasons, or if the patient is experiencing a severe depression, new generation antidepressants are used. The two principal antidepressants in this class

used to treat pain are venlafaxine (Effexor) and duloxetine (Cymbalta). In general, one person out of three will note an improvement in their pain after taking antidepressants.

Antidepressants have many side effects: dry mouth, constipation, drowsiness, low blood pressure, weight gain, arrythmia, etc. Moreover, they are contraindicated in the case of patients with glaucoma, prostatism, severe arrhythmia or those for whom a high suicide risk has been identified. Antidepressants can interact with other medications, including monoamine oxidase inhibiters (MAOI).

## ANTICONVULSANTS

- Almost all anticonvulsants can reduce pain. They act on pain in several manners. They can stabilize the irritability of the membranes of the peripheral nerves and the spinal cord (transduction and transmission) and improve modulation (by means of gamma-aminobutyric acid, a neurotransmitter).
- The principal anticonvulsants prescribed for pain include: gabapentin (Neurontin), pregabalin (Lyrica), carbamazepine (Tegretol), lamotrigine (Lamictal), topiramate (Topamax) and valproic acid (Epival).
- Since most act in different manners, it should come as no surprise if a molecule that is not effective for a given individual is replaced by another. It is also possible to combine two anticonvulsants so as to benefit from two different modes of action and improve pain control. As in the case of antidepressants, anticonvulsants are not effective for all individuals. Generally, an anticonvulsant can reduce pain in one out of three people.
- Generally, the side effects of anticonvulsants include drowsiness and dizziness, but some of them can also cause harmful side effects that require medical supervision in the case of a small proportion of patients. These include: liver toxicity (carbamazepine, valproic acid), hematologic toxicity (carbamazepine) and dermatologic toxicity (lamotrigine).

## 4. CANNABINOIDS

Cannabis has been used for therapeutic purposes for thousands of years. At the beginning of the 20th century, cannabis use declined considerably as a result of the risk of dependency and the increasing popularity of products produced in the laboratory. Nevertheless, research has highlighted the analgesic properties of cannabinoids and resuscitated clinical interest in these products. **Cannabinoids act on pain by decreasing the transmission of pain and improving modulation capacity.**

There are more than 60 cannabinoids; the principal ones are: delta-9-tetrahydrocannabinol (THC), cannabidiol, etc. The cannabinoids produced in the laboratory can be as powerful and effective as morphine.

Three preparations are currently available on the Canadian market. Two of them are derivatives of cannabinoids produced in the laboratory:
- Nabilone (Cesamet);
- Dronabinol (Marinol); and
- The third is a spray containing primarily two natural cannabinoid derivatives, THC and cannabidiol (Sativex).

Finally, on July 30, 2001, Canada adopted a regulation on access to marijuana for medicinal purposes, thereby allowing certain patients to use cannabis. In order to have access, the patient must complete the forms prepared by Health Canada, indicating the daily dosage used, and a specialist doctor must confirm that the individual has not experienced adequate relief with other common medications. Moreover, since cannabis is not actually a medication, the individual who uses it through the governmental medical marijuana access service must sign a waiver acknowledging that he/she will not sue the physician who completed the documents, in the event that there is a complication associated with the use of marijuana.

The principal side effects associated with cannabinoids are drowsiness and reduced vigilance. Cannabinoid derivatives are contraindicated in the case of patients with serious liver or kidney failure, who have a serious cardio-vascular disease (ischemic heart disease, arrhythmia, poorly controlled high blood pressure or serious heart failure), who have a history of schizophrenia or any other psychotic disorders, and who are under the age of 18, as well as well as for pregnant or breast-feeding women.

Additional studies are required in order to evaluate the long-term effects of cannabinoids. Among other things, we must further document the analgesic benefits in the case of people, identify the populations that could benefit the most, explore the impact on the ability to concentrate and better detect the risks of psychological dependency.

## 5. FORMULATIONS

### ORAL MEDICATION

#### Tablets

Tablets, which are well tolerated by patients, are generally preferred as a result of their simplicity and their effectiveness. There are two formulations: short action and slow release.

Short-action tablets are indicated for relieving acute, short-term pain and chronic pain that occurs only when an effort is made. Determining the dosage needed to relieve the pain of a patient suffering from persistent chronic pain when the physician wants to replace the treatment with a long-acting medication, and controlling pain, excesses in the case of a patient taking a long-acting medication.

The advantage of slow release or long-acting tablets is that they provide stable blood levels. They are indicated in the case of patients with constant pain.

## ELIXIRS, SUPPOSITORIES, PATCHES AND INJECTIONS

Elixirs and suppositories are seldom prescribed, but they can be useful in the case of patients who have problems swallowing. Certain opioids (such as fentanyl and buprenorphine) are absorbed well through the skin. Patches, which can be applied on the skin, are available for these two analgesics. Injections (sub-cutaneous, intramuscular and intravenous) are rarely prescribed for patients with non-cancerous chronic pain. They are reserved for patients who are unable to take opioids in other formulations.

## TOPICAL PREPARATIONS

Taking medication by mouth can have significant side effects. Since systemic absorption is slow and side effects are minimal, using a cream can be effective and safer.

The most frequently used topical preparation contains local anaesthetics. It has also been reported that creams made from antidepressants, anticonvulsants and ketamine (a molecule that blocks pain by means of a receptor localized in the spinal cord: NMDA receptor) have been useful in certain cases. The use of a cream is most justified in the case of localized neuropathic pain, such as neuralgia that occurs following shingles.

# 6. RULES FOR PRESCRIBING MEDICATION

Some prescription principles serve to provide better results with these products.

### 1. PERSONALIZE THE DOSAGE

Every one responds differently to the same medication. It should come as no surprise that two people experiencing the same comparable intensity of pain can take different dosages of medication.

### 2. INCREASE DOSAGES GRADUALLY

Most of the medications prescribed to relieve pain have side effects. It is recommended that you start with small dosages and increase them gradually so as to avoid side effects.

### 3. PREVENT AND TREAT SIDE EFFECTS

The side effects caused by analgesics can become as problematic as the pain itself. The analgesic prescription is generally accompanied with by a protocol for treating undesirable effects.

### 4. USE A MULTIMODAL ANALGESIC TREATMENT

Multimodal analgesia involves combining various medications such as acetaminophen, anti-inflammatories, opioids and adjuvant medications or co-analgesics (antidepressants, anticonvulsants and others) described together to relieve pain. By using medications from different families, greater pain relief can be used, despite the fact that small dosages of each of the products are prescribed.

### 5. PERSEVERE

Acetaminophen, anti-inflammatories, opioids and cannabinoids generally have rapid effects on pain. Nevertheless, since they have side effects, the dosages must be increased slowly. As for co-analgesics, it is generally necessary to administer the agent on a continuous basis for two to three weeks in order to see the clinical effects. All in all, regardless of the type of medications prescribed, the patient must be patient and perseverant, and follow the doctor's recommendations.

### 6. STOP TAKING MEDICATIONS

After making a valid test, when a medication does not appear to provide any significant relief, or when the side effects are too serious, the patient should stop taking the medication. For most of these products, and in order to avoid withdrawal, it is important to reduce the dosages progressively, in keeping with the doctor's recommendations.

# MORRIS' STORY

**Morris K.,** Montreal, Quebec, Canada

(See other testimonials, pages 100, 300, 310, 372 and 382.)

*Morris survived a plane crash, and recuperated from a broken jaw and ankle, as well as fractures to the spine.*

During a routine visit to my family physician, he asked many questions about how things were going. He would not hear of me carrying this, all bottled up inside of me. I needed to talk about it. I saw a psychologist who, after three or four months, recommended that I see a psychiatrist, as she had done all that she could to get me to empty the extra large sack full of feelings and stories. She felt that I needed some medication to help deal with underlying feelings of anxiety and depression, and psychologists could not prescribe medications.

My wife took the lead on this massive journey to find the right psychiatrist in the public system to treat me. It was a frustrating journey but she did succeed. This psychiatrist first saw us as a couple, then separately for a few times and finally saw me separately on a regular basis. At some point he prescribed some antianxiety and antidepression medications. This was a trip of its own. Everything was largely experimental, to the degree of what would work best for me and what would agree with my body. Eventually, we found what would do the job for me.

Now 22 and a half years after the trauma, I still see my psychiatrist for a yearly evaluation so that he can continue to prescribe me the medications I need.

# MEDICATIONS FOR THE PEDIATRIC
# **PATIENT IN CHRONIC PAIN**

**Janice Sumpton**, RPh, BSc Phm, London, Ontario, Canada
Read by Roxane Therrien, BPharm, MSc, pharmacist, Centre hospitalier universitaire Ste-Justine,
Montreal, Quebec, Canada

**31**

## ABSTRACT

Non-pharmacological interventions should always accompany medications in the treatment of chronic pain. Chronic pain in children significantly impacts the quality of life of the child, and functioning of the family. It affects the child's ability to attend school, perform to the best of their ability and develop socialization skills[1,2,3]. However, the medications themselves may affect the child's ability to function.

This chapter will discuss the challenges in pain management for chronic pain in children, and review the medications used to treat these patients. The most common chronic pain conditions in pediatrics and the pharmacological approach will be outlined.

### Disclaimer
**The content of this chapter does not replace a pharmacist's advice. Before administering any medication to children, or changing the dosage, speak with your pharmacist.**

# 1. INTRODUCTION

Chronic pain in children is prevalent and most troublesome to the child and their caregivers. The incidence reported in the literature varies, and is likely a conservative estimate. A Canadian study of 495 children (9 to 13 years old) found 57% reported 1 or more recurrent pain, and 6% stated chronic pain.[1] A Dutch survey of over 5,000 school children living with pain lasting longer than 3 months found an incidence of 25%.[1] The frequency of chronic pain in adolescents is similar to that reported in adults.[2]

# 2. THE CHALLENGES INHERENT TO PEDIATRIC PHARMACOLOGY

## DEVELOPMENTAL CHANGES AND EFFECTS ON DRUG RESPONSE

Developmental changes have an impact on drug response in children. Maturation of organs occurs rapidly after birth. The effects of drugs change with these body changes, resulting in drug dosing according to age and weight. Kidney function increases from the first day of life, rapidly during the first month, and is at adult capacity by 24 months. The kidneys remove most drugs from the body in the urine, affecting the dosage for children. From birth onward the percentage of body water and protein available for drug binding changes the amount of active drug available. All of these quickly changing processes affect the drug dose and frequency of administration.[1,4,5] This adds to the complexity of adequate pain relief in children with chronic pain.

## INADEQUATE DOSAGE FORMS

### Always check dosage and medications with your pharmacist.

Some pain medications are marketed in solid oral dosage forms only (e.g. Pills) that do not necessarily correlate with the doses needed by children. For example, cutting a pill in an attempt to obtain a smaller dose can often lead to inaccurate dosing. There are recipes for the pharmacist to use when preparing liquid dosage forms for some medications.

- When cutting a suppository in half, it is more accurate to split from end to tip rather than a cross-section cut.
- Fentanyl patches were available until recently with 25 µg/hour as the lowest strength. A 12.5 µg/hr patch is now available in many countries. If a partial dose is required, do not cut the patch. If one-half the dose is needed then apply an occlusive dressing (e.g. Tegaderm™) to the skin first, then the fentanyl patch on top with half the fentanyl on top of the dressing (this portion will not be absorbed by the skin).[6]

## DILEMMAS IN PEDIATRIC RESEARCH

Ideally, in this evidence-based era, one should have sufficient published data to design guidelines for analgesic use in pediatrics. However, chronic pain is a specialty within the specialty of pediatrics, making this task extremely difficult.

Ethical considerations, age-appropriate pain assessment tools and low patient numbers add to the challenge.[7] Often, the dosing must be extrapolated from adult data[1] even if this is inappropriate for pediatrics.

## DOSING CAUTIONS

When available, mg/kg dosing should be utilized in children. But the dose should not exceed the normal adult dose (this becomes important in older children who are adult size). Whichever dose is lower should be used. One should not to exceed the total daily recommended dose when giving the drug on a regular schedule for chronic pain.

## ERRORS IN DOSE MEASUREMENT

Inadvertent dosing errors (under- or overdosing) can frequently occur with medications in liquid forms. Acetaminophen is available in different strengths. Parents are most familiar with the dose in a given amount to measure, (number of millilitres or teaspoonful), but if a different strength is purchased by mistake and administrated to the child, he/she is at risk for decreased efficacy or toxicity. It is mandatory to use an accurate measuring device such as a small-volume oral syringe in infants and young children, and medication cup/tube with accurate markings for older children. The household teaspoon is very inaccurate for medications.

Inadvertent overdosing of acetaminophen can occur if the child is taking other products containing acetaminophen such as common cold products and some pain relievers (including Percocet® and Tramacet®).

A study of 100 caregivers showed only 30% were able to state the correct acetaminophen dose to administer to their child, and accurately measure the dose they intended to give.[8]

## 3. BASIC PRINCIPLES IN PEDIATRIC PAIN MEDICATION

The basic principles in pain medication management for children are as follows:
- The oral route is most preferred in infants and children.
- The rectal route is an alternative if the child is unable to tolerate oral administration, and a rectal dosage form is available.
- Intramuscular injections should not be used because of pain on injection and children's varied muscle mass affecting the amount of drug absorbed.
- Subcutaneous and intravenous routes are options for patients in severe pain with a line for access.
- Patient controlled analgesia (pca) in children six years or older is supported in the literature[5], and gives the patient some control in their own pain management.
- Acetylsalicylic acid or asa (aspirin®) is reserved for children with rheumatic diseases, or who require platelet inhibition. This reservation is a result of the potentially fatal risk of Reye's Syndrome which is possibly associated with asa use[5] in children under 18 years of age.

A general guideline for chronic pain is adapted from the World Health Organization's approach to pediatric cancer pain.[9] A numerical score of 0 for no pain and 10 for worst pain is used.

| SEVERITY OF PAIN | ANALGESIC CHOICES |
|---|---|
| **Mild (score 1 to 3)** | Acetaminophen, non-steroidal anti-inflammatory drugs (NSAIDs) |
| **Moderate (score 4 to 6)** | NSAIDs, acetaminophen/opioid combination products |
| **Severe (score 7 to 10)** | Opioids (avoid meperidine) |

### ACETAMINOPHEN

Acetaminophen is commonly used in infants and children, and has the advantage of multiple variations in dosage form. Absorption is delayed and erratic when given rectally.[5] The dose in children is 10 to 15 mg/kg/dose every 4 to 6 hours to a maximum total of 60 to 75 mg/kg/day. An adult dose of 1 g every 6 hours (or 4 g per day)[5,6,10,11] should not be exceeded. Because of the risk of liver toxicity, some experts recommend 2 to 2.5 g per day as the maximum (rather than 4 g) when given every day for chronic pain. How acetaminophen works against pain is multi-factorial. It blocks pain impulses, and inhibits chemicals in the brain and spinal cord, that are responsible for pain perception.[12]

Toxicity has been reported in children receiving one therapeutic dose of acetaminophen with repeated dosing.[11,12] Toxicity stems from the metabolism of acetaminophen. Acetaminophen is metabolized by the liver.[11,12] One of the resultant products is toxic and binds to a substance rendering it non-toxic.[11] If there isn't enough of this substance then the toxic form kills liver cells.[6,11] Resulting in liver failure. Acute kidney failure is reported following therapeutic dosing of acetaminophen.[13,14] Several reports of liver failure after supra-therapeutic dosing (higher doses than recommended) of acetaminophen exists in children.[15,16]

Risk factors for toxicity include inappropriate dosing of acetaminophen, reported in 15% of cases in one report.[17] Other contributing factors to toxicity include fasting, decreased substance to make the metabolite non-toxic, drug interactions with concomitant medication competing for metabolism in the liver, fever in the child, and genetic factors affecting the amount of liver enzymes.[11,12]

## IBUPROFEN

Ibuprofen is used commonly as a pain reliever in infants and children. It belongs to a class of drugs referred to as non-steroidal anti-inflammatory drugs (NSAIDs). Other drugs in this group include naproxen, diclofenac and piroxicam. NSAIDs work by decreasing the formation of prostaglandins, a substance that causes inflammation. By decreasing the inflammation, the pain is reduced.[6,10,12] The drug also has fever-reducing effects.[12]

Ibuprofen has advantages compared to acetaminophen of having a longer duration of action needing less frequent dosing and a direct effect on decreasing inflammation.[6] The dose in infants and children older than 6 months is 5 to 10 mg/kg/dose every 6 to 8 hours to a maximum total of 40 mg/kg/day. Do not exceed the usual adult dose of 1,200 to 2,400 mg per day, depending on the reason for use.[5,6,10,18] Ibuprofen and acetaminophen can be used together for pain.[10,18] The literature has not found any increased benefit for treating a fever by alternating doses of acetaminophen and ibuprofen, compared to each drug used alone. In fact, there is more risk of harm to the child, because the different frequency to give the two drugs is confusing to follow. This can lead to under- or overdosing.[19]

Ibuprofen is generally well tolerated. The most common side effect is stomach upset, which is decreased when given with food. Ibuprofen use in children can cause acute renal failure. The decrease in prostaglandins by nsaids decreases blood flow to the kidney. Alternatively, inflammation of the working areas of the kidney can result in kidney failure.[12] Ibuprofen must be used with caution in children under 6 months of age or weighing less than 10 kg, children with a medical history of stomach ulcer, kidney impairment, dehydration or allergy to asa; or who are taking blood thinners.[6,10,18]

## 4. CHRONIC MUSCULOSKELETAL PAIN

A study of school-aged children found that 30.8% Had pain that lasted longer than 6 months. The same study indicated that 64% of all the pains reported were musculoskeletal pains.[3] The types of pain in children and adolescents include diffuse idiopathic pain syndromes (juvenile fibromyalgia), complex regional pain syndrome (CRPS), juvenile hypermobility with pain, back pain, and childhood disease with chronic pain features.[3]

There is little literature support for the medications used in musculoskeletal pain compared to placebo (sugar pill) to scientifically evaluate the effectiveness and side effects of the medications in children and adolescents. Depending on the type of musculoskeletal pain, different drugs have been used with some success. These include antidepressants (for their analgesic effects), NSAIDs, opioids, nerve blocks and anti-seizure medication (anticonvulsants, used for their analgesic effects in nerve pain).[3] Drug specifics are covered in the other pain sections of this chapter.

## 5. MENSTRUAL PAIN

Painful menstruation (or dysmenorrhea) is common in female adolescents with a reported incidence of 20 to 90%. The pain usually starts just before, or at the start of menstruation and continues for 12 to 48 hours of flow.[20]

The pain is caused by prostaglandins, which cause the uterus to contract and spasm. The pain responds well to NSAIDs since they decrease the amount of prostaglandins available. The nsaids are taken for short intervals during the time of menstrual pain, which helps to decrease side effects. Significant pain relief is found in 60 to 90% with NSAIDs.[20] Ibuprofen, naproxen and others have been well tolerated. Some experience stomach upset and other gi symptoms.[6,20]

The ibuprofen dose recommended in menstrual pain is 200 to 400 mg/dose every 4 to 6 hours, not to exceed 1,200 mg total in a 24-hour period. The naproxen dose is one dose of 500 mg, then 250 mg every 6 to 8 hours, not to exceed 1,250 mg total for the first 24 hours, then a daily maximum of 1,000 mg thereafter.[6]

Oral contraceptives are commonly used, and reports have indicated complete pain relief in 50%.[20] Oral contraceptives have advantages and disadvantages beyond the scope of this review.

# 6. JUVENILE IDIOPATHIC ARTHRITIS (JIA)

Pain is common in children with arthritis. In a two-month period, children with arthritis in more than one joint experienced pain about 73% of the days. Approximately one third described their pain as severe.[21]

The approach to management of chronic pain with arthritis has traditionally involved treatment of the underlying reason for pain, which is the arthritis itself.[21] Despite treatment with drugs targeted at treating the arthritis including methotrexate and biologic-modifying drugs, 66% of children still experienced pain.[21]

A survey of North American rheumatologists revealed no consensus on the use of opioids in children with severe pain with arthritis.[22] The cause of pain is a result of many factors including changes to the peripheral and central nervous systems. Pain may be present despite lack of tissue damage.[23]

Nsaids are the most commonly used drugs in arthritis. Unfortunately, these drugs have a "ceiling effect," which means that as the dose is increased, at a certain point the increased dose will not have added pain relief; however, it does produce more side effects at this higher dose. [23] The ibuprofen dose recommended is as mentioned earlier in this chapter.[6] The usual naproxen dose in juvenile arthritis is 10 to 15 mg/kg/day divided into two doses, not to exceed 1,000 mg per day.[6,24]

Prednisone is a corticosteroid with anti-inflammatory effects. It is given in doses of 0.05 to 2 mg/kg/day to a usual maximum dose of 60 mg/day given with food, once daily or divided doses.[6] Long-term prednisone use has many side effects. Serious side effects are bone thinning, and stunting growth. Weight gain and increased risk of infection are common.[6,22]

Opioids display anti-inflammatory effects that may reduce pain in arthritis. Antidepressants and anticonvulsants can have effects on nerve pain, which is of benefit if there is a component of neuropathic pain (nerve pain).[23]

# 7. CHRONIC HEADACHE

Chronic daily headache (CDH) in children has been listed as high as 1.5%. Cdh occurs in younger children (under 6 years old) as well as in the adolescent age group. A Cochrane Review found migraines affect 10% of children from ages 6 to 20 years. This significantly affects their ability to attend school, on average missing 1.5 weeks of school compared to their healthy classmates.[26] The most common types of headache in children are tension headaches and migraines (with or without an aura).[27]

CDH is defined as a headache for more than 15 days per month that is not a tension headache or migraine, or caused by an underlying medical condition.[25,27]

## GENERAL PRINCIPLES OF HEADACHE TREATMENT

It is important to start treatment as soon as the headache starts to achieve the best results.[25] Medication overuse should be avoided since this leads to rebound headaches. If the child is experiencing two or more headaches a week requiring medication, they are at a higher risk of medication overuse.[25,27] Rebound headaches are insidious in nature, and a difficult cyclic headache pattern to eliminate.[28]

## TREATMENT OF MIGRAINES

Acetaminophen, nsaids and triptans have been used in children for acute treatment.[25,28,29] One study comparing acetaminophen to ibuprofen to placebo, in 88 children (ages 4 to 15[8] years) showed that ibuprofen was twice as effective as acetaminophen, and three times more than placebo, to abort the headache in two hours.[29]

Sumatriptan is a specific migraine drug that works by constricting (narrowing) the dilated blood vessels, and decreasing inflammation causing the migraine. Single oral doses of 25 to 100 mg have been used in children 12 to 17 years of age. Side effects were more common in the younger children. The usual onset of action is 1 to 1.5 hours with the maximum effect 2 to 4 hours after the dose. Side effects include high blood pressure, chest tightness (and rarely heart attacks), flushing, dizziness, drowsiness, headache, nausea and vomiting.[6]

## PREVENTION OF MIGRAINES

Preventive treatment is considered when headaches occur frequently.[25] Reasonable expectations of the preventive treatment are key. The goal is to reduce the number of headaches (rather than the severity of a headache). An adequate trial of at least one month of an individual drug (if tolerated) should be given before trying a different agent. There are few well-conducted studies comparing drugs for the treatment of migraine in children. In turn, there are no guidelines as to which drug to try first, or well-defined dosing specific to children.[28]

One study showed propranolol to be more effective than placebo in preventing migraines in children.[26] Propranolol reduced headaches by at least 60%[30] propranolol doses range from 0.6 to 1.5 mg/kg/day divided three times daily.[6] Propranolol is contraindicated in children with asthma or reactive airways, certain heart diseases and diabetes.[6,28]

More scientific studies are necessary on drugs for migraine prevention in children. Listed below are drugs that have been used, suggested dosing and common side effects. If the child has other medical conditions, the choice of drug may be guided by the benefits in those co-existent conditions.[28]

Amitriptyline (a tricyclic antidepressant) has been successful in children, and has the benefit of night-time sedation. The dose is given with supper or a few hours before bed.[28] A study of 192 children ages 9 to 15 years with 3 or more headaches per month received amitriptyline at an initial dose of 0.25 mg/kg/day. The dose was increased by 0.25 mg/kg every 2 weeks to a maximum of 1mg/kg/day. Amitriptyline effectively decreased the frequency, severity and length of headache, and was well tolerated.[31] Amitriptyline may cause constipation, dry mouth, increased heart rate, dizziness and weight gain.[6,28] Caution should be heeded in adolescents taking other antidepressants or suffering from depression secondary to pain. The possible risk of suicidal ideation should be considered when choosing which drug to use.[6,25]

Some anticonvulsants have been used in children including valproic acid, in doses of 10 to 30 mg/kg/day, divided twice daily. It is recommended to begin with a night-time dose and increase the dose as tolerated once a week.[24,27] Common side effects are weight gain, drowsiness and nausea (take with food). Rarely, valproic acid may cause serious liver dysfunction and pancreatitis. Topiramate has been used in doses starting at 0.5 To 1 mg/kg/day or 12.5 mg per day, and increased as tolerated weekly, to 50 mg twice daily (or a maximum of 200 mg/day). Most common side effects are weight loss, thinking problems, paresthesia (pins and needles), decreased sweating and drowsiness. It is important to drink plenty of fluids to prevent dehydration and kidney stones. Caution should be also heeded in hot temperatures or during exercise since one is less able to sweat and maintain normal body temperature.[6,25,28]

Cyproheptadine has been used for many years in children. Doses vary from 4 mg two or three times daily with food or milk. Generally it is well tolerated, but may cause weight gain and drowsiness.[6,25,28]

## 8 ABDOMINAL PAIN

Repeated abdominal pain occurs in 10 to 20% of children. While often benign, it is very disruptive to the child, their schooling and the family as a whole.[32] Chronic abdominal pain makes up 2 to 4% of visits to pediatricians.[33] Examples include constipation, gastritis and intestinal infections.[9]

Abdominal migraines in children have been treated with pizotifen.[33,34,35] One study in 14 children used doses of 0.25 mg twice daily, and had fewer days of abdominal pain in addition to less severe pain. Side effects may include drowsiness, dizziness and weight gain.[31]

Famotidine decreases the amount of acid secreted by the stomach.[6] Doses of 0.5 mg/kg/dose given twice daily to a maximum daily dose of 40 mg was studied in 25 children. While there was general improvement, there was no difference in pain scores compared to the placebo group. There may be a subgroup with upper tract symptoms that may benefit from famotidine.[36] It is difficult to make a general statement on effectiveness, and more study is needed.

## 9 NEUROPATHIC PAIN

Neuropathic pain comes from damage to the nerve itself, rather than damaged tissue affecting the nerves around it. Neuropathic pain is more difficult to treat, and may be underrecognized (and undertreated) because it is difficult to describe, especially for younger children.[9] Neuropathic pain can be secondary to surgery or trauma, or from various treatments for cancer.[1] A survey of children up to 14 years of age showed the incidence of various types of neuropathic pain (phantom limb pain, trigeminal neuralgia, postherpetic neuralgia) increased with age. No child under 14 years of age had diabetic neuropathy.[37]

Amitriptyline (an antidepressant) is used for its effect on nerve pain and has the advantage of once daily dosing at night, to use its sedative qualities.[38] It works by increasing neurotransmitters (chemicals in the brain) that decrease the perception of pain. The initial dose is low (0.1 mg/kg at bedtime), and increased as tolerated over 2 to 3 weeks to 0.5 To 2 mg/kg at bedtime (not to exceed an adult dose).[6] The side effects are described above in the headache section.

Gabapentin has been used successfully in neuropathic pain.[38] The suggested initial dose is 5 mg/kg at bedtime on day 1, 5 mg/kg/dose twice daily on day 2, then 5 mg/kg/dose three times daily, followed by increasing the dose as tolerated to 8 to 35 mg/kg/day divided three times daily.[6] Some patients may require the dose divided four times daily.[18] The capsules may be opened up, and the contents sprinkled and mixed in soft food (applesauce) or drinks (orange juice).[6,18] Most common side effects are drowsiness, dizziness, headache, nausea (take with meals to decrease) and diarrhea.[6,39]

Tramadol is used extensively for chronic pain. It is considered to be a "medium strength" analgesic in potency. It has very weak opioid activity and also increases some of the neurotransmitters that decrease the perception of pain.[40] Available dosage forms limit its use to older children. Studies in children are limited, but so far side effects are similar to those in adults. A postoperative study in children found the most common side effects were nausea, vomiting, itchiness and rash.[41] One study used tramadol for chronic pain for up to 30 days in 113 children ages 7 to 16 years old. Doses used were 1 to 2 mg/kg/dose every 4 to 6 hours to a maximum of 8 mg/kg/day (not exceeding 400 mg/day). Pain relief was very good to excellent in 69%, as rated by the parents. The children had a variety of types of chronic pain. Tramadol was well tolerated with only 12 patients stopping the study early because of side effects.[42] This medication must be used with caution in patients at risk for seizures and patients on antidepressants.[6]

## 10. COMPLEX REGIONAL PAIN SYNDROME (CRPS)

Crps is continuous pain in part of an extremity frequently experienced following trauma. The pain often continues beyond the time of tissue inflammation or injury.[9] It is most common in adolescent females, and the lower limb is much more likely involved compared to an upper limb. Treatment in children is extrapolated from the adult population.[1] (See **Chapter 4**).

## 11. SICKLE CELL CRISIS

Vaso-occlusive crisis (VOC) is a very painful occurrence in patients with sickle cell disease. The pain is a result of ischemia (no blood flow or oxygen to an area). Misshapen red blood cells stick to the blood vessels, and blood flow is decreased. The pain may last from days to weeks and is unpredictable.[43]

A step-wise approach to choice of analgesic is recommended according to the severity of pain the child is experiencing. For mild pain, acetaminophen or NSAIDs are given, for moderate pain, NSAIDs and a weak opioid and for severe pain, a stronger opioid. In some cases, combining acetaminophen with an NSAID and an opioid is needed. Extreme cases (about 10%) require admission to the hospital for high doses of drugs that require medical monitoring or intravenous opioids for optimum pain control.[43]

## 12. CANCER

Pain in children with cancer is a result of procedures, cancer treatment, the tumour itself the spreading of the tumour, or a combination of the above.[38] The incidence of pain in children at the time of their diagnosis of cancer is quoted to be 50%.[44] In the more advanced stages of cancer, pain needing regularly scheduled pain medication occurs in up to 89% of children.[45] The child may not voice their pain in attempts to avoid more painful procedures.[44] Studies indicate that the risk of side effects and opioid addiction is low in children with severe pain.[46] Addiction to opioids happens in less than 1% of patients in pain, and usually there is a history of substance abuse.[9] A study in terminally ill children showed that all children with solid tumours needed opioids.[47] Infants, once they reach an age of three to six months, experience the same pain control and degree of respiratory depression (decrease in breathing) when given morphine or fentanyl (two common opioids) as the adult population.[5]

The use of suppositories is generally avoided in cancer patients because of mucous membrane injury that may occur on insertion. This could result in dangerous bleeding, especially when platelets are low.[44]

The use of any fever-reducing drug (acetaminophen, NSAIDs) is avoided until the doctor is contacted, since fever is a very important sign of infection. Masking this sign and infection left untreated could have very dire consequences, especially in a patient with decreased white cells to fight infections.

The World Health Organization's (WHO) Practice Guidelines for Cancer Pain Management is a step-wise approach to pain treatment.[9,45,48] The general guideline is outlined earlier in the chapter. Adjuvant medications are added when needed for prevention of nausea, vomiting and constipation; treatment of neuropathic pain; and anxiety.[48]

## OPIOIDS FOR CANCER PAIN

The name "opioid" refers to any substance that has morphine-like actions.[27] Opioids work by several different mechanisms that affect pain signals to reduce pain.[24,48] Usually a weak opioid such as codeine is used for moderate pain. For severe pain, a stronger opioid such as morphine, fentanyl or hydromorphine is needed. Opioids for pain do not have a ceiling effect. The side effects of the particular opioid is what limits how high the dose can go and be tolerated.[27] Side effects include sedation, decreased breathing, nausea, vomiting and constipation, effects on mood, itchiness, urinary retention and small pupils.[27,48] The body builds tolerance to most of the side effects (the body gets used to them) with continued treatment, except for constipation and miosis (decrease in pupil size of the eyes).[27]

If a strong opioid is required for severe pain, it should be scheduled to be delivered around the clock.[18,45] The initial dose will be much lower in an opioid-naive patient (has not been on opioids). A much higher dose is needed when the child is not opioid-naive.[18] If pain is not controlled with maximum-tolerated regular-dose opioids, a "breakthrough dose" (dose given if pain occurs between the last and next scheduled dose) is ordered. The amount of opioid used per 24 hours is closely monitored for effectiveness and side effects. If more than a few (number determined by the doctor) breakthrough doses are needed, the regularly scheduled dose is reassessed.[18,45] When switching from one opioid to another, choose the new dose at 25% less than the equipotent dose. This accounts for the tolerance obtained with the first opioid, which is not present when starting the alternative opioid.[45]

> **Codeine** is used primarily for moderate pain. Codeine needs to be converted in the liver to morphine in order to be effective. Ten percent of individuals lack this enzyme to convert the codeine to active drug.[24,48,49] Also, there are people who convert codeine to active drug faster than usual.[49] This makes predictability of dosing difficult, and can result in serious toxicity.

**Morphine** is the standard opioid to which others in this group are compared.[24,44,45] It is the opioid that has been most studied in children.[45] It is available orally in immediate action and sustained action tablets, liquid form and injectable form. M-Eslon® and Kadian® capsules can be opened up and sprinkled on a spoonful of soft food.[49] The usual oral starting dose is 0.2 to 0.4 mg/kg/dose every 3 to 4 hours for the immediate action dosage form.[5,27] If the child weighs at least 50 kg then begin with 10 to 15 mg every 3 to 4 hours.[48] Once stabilized on the immediate action form, the total daily dose can be converted to the sustained action form divided every 12 hours if necessary. In some children using the controlled-release morphine, a dose every 8 hours is needed. Side effects are similar to those seen in adults (and described above). However, it is less common in children to need an antiemetic (antivomit) drug to counteract the side effect of the opioid. Constipation is prevalent, and because the opioid causes a decrease in bowel motility (motion, movement), a stimulant-action laxative may be needed (e.g. Senna). Children seem more apt to have urinary retention (bladder not completely empty after urination). If present, it might be necessary to switch to a different opioid.[45]

> **Hydromorphone** is available orally as immediate-action and sustained-action tablets, and in liquid and injectable form. The usual oral starting dose is 0.03 to 0.08 mg/kg/dose every 3 to 4 hours of the immediate release form.[5,27,48] In children weighing at least 50 kg, start with 2 to 4 mg every 3 to 4 hours.[5] It is about five times more potent than morphine in adults.[45] It works similar to morphine, and there is less experience in children.[48]

**Oxycodone** is available orally as immediate action and sustained action tablets. It is 1.5 to 2 times more potent than oral morphine.[48] It works similar to morphine, and there is less experience when used on a chronic basis in children.[45,48]

> **Fentanyl** is available as a transdermal (absorbed through the skin) patch and in injectable form. The patch offers the advantage of an alternative to oral administration. When the oral route is not possible, subcutaneous (injection under the skin) or intravenous (injection into a vein) routes, which are more invasive, are avoided.[44,45] The patch has the advantage of providing a constant release of fentanyl, 24 hours a day. The dose absorbed from the patch may vary amongst children because of the variation in skin thickness and blood flow to the skin. The thinner the skin and greater the blood supply to the area, the greater the effect.[50] In children it is best to apply the patch to the back in an area where the child will not pull it off. Fentanyl should be used only in children who have already received opioids.[48,51] To decrease the risk of decreased breathing, the patch should be considered only in children stabilized on at least 30 mg oral morphine per day (equivalent to the 12.5 g/hour fentanyl patch).[52] Fentanyl may cause less itchiness, urinary retention and constipation compared to morphine.[45] Studies in children indicate that children 1 to 5 years of age clear fentanyl faster when the patch is dosed by weight. Older children (7 to 16 years old) took longer for the full effect when starting fentanyl patches compared to adults. In some children there were difficulties in the patch not staying well-adhered to the skin, resulting in less drug delivered. One group found that 40% needed supplemental adhesive to keep the fentanyl patch attached to the skin. Some children may require the patch being replaced every 48 hours rather than the usual 72 hours.[52]

**Methadone** is available as tablets and liquid. Methadone is unique in the opioid group of drugs because in addition to the usual opioid action, it works on another pathway to decrease pain. It has a very long duration of action in the body, but the analgesic activity itself is much shorter. Dosing and effect can be unpredictable.[48] There is little published on the use of methadone for chronic pain in children.[45]

> **Meperidine** (pethidine) is not used in chronic pain in children. It is a weaker pain reliever than morphine, and its absorption is highly variable.[45] Also, the metabolite can cause seizures.[5]

## 13. CONCLUSION

The need for further research of chronic pain in infants and children is necessary. This vulnerable population is in need of better pain management guidelines. It is a child's basic right not to endure pain.

As a medical community, we need to further advance our understanding and management of chronic pain. Specific drug dosing for infants and children suffering with chronic pain continues to require further study. In many instances the drug dose and side effect profile is extrapolated from adult data. Infants and children are not little adults. They respond differently to medication. The golden rule applies, "first, do no harm."

## REFERENCES

1. WALKER, SM. Pain in children: recent advances and ongoing challenges. Br J Anaesth, 2008; 101:101-10.
2. ECCLESTON, C., J. Clinch. Adolescent chronic pain and disability: A review of the current evidence in assessment and treatment. Paediatr Child Health 2007; 12(2): 117-20.
3. CLINCH, J., C. Eccleston. Chronic musculoskeletal pain in children: assessment and management. Rheumatology, 2009; 48: 466-74.
4. ATIYEH, BA, SS Dabbagh, AB Gruskin. Evaluation of renal function during childhood. Pediatrics in Review, 1996; 17(5):175-80.
5. BERDE, C., NF Sethna. Analgesics for the treatment of pain in children. N Engl J Med, 2002; 347(14): 1094-1103.
6. TAKETOMO, CK, JH Hodding, DM Kraus. Pediatric Dosage Handbook. 15th ed.© 2008. Lexi-Comp Inc. Hudson, Ohio.
7. BIRENBAUM, D., DR Mattison. Letter to editor, Analgesics for the treatment of pain in children. N Engl J Med, 2003; 348(10): 959-60.
8. SIMON, HK, DA Weinkle. Over-the-counter medications. Do parents give what they intend to give? Arch Pediatr Adolesc Med, 1997; 151(7): 654-6.
9. DAABISS, M. Management of chronic pain conditions in pediatric population. The Internet Journal of Health, 2008; 7(1): 1-13.
10. REGIER, L., B. Jensen, B. Kessler. Pediatric pain: Treatment considerations, Q&As. 2008 Apr. © RxFiles, Saskatoon Health Region, www.RxFiles.ca
11. KOZER, E. et al. Repeated supratherapeutic doses of paracetamol in children – a literature review and suggested clinical approach. Acta Paediatrica, 2006; 95: 1165-71.
12. ONAY, OS et al. Acute, reversible nonoliguric renal failure in two children associated with analgesic-antipyretic drugs. Pediatr Emer Care 2009; 25: 263-6.
13. SATIRAPOJ, B., P. Lohachit, T. Ruamvang. Therapeutic dose of acetaminophen with fatal hepatic necrosis and acute renal failure. J Med Assoc Thai 2007; 90(6): 1244-7.
14. SHAHROOR, S. et al. Acetaminophen toxicity in children as a "therapeutic misadventure". Harefuah 2000; 138(8): 654-7,710.
15. HEUBI, JE, MB Barbacci, HJ Zimmerman. Therapeutic misadventures with acetaminophen: hepatotoxicity after multiple doses in children. J Pediatr, 1998;132(1): 22-7.
16. MILES, FK et al. Accidental paracetamol overdosing and fulminant hepatic failure in children. Med J Aust, 1999; 171(9): 472-5.
17. CROCETTI, M, .N Moghbeli, J. Serwint. Fever phobia revisited: have parental misconceptions about fever changed in 20 years? Pediatrics, 2001; 107(6): 1241-6.
18. CURRIE, JM. Management of chronic pain in children. Arch Dis Child Ed Pract, 2006; 91: ep111-14.
19. SHORTRIDGE, L, V. Harris. Alternating acetaminophen and ibuprofen. Paediatr Child Health, 2007; 12(2): 127-8.
20. TZAFETTAS, J. Painful Menstruation. Ped Endocrinol Rev, 2006; 1: 160-3.
21. SCHANBERG, LE et al. Daily pain and symptoms in children with polyarticular arthritis. Arthritis Rheum, 2003; 48(5): 1390-7.
22. KIMURA, Y. et al. Treatment of pain in juvenile idiopathic arthritis: a survey of pediatric rheumatologists. Arthritis & Rheumatism (Arthritis Care & Research) 2006; 55(1): 81-5.
23. KIMURA, Y, Walco GA. Treatment of chronic pain in pediatric rheumatic disease. Nature Clinical Practice Rheumatology 2007; 3(4): 210-8.
24. CHAMBLISS, CR et al. The assessment and management of chronic pain in children. Pediatr Drugs, 2002; 4(11): 737-46.
25. HERSHEY, AD, MA Kabbouche, SW Powers. Chronic daily headaches in children. Current Pain and Headache Reports, 2006; 10: 370-6.
26. VICTOR, S, SW Ryan. Drugs for preventing migraine headaches in children. Cochrane Database of Systematic Reviews 2003, Issue 4. At. No.: CD2761. DOI: 10.1002/14651858.CD002761.
27. Managing pain in children: A clinical guide. Ed. Twycross, A., SJ Dowden, E. Bruce . © 2009. Blackwell Publishing Ltd, Oxford, United Kingdom.
28. MACK, KJ, J. Gladstein. Management of chronic daily headache in children and adolescents. Paediatr Drugs, 2008; 10(1): 23-9.
29. HAMALAINEN, ML et al. Ibuprofen or acetaminophen for the acute treatment of migraine in children: a double-blind, randomized, placebo-controlled crossover study. Neurology, 1997; 48: 103-7.
30. LUDVIGSSON, J. Propranolol used for prophylaxis of migraine in children. Acta Neurologica Scandinavica, 1974; 50: 109-15.

31. HERSHEY, AD et al. Effectiveness of amitriptyline in the prophylactic management of childhood headaches. Headache, 2000; 40: 539-49.

32. ROSE, JB. Pharmacologic interventions for chronic pain in children, an evidence based review. SPA 20th Annual meeting, Chicago, IL, 2006.

33. CAMPO, JV. Coping with ignorance: exploring pharmacologic management for pediatric functional abdominal pain. J of Pediatric Gastroenterology and Nutrition, 2005; 41: 569-74.

34. SYMON, DN, G. Russell. Double-blind, placebo-controlled trial of pizotifen in the treatment of abdominal migraines. Arch Dis Child, 1995; 72: 48-50.

35. Subcommittee on Chronic Abdominal Pain, American Academy of Pediatrics, Technical report. Pediatrics, 2005; 115: e370-e381.

36. SEE, MC et al. Double-blind, placebo-controlled trial of famotidine in children with abdominal pain and dyspepsia. Dig Dis Sci, 2001; 46: 985-992.

37. HALL, GC et al. Epidemiology and treatment of neuropathic pain: the UK primary care perspective. Pain, 2006; 122: 156-62.

38. ANDERSON, BJ, GM Palmer. Recent developments in the pharmacological management of pain in children. Curr Opin Anaesthesiol, 2006; 19: 285-92.

39. REGIER, L. Table 2: Overview of drugs used in treatment of chronic non-malignant pain (CNMP), p. 47, 2007 Feb.© RxFiles, Saskatoon Health Region. www.RxFiles.ca

40. BOZKURT, P. Use of tramadol in children. Pediatric Anesthesia 2005; 15: 1041-7.

41. FINKEL, JC et al. An evaluation of the efficacy and tolerability of oral tramadol hydrochloride tablets for the treatment of postsurgical pain in children. Anesth Analg, 2002; 94: 1469-73.

42. ROSE, JB et al. Oral tramadol for the treatment of pain of 7-30 days' duration in children. Anesth Analg, 2003; 96: 78-81.

43. STINSON, J, B. Naser. Pain management in children with sickle cell disease. Pediatr Drugs, 2003;5(4): 229-41.

44. MERCADANTE, S. Cancer pain management in children. Palliative Medicine, 2004; 18: 654-62.

45. HAIN, RDW et al. Strong opioids in pediatric palliative medicine. Pediatr Drugs, 2005; 7(1): 1-9.

46. DESPARMET, J, P. Guelen, L. Brasseur. Opioids for the management of severe pain in children and infants. Clin Drug Invest, 1997; 14 Suppl.1: 15-21.

47. SIRKIA, K et al. Pain medication during terminal care of children with cancer. J Pain Symptom Manage, 1998; 15: 220-6.

48. FRIEDRICHSDORF, SJ, TI Kang. The management of pain in children with life-limiting illnesses. Pediatr Clin N Am, 2007; 54: 645-72.

49. REGIER, L. Opioid analgesic: Comparison chart. P49, 2007 Feb. © RxFiles, Saskatoon Health Region. www.RxFiles.ca

50. Committee on Drugs, American Academy of Pediatrics. Alternative routes of drug administration- advantages and disadvantages. Pediatrics, 1997; 100(1): 143-52.

51. New Indication. Fentanyl patch for stable chronic pain in children. Translated from Rev Prescrire, 2008; 28(292): 101.

52. ZERNIKOW, B, E. Michel, B. Anderson. Transdermal fentanyl in childhood and adolescence: a comprehensive literature review. The Journal of Pain, 2007; 8(3): 187-207.

# THE ROLE OF THE PHARMACIST
## IN CHRONIC PAIN MANAGEMENT

**Andrée Néron**, BPharm, DPH, pharmacist,
Pelviperineology team, Palliative care team, Centre hospitalier universitaire de Sherbrooke - CHUS,
Sherbrooke, Quebec, Canada
Read by Janice Sumpton, RPh, BSc Phm, London, Ontario, Canada

# 32

## ABSTRACT

Unique and specialized university training makes the pharmacist the health professional who is a "medication expert". The pharmacist is probably the health professional with whom the average individual has the most contact; he/she is accessible almost all of the time, and regularly serves as a link between the patient and the doctor or with the other health professionals.

The pharmacist has the expertise and knowledge to monitor the pharmacotherapy, namely anticipating, detecting, preventing and treating problems related to drug therapy (notion of effectiveness and safety). His/her interventions often take place in obscurity, behind the counter and, as a result, the patient does not necessarily realize that the pharmacist will contact the physician to modify a prescription, for the patient's safety.

Pharmaceutical care activities include drug monitoring. However, the pharmacist can also initiate or adjust medication therapy, depending on prescription by protocol, asking for the appropriate laboratory tests to be done, if needed (Bill 90 in Quebec).

In specialized settings (and also occasionally in the community), the pharmacist can play a pivotal role as a member of the pain team. He/she can also participate in clinical research on pain.

The role of the pharmacist is to advise, recommend or suggest (to your physician or other health team professionals) medication treatments, based on a comprehensive evaluation he/she has made, the symptoms described by the patients or their loved ones, the patient's age and physical condition (heart, liver, kidney, stomach and so on) and the medication history (including prior drug response). Pharmacists help in patient follow-up and make sure, along with the physician and the other members of the team, that the analgesic treatment works (efficacy, effectiveness, side effects, drug interactions, allergies, and so on).

For drug management to be effective, pharmacists interact proactively with other team players making sure that the patient, the caregivers, and the other professionals involved with the patient understand the key idea of the care plan. Working with the health care teams, pharmacists can re-evaluate the plan on a regular basis to make sure the benefits persist over time, and that a balance is maintained between the benefits, the undesirable effects, quality of life and functionality.

Pain and suffering are two inseparable partners in the case of a pain that persists beyond its mission as an alarm.

When your eyes are sad, your heart is filled with sorrow.

## 1. PHARMACISTS IN MY ENVIRONMENT – WHERE DO THEY COME FROM AND WHAT DO THEY DO?

Unique and specialized university training makes the pharmacist the health professional who is a "medication expert". With the new university curriculum, pharmacy students will be even closer to the patients, and prepared to exercise their skills by offering quality pharmaceutical care. The new doctoral programme in pharmacy allows students to acquire target skills and knowledge.

Pharmacists share the following skills with other health professionals: professionalism, excellent communication and interpersonal skills, team work and interdisciplinarity, scientific reasoning and critical thinking, learning autonomy and leadership.

The skills specific to the profession of pharmacist include: comprehensive pharmaceutical care, ambulatory community service, and management of the practice and operations.

## 2. WHERE DO PHARMACISTS WORK?

### HOSPITAL PHARMACISTS

Few people know that there are pharmacists working in the health facilities (moreover, Mr. John Doe never really knows quite how to refer to them: doctor, nurse, Sir, Madam, the pharmacist, etc.) and the general public is always surprised to learn that this professional plays a very important role in such facilities. The pharmacist's practice is very different in a facility than in a private setting, specifically as a result of the following elements: most institutional pharmacists have either done postgraduate studies or have a specialization in hospital pharmacy (which requires additional studies). Institutional pharmacists do not sell medications to the public; they are responsible (alone or as a member of a team) for everything that concerns medications in the hospital setting.

Institutional pharmacists spend close to 40-60% of their time providing direct care to the patients, excluding their dispensing activities; they can be found in care units and out-patient clinics, where they work in close cooperation with physicians and other health professionals. The pharmacist is involved in various fields of expertise and can be found, for example, at the information drug centre, with the pain team, in internal medicine, intensive care, cardiology, nephrology, diabetes, asthma, anticoagulant follow-up, infectiology, medication blood level follow-up, psychiatry, paediatrics, the transplant team, etc.

Institutional pharmacists take part in medical rounds and give pharmacotherapeutic advice concerning the choice of medications for a given patient. They analyze patient charts (studying the medical history, the progress notes, laboratory test results, prescriptions, etc.), meet with patients (spontaneously, or following a request for a consultation), and guide the treatment.

Pharmaceutical practice in an institution is very different from pharmaceutical practice elsewhere since it is more varied, more complex and more specialized.

### PHARMACISTS IN THE COMMUNITY ENVIRONMENT

Community pharmacists also develop their fields of expertise through preparing antibiotics to be used at home, emergency oral contraception, drug compounding, as well as through their direct involvement with shelters, residential and long-term care centres, for integral follow-up of pharmacotherapy for patients, their involvement at themed conferences for the general public, their follow-up of oral anticoagulant treatments, etc. Outside the hospital walls, these are probably the health professionals with whom you have the most contact; they are accessible at all times and serve as a link between the patients and their physicians, or with the other health professionals such as the dentist, the nurse, the social worker, the dietician, the psychologist and the physiotherapist.

## 3. PHARMACISTS PROVIDE PHARMACEUTICAL CARE: WHAT DOES THIS MEAN?

In Quebec, Bill 90 recognized the evolution that has occurred with respect to the role of pharmacists in recent years, specifically their expertise with respect to pharmacotherapy follow-up, namely the anticipation, detection, prevention and treatment of problems related to drug therapy (notions of effectiveness and safety). Pharmacotherapies for patients affected by serious or chronic health problems are increasingly complex, requiring skills, knowledge and accessibility on the part of pharmacists.

In Canada, on average, a new medication is marketed every 10 days; the pharmacist is an expert in a pharmacopeia that includes more than 20,000 pharmaceutical entities.

# 4. PHARMACISTS AND PAIN

When dealing with patients in pain, the pharmacist's objective is to define a therapeutic strategy that is adapted to the patient, and serves to improve the patient's overall quality of life and functionality.

When providing pharmaceutical care, pharmacists are concerned about providing the benefits of pharmacotherapy while respecting ethical principles.

## PHARMACISTS AND PAIN TEAMS

In specialized settings as well as in the community, pharmacists can play a pivotal role as members of pain teams. They can also participate in clinical research on pain. Pharmacists who want to develop a particular interest in pain management have access to a wide variety of information about the subject, as well as to various training programmes (continuing education, professional refresher courses, meetings and symposia, specialized literature).

Pharmacists are essential partners for physicians. Their role is to advise, recommend or suggest medication treatments, or changes in drug therapy to the physician. The pharmacists' suggestions are based on the evaluation they have made, the symptoms described by the patients or their loved ones, the patient's age, physical condition (heart, liver, kidney, stomach and so on), vulnerabilities, prior response to drug therapy and medication history. Pharmacists help in patient follow-up, and make sure, along with the physician and the other members of the team, that the analgesic treatment works (effectiveness, side effects, drug interactions, allergies, and so on).

Chronic pain is not a mindset, but because it endures, it cannot be dissociated from suffering. The biopsychosocial factors intervene and complicate this treacherous "disease". Pharmacists help patients in their undertakings with the other members of the care team. Since pain is a whole, the entire therapeutic approach includes not only medication, but also a focused approach that can avoid the pitfalls of increasing dosages, or the number of medication entities. The pharmacist is also responsible for suggesting the withdrawal of or a decrease in the dosage of a therapeutic agent when everything seems to indicate that the benefits have levelled off or disappeared.

Pharmacists like to learn, to grow, to discover, and to innovate. The fact that they work closely with colleagues, patients and their families also inspires suggestions and choices that they adapt to meet their patients' needs. Since they are human, and therefore fallible, they strive to achieve clinical benefits without causing harm (*"primum non nocere"*).

## LISTENING TO THE INDIVIDUAL SUFFERING FROM CHRONIC PAIN

Pharmacists listen to their patients, and are always at their posts, ready to make adjustments, to start over, to understand and to search for solutions. As the secular heirs to the art of pharmacology, they make their knowledge and pharmaceutical intuition available. Their objective is to defeat the disharmony that pain as a "disease" brings into the lives of patients who must cope with this problem. Pharmacists cannot do just anything. They must respect the guidelines (with a certain amount of flexibility), standards and local, provincial and federal laws that govern the management of medications. This is not always easy…

From the outset, pharmacists try to establish relationships built on honesty, explaining the issues and the expectations with respect to the chances of success; they may verify their patients' own expectations so as to limit the damage caused by the profound disappointment that may occur if the benefits obtained are less than they had silently hoped for. Pharmacists must welcome their patients, and believe them; they must have the honesty to recommend them to another professional if the initial game plan does not fit in with their personal convictions.

Pharmacists make sure that the patient, the caregivers and the other professionals involved with the patient understand the key idea of the care plan. Working with the health care teams, pharmacists can re-evaluate the plan on a regular basis to make sure the benefits persist over time, and that a balance is maintained between the benefits, the undesirable effects, quality of life and functionality.

The main issue of chronic pain management in an ambulatory care setting is patient's lack of adherence. Pharmacists make sure that the patient clearly understands the message that is transmitted focusing on therapeutic goals and how the medication is to be taken (this is particularly relevant and crucial if the drug has to be administered by an unconventional route, such as a preparation of medications to be injected under the skin).

Through effective education on drug therapy, pharmacists must be able to guide patients toward imperative goal: a balance between pain relief, other outcomes and bearable side effects.

Pharmacists also re-evaluate the treatment plan with patients and their prescribers when the patients have obtained optimal relief for an extended period of time (three to six months), so as to avoid continuing the use of medications that may no longer be useful (evanescent pain, changing pain). **Therefore, the pharmacist is responsible for ensuring that the treatment plan is balanced.**

FIGURE 1: Balance between drug adjustments over time, pain intensity and appearance if side effects
The pharmacist is responsible for achieving a balance.

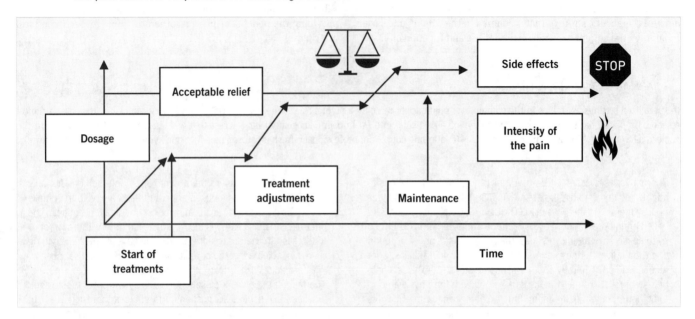

The main principles that govern the activities of a pharmacist involved directly or indirectly with pain teams are the general principles of pain relief, as well as the general principles of pain relief and pain management.

## GENERAL PRINCIPLES OF PAIN RELIEF FOR ALL HEALTH PROFESSIONALS

- Respect and believe the patient and his/her pain (unique character and relativity);
- Know when to suggest a treatment;
- Treat the underlying cause or pain "as a disease" in keeping with the prescription, knowledge and expertise;
- Regularly re-evaluate the treatment and adapt it (efficacy, effectiveness, harmlessness).

## GENERAL PRINCIPLES OF PAIN RELIEF AND PAIN MANAGEMENT

- Integrate analgesia in an overall evaluation and treatment plan;
- Consider and treat the emotional and cognitive aspects;
- Do not undertreat pain; it is more often under-treated than vice versa;
- «Individualize» the pain management plan (patient specific);
- Consider a multimodal approach by using pharmacological and non-pharmacological approach;
- Optimize drug administration by selecting a drug product and route of administration that are appropriate for the situation, when a pharmacological treatment is considered;
- Anticipate, prevent if possible and palliate undesirable side effects;
- Discuss and demystify the patient's concerns about opiate analgesia, or other agents used to relieve pain (ex.: antidepressants prescribed for their analgesic properties);
- NEVER use a placebo to treat pain.

## INDIVIDUALIZATION OF DRUG TREATMENT

Individualizing the treatment means that the pharmacist must consider the following elements:

- The collection of analgesic drug history and other medications (prescription medications, over-the-counter medications, street drugs, alcohol, tobacco, etc.);
- The appropriate pharmaceutical dosage form;
- The costs;
- The side effects, allergies;
- The relative and absolute contra-indications;
- The effects of concomitant medications – that can sometimes be beneficial (drug interactions);
- The patient's wishes: degree of relief desired vs. side effects;
- The consideration of the past response to medications and the patient's preference;
- The information to be transmitted depending on the general condition, autonomy, and the complexity of the treatment;
- The implementation of only one treatment at a time if possible (depending on the medical prescription) to maximize the effect;
- Progressive withdrawal of the treatment in case of inefficacy (with the physician's authorization); combination if the effect levels out (according to medical prescription protocol).

## PHARMACOLOGICAL APPROACH

The pharmacological approach includes:

- The implementation of the simplest plan for the patient, loved ones, caregivers, health care providers;
- Oral administration (by mouth) when possible;
- A regular drug schedule, but flexible enough to be adapted to the patient's reality;
- Frequency of administration adapted first for the patient, but also feasible for the health care personnel;
- Respect for the philosophy of consensus and guidelines of scientific societies (when opportune);
- Individualized prescription;
- Patient's cooperation.

## SUGGESTIONS BY A PHARMACIST TO HIS/HER PATIENT

What can the pharmacist who specifically takes part in monitoring pain relief suggest to the patient?

### 1. A log (see next page)
Attention: This log must serve as a **guide** for the patient and the clinician to help them find means to better identify the nature and the behaviour of the pain; keeping a log should not become an obsession that takes over daily life.

### 2. A dosette, a pillbox, or a weekly system such as the dispill packaging system
It is essential that everyone understands the dynamics of a drug treatment plan, and the appropriate use of medication. If the patient does not understand the directions, and the pharmacist and the physician imagine something other than what the patient is actually taking, there may be a misunderstanding that could endanger the patient. Although they do not resolve all problems, the medication boxes (prepared by the pharmacist) are tools that facilitate adherence to drug regimen for pills that must be used on a regular basis, and at the right time. Analgesic agents must be taken on a regular basis in order to provide sustained relief of pain. If the patient does not take the medication as planned, or as thought, or if he/she does not remember how or when to take medication, it will be difficult to readjust the care plan.

### 3. One single community drug store in as much as possible

Pharmacists from different settings (hospital and community) communicate among themselves in case of complex situations (in keeping with professional ethics and the patient's approval). This is also very helpful for clarifying any misunderstanding related to a patient's drug profile.

We cannot insist too much on the importance of being faithful to your pharmacist and providing a good medication history when you are asked questions; this could save your life. Here is an example.

When he was hospitalized, Philip brought all of the medications he was taking with him. Some products came from different drug stores, but all had been prescribed. Philip brought everything with him without indicating which prescriptions were active and which were not. Philip became agitated and confused until the pharmacist for the pain team was called in and took note of the situation. The pharmacist immediately recommended that Philip stop taking all useless medications and Philip rapidly recovered. The situation could have ended on a more tragic note.

SAMPLE LOG

## PAIN PARAMETERS TO BE EVALUATED

| | Date: Sept. 24 | Date: Sept. 25 | Date: | Date: |
|---|---|---|---|---|
| Where? | Ex.: sacrum | Ex.: buttock and thigh | | |
| When? | Ex.: always | Ex.: morning | | |
| Pain quality and characteristics | Ex.: deep | Ex.: tingling, stinging | | |
| Duration | Ex.: 10 hours | Ex.: 3 minutes | | |
| Relief factors | | | | |
| Exacerbation factors | Ex.: movement | Ex.: movement | | |
| Irradiation | | Yes | | |

## NUMERIC PAIN SCALE FROM 0 TO 10

| | Date: Sept. 24 | Date: Sept. 25 | Date: | Date: |
|---|---|---|---|---|
| Average intensity during the last week | Ex.: 3 | Ex.: 3 | | |
| Intensity in the last 24 hours | Ex.: 2 | Ex.: 3 | | |
| Intensity at the worst moment | Ex.: 5 | Ex.: 5 | | |
| Intensity at the best moment | Ex.: 1 | Ex.: 0 | | |

**Comments** (Indicate specific characteristics, impact of the quality of life and any side effects, and date your comments.):

_____

_____

_____

_____

### A TREATMENT PLAN FOR CHRONIC PAIN

When dealing with chronic pain, when relief is achieved, the same plan is usually kept for a few months. If there is optimal relief for a continuous period of a few months, the prescriber may authorize his/her patient to progressively stop the treatment (withdrawing one medication at a time). If there is a failure when one of the medications is withdrawn, the patient might be advised to progressively reduce the dosage of another one of the medications. If it is impossible to completely withdraw the medication, it is important to maintain the dosage at the minimum tolerated by the patient and consider making another attempt in a year or so. It is essential to focus on the patient's quality of life and functionality.

There is no magic solution. The success rate varies according to the situation; despite efforts to achieve relief, perfect control is not always feasible.

## 5. THE RATIONALE BEHIND POLYPHARMACOLOGY

Is it logical to take more than one medication in order to relieve pain? The specific situation of the patient who is in pain and suffering may make polypharmacology necessary. The rationale behind polypharmacology is illustrated in **Figure 2** and **3**.

FIGURE 2: The rationale behind polypharmacology I

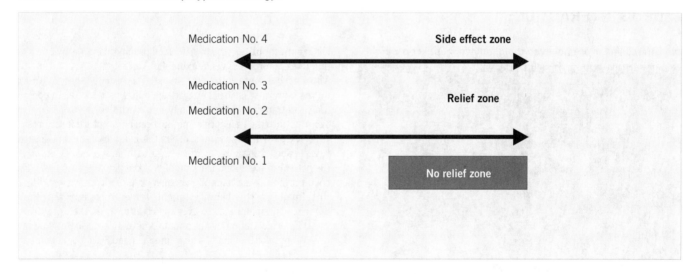

FIGURE 3: The rationale behind polypharmacology II

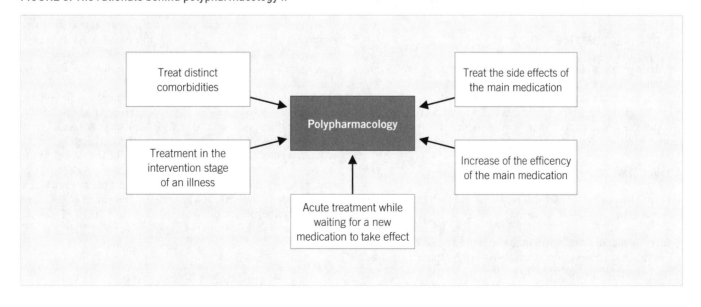

## PAIN AS AN ILLNESS: A JUDICIOUS DRUG COMBINATION

In addition to the reasons provided in **Figure 3**, particularly for pain as a disease, the physician may opt for a combination of medications (polypharmacology) when:

- The patient's response to a first-line treatment at an optimal or tolerated dosage is partial or unsatisfactory;
- The assessment of the type of pain or the intensity of the pain is such that it is preferable to consider a combination of medications at least for a certain amount of time;
- The complementary mechanisms for action on the human body are taken into consideration.

**The medication acts on:**
- A receptor (ex.: an opiate such as morphine anchors itself to the opiate receptors in the human body in order to act);
- A drug channel (ex.: injection of a local anaesthetic (called a nerve block) that blocks a certain type of sodium channel and, by reducing their discharge frequency, relieves pain);
- Monoamines (ex.: antidepressants short-circuit pain by increasing the availability of serotonin and noradrenaline);
- Peptides (ex.: capsaicine affects the substance P - P for pain);
- A system (ex.: cannabinoids such as nabilone and dronabinol anchor themselves to specific receptors in the human body);
- Substances derived from membranes (ex.: anti-inflammatories act on the prostaglandins involved in pain and inflammation).

## THE INCONVENIENCES OF POLYPHARMACOLOGY

**Polypharmacology** has the following inconveniences: the risks of medication-medication, medication-food, medication-tobacco, medication-alcohol, medication-natural products, and medication-street drug interactions.

# 6. DRUG INTERACTIONS

**We cannot see or predict everything, but we must keep watch!**

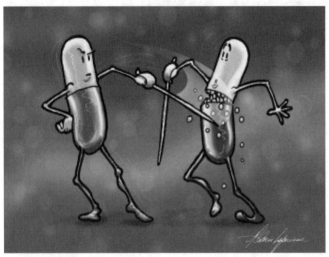

## BIOTRANSFORMATION

Metabolic reactions allow the organism to transform a medication into substances that are still active, or components that are inactive from a pharmacological point of view. To do this, the body uses enzymatic reactions, and calls on numerous tissues such as the skin, the lungs, the kidneys, the intestines, the brain, etc. The principal site of biotransformation is the liver.

## THE CONSEQUENCES OF DRUG METABOLISM

What happens to the product that is transformed by the body (called metabolite)?

- **Inactive metabolites** (the transformed product is no longer active): ex.: anti-inflammatories (ex.: ibuprofen: Advil™, Motrin™; gabapentin: Neurontin™; pregabaline: Lyrica ™).

- **Active metabolites** (the transformed product has an effect on the body): ex.: morphine; venlafaxine: Effexor XR™.
- **More active metabolite** (the transformed product has an effect on the body that is stronger than the initial product): ex.: codeine (partially transformed by the body into morphine).
- **Toxic action** (the transformed product can be harmful if it accumulates in the patient's body; most often, this happens if the safe dosage is exceeded, if there is an interaction with another medication, if the patient drinks too much alcohol or if the patient has a particular condition): ex.: acetaminophen in high doses: Tylenol™: most often, this situation occurs because patients forget to mention that they buy acetaminophen tablets over the counter when their physician prescribes a medication that also contains acetaminophen (ex.: Empracet -30 contains 325 mg of acetaminophen and 30 mg of codeine).

## THE CONSEQUENCES OF A DRUG INTERACTION

The body's objective is to defend itself against toxins, although it does not always succeed.

Some people have genetic variations; this means that their metabolic system does not work like those of most other people. When they have to take a medication that requires that metabolic path, they experience an unexpected response since their capacity to transform the medication is different.

In a different manner, the body's capacity to transform medications may be modified when a patient takes several medications that interact with one another; this can also occur if a medication interacts with food, alcohol, so-called natural products, street drugs or tobacco.

An interaction occurs when the properties of the medication(s) involved are modified when two or more medications are associated, or under the influence of a substance that the patient has stopped taking (the medication in question still has an effect because it is eliminated very slowly). The modification may be immediate or delayed, and can change the overall therapeutic response.

An interaction may also occur, and lead to a modification in the overall pharmacological response (effect desired, undesirable effect or toxic effect) when two medications (or more), which affect the same system, the same transmitter or the same receptor, are associated. The interaction may be quick and predictable (ex.: similar undesirable effects) or unpredictable, rare and even very serious. A judicious therapeutic choice will prevent the concomitant administration of medications that are transformed by the same metabolic pathway, so as to reduce the risk of metabolic drug interactions.

It should be noted that a particular individual will not necessarily suffer a drug interaction even though it has been reported in the scientific documentation. It should also be noted that, even though this situation is rare, an interaction could be beneficial (desired effect of a medication interaction). Once again, it is important to overemphasize the necessity to keep going to the same community drug store, to trust the pharmacist, and to give the pharmacist as much information as possible about all prescription and non-prescription medications (over the counter medications, homeopathy, etc.).

**Patients who browse the Internet and reach their own interpretations should also take care – the pharmacists are still the professionals to be consulted in order to determine the pertinence of an interaction, since they consider and analyze all of the elements of a particular situation (they take stock of and assess determinants of drug interaction).**

**In the case of drug interactions, the pharmacist is proactive in order to prevent or clear up this type of problem.**

In the pharmacopeia of analgesic medications, codeine, methadone, fentanyl, antidepressants (with analgesic properties), dextromethorphane, tramadol (Tramacet™, Tridural™, Zytram™, Ralivia™), antiarrhythmics (prescribed to relieve pain), grapefruit juice and St. John's wort are more likely to be involved in drug interactions.

# 7. ROUTES OF DRUG ADMINISTRATION

The pharmacist has the knowledge required to consider other routes of drug administration when oral administration (by mouth) is not possible or not desired. In the field of analgesia, when the pain is localized and accessible, the application of a topical drug preparation that can penetrate the mucous membranes or the cutaneous tissues may allow for targeted activity of the prescribed substance, thereby bypassing the inconveniences of oral administration. Local measures may be perceived as focusing on the source of the pain and generally include fewer risks of side effects compared with other routes of drug administration. For example, the pharmacist may suggest the preparation of an analgesic cream or gel to apply to the skin at the site of the pain if the application surface is not too large (ex.: preparation of baclofen, an anti-inflammatory, ketamine, etc.).

When choosing or changing the route of drug administration, the pharmacist must consider the following factors:

- The properties of the medication;
- The medication be administered by this new route; (if not certified for that mode of administration, the pharmacist will collect scientific information to ensure that the data indicates we can do so);
- The patient's preference;
- The cooperation of the patient and family members;
- The skill and time required for administration;
- The potential pharmacological options;
- The presence of nausea and vomiting;

- Difficulty swallowing;
- The obstruction of the oesophagus or the intestine;
- The level of consciousness and psychiatric condition;
- The urgency with which the symptoms need to be relieved;
- The possibility and ease of administration;
- The cost of the medication;
- The possibility of continuing the treatment at home if the patient was initially hospitalized.

# 8. CONCLUSION

**Your pharmacist is an ally. Pharmacists do not claim to know everything but they do have the knowledge to work with you in matters of medication. Trust your pharmacist!**

# I FORGIVE YOU

Louise O'Donnell-Jasmin, BEd. Laval, Quebec, Canada

(See other testimonials, pages 84 and 328. See Chapter 1, page 3.)

When justice can never remedy all of the wrongs that have been done to me and mine, only forgiveness can release both of us from this nightmare. The medical act that led me into chronic pain could have been avoided... Since it is impossible to change the past, I can at least change the present and all of the remaining days of my life. And this renewal starts with forgiveness.

I have no bitterness, no desire for vengeance with respect to you. I am taking the most courageous act of my life: forgiving you. You can only be released from the sense of guilt you no doubt feel through my forgiveness. This book that you are holding in your hands is the result of a promise I made to help other people who are living with chronic pain. It is a consequence of my forgiveness for you, of my leap into the future and of my faith in life.

I forgive you for injuring me, for not referring me to a specialist immediately, for hampering my chances of receiving emergency treatment that could have reduced the impact of the injury. I forgive you for failing to note the injury in my file, for protecting yourself. I forgive you for not helping me when I was in danger. I forgive you for not having the courage to find out about my condition in the following months, for lacking the courage to face the consequences of your actions, for your professional errors as well as the fear you felt when faced with the scope of the problem you created. I forgive you for never apologizing, for not admitting the facts that we both know.

Following this injury, the disease progressively destroyed my quality of life and the lives of all those around me. Although you are responsible for everything that this disease changed in my life, while you were informed and fully aware of it, I forgive you.

The most difficult thing to forgive is the following: the emotional consequences of the pain on the people I love and who love me. As a result of the chronic pain that settled in for very long years, they had to live through many dramatic situations. They saw me suffering, transformed by the medications I took and the stranglehold of the pain, unrecognizable. My children were deprived of a normal relationship with their mother, but never of my love. The pain caused them distress and terror at the thought of losing me. It destroyed a major part of their childhood. They were deprived of peace of mind and experienced the constant threat of my suffering as much as their powerlessness to deal with my condition. My life as a couple was handicapped for a long time as a result of the perverse effects of the pain on my personality, the depression caused by the pain and the side effects of numerous medications. We dealt with emotions frozen to ensure survival, by a lengthy wait shaded with hope, the hope that I would one day return to normal. Being deprived of a normal love life had serious consequences. We did our best. One day these injuries will be healed for good. But our memories will never heal... On behalf of all those who love me unconditionally, I forgive you.

Make the most of this new chance for truth, integrity and the pursuit of medical ideals provided by relieving suffering and preventing disease. I hope that you find peace in your soul one day and that you then find and take all of the means possible to ensure you never injure anyone again. You will have to walk the rest of the road to peace in your soul on your own. I hope that you are surrounded by a lot of love when you take that walk, **and that one day you forgive yourself.**

# MANAGING CHRONIC PAIN:
## THE ROLE OF THE NURSE

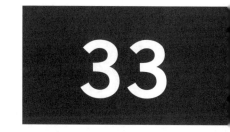

**Patricia Bourgault** RN, PhD, Associate Professor, École des sciences infirmières, Faculté de médecine et des sciences de la santé, Université de Sherbrooke, Quebec, Canada
**Dave Bergeron** RN, BSc, Master's student in Clinical Sciences, Université de Sherbrooke, Quebec, Canada

The authors would like to thank Robin Marie Coleman RN, BSc, Master's student in clinical sciences, Université de Sherbrooke, Quebec, Canada

## ABSTRACT

Since managing chronic pain requires an interdisciplinary approach, each professional may have a positive impact on the patient and enhance his/her well-being. As a result of their training and the expertise they develop, nurses can intervene in a concrete manner with people suffering from chronic pain in order to optimize their relief. Considering their proximity to the patient and family, and as a result of their global vision of care, nurses are able to provide care based on a holistic approach, involving both a traditional medical approach and an alternative focus, including psychosocial and non-pharmacological interventions. This characteristic of the nursing profession promotes continuity of care and empowerment of the patient, and increases the well-being and quality of life of people dealing with chronic health problems.

ABSTRACT

1. INTRODUCTION

2. PAIN ASSESSMENT

   Pain scales
   Assessment and analysis of all components of chronic pain
   Pharmacological treatment
   Teaching pain management
   Clinical monitoring

3. FOR THE DEVELOPMENT OF AN INTEGRATED AND GLOBAL APPROACH FOR DEALING WITH CHRONIC PAIN

   Treatment models for the nursing personnel
   Interventions by the nursing personnel in the pain clinic
   Support from nursing personnel: an element that facilitates the management of pain

4. CONCLUSION

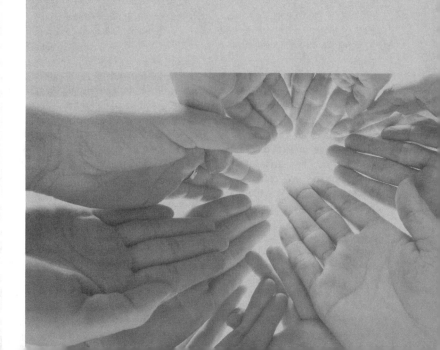

# 1. INTRODUCTION

In Quebec, following the adoption of Bill 90 modifying the *professional code*, the role of the nurse has been enhanced. Nurses are now responsible for the assessment of the physical and mental condition of the individua**l**s they care for. This evaluation involves gathering and analyzing data concerning the individual's health situation, and includes, among other things, an evaluation of the social dimension and potential of the patient. Once the initial evaluation has been made, the nursing personnel must ensure the monitoring of individuals with complex health issues such as diabetes, hypertension and chronic obstructive pulmonary disease.

Over the past two years, this enhancement of the nurse's role has concretely translated into action through the introduction of the therapeutic nursing plan (tnp). In this plan, nurses must determine nursing guidelines pertaining to elements of monitoring of health issues they consider priorities. The tnp also helps nursing personnel note any adjustments made in accordance with changes in the individual's condition, as well as the effectiveness of the pre-determined approaches (*OIIQ*, 2006).

In Quebec, the role of the nursing personnel in the assessment and management of acute and chronic pain is determined by the *Ordre des infirmières et infirmiers du québec* (*OIIQ*). The order has indicated that nursing personnel must evaluate the patient's pain regardless of whether he/she is in front-line centres, such as the *CLSCS* (local community service centres), a hospital or in a long-term care facility (*OIIQ*, 2009; 2004; 2003; 2000; 1996). In the presence of pain, the nursing personnel must administer an analgesic in accordance with the medical prescription, and then teach patients and their families how to manage pain while respecting and considering their own capacities.

# 2. PAIN ASSESSMENT

When assessing pain, nurses must use standardized measurement tools such as one-dimensional scales that measure the intensity of pain (*OIIQ*, 2009). As well, it should be noted that pain assessment is increasingly recognized as the 5th vital sign that nursing personnel must evaluate in patients; the others are blood pressure, pulse, respiration and body temperature (Fishman, 2005).

Overall, pain assessment by nursing personnel, regardless of whether the pain is acute or chronic, should include the following elements, which are identified by the acronym **PQRSTU**:

**PQRSTU:**
[P]    provocative/palliative;
[Q]    quality and quantity;
[R]    region and radiation;
[S]    severity scale;
[T]    timing – onset, duration and frequency;
[U]    understanding the patient's perception.
(Jarvis, 2009)

### PAIN SCALES

Several standardized and validated scales can be used to quickly, and systematically measure the intensity of pain, including: the visual analog scale, the numerical scale, the verbal descriptive scale and the faces scale (See page 118.). All of these tools are quick and easy to use, and serve to facilitate documenting the effectiveness of the therapeutic measures implemented to relieve the pain. All of these scales are based on the idea that the individual holds the authority when it comes to evaluating his/her own pain.

However, most of these tools become less reliable when used with individuals at both age extremes (infants and elderly people), as well as with individuals who cannot communicate, and who have hearing, visual or cognitive deficits. In order to overcome this problem, a hetero-evaluation of pain (evaluation made by another person by observing behaviour) may be used. In this respect, there are several tools that can be used to standardize the pain assessment of patients who are unable to use the one-dimensional tools listed above. For example, for elderly people, the "Pain Assessment Checklist for Seniors with Limited Ability to Communicate (PACSLAC) (See page 121), the Abbey Pain Scale (APS) and the Doloplus-2 scale have already undergone an advanced validation process, and are promising tools for this group. For children who have difficulty communicating, for example children with polyhandicap, the San Salvador Children's Scale or the Non-Communicating Children Pain Checklist-Revised (Breau, Mcgrath, Camfield & Finley, 2002; http://www.aboutkidshealth.ca/shared/.../akh_breau_post-op.pdf) can be used to estimate pain, while the Gustave Roussy Child Pain Scale (Gauvain-Piquard, Rodary, Rezvani, & Serbouti, 1999; www.cebp.nl/vault_public/filesystem/?Id=1306) was developed to evaluate paediatric cancer pain. Finally, the behavioural observation of pain checklist is another tool that nursing personnel can use for people who are hospitalized and intubated in intensive care (Gélinas & Johnston, 2007). These are just a few examples of measurement scales that can be applicable to both acute and chronic pain, that must be used when assessing the pain experienced by particular groups of patients.

### ASSESSMENT AND ANALYSIS OF ALL COMPONENTS OF CHRONIC PAIN

It is important to consider the fact that, in the presence of chronic pain, a one-dimensional evaluation may neglect other significant aspects of the health problem, including functional status and quality of life. As a result, treatment may not be optimal (Gottrup & Jensen, 2008). In such a situation, the nursing personnel must perform a detailed evaluation and analysis of all the components of chronic pain. To do this, the nursing personnel must note other parameters: the knowledge of the disease and the treatments, the perceptions and expectations of the individual and his/her family, the impacts of the pain on the biopsychosocial, cultural and spiritual spheres, the occurrence of events that have an impact on the patient's life, as well as the reactions of the patient and the family to the treatments. The use of multidimensional tools, as well as related measurement tools, may be very pertinent in this case, and can be used by the nursing personnel. The following tools are noteworthy: the Beck Depression Inventory (Beck & Steer, 1996; www.fpnotebook.com/psych/exam/bckdprsninvntry.htm), which is used to measure depression, a health problem that is closely related to chronic pain, and the State-Trait Anxiety Inventory (Spielberger, 1985; http://faculty. Sjcny.Edu/~treboux/documents/State%20Trait%20Anxiety%20Inventory.Doc), which measures state-trait anxiety, common components in the case of people for which the cause of pain is uncertain (ASPMN, 2002; Lebovits, 2008). For its part, the Coping Strategies Questionnaire helps nursing personnel better identify the cognitive and behaviour strategies that individuals use to manage their pain (Robinson et al., 1997; Lebovits, 2008), while the Brief Pain Inventory (Cleeland & Ryan, 1994) deals with several dimensions of pain, including the patient's beliefs concerning the pain condition, as well as the effect the pain has on quality of life and functionality (ASPMN, 2002). It should be noted that these questionnaires provide an overall assessment of the repercussions of chronic pain on the individual, and serve to guide the treatment. The results may also be used to confirm the necessity of consulting other professionals, or may be covered by a directive in the therapeutic nursing plan.

## PHARMACOLOGICAL TREATMENT

Nursing personnel, in collaboration with the medical team, play an important role in the pharmacological treatment of chronic pain. In respect with the medical prescription, nursing personnel may choose the analgesic, the route of administration, as well as the appropriate dosage for the patient's condition. In addition to anticipating and preventing the side effects of the pharmacological measures chosen, they must closely monitor the safety and the effectiveness of the treatment (*RNAO*, 2002). In a context of first-line care, nurses may, always in keeping with the medical prescription issued, adjust the pharmacological treatment, contact the physician in order to have the prescription changed, or even notify the physician about the patient's reactions to the treatment (*OIIQ*, 2003a). Nevertheless, in order to correctly fulfil their role, nurses must have a solid understanding of the pharmacokinetics and pharmacodynamics of all the analgesics and co-analgesics used to manage chronic pain (*RNAO*, 2002).

## TEACHING PAIN MANAGEMENT

Teaching is one of the primary roles of the nursing personnel. Thus, with respect to the management of pain, the *OIIQ* states that the nurse must show the patient how to optimize the pharmacological treatment prescribed by the physician, as well as teach non-pharmacological methods of pain relief, such as respiration techniques, massages, visualization techniques, the application of heat or cold, relaxation techniques, etc. (*OIIQ*, 2000, 2003a). This education should not take the form of the simple reading of a list of information, but must be based on the patient's knowledge, take into consideration his/her desire to learn, and respect the treatment objectives. This will ultimately serve to establish a true partnership between the nurse and the individual in chronic pain (gottlieb & feeley, 2007). Moreover, this education process must be provided to patients as well as their families, and those people important to them. This partnership will ensure the integration of the actions taken to manage pain and is in conformity with the recommendations of the *Société québécoise de la douleur* (2005), which insist on involving families in the pain management process. The nursing personnel must rally the family and people close to the individual suffering from chronic pain, since their support is viewed as a facilitating factor in the successful management of the patient's pain (Bair *et al.*, 2009; Sylvain & Talbot, 2002). It is also important for the nursing personnel to ensure smooth communication with families and their loved ones, in order to evaluate their acceptance and satisfaction with respect to the treatment plan (*RNAO*, 2002).

## CLINICAL MONITORING

Clinical monitoring is essential in the case of individuals who are given opiates, or any other medication that has a depressive effect on the central nervous system, such as anxiolytics, antiemetics, muscular relaxants, etc. It is of prime importance that this includes an evaluation of the levels of sedation, and the respiratory condition of patients receiving opiates, or any other medication that has a depressive effect on the central nervous system (*OIIQ*, 2009). More specifically, the patient's level of sedation and respiratory condition must be evaluated in accordance with the peak effect, and selected route of administration of the administered opiate. The peak effect of an opiate represents the time when the individual is most likely to suffer a depression of the central nervous system. It is also necessary to pay particular attention to individuals who are most at risk of experiencing respiratory depression, such as elderly people, patients with kidney or liver failure, chronic obstructive pulmonary disease, sleep apnea or obesity, or those taking other medication having a depressive effect on the central nervous system (*OIIQ*, 2009; Gélinas, 2004). This monitoring doesn't only concern hospitalized patients, it also applies to patients seen in out-patient and chronic pain clinics, when their dosage is being modified, or a new opiate is being introduced.

## 3. FOR THE DEVELOPMENT OF AN INTEGRATED AND GLOBAL APPROACH FOR DEALING WITH CHRONIC PAIN

In comparison with Canadian, American and British guidelines, the role Quebec nurses play in chronic pain management could be broadened and more clearly defined, promoting the development of an integrated and global approach that would facilitate the treatment of people suffering from chronic pain. The management of chronic pain is generating notable interest in institutions throughout the world, which has led to the development of several recommendations intended to improve the management of this health issue. As a result of the omnipresence of medical discourse in the development of exemplary practices for pain management, few pain management guidelines have been specifically developed for nursing personnel (Price & Cheek, 1996). Nevertheless, some of these guidelines do provide interesting benchmarks for the actions taken by nurses with respect to pain management, and serve to better identify their role (*JCAHO*, 2000; VHA, 1998; *RNAO*, 2002). **Table 2** summarizes the interventions that arise out of these guidelines.

TABLE 2: Summary of nursing interventions for the monitoring and treatment of chronic pain

### SUMMARY OF NURSING INTERVENTIONS FOR THE MONITORING AND TREATMENT OF CHRONIC PAIN

**1) Pain screening**

**2) Presence of pain requiring a more detailed assessment**
a) Assess the pain using standardized tools
b) Assess the pain on an on-going basis

**3) Documentation and communication**
a) Ensure systematic, concise and clear documentation of the pain
b) Ensure communication with the patient, family and other health professionals

**4) Treatment plan**
a) Apply pharmacological measures (in respect to medical prescriptions or protocols)
b) Apply non-pharmacological measures
i) Optimize the patient's relief
ii) Ensure the patient's safety (clinical monitoring of patients taking opiates)
iii) Effectively manage the side effects of analgesics
iv) Evaluate the acceptance, the response and the satisfaction of the patient and the family

**5) Cooperation with patient and family**

**6) Adapted and personalized treatment for patient and family**

**7) Verification of patient's and family's satisfaction with the intervention process**

**8) Interventions performed throughout patient's care**

## TREATMENT MODELS FOR THE NURSING PERSONNEL

Despite articles written in Quebec reporting the importance of an interdisciplinary approach involving several health professionals, including nursing personnel, nurses seem to have very little involvement, in fact, in the management and assessment of chronic pain in interdisciplinary pain clinics (*AÉTMIS*, 2006; *SQD*, 2005). However, a few initiatives taken in Quebec do reveal the added value provided by nurses in interdisciplinary clinics, and as part of first-line treatment in the management of chronic pain, particularly in relation to the support and teaching provided to patients, their families and their loved ones. Elsewhere in the world, several models for treating people with chronic pain place a great deal of importance on the role of nurses. This is evident in the introduction of the nurse led pain clinics in the united kingdom (http://www.Nursingtimes.Net/nursing-practice-clinical-research/nurse-led-community-pain-management-clinic/207737.Article) and of the nurse pain clinics of the Veteran Health Administration (VHA) in the United States.

In general, nurses working in these clinics assume a pivotal role by performing complete evaluations of the patients, by taking part in the adjustment and evaluation of their pharmacological and non-pharmacological treatments, as well as by ensuring subsequent follow-ups, while implementing an individual education plan for each patient that satisfies the role expected of them by the *OIIQ*.

## INTERVENTIONS BY THE NURSING PERSONNEL IN THE PAIN CLINIC

The primary objective of the interventions of nursing personnel in a pain clinic is to help patients learn to live with their pain, and adapt to it, which will ultimately increase their sense of control, reduce the catastrophization and severity of the pain, without healing them. With the assistance of a psychologist, the nurse can also initiate a cognitive-behavioural therapy with the patient, which includes the development of new coping strategies, such as stress management, relaxation, cognitive restructuring, distraction, problem solving, and the establishment of objectives. These techniques help the patient become self-sufficient with respect to managing the pain condition.

## SUPPORT FROM NURSING PERSONNEL: AN ELEMENT THAT FACILITATES THE MANAGEMENT OF PAIN

The presence of nursing personnel close to people suffering from chronic pain generally reduces the intensity of their pain, and helps them to better master the exacerbations, increasing their satisfaction with the treatment, and improving both their quality of life and their level of functioning. Moreover, patients who receive nursing care generally describe the nursing personnel as a facilitating element in the management of their chronic pain.

# 4. CONCLUSION

In conclusion, nurses can play an increased role in the treatment of people suffering from chronic pain. As a result of their training and their expertise, nurses have the skills to make overall global assessments of suffering individuals, and work with them, their families or loved ones, as well as other health care professionals, to ensure optimal management of the pain. This role is in the process of being developed in Quebec; over the next few years, the "added value" of the contribution of nursing personnel in the management of chronic pain should be confirmed, enhancing the well-being of patients.

# REFERENCES

1. Abbey, J., N. Piller, A. De Bellis, A. Esterman, D. Parker, L. Giles et coll. (2004). The Abbey pain scale: A 1-minute numerical indicator for people with end-stage dementia. International Journal of Palliative Nursing, 10(1), 6.
2. Agence d'évaluation des technologies et des méthodes d'intervention en santé (AÉTMIS). (2006). Prise en charge de la douleur chronique (non cancéreuse): Organisation des services de santé. Montréal: AÉTMIS.
3. American Society of Pain Management Nurses (ASPMN). (2002). Core curriculum for pain management nursing. Philadelphia, Pennsylvania: Elsevier Science W.B. Saunders Company.
4. Aubin, M., A. Giguère, T. Hadjistavropoulos et R. Verreault. (2007). L'évaluation systématique des instruments pour mesurer la douleur chez les personnes âgées ayant des capacités réduites à communiquer. Pain Research & Management, 12(3), 195-203.
5. Aubin, M., R. Verreault, M. Savoie, S. Lemay, T. Hadjistavropoulos, L. Fillion et coll. (2008). Validité et utilité clinique d'une grille d'observation (PACSLAC-F) pour évaluer la douleur chez des aînés atteints de démence vivant en milieu de soins de longue durée. Canadian Journal on Aging, 27(1), 45-55.
6. Bair, MJ, MS Matthias, KA Nyland, MA Huffman, D. Stubbs, K. Kroenke et coll. (2009). Barriers and facilitators to chronic pain self-management: A qualitative study of primary care patients with comorbid musculoskeletal pain and depression. Pain Medicine, 10(7), 1280-1290.
7. Boulard, M. et S. Le May. (2009). Pratique avancée en gestion de la douleur chronique: exploration d'un modèle de rôle anglais en sciences infirmières. L'infirmière clinicienne, 5(1), 11-18.

8.  Bourque, P., et D. Beaudette. (1982). Étude psychometrique du questionnaire de dépression de Beck auprès d'un échantillon d'étudiants universitaires francophones. Canadian Journal of Behavioural Science/Revue Canadienne Des Sciences Du Comportement, 14(3), 211-218.

9.  Brooks, E. et J. Younce. (2007). A case management model for the ambulatory care patient experiencing chronic pain. AAACN Viewpoint, 29(1), 3-5.

10. Cleeland, CS et KM Ryan. (1994). Pain assessment: Global use of the brief pain inventory. Annals of the Academy of Medicine, Singapore, 23(2), 129-138.

11. Collignon, R., B. Giusiano, AM Boutin et J. Combes. (1997). Utilisation d'une échelle d'hétéro-evaluation de la douleur chez le sujet sévèrement polyhandicapé. Douleur et analgésie, 10(1), 27-32.

12. Courtenay, M. et N. Carey. (2008). The impact and effectiveness of nurse-led care in the management of acute and chronic pain: A review of the literature. Journal of Clinical Nursing, 17(15), 2001-2013.

13. Fishman, SM (2005). Pain as the fifth vital sign. Journal of Pain & Palliative Care Pharmacotherapy, 19(4), 77-79.

14. Gauthier, J., & S. Bouchard (1993). Adaptation canadienne-française de la forme révisée du State–Trait anxiety inventory de Spielberger. Canadian Journal of Behavioural Science/Revue Canadienne Des Sciences Du Comportement, 25(4), 559-578.

15. Gauvain-Piquard, A., C. Rodary, A. Rezvani, et J. Lemerle. (1988). La douleur chez l'enfant de 2 à 6 ans: Mise au point d'une échelle d'évaluation utilisant l'observation du comportement. Douleur et analgésie, 1(3), 127-133.

16. Gélinas, C. (2004). Prévenir la dépression respiratoire liée à certains médicaments. Perspective infirmière, 2(2), 1-5.

17. Gélinas, C., et C. Johnston. (2007). Pain assessment in the critically ill ventilated adult: Validation of the critical-care pain observation tool and physiologic indicators. The Clinical Journal of Pain, 23(6), 497-505.

18. Gottlieb, LN, et N. Feeley. (2007). La collaboration infirmière-patient: un partenariat complexe (MC Désorcy, trad.). Montréal, Beauchemin.

19. Gottrup, H., et TS Jensen. (2008). Assessment of the patient with neuroptahic pain. In PR Wilson, PJ Watson, JA Haythornthwaite & TS Jensen (Eds.), Clinical pain management: Chronic pain, 2e édition, Londres: Hodder Arnold, 132-144.

20. Loi modifiant le Code des professions et d'autres dispositions législatives dans le Domaine de la santé. Projet de Loi 90, Chapitre 33, Québec (2002).

21. Irachabal, S., M. Koleck, N. Rascle & M. Bruchon-Schweitzer. (2008). Stratégies de coping des patients douloureux: Adaptation française du coping strategies questionnaire (CSQ-F). L'Encéphale: Revue de psychiatrie clinique biologique et thérapeutique, 34(1), 47-53.

22. Jarvis, C. (2009). Évaluation de la douleur: autre signe vital. In C. Jarvis (Ed.), L'examen clinique et l'évaluation de la santé (C. Gélinas Trad.). Montréal: Beauchemin, 189-208.

23. Joint Commission on the Accreditation of Healthcare Organisations (JCAHO). (2000). Pain assessment and management: An organisational approach. Oakbrook Terrace, IL: JCAHO.

24. Lamb, L., JX Pereira & Y. Shir. (2007). Nurse case management program of chronic pain patients treated with methadone. Pain Management Nursing, 8(3), 130-138.

25. Lebovits, A. (2008). The psychological assessment of pain in patients with chronic pain. In P. R. Wilson, P. J. Watson, J. A. Haythornthwaite & T. S. Jensen (Eds.), Clinical pain management: Chronic pain, 2e édition, Londres: Hodder Arnold, 122-131.

26. Metzger, C., M. Schwetta et C. Walter. (2007). Évaluation de la douleur. In A. Muller, C. Metzger, M. Schwetta et C. Walter (Eds.), Soins infirmiers et douleur, Paris: Masson, 3e édition, 174-195

27. Ordre des infirmières et infirmiers du Québec (OIIQ). (1996). L'exercice infirmier en soins critiques. Montréal: OIIQ.

28. Ordre des infirmières et infirmiers du Québec (OIIQ). (2000). L'exercice infirmier en soins de longue durée. Au carrefour du milieu de soins et du milieu de vie. Montréal: OIIQ.

29. Ordre des infirmières et infirmiers du Québec (OIIQ). (2003a). L'exercice infirmier en santé communautaire. Soutien à domicile. Montréal: OIIQ.

30. Ordre des infirmières et infirmiers du Québec (OIIQ). (2003b). Notre profession prend une nouvelle dimension - des pistes pour mieux comprendre la loi sur les infirmières et infirmiers et en tirer avantage dans notre pratique. Montréal: OIIQ.

31. Ordre des infirmières et infirmiers du Québec (OIIQ). (2004). Avis sur la surveillance clinique des clients qui reçoivent des médicaments ayant un effet dépressif sur le système nerveux central (SNC). Montréal: OIIQ.

32. Ordre des infirmières et infirmiers du Québec (OIIQ). (2006). Le plan thérapeutique infirmier: La trace des décisions cliniques de l'infirmière. Montréal: OIIQ.

33. Ordre des infirmières et infirmiers du Québec (OIIQ). (2009). Surveillance clinique des clients qui reçoivent des médicaments ayant un effet dépressif sur le système nerveux central. Montréal: OIIQ.

34. Price, K. et J. Cheek. (1996). Exploring the nursing role in pain management from a post-structuralist perspective. Journal of Advanced Nursing, 24(5), 899-904.

35. Registered Nurses Association of Ontario (RNAO). (2002). Nursing best practice guideline - assessment and management of pain. Toronto: RNAO.

36. Richardson, C., N. Adams et H. Poole. (2006). Psychological approaches for the nursing management of chronic pain: Part 2. Journal of Clinical Nursing, 15(9), 1196-1202.

37. Richardson, C. et H. Poole. (2001). Chronic pain and coping: A proposed role for nurses and nursing models. Journal of Advanced Nursing, 34(5), 659-667.

38. Société québécoise de la douleur (SQD). (2005). Projet de développement d'un programme national d'évaluation, de traitement et de gestion de la douleur chronique. Montréal: SQD.

39. Stanos, S. et TT Houle. (2006). Multidisciplinary and interdisciplinary management of chronic pain. Physical Medicine & Rehabilitation Clinics of North America, 17(2), 435-450.

40. Sylvain, H. et LR Talbot. (2002). Synergy towards health: A nursing intervention model for women living with fibromyalgia, and their spouses. Journal of Advanced Nursing, 38(3), 264-273.

41. Veillette, Y., D. Dion, N. Altier et M. Choinière. (2005). The treatment of chronic pain in Quebec: A study of hospital-based services offered within anesthesia departments. Canadian Journal of Anaesthesia, 52(6), 600-606.

42. Veterans Health Administration (VHA). (1998). VHA national pain management strategy. Washington, D.C.: VHA.

43. Wary, B. et C. Doloplus. (1999). Doloplus-2, une échelle pour évaluer la douleur. Soins Gérontologie, (19), 25-27.

44. Watson, J. (1998). Le caring: Philosophie et science des soins infirmiers (J. Bonnet Trad.). Paris: Seli Arslan.

# INVASIVE TECHNIQUES:
# **NEUROMODULATION**

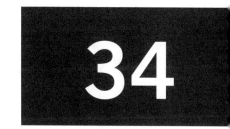

## 34

**Christian Cloutier** BSc, MD, FRCPC, neurosurgeon
Clinical Professor, Department of Surgery, Centre hospitalier universitaire de Sherbrooke - CHUS,
President, Quebec Pain Society, Medical officer, RUIS Sherbrooke, Pain Expertise Centre,
Sherbrooke, Quebec, Canada

## ABSTRACT

There are many approaches for dealing with pain: drug therapy, physical therapy, psychological therapy, alternative and complementary forms of medicine, etc. Occasionally, used individually, or in combination, these approaches do not successfully relieve certain painful conditions, particularly those of a neuropathic nature. For this reason, it is necessary to refer to an interventionist doctor who provides 'invasive' treatment. Occasionally, curative surgery is indicated (herniated disk, vascular loop causing a painful tic, etc.), or sometimes the insertion of a neuromodulation device, such as a neurostimulator or an intrathecal pump, is indicated in the cases of certain types of refractory pain, and in patients who have been selected and prepared well. These treatments may appear risky, yet, since they are known to be effective, they may be less dangerous than the over-use of conventional approaches. Above all, they can be very beneficial for the individual who is dealing with severe, incapacitating pain that is destroying his/her life.

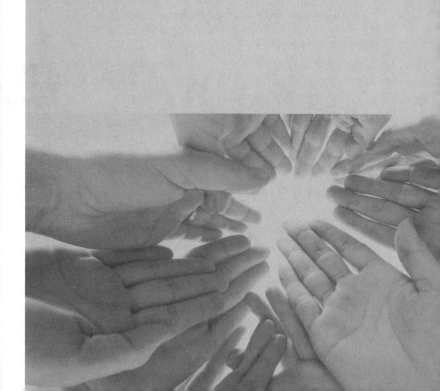

# 1. INTRODUCTION

Up to this point, we have been able to read about a multitude of medical approaches involving the use of medication, physical intervention, psychological approaches, anaesthetic techniques, etc., all in keeping with a treatment scale that could be qualified on a continuum… from the simplest to the most complex.

When medical treatment, often called conservative, fails, it is occasionally possible and necessary to have recourse to so-called invasive techniques, namely surgical techniques. It should be noted that any treatment for chronic pain must be multimodal. In 1990, Health Canada warned that no speciality or therapeutic intervention is capable of remedying this problem on its own. It is only through calling on the skills of specialists in several fields that a solution will be found.

«… no specialty of therapeutic intervention can remedy this problem on its own. Only by using the skills of specialists in several disciplines can we overcome it…»

In certain situations of severe, rebellious and refractory pain, the patient must be referred to an interventionist surgeon. Most often, this will be a neurosurgeon.

# 2. SURGICAL APPROACHES

**The surgical approaches can be divided into three categories: curative, destructive or augmentive.**

## Curative surgical approaches

Occasionally, there is a clear indication for surgery to correct the cause of the pain, as in the case of a herniated disc, lumbar spinal stenosis (compression on nerve roots in the spinal column), a tumorous mass, a vascular loop compressing the trigeminal nerve (causing facial pain as an electrical discharge of the painful tic), etc. These possible surgical treatments remedy the anomaly and, more often, also eliminate the pain completely (which is why the approach is referred to as curative).

## Destructive surgical approaches

In the past, recourse to destructive surgical interventions was common. For a long time, it was believed that cutting off the painful nerve impulse was the only effective solution. For example, the nerve or the nerve bundle would be cut in the spinal cord, which corresponded to the painful zone. Now, it is acknowledged that the central nervous system reacts very poorly to such an insult, that the pain both returns within 6 to 12 months and is often intensified, and the consequences of a loss of function can be devastating. These approaches are rarely used, except in the case of palliative care provided to patients in a terminal phase, with a life expectancy of less than three to six months. However, certain types of interventions that create lesions (destructive) are very useful in certain situations, such as irradiating the Gasserian ganglion (trigeminal ganglion) of the sensitive facial nerve (trigeminal nerve), with a Gamma Knife. This device creates a partial lesion through concentrating ionizing gamma irradiation on the ganglion (**Figure 1**).

**FIGURE 1: Gamma Knife**

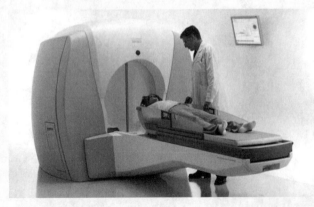

Courtesy of Elekta

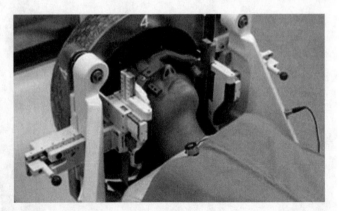

Courtesy of Elekta

Also, in order to relieve facet pain (one of the causes of neck pain and non-specific lower back pain), thermolesion (or 'burning' lesion) can be applied to the posterior-median branch of the nerve of the zygoapophyseal joint (the posterior joint of the vertebra, called the facet). Such a procedure is indicated for patients who experienced adequate but temporary relief (lasting only a few weeks) following an injection (xylocaine and cortisone) of this or these facets. The effect of thermolesion is extended but highly variable, lasting from a few months to years.

## Augmentive surgical approaches

Finally, there are the augmentive surgical approaches, which are called that since they involve the addition of a system (specialized equipment). If no beneficial analgesic effect is obtained, the equipment is removed and the patient returns to his initial preoperative state. Usually, there are no consequences for the patient and, above all, no damage to the central nervous system.

# 3. NEUROMODULATION

The term 'neuromodulation' refers to a specialized medical treatment, used to modulate the functioning (and not to alter the anatomy) of the nervous system and, by doing so, alleviate pain. This is done by surgically implanting a device that either stimulates the transmission of the signal and/or neuron activity electrically, or inhibits them chemically, in order to produce a therapeutic effect. Two very different systems are used.

- The first system stimulates certain parts of the nervous system (the spinal cord or the brain); it is called neurostimulation.

- The second system involves injecting substances into the cerebrospinal fluid in the spinal column using an intrathecal pump. Compared to the destructive techniques, the neuromodulation systems are clearly much more beneficial in clinical terms.

Before an internal neuromodulation system is installed, care must be taken to identify the medical pathology clearly, as well as to ensure that the patient is a good candidate for this invasive surgical approach (indication and risks), that he/she is psychologically prepared to undergo this type of surgery (profile, expectations) and that he/she has a clear understanding of the consequences of the surgery, meaning difficulties, and even the improvement.

## Neurostimulation of the spinal cord and the brain

The exact mechanisms involved in neuromodulation through the stimulation of the posterior cords of the spinal cord remain unknown: does it affect the gate control of pain mechanism or the neurotransmitters of the posterior horn or activate the long ascending and/or descending bundles (**Figure 2**) of the spinal cord.

FIGURE 2: Neurostimulation of the posterior cords of the spinal cord

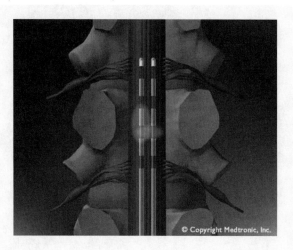

© Copyright Medtronic, Inc.

Does the effect occur at the spinal level, where the electrode is placed, or the supra spinal level, at a distance at the cerebral level? Research attempting to understand the mechanisms of the therapeutic electric action will be published soon at the *Université de Sherbrooke* (Sherbrooke, Quebec, Canada), as part of a master's degree undertaken by the author of this chapter (Dr. Christian Cloutier) in cooperation with Dr. Serge Marchand, neurophysiologist.

Traditionally, old articles provided evidence that the stimulation was only 50% effective on a long-term basis.[1] Recently, in 2007, a group of researchers, the European Federation of Neurological Societies (EFNS), published a complete literature review of the most recent articles based on the evidence.[2] This review attributes a level B effectiveness, namely probable effectiveness, to neurostimulation for:

- Cases of failed back surgery syndrome, namely for patients who have had one and, above all, several lower back operations);

- Cases of Type 1 complex regional pain syndrome (CRPS), which means that there is no neurological lesion causing the syndrome.

The review attributed a Level D effectiveness, namely effectiveness based on descriptive, non-comparative studies, for relieving pain caused by:

- A type 2 CRPS (presence of nerve damage);
- A diabetic or postherpetic traumatic neuropathy;
- Plexopathy;
- An amputation (phantom limb);
- A partial spinal injury.

To summarize, this treatment is acknowledged to be effective with neuropathic lesions, particularly those that are peripheral, which result in neuropathic pain that is clearly identified by means of the DN4[3] questionnaire, and which must be accompanied by a sensitive deficit, a state of deafferation. On the other hand, purely nociceptive pain (somatic and visceral, namely not neurological) does not respond to this technique, unless the cause is vascular, as in the case of chronic ischemia of the lower limbs, and serious refractory angina. Once again, the mechanism is still unknown, probably managed by interaction via the autonomic sympathetic system, since neurostimulation serves to improve vascularization. The results for these vascular patients are excellent, the best in fact, but as they have progressive diseases, the condition may improve initially, but as the disease progresses and deteriorates on a long-term basis, the patient will experience much less pain.

It is difficult to conduct comparative studies with a placebo on surgical treatments that involve the insertion of equipment. As a result, such randomized studies are rather rare. Yet, it should not be forgotten that the lack of evidence does not necessarily mean the absence of effectiveness. The relief rate is 70% to 85% for well selected cases. In a review of 101 patients, conducted by the author, the effectiveness rate was 85% (article in the process of being prepared). It should not be forgotten that we are at the top of the ladder in terms of pain treatment. It is a question of selected refractory cases, which are difficult to treat.

These interventions are called invasive since there is a risk of complications. The most common one is epidural hematoma (rare: 1 chance out of 700 cases) along with paraparesis, and even paraplegia, which means the paralysis of the lower limbs with urinary incontinence. Most often, it can be reversed through the exeresis (removal) of the accumulated blood, but there is a slight possibility of irreversible damage.

In the most refractory situations, it is possible to place the electrode in the cortical motor epidural region in the brain, in the case of neuropathic pain, or to insert the electrode in the thalamus for nociceptive pain. Motor cortex stimulation or MCS, the type most commonly used at present, produces good results[4] for neuropathic pain of the face and arms, and for pain secondary to a cerebral vascular accident (CVA), formerly referred to as thalamic syndrome. Neuropathic pain of the lower limb is excluded since there is a problem concerning accessibility and the procedure for inserting the electrode on the median line (of the brain) in the falx cerebri.

## Intrathecal pump

The intrathecal pump (**Figure 3**) is exceptionally effective in the case of spasticity (using baclofen), and significantly effective in cases of refractory pain, particularly neuropathic pain (using an anaesthetic substance, an opiate or clonidine). It is possible to insert a catheter in the spinal column and the pump under the skin of the abdomen without too great a risk. The principal inconveniences for the patient is the need to return to the out-patient clinic every three months in order to fill the pump with the medication, except in the case of baclofen, when this can be done every six months if the amount to be injected does exceed the capacity of the pump. This localized and targeted pharmacotherapy[5] permits a gradient of 100:1, on average, for the dosage the patient is to receive. As a result, the systemic secondary effects can be reduced considerably, except in the case of opiates that deregulate the hypothalomo-hypophyseal axis or, in others word, create a series of endocrinal problems, primarily hypogonadism, which essentially affects sexual function in the case of men.

FIGURE 3:

Intrathecal pump and catheter placed in the spine

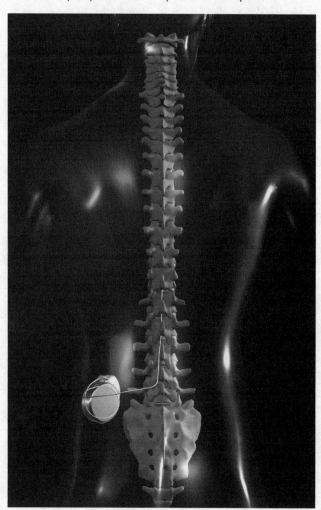

© Copyright Medtronic, Inc. 2010.

## 4. CONCLUSION

Like any other surgical intervention, these techniques can result in complications which are for the most part peri-operatory, yet rarely significant and permanent. For this reason, these invasive approaches are reserved for clearly selected clinical conditions, for which the patient must undergo a very complete assessment. But, in a therapeutic context, this approach serves not only to reduce the pain but also to increase the physical capacities and activities of the patient, improving his life quality and decreasing the quantities of drugs taken while also decreasing their adverse reactions.

## REFERENCES

1. Day, M. *Neuromodulation: spinal cord and peripheral nerve stimulation*. Current Review of Pain. 2000; 4(5): 374-382.

2. Bouhassira D et al. *Comparison of pain syndromes associated with nervous or somatic lesions and development of a new neuropathic pain diagnostic questionnaire (DN4)*. Pain, 2005; 114: 29-36.

3. Cruccu G, Aziz TZ, Garcia-Larrea L, Hansson P, Jensen TS, Lefaucheur JP, Simpson BA, Taylor RS. *EFNS guidelines on neurostimulation therapy for neuropathic pain*. Eur J Neurol, 2007; 14(9): 952-970.

4. Richard K. Osenbach, M.D. Motor Cortex Stimulation for Intractable Pain, Neurosurgical Focus, Published: 2007-02-05.

5. Polyanalgesic Consensus Conference 2007. *Recommendations for the Management of Pain by Intrathecal (Intraspinal) Drug Delivery: Report of an Interdisciplinary Expert Panel*. Deer, Timothy MD et al; Neuromodulation. 10(4): 300-328, October 2007.

# TEAMWORK IN PHYSICAL REHABILITATION...
## WHEN DEALING WITH CHRONIC PAIN

**Lucette Chabot** Pht, Quebec City, Quebec, Canada
**Marie-Josée Gobeil** OT, Quebec City, Quebec, Canada
Institut de réadaptation en déficience physique de Québec, Quebec, Canada

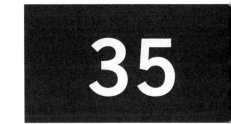

**35**

## ABSTRACT

Over the years, we have observed the evolution of knowledge and philosophies concerning pain. We have discovered a complex problem that is gradually changing and requires adjustments on the part of both those who suffer from pain and the health professionals. Thus, a better understanding of this phenomenon will enable both the clinician and the patient to replace the sense of powerlessness that leads to frustration and anger, with active strategies that can have an impact on the occasionally disastrous consequences of this problem. This chapter is intended to provide an overview of clinical practice in physical rehabilitation, and then illustrate the principles through clinical case studies.

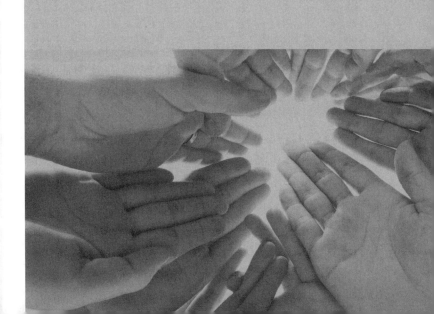

# 1.INTRODUCTION

For people dealing with chronic pain, *physical rehabilitation* is experienced in partnership with the team of clinicians. It is in this respect that we were invited to take part in writing this section of the book (**Working together when facing chronic pain**), which focuses on team work. In this chapter, we will describe our daily life as part of an interdisciplinary rehabilitation process[1], both as a clinic coordinator and as a clinician working as part of a team that has been dedicated to chronic pain for several years at the *Institut de réadaptation en déficience physique de Québec (IRDPQ), PERT*, implemented in 1989.

Each of us will experience pain during the course of our lives. Some people, unfortunately, will have to deal with a physical problem that may lead to disabilities related to that pain. Whether pain occurs as a result of an illness, an accident, a trauma or a surgery, the person in pain will experience, to various degrees, difficulties, and possibly even an inability to return to his/her life habits or living environment. When that individual has a handicap, rehabilitation may provide support throughout the adaptation/rehabilitation process intended to ensure a return to autonomy, the optimal recovery of abilities, and a reduction in the environmental obstacles that prevent a return to ordinary activities and social roles (family and community life, education, work, leisure activities, interpersonal relations).

# 2. REHABILITATION AND CHRONIC PAIN, AN EVOLVING REALITY

Physical rehabilitation for people suffering from persistent or chronic pain of a non-cancerous origin is a relatively recent phenomenon compared to other approaches for managing pain (rest, surgery, medication or others). In fact, the notion of chronic pain in rehabilitation has evolved significantly in recent decades. Clinicians working with patients with this type of problem have had to change their viewpoints, and adjust their knowledge and their skills as scientific data develops. Whereas, in the past, interventions focused on finding and treating the musculoskeletal structure responsible for the original pain, health

professionals now intervene in terms of preventing chronicity, and treating the disability associated with the persistent pain. In recent years, clinicians and scientific researchers have demonstrated that pain, and the disabilities that result from, are caused by multiple factors. In fact, the biological aspect of the injury is not the most important in the persistence of pain. Despite the scarring and remodelling of the tissues that were initially injured, the pain persists, and other factors must be examined to account for this persistence.

# 3. THE BEGINNINGS

In the 1980s, considering the prevalence of **lower back** pain, the disparity of the treatments available, and the associated costs, experts[2] examined how this problem was treated in the case of workers, so as to develop guidelines and issue recommendations. Following this, studies were also conducted with respect to persistent **neck pain**. These studies made with respect to these pathologies are currently considered references when referring to persistent pain. The evolution of knowledge in rehabilitation was principally supported by the *Commission de la santé et de la sécurité au travail (CSST, in Quebec)*. *The Société de l'assurance automobile du Québec (SAAQ, in Quebec)* also took part in this development. Their common interest grew out of a desire to develop services that would limit the social and economic losses resulting from neck and back problems.

All of this work led to the development of a new **treatment for back and neck pain**; it also led to changes in the perceptions of disability at work and chronicity. It was also used to evaluate the various therapeutic means by validating their effectiveness, and their pertinence

in keeping with the real impact obtained on progress in the patient's condition. Various decision-making trees and clinical guides were also developed from this same viewpoint, and in an effort to reduce the risk of chronicity. Let us take, for example, the *CLIP*[3] intended for clinicians treating back pain. It was designed and distributed in 2005-2006. This guide is an example of practice based on conclusive evidence, as well as the clinical expertise and knowledge of various health professionals. The CLIP is intended to be a clinical tool for the health professional who is treating people with back pain, regardless of the discipline. It facilitates communication among the various health professionals, and promotes continuity in care. This guide can be used by the first responders in the private sector of the health and social services network to identify clients who are at risk for chronicization and, as a result, can serve to guide their intervention judiciously. The notion of duration is decisive with respect to pain. It is a factor that will influence clinical reasoning and the resulting decisions.

- With respect to back pain, **a first transition period occurs during the fourth week of disability** and identifies the transition from acute to sub-acute pain. When patients cannot return to their activities, and they describe no significant improvement in their perception

of the disability, the clinician should be concerned about a risk of chronicity. In this case, it is necessary to work with the patient to identify elements that could be contributing to the persistence of the symptoms and the disability, in keeping with the rules and the protocols, so as to prevent the condition from evolving into chronic back pain. If the clinician and the patient feel that they are able to take action with respect to the factors of chronicity, there is no indication for referral to an interdisciplinary team.

- **The second transition period takes place three months after the appearance of the first symptoms**. This is the transition from the sub-acute phase to the chronic phase in the case of back pain.

- In all cases, the chronic state is defined as **back pain that persists beyond the time normally required for the healing of tissues, which is generally set at three months**, but can also vary depending on the pathology. At this stage, if the condition of the person with the pain has not evolved despite the fact that he/she has received the care recommended in the guides (such as the *CLIP*) supported by evidence-based treatments, it is suggested that the clinician and the patient discuss the possibility of a referral to an interdisciplinary team specialized in the treatment of chronic pain.

# 4. REHABILITATION IN THE CASE OF CHRONIC PAIN

The biomedical model is very effective for treating acute pain conditions in the early stages, namely the first few days, following an injury. The thinking behind this model is focused on the following model, and completely suitable for it:

| The signs and symptoms of the acute condition | → | the diagnosis | → | the treatment | → | healing |
|---|---|---|---|---|---|---|

## THE PAIN SYNDROME

However, research has highlighted the fact that this so-called conventional model fails in the case of the rehabilitation of patients suffering from chronic pain. Research has also identified factors other than biological that can contribute to the persistence of pain. Various studies have demonstrated that, in the case of a musculoskeletal problem, when the pain lasts more than six months, **the pain phenomenon becomes an entity on its own, called the pain syndrome.**

In fact, the complexity of the symptoms and the disability observed in the individual suffering from chronic pain are not caused by the original condition, but by various closely related factors that are biological, psychological and social in nature. Individuals suffering from pain that does not respond to various treatments develop an increasingly complex painful existence that has repercussions on those around them, and affects the way in which they interact with others. Simultaneously, the different ways in which the environment responds will, in turn, affect the adaptation of the person suffering from chronic pain, and could unfortunately support the chronicization of poorly adapted attitudes and behaviours. **This is a truly complex interaction that concerns the individual and his/her environment.**

Considering these factors, various theoretical models for biopsychosocial interventions have been developed to guide people suffering from chronic pain. They include the cognitive-behavioural[4] approaches which focus more on managing the pain, and increasing the level of physical and functional activity than on the disappearance of symptoms. **The ultimate goal is to reduce people's disabilities so that their lives can be more satisfactory, and not focused solely on their pain.** It is the individual who controls his/her own pain, and not the pain that controls the individual's life.

In keeping with this vision, various theoretical models for treatment were developed, including: *École interactionnelle du dos*[5], Sherbrooke model[6], *Programme d'évaluation et de rééducation des travailleurs aux prises avec des maux de dos chroniques (PERT)*[7], and many others. **They all share a global team approach for treating the individual** — which focuses on physical, cognitive and behavioural rehabilitation for patients with specific problems (back pain, neck pain, fibromyalgia, headaches, etc.).

The *PRÉVICAP*[8] approach demonstrates the importance of an environmental approach that can support workers <u>directly</u> in their environment. This approach takes into account the overall intervention of an individual with his/her environment in various aspects of his/her life.

The *PEGAP*[9] programme is also intended for people who have developed a disability following a pain problem. This programme was the first to offer training to health professionals and referring organizations (*SAAQ* and *CSST* in Quebec) in order to prepare them to target, and then take action with respect to the psychological risk factors such as catastrophic thinking, the fear of moving (kinesiophobia), perceived disabilities and depressive elements. This uni-disciplinary approach involves university professionals from various disciplines who have been trained to use this model. The PEGAP programme focuses on facilitating the return to work through the reduction of the risk factors that lead to extended disability, the progressive management of activity and the improvement of functional ability.

## 5. THE CURRENT VISION

In order to harmonize the services offered to patients suffering from chronic or persistent pain, and in keeping with the work started in the 1980s, more recent recommendations (May 2006) were issued by the *Agence d'évaluation des technologies et des modes d'intervention en santé* (AETMIS)[10] with respect to the treatment of non-cancer chronic pain. The treatment of chronic pain[11] should involve the following key elements: professional knowledge, hierarchical and organized services, interdisciplinary care, on-going evaluation of the quality of the care and the results, all in partnership with the individual suffering from the pain.

> Following an illness, a trauma or an accident, the individual receives common services, medical consultations and appropriate treatments. If these treatments fail and the problem persists, treatment will continue with specialized services, including specific rehabilitation services. Obviously, the services offered will be adapted in keeping with the evolution, and the resolution of the factors that prevented the individual from returning to his/her life habits.

As in the case of any other form of physical disability, rehabilitation for chronic pain will initially attack the **loss of autonomy**, and the **disabilities** that result from the painful condition. Professionals specializing in rehabilitation for chronic pain will help their patients attain their objectives, and recover their potential. Moreover, adjusting the intervention for this clientele demonstrates the importance of the patients' involvement in and responsibility for their rehabilitation. With an active approach, it is easier for the patient to learn and take control of his/her treatment, and then continue the work started during rehabilitation autonomously.

> **The individual must agree with and take part in the intervention plan developed with the rehabilitation team if the desired results are to be attained.**

Rehabilitation will require, on the part of those working in this field, a knowledge of both the phenomenon of chronic pain and human functioning (physical, psychological and within the individual's environment). Considering the importance of this overall vision, it is easy to see the **pertinence of team work** involving health professionals from various fields who fulfil these conditions and intervene with respect to the various specific problems related to the roles the individual plays in his/her life.

Also, depending on the situation, the vocation of the facility, and the specific needs of the individual to be treated, physical rehabilitation teams will include representatives of several disciplines (occupational therapist, physiotherapist, rehabilitation technician, physical educator, kinesiologist, guidance counsellor, ergonomist, nurse, pharmacist and others) who will complement the physicians and psychologists traditionally involved in resolving the problem of chronic pain. At present, there are several programmes involving health professionals working in teams dedicated to patients that suffer from chronic pain. Depending on the regions, these teams work in hospitals, rehabilitation centres or private clinics.

## 6. WORK AND PHYSICAL REHABILITATION

Following a problem involving the musculoskeletal system, individuals who are suffering from chronic or persistent pain, and are admitted for physical rehabilitation, have several physical disabilities and coping difficulties with respect to several daily living activities in their lives (family life, work, leisure activities, home maintenance, personal care). Such people have experienced several therapeutic failures, and must face the fact that they cannot assume their responsibilities. It is in this context that various problems associated with the painful syndrome may appear, including sleep disorders, anxiety or depression, which should also be treated with a combined biopsychosocial approach.

Admission into the chronic pain socioprofessional rehabilitation programme offered by the *Institut de réadaptation en déficience physique de Québec (IRDPQ)*[12] combining **de-sensitization and retraining for effort** requires the physician's authorization. Programme participation may be hampered by cardio-vascular deconditioning, or any other uncontrolled associated condition that can interfere with a return to activity (high blood pressure, diabetes, substance abuse, non-compliance with prescribed medication therapy, etc.).

When going into rehabilitation, individuals suffering from chronic pain are first evaluated, so as to identify all aspects of their problems, their needs and their objectives. Each professional, depending on his/her field of expertise, should evaluate the potential for rehabilitation or improvement in a realistic manner since, all too often, the legitimate desire expressed by the individual is to be free of pain, and go back to the way things were. **The individual in pain often expects complete relief of his/her pain before returning to his/her usual activities. This expectation or this human reflex to avoid pain, while understandable, contributes to chronicity and persistent disability by causing the individual to avoid activity in general.** Pain that has lasted several months or years may take months and even years to disappear.

> As a result, patients must be able to judiciously analyze, with treatment team, their situation in terms of the importance of gradually returning to activity despite the persistence of pain.

# 7. THE USER/CLINICIAN RELATIONSHIP FOR A GOOD START

## 1. LISTEN CAREFULLY TO IDENTIFY THE CONDITION

**Listening to the individual's history** will enable you to evaluate the symptoms and identify the perceptions and representations (knowledge, understanding and beliefs) that can contribute to the maintenance of chronicity. Active listening will initially serve to determine how the individual represents the disease, and then enable the clinician to reassure and gradually rectify the elements of the patient's knowledge and understanding that impeded a return to activity.

## 2. EVALUATE IN ORDER TO BETTER UNDERSTAND THE PAINFUL EXPERIENCE

First, the clinicians will try to **make an accurate evaluation of the individual, his/her environment and his/her life habits** so as to clearly understand the situation. The evaluation tools used at this point should have sufficient *metrological qualities* (reliability and validity) to limit the interpretations or perceptions specific to the clinician.

**The psychological evaluation will initially identify the individual's expectations and willingness to take part in this type of approach.** This interview will validate the fact that the individual wishes to return to a more active life despite the presence of persistent pain. Second, the psychologist will evaluate the extent to which the elements of psychological distress contribute to the persistence of the pain. For example, this includes a search for elements of depression or anxiety, a sleep disorder, loss of interest and motivation, coping strategies and difficulties, family and conjugal problems, an unresolved grieving process, elements of post-traumatic stress that are still active, among others.

The other members of the rehabilitation team will help to determine the prognosis for improving the individual's physical capacities and enabling him/her to return to significant activities (life habits, leisure activities, work, etc.). All of the professionals involved should determine the individual's potential for change (habits, attitudes) in order to deal with the requirement of his/her work environment or life.

## 3. IDENTIFY OBJECTIVES THAT CAN BE ACHIEVED IN THE SHORT TERM

**The in-depth evaluation of the painful experience by understanding clinicians will enable the individual to identify objectives that can be achieved in the short term.** This is very important. The clinicians will provide close supervision at the start so that the individual does not experience another therapeutic failure. The objectives will be revised and adapted throughout the rehabilitation process, and will be intended to achieve the life project or goal pursued in the medium and long term. For example, the goal may be to return to a previous job, to return to the job market in another sector, or to return to life habits. By experimenting with new strategies and, above all, by integrating new tools in a safe context, the individual may acquire more confidence in his/her movements, and will be better able to develop his/her full potential based on a series of positive events.

These evaluations will serve to identify the physical elements, the perceptions, the emotions, the behaviours, and the context associated with a painful syndrome. They will guide the choices made by the rehabilitation team and the patient, who will be exposed to gestures, activities or other elements that he/she has learned to avoid. This exposure and the development of the ability to act (behaviour) are necessary if the objectives are to be attained.

# 8. THE INTERVENTION PLAN

Sharing various strategies for improvement should lead to the development of an **individualized, interdisciplinary intervention plan** that takes the context of the individual suffering from chronic pain into account. The intervention plan will be based on the individual's expectations and objectives in terms of the rehabilitation process. It will also enable discussion between the individual and the rehabilitation team concerning the prognosis for improvement, and the activities proposed to attain it.

The principal challenges for the individual will be maintaining motivation, persevering and demonstrating an ability to change radically on occasion in order to attain the objectives.

Acceptance of the intervention plan is an essential factor. The user must be satisfied with the plan and agree with the measures proposed. The individual must not submit to the interventions but feel responsible for the evolution of his/her condition. He/she will indicate the direction he/she wants to take, and the treatment team members will indicate the parameters and the actions to be taken to make the rehabilitation experience a success. Often, this success will be the most wonderful treatment experience the individual has known. It is based on a coherent and concerted team approach that is dedicated to this specific clientele.

# 9. THE INTERVENTIONS

Current knowledge has validated the following fact: when people suffer from persistent pain, returning to their activities and a more active lifestyle will help them to develop better control over their pain.

As part of the intervention plan discussed with the team, the initial interventions will focus on instructing the individual about his/her condition and the mechanisms involved in his/her pain and disabilities. With this new understanding, the individual will gradually be able to make his/her way to effective management and self-treatment, based on the objectives set. **Participation in various types of interventions such as training sessions, personalized physical training periods, an specific exercise programme to the painful condition, relaxation training, and supervised role playing will help the individual have a better understanding of the painful condition and develop his/her capacities and skills.**

Thus, certain people will indicate that they have to modify their life habits or movement patterns that serve to maintain their pain. For others, better knowledge of their condition, the pacing of the activity and learning techniques for the healthy management of their energy will help them gradually return to a more satisfying life. **In this way, they will be able to break the cycles of "too much activity" to "complete rest for several days".**

Several elements have been identified as key factors in the success of the rehabilitation process. They include communication and constant support that are intended to be reassuring, and may occasionally confront the individual, but always provide support throughout the process so as to ensure his/her cooperation and progress. The vocabulary used by all of the professionals must also be consistent in order to indicate a shared philosophy and common objectives, and ensure daily clinical discussions.

# 10. TEAM WORK: THE KEY ELEMENTS OF SUCCESS

Since the outset of this great journey on the road to interdisciplinarity for the treatment and management of chronic pain, team work has demonstrated the importance of the following elements, considering the complexity of this problem.

- Cooperation and partnership of all those involved, including the patient;
- Sharing of common values and final goals with respect to rehabilitation;
- Coordination of clinical interventions;
- Constant communication (daily clinical meeting);
- Consistency in the instruction and information provided (same vocabulary);
- Support for learning;
- Confidence in oneself and others;
- Respect for the other's field of expertise;
- Updating of knowledge; and
- Creativity and openness.

All of these elements are major, even fundamental. Moreover, in the complex cases of painful syndromes, creativity and openness are even more significant for clinicians who will be required to evolve and surpass themselves when faced with this complexity. These key elements bring out the strengths of all, since complementarity makes the team strong (one for all, all for one). **A combined intervention is more than the sum of each of the disciplines involved.**

### The most important member of the team

The most important member of the team is still the person suffering from chronic pain. It is through this individual that we evolve constantly in interdisciplinarity. When we lose sight of this individual, it is easy to return to the automatic responses associated with our professional sector. That is when we can return to the value our field of professional expertise gives us by giving us the illusion that we alone have the power to "heal" a very complex condition. Generally, reality will bring us back into line, and make us a little more modest.

Team work requires professional assurance based on knowledge and experience, but also on the humility to recognize that, on our own, we will not be able to resolve the problem of complex pain. Just like the individual being treated, the professionals need an outside look and the cooperation of other clinicians to get out of the impasse. This constant interaction involving all of the professionals, namely the attending physician, the general practitioner, the physiatrist, the psychologist, the occupational therapist, the physiotherapist, the kinesiologist, the guidance counsellor and the clinic coordinator, will enable us to consider all of the solutions possible.

In order to make the notions discussed so far more concrete, we will now relate three therapeutic processes representative of our clientele. We will describe the socioprofessional rehabilitation process in a context of chronic or persistent pain.

# 11. THREE THERAPEUTIC PROCESSES

## JULES

Note from the authors: This first case study describes a critical situation. The path chosen was exceptional in terms of physical, psychological and social elements.

Jules was 39 years old. He had been married for 15 years and had two children. This welder/machine operator had been off work for five years after having handled a steel plate. He experienced back pain and numbness of the left arm. Here are the diagnostic impressions noted in the file:
- Results of a cervical sprain;
- Herniated disk , C5-C6 left, D1-D2 left, with no radicular compression;
- Reduced sensitivity of the fifth finger on the left hand;
- Multi-stage degeneration of D4-D5 to D10-D11;
- Myalgia of the left trapezium;

- History of back pain, muscular and cardiac deconditioning, vertigo; and
- Major depression treated.

Here are the treatments he had received: 202 physiotherapy treatments, osteopathy, multiple consultations with numerous specialists (orthopedists, neurologist, neurosurgeon, physiatrist). He had tried several medications, which had been recently replaced by methadone. The patient said that he experienced less relief with this medication. When he arrived, he was still receiving psychotherapy treatments.

### Questions asked by the physical rehabilitation team

Can we help him? It would be easy to say: "Learn to live with your pain." The rehabilitation team would take care to try everything else before suggesting this.

### Identification of the problems

A rehabilitation process was initiated with interdisciplinary evaluations. The various physical evaluations demonstrated good cooperation, and enabled us to identify the following problems.

- Severe neck and back pain irradiating to the fifth finger of the left hand;
- Overprotection of the left arm and neck, under use of the left arm; the patient indicated that his physician had told him to stop using his upper left arm;
- Major functional loss of neck, left shoulder and left arm; mobility reduced by avoidance and persistent pain;
- Beginning of transfer of dominance to upper right arm (was left-handed);
- Severe postural deficit when sitting, standing and walking;
- Deficient postural hygiene, unsafe work techniques;
- Severe deconditioning with respect to maximal stress test on treadmill, placing him in the lowest percentile for his age group;

- Sedentarity ++ since the accident, lack of leisure activities, despite a sports past;
- Severe interference with his activities; he often lay down during the day;
- Serious fears that his condition would be aggravated when he returned to physical activity;
- Sensation of fatigue in all four limbs;
- Lack of endurance, difficulty handling light loads;
- Difficulty performing daily living activities;
- Marked deterioration in couple's life;
- Unemployed, loss of employment link, uncertainty concerning the future +++;
- Lack of knowledge concerning his condition and his prognosis for recovery;
- Passive management focused on rest while lying, medication and heat; and
- Sleep disturbed by pain: he slept two hours a night, lying on his left side.

### Psychological condition

The psychological evaluation highlighted a desperate need for assistance and a non-dynamic appearance. We noted elements of psychological distress (strong elements of depression and anxiety), the presence of anger with respect to the situation; he described himself as passionate about his work prior to the accident. Indications of kinesiophobia, catastrophic thoughts, the impression of disability and depression were all very high.

## Interventions

Our first intervention took place during the evaluation period, since it seemed to be a priority to us. We suggested that he change his sleeping position (adequate position and pillows) and provided the necessary equipment. The patient was attentive to the instruction; he applied the recommendations that same night. He noted a radical chance in the duration and the quality of his sleep, which was a first therapeutic success and helped develop his trust in the team. Throughout his six-week stay, he was highly motivated and very cooperative.

## Intense de-sensitization and retraining programme

He took part in the intense de-sensitization and retraining programme 35 hours per week, from 8:00 a.m. to 4:00 p.m., including two breaks per day, and one hour for lunch. He got involved quickly. He participated regularly, and respected the intensity, exercise quota and progression requested. He acquired the knowledge he needed to take action with respect to the factors that influenced his pain. Moreover, he integrated means for managing his pain in the various sectors of activity during his stay.

## Results and final evaluations

Jules kept a large quantity of medication which he eventually intended to use to finish it all if he couldn't find a way out of his situation. He turned this medication over in the middle of the programme, explaining that he no longer wanted to end things, and that he was regaining his taste for life. He learned to control his pain through exercise and relaxation. He understood the importance of gradually returning to his activities. He interpreted his many successes as **"the more I move the better I feel"**. At the end of the programme, the results obtained in the various tests evaluating kinesiophobia, catastrophism, the index of pain-related disability and the depressive elements — which were severe at the time of his arrival — had become insignificant. The final evaluations indicated the following improvements.

- Disappearance of protective and avoidance behaviours;
- Marked improvement in posture while resting and active;
- Mobility and muscular strength of upper left arm close to normal, disappearance of irradiation to the left arm;
- Persistence of slowness in left arm but normal movement;

- No longer perceived himself as limited with respect to daily and leisure activities;
- Evaluation of cardio-vascular condition indicated a significantly improved physical condition (10th percentile of a healthy population);
- He developed active and effective management techniques (exercises, muscular relaxation of neck and shoulders, relaxation);
- He described a significant return to his activities;
- His marital life had improved greatly;
- He had specific projects to return to the job market; and
- He had joined a physical training centre and wished to return to his sports activities gradually, while respecting certain parameters.

His repeated successes contributed to the development of a high sense of personal efficiency with respect to returning to his life habits. **At the end of the process, the patient said that he was ready to take control of his life and felt capable of doing so.**

## LUCIE

Note from the authors: This second case study demonstrates the importance of accepting the intervention plan, without which there can be no therapeutic process leading to the expected behavioural changes.

Lucie was 42 years old and lived in the country (about an 8-hour drive from Quebec City). She has been with her partner for 23 years, and had three children at home. The victim of a car accident that occurred three years ago, she had not returned to work since. She had performed several kinds of work while self-employed. At the time of her accident, she had been working as a receptionist for two years. She was right-handed.

Her history described no loss of consciousness during the accident. The diagnoses in the file indicated a cervical sprain and a fracture of the right humerus (open reduction). Imaging later demonstrated degenerative cervical diskopathy. Considering the persistence of her inability to lift her arm and the severe pain she described in her right shoulder and the cervical region, she saw five specialists (orthopedist, physiatrist), sought consultations in anaesthesia (pain clinic). She also consulted specialists on two occasions, and was advised not to lift more than five kilograms with her right arm. She was given several injections in her right shoulder and neck area without any relief. She mentioned that the various therapists could not touch her since she experienced too much pain, which limited the scope of the interventions.

## Questions of the physical rehabilitation team

Had the patient adapted to her situation? Could she leave her family and focus on the rehabilitation context proposed to her?

## Identification of the problems

The patient had help at home for domestic chores. She viewed herself as incapable of making meals, or doing any other kind of housework. Her objective when she arrived was to become the person she had been before the accident. The diagnosis made when she was admitted was: chronic pain syndrome following a fracture of the right humerus. The evaluations and interviews uncovered the following problems.

- Marked protectiveness with respect to the upper right limb;
- Absence of vaso-motors or trophic signs in the right arm;
- Serious deterioration in posture, reduction in weight-bearing on the entire right side when seated, standing and walking;
- She said that she was involved in sports in the past and her performance on the maximum effort test (treadmill) placed her in the 45th percentile for women of her age;
- She did not describe any fear of movement in her responses to specific tests, but when taking part in activities, she expressed a high degree of fear with respect to sports activities;
- She described herself as unfit for any employment and reported that the pain had a very severe impact (disabling) on her functional activities;

- Serious anger against her former employer;
- She demonstrated severe slowing during a functional activity circuit, under-used the right arm, blocked her respiration, used poor body techniques when making an effort;
- The evaluation of the psychological factors indicated that she was still waiting for a miracle treatment and no anxiety or depression was noted during the specific evaluations; and
- She wanted to put a positive perception on everything, denied the psychological aspects of her pain, declared that she had no personal problems and that everything was going well in her environment.

Despite the information she received during the first few days of the intervention concerning her chronic pain and rehabilitation, the patient indicated that she did not feel concerned by it. Her lack of openness with respect to the analysis of her psychosocial situation seriously limited the possibilities of rehabilitation. Moreover, she continued to wait for a "miracle" solution that would enable her to be what she used to be without having to get more involved in her rehabilitation process, and without having to change her habits.

## Results and final evaluations

The only support we were able to offer her was the recommendation of certain adaptations such as an adequate pillow to facilitate her sleep, and a "sports support" for the right shoulder, to make it slightly more functional while reducing her protectiveness of her arm. She put an end to the process after one week. She was happy to go home. The patient was not prepared to take part in rehabilitation.

## SUZANNE

Note from the authors: In this case, we will show that close monitoring of this woman enabled her to continue with her rehabilitation process despite the appearance of a new painful condition affecting her knees. A consultation and timely follow-up resulted in changes to her programme so that she could complete the process successfully.

Suzanne was 51 years old. She had been married for 32 years, had two children and two grandchildren. She had been working as a nurse in a hospital for 25 years. Eighteen months ago, she experienced sudden back pain when transferring a patient from a bed; the patient grabbed her to keep from falling. She was off work for two weeks as a result of a back sprain. She took a temporary assignment two days per week. She was not able to increase her work load as a result of back pain.

When she came to us for treatment, she was experiencing a left side low back pain, with irradiation to her left leg that had persisted for more than a year. Suzanne was directed to a work rehabilitation programme lasting nine weeks that focused on a sustainable and full-time return to her work as nursing assistant working the night shift. The patient's principal expectation was to become physically capable of returning to work.

## Questions asked by the physical rehabilitation team

We felt the context was favourable for rehabilitation. Was physical deconditioning the only factor involved in her inability to return to her normal tasks? Were there any environmental obstacles? Was the work environment open to meeting with the rehabilitation team as part of an ecological approach?

## Identification of the problems

The interviews and evaluations conducted at the start of the process enabled us to identify the following problems pertaining to the persistent pain and disability.

- History of a condition of musculo-skeletal origin that resulted in a work stoppage lasting six months;
- The intensity of the pain varied from moderate to severe;
- Posture change, reduction of weight bearing on the left leg when standing;
- Reduced mobility in the back region and the lower left leg, reduced muscular control of the lower left leg;
- Persistent and disabling pain syndrome lasting more than one year and irradiating to the left knee;
- Reduced balance when crouched;
- Difficulty lifting a load, biomechanical compensation when handling a load;
- Stress test on treadmill (55th percentile for women of her age);
- Reduced tolerance sitting and standing;
- Lack of knowledge about her condition and means for managing pain, primarily concerning the irradiations she experienced, few active management strategies;
- She had given up several household chores, both inside and outside (gardening, shovelling);
- Her leisure and family activities had been disrupted significantly;
- Great fear of a relapse of a deterioration associated with a return to activity;
- Conjugal and family difficulties;
- Sleep disturbed and not restorative as a result of the pain;
- Extended absences from her regular tasks at work; and
- Absence of elements of anxiety or depression

## Physical training programme

Suzanne was monitored for two weeks in a clinical setting. During this period, she took part in a physical training programme intended to help her progressively get back in shape and gradually increase her capacity for postural efforts and tolerances. Her work station was inspected, along with the paying agent and her immediate supervisor. This meeting served to identify the obstacles in her work environment, and prepare for a progressive return to her duties.

During the re-training, Suzanne demonstrated a good ability to integrate work techniques, and modified the inappropriate movements associated with her spinal problem. She reported pain in both knees. A femoro-patellary syndrome was diagnosed by the team physician. She was given physiotherapy treatments in the following days, and took part in a muscular strengthening programme specific to her condition, in addition to a programme concerning the rehabilitation of her vertebral column which she took part in at our clinic setting, and following that as part of her work activities.

## Results and final evaluations

A progressive reduction in pain in both knees was reported and controlled after two weeks. At the end of this two-week rehabilitation programme in the clinic, she returned to work under supervision. Several visits were made during this period and improvements in her condition were noted from the very first weeks. She integrated the appropriate posture and vertebral protection principles taught, along with the principles for the active management of her symptoms at work. After being exposed to several situations involving greater risk and dealing with them successfully, she viewed herself as fit to go back to providing services to unpredictable residents or in situations involving a high risk of relapse. Progressively, Suzanne was able to return to work four consecutive days, which was her regular schedule. She also went back to performing all of the tasks associated with her work.

Suzanne reported occasional pain in her left hip, which she managed to control using the management mechanisms she was taught. In order to support her in this management, she was given physiotherapy treatments so as to verify the irritability of her condition, and teach her adequate management mechanisms. During this period, she also asked her colleagues for help so that she would not compromise her presence at work. She had her pain under control in three days. She also returned to her outdoor sports activities: snowshoeing and cross-country skiing. She mentioned that her family relationships had improved since she had returned to her leisure activities. She reported that she felt confident in her professional future, and perceived herself as capable of performing her work duties.

At the end of her work rehabilitation programme, Suzanne demonstrated significant improvements with respect to the principal factors that formed an obstacle to her return to work (intensity of her symptoms, management of her symptoms and psychosocial factors).

## HOW DO WE ANALYZE THESE RESULTS?

The three case studies presented illustrate one spectacular success, and one more moderate success. Certain rehabilitation processes can have mitigated results when the patient perceives more inconveniences than advantages in taking action for change, or when he/she continues to expect an exterior solution or a new medical treatment. Thus, the objectives, the progress and the results are different for each individual. **But the key to success still depends on the cooperation and team work of the user and the rehabilitation professionals, as well as on joint efforts with the various partners involved in the rehabilitation process.**

# REFERENCES

1. Tel que vécu à l'Institut de réadaptation en déficience physique de Québec, au Programme de réadaptation socioprofessionnelle (volet douleur chronique).
2. Rapport Walter O. Spitzer. Les aspects cliniques des affections vertébrales chez les travailleurs, février 1986.
3. Rossignol, Michel, Bertrand Arsenault. Clinique de lombalgie interdisciplinaire de première ligne 2006. Ce guide pratique a été fait en collaboration avec 5 organismes représentant les professionnels de la santé de première ligne. www.santepub.mtl.qc.ca/dep/index.html
4. Waddell, G., Vlaeyen, J.W.S., Kori, S.H.
5. http://ecoledudos.uqat.ca/
6. Loisel, P., Durand, P., Abenhaim, I. Management of occupational back pain: the Sherbrooke model. Results of a pilot and feasibility study. Occup. Environ. Med. 1994, 51: 597-602.
7. http://www.irdpq.qc.ca/services_clientele/programmations/adultes/integration_scolaire_professionnelle.html
8. http://www.previcap.com/, www.caprit.ca
9. PEGAP: Programme de gestion de l'activité progressive (PDP-PGAP.com)
10. Agence d'évaluation des technologies et des modes d'intervention en santé (AETMIS). Document sur la prise en charge de la douleur chronique (non cancéreuse), Organisation des services de santé, mai 2006: volume 2, numéro 4.
11. Douleur chronique: douleur persistante au-delà de 3 à 6 mois et rebelle au traitement.
12. http://www.irdpq.qc.ca/services_clientele/programmations/adultes/integration_scolaire_professionnelle.html

# BIBLIOGRAPHY

- Bradley, K. & MD Weiner. The Biopsychosocial Model and Spine Care. Spine Update. Spine, 2008; 33 : 219-223.
- Butler, David S. & Lorimer G. Moseley. Explain Pain, Noigroup publications, 2004.
- Charest, Jacques, Jean-René Chenard, Benoît Lavignolle & Serge Marchand. Lombalgie, École interactionnelle du dos, Masson, Paris, 1996.
- Chown, Marjorie, Lynne Whittamore, Mark Rush, Sally Allan, David Stott & Archer Mark. A prospective study of patients with chronic back pain randomised to group exercise, physiotherapy or osteopathy. Physiotherapy, 94, 2008; 21-28.
- Core Curriculum for Professional Education in Pain, edited by Edmond Charlton. Physical Medicine and rehabilitation. IASP Press, Seattle, 2005 (22).
- Duval, Luc & Alain Dubois. La douleur et l'expression du vécu douloureux vers une approche globale. L'orientation Professionnelle, volume 21, numéro 1, 1985 : 97-119.
- Duplan, B. & JM Guillet. Approches multidisciplinaires de la douleur lombaire : l'expérience française. Du conditionnement à l'effort à l'approche psychosomatique. Rev Rhum, 2001; 6, 8 (2) : 170-174.
- Gross, AR., C. Goldsmith, JL Hoving et al. Conservative Management of Management of Mechanical Neck Disorders: A Systematic Review. J Rheumatol, 2007; 34 (30) : 1083-1102.
- Godges, JJ, MA Anger, G. Zimmerman & A. Delitto (2008). Effects of education on return-to-work status for people with fear avoidance beliefs and acute low back pain. American physical therapy, 88(2) :231-239.
- Guzmán, Jaime, R. Esmail, K. Karjalainen, A. Malmivaara, E. Irvin & C. Bombardier (2007). Multidisciplinary bio-psycho-social rehabilitation for chronic low-back pain. Cochrane Database Syst, Rev, 2007, Jul 18; (2) : CD000963.
- Hildebrandt, Jan, Michael Pfingsten, Petra Saur & Jürgen Jansen. Prediction of Success from a Multidisciplinary Treatment Program for Chronic Low Back Pain. Spine, May 1997 (22)-9, 990-1001.
- Hlobil, H., JB Stall, J. Twisk, J. KÖke, A. Arl, G. Ens, T. Smid & W. Van Meclelen (2005). The effects of a graded activity intervention for Low-back-pain in occupational health on sick-leave, functional status and pain: 12 months result of a randomised controlled trial. Journal of Occupational Rehabilitation, 15(4,) 569-579.
- Hurwitz, EL, EJ Carragee, G. Van Der Velde, LJ Carroll, M. Nordin, J. Guzman, PM Peloso, LW Holm, P. Côté, S. Hogg-Johnson, JD Cassidy & S. Haldeman. Bone and Joint Decade 2000-2010 Task Force on Neck Pain and its Associated Disorders. J. Manipulative Physiol Ther, 2009 Feb; 32 (2 suppl) : S141-175.
- Keer, M.S., JW Frank, HS Shannon, RWK Norman, RP Wells, WP Neumann & C. Bombardier (2001). Biomechanical and psychosocial risk factors for low back pain. American journal of public health, 91(7), 1069-1075.

## BIBLIOGRAPHY (CONT'D)

- Kori, SH, RP Miller & DD Todd. Kinesiophobia a new view of chronic pain behavior. Pain Management, Jun/Feb; 1990 : 35-43.
- Loisel, P., MJ Durand, D. Berthelette, N. Vézina, R. Baril, D. Gagnon, C. Larivière & C. Tremblay (2001). Disability Prevention - New Paradigm for the Management of Occupational Back Pain. Disease Management and Health Outcomes, 9 (7), 351-360.
- Loisel, P. & MJ Durand. La douleur persistante : un défi pour la réinsertion socioprofessionnelle. La Lettre de l'institut UPSA de la douleur. Septembre 2006, (24).
- Loisel, P., MJ Durand et al. From evidence to community practice in work rehabilitation: The Quebec experience. The Clinical Journal of Pain, (2003) 19, 105-113.
- Loisel P., QN Hong, D. Imbeau, K. Lippel , J. Guzman, E. Maceachen, M. Corbière, BR Santos & JR Anema. The work Disability Prevention CIHR Strategic Training Program: Program Performance after 5 years of implantation. J Occup Rehabil, March 2009; 19 (1) : 1-7.
- McWilliams, LA, BJ Cox & MW Enns. Mood and anxiety disorders associated with chronic pain: An examination in a nationally representative sample. Pain, 2003; 106(1-2) : 127-133.
- Morel-Fatio, M. & F. Boureau. Aspects comportementaux de la douleur chronique, implications pour la prise en charge en rééducation. J Réadapt Med, 1997; 17(3) : 112-116.
- Moseley, Lorimer G. I can't find it! Distorted body image and tactile dysfunction in patients with chronic back pain. Pain, 140, 2008; 239-243.
- Nicholas, M., A. Molloy, L. Tonkin & L. Beeston. Manage your pain. Practical and positive ways of adapting to chronic pain. Sydney, Australia: ABC Books; 2000.
- O'Sullivan, Peter. Diagnosis and classification of chronic low back pain disorders: Maladaptive movement and motor control impairments as underlying mechanism. Manual Therapy, 10, 2005 : 242-255.
- Ostelo, RW, MW Tulder, JW Vlaeyen, SJ Linton, SJ Morley & WJ Assendelft. Behavioural treatment for chronic low-back pain. Cochrane Database Syst Rev, 2005; (1) : CD002014.
- Perreault, Kadija & Clermont E. Dionne. Does patient-physiotherapist agreement influence the outcome of low back pain? A prospective cohort study. BMC Musculoskeletal Disorders, 2006, 7:76.
- Philips, H.C. Avoidance behaviour and its role in sustaining chronic pain. Behav Res Ther, 1987; (25) : 273-279.
- Selander, J., SU Mametoff, & M. Asell (2007). Predictors for successful vocational rehabilitation for clients with back pain problems. Disability and Rehabilitation, 29(3), 215-220.
- Shaw WS, SJ Linton & G. Pransky (2006). Reducing sickness absence from work due to low back pain: how well do interventions strategies match modifiable risk factors? Journal of Occupational Rehabilitation, 16, 591-605.
- Swanson, David W, MD. Clinique Mayo, La douleur Chronique, Approche Globale. Bibliothèque nationale du Québec, 1er trimestre 2000.
- Udermann, BE, KF Spratt, RG Donelson, J. Mayer, JE Graves & J. Tillotson. Can a patient educational book change behaviour and reduce pain in chronic low back pain patients? Spine J, 2004; 4(4) : 425-435.
- Veillette, Y. L'interdisciplinarité dans la gestion de la douleur chronique. Congrès annuel de la Société québécoise de la douleur, Montréal, 22 octobre 2004. Montréal, Québec : OPPQ; 2004.
- Vlaeyen, JWS, AMJ Kole-Snijders, GB Boeren & H. Van Eek. Fear of movement/(re)injury in chronic low back pain and its relation to behavioural performance. Pain, 1995; (62) : 363-372.
- Waddel, G. A new clinical model for treatment of low back pain. Spine, 1987, (12), 632-644.

# THE PLACE OF PHYSIOTHERAPY
## IN THE TREATMENT OF NOCICEPTIVE, NEUROPATHIC AND CHRONIC PAIN

**36**

**Paul Castonguay** Pht, MSc, FCAMT, ISTP, physical therapist and consultant, Montreal, Quebec, Canada

Email: paulcastonguay@bellnet.ca
paulcastonguay2009@hotmail.com

## ABSTRACT

The physiotherapist makes a physiotherapeutic diagnosis after evaluating the individual's disabilities and incapacities. Evaluating pain is one component of this diagnosis, and physiotherapy remains an essential approach in the treatment of a painful condition. As a result of their molecular effects, physical agents can complement or replace anti-inflammatory or analgesic medication. Partial or complete relief of pain by means of these invasive forms of energy will, in most cases, improve quality of life, but will also enable the individual to undertake functional rehabilitation that will restore functional losses, so that he/she can attain his/her maximum functional performance, and consolidate the physical skills acquired for an active and fulfilling life.

ABSTRACT

1. ROLES OF PHYSIOTHERAPY AND THE TREATMENT OF PAIN

2. PHYSIOLOGICAL EFFECTS OF VARIOUS PHYSICAL AGENTS

3. THERAPEUTIC EFFECTS

The immediate post-traumatic phase
Acute phase (0 to 4 weeks)
Sub-acute phase (4 to 12 weeks)
Tissue re-modelling and functional gain phases
Chronic phase

4. PHYSIOTHERAPY AND MEDICATION

Physiotherapy treatments
Simple analgesics and non-steroidal anti-inflammatories
Opioids
Co-analgesics such as anti-convulsants and anti-depressants

5. CONCLUSION

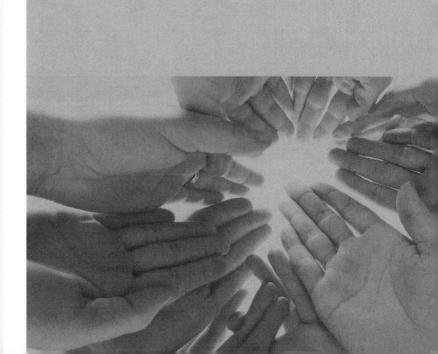

# 1. ROLES OF PHYSIOTHERAPY AND THE TREATMENT OF PAIN

The indications for physiotherapy treatment are diverse, numerous and often unknown to the general public and health professionals. In the field of physiotherapy, we know that one of the major indications and one of the most frequent reasons for consulting is to treat pain, at all stages in the pathological process, from the post-trauma to the chronic phase. In all stages, physiotherapists must adapt their treatment to those of the care team, since certain treatment means could work against the medication or objectives.

The treatment and relief of pain serve to start a functional re-education programme and treat physical deficits and incapacities. **It is essential for people to understand that pain control is used to minimize and restore functional losses that arise out of weakness, muscular imbalance, or loss of joint amplitude, as well as to soften scar tissue or adherences.** Certain pain clinics offer relatively complete treatments including an approach in physiotherapy and psychology. The patient must participate in the entire approach offered, from the use of medication to relieve pain to re-education of the body and mind.

Several published articles and books document the scientific aspect of a physiotherapy approach.[1, 2, 3] However, it is acknowledged that there is no scientific evidence concerning the exclusive use of physical agents or medication for the purpose of re-education.

**For the physiotherapist, pain relief should be used as part of a global approach including, as the case may be, manual techniques, ergonomic advice, general or specific exercises, and a return to functional activities.**

# 2. PHYSIOLOGICAL EFFECTS OF VARIOUS PHYSICAL AGENTS

Several studies documenting the physiological effects observed have served to explain the therapeutic applications of the various physical agents. Physiotherapy and the physical agents can act on pain by means of various mechanisms in the same manner, or as a complement to medication. This chapter will not discuss the physiological or molecular effects of physical agents in detail. **Table 1** lists those that are proposed most often in literature.

TABLE 1: Physiological effects proposed by the various physical agents

| PHYSIOLOGICAL EFFECTS | PHYSICAL AGENTS |
|---|---|
| Increase or decrease in the activity of the sensitive receptors and nerve depolarization of sensitive fibres by:<br>· Closing of the Melzack Wall gate<br>· Stimulation of Golgi tendon organs<br>· Inhibition of the neuromuscular spindle | Thermotherapy<br>Vibratory stimulations<br>Electric currents such as TENS and other related currents<br>Cryotherapy<br>Endermotherapy |
| Release of neurotransmitters such as endorphins and enkephalins | Cryotherapy and alternating hot/cold baths<br>TENS<br>Extracorporal and radial shocks |
| Slowing of nerve conduction | Cryotherapy |
| Action on motor unit recruitment:<br>· By nerve depolarization<br>· By reducing pain inhibition<br>· By direct stimulation of the muscle without the intermediary of the motorneuron<br>· Through awareness of the muscle contraction | Low or medium frequency neuromuscular stimulator (ex.: Russian current)<br>Cryotherapy, electroanalgesia (ex.: TENS and related techniques)<br>Low frequency muscular stimulator with broad impulse duration<br>Biofeedback |

TABLE 1: Physiological effects proposed by the various physical agents (continued)

| PHYSIOLOGICAL EFFECTS | PHYSICAL AGENTS |
| --- | --- |
| Action on the cellular metabolism<br>· Increase<br>· Decrease | Thermotherapy<br>Cryotherapy |
| Activation of growth factors (cytokines) | Ultrasound<br>Polarized electric currents<br>(ex.: MET, HVPC*)<br>Laser<br>Radial and extracorporeal shocks<br>* MET: micro-current, HVPC: high-voltage current |
| Re-establishment of the electric potential of damaged cells needed for healing tissues (injury current) | Polarized currents (HVPC, MET, CEMP*), monophasic current<br><br>* CEMP: pulsed electromagnetic fields |
| Increase in ATP* production<br><br>*ATP: adenosine triphosphate | Low-energy techniques: laser, MET, CEMP |
| Increase in transmembrane ion exchanges: direct effect (ex.: mechanical) or indirect (ex.: by local increase of ATP) | Ultrasound<br>MET<br>Diathermy (dielectric heating)<br>CEMP |
| Reproduction of a current similar to that produced by the piszo-electric effect present in the various collagen tissues | Devices producing mechanical constraints (ultrasound)<br>Low-intensity electric currents such as MET and CEMP that produce this type of current |
| Modification of vascularisation (for all means) by:<br>· Vasodilatation<br>· Vasoconstriction<br>· Increase in blood flow back to the heart | Thermotherapy<br>Electroanalgesia: TENS and related currents<br>Cryotherapy<br>Intermittent compression devices<br>Endermotherapy<br>Rhythmic neuromuscular stimulation, including low-frequency or slow-frequency pulsed TENS type devices |
| Migration of ionized particles or cells by:<br>· Migration to the cathode: fibroblasts<br>· Migration to the anode: albumin, epithelial cells, macrophages, leucocytes | Polarized electric current (MET, HVPC) |
| Modification of viscoelastic properties of collagen tissue | Ultrasound, diathermy before or during stretching<br>Cryotherapy for a collagen tissue in stretched position after mobility exercises<br>Endermotherapy |
| Modification of the shape of a protein, such as an enzyme, by resonance between the protein and the energy spent to activate or inhibit the protein | Ultrasound<br>Laser |
| Cutaneous penetration of a medicinal substance (ex.: dexamethasone, topical NSAID) | Iontophoresis: constant continuous current<br>Phonophoresis: ultrasound |
| Modulation of medication effectiveness (ex.: chemotherapeutic agents, thrombolytics, DNA based) | Ultrasound |

# 3. THERAPEUTIC EFFECTS

Pain starts with primary hyperalgesia at the site of the lesion. This hyperalgesia is the consequence of a tissue lesion, a haemorrhage, or an inflammatory reaction. Inadequate pain control, from the outset, will result in a cascade of events that occasionally lead to chronic pain. A chronic lesion can go back into an acute phase during a relapse. For

this reason, we are presenting the most conclusive therapeutic effects for the relief of pain, obtained from therapies using physical agents, in keeping with healing stages.

## THE IMMEDIATE POST-TRAUMATIC PHASE

During the immediate post-traumatic phase, the therapeutic effects desired are the reduction of the haemorrhage, the restriction of the development of oedema, and the prevention of hypoxic lesions secondary to the compression caused by the oedema, vascular breaks or tissue debris.[4]

Quite soon after the trauma, the state of the capillaries is altered. This alteration is a process that is necessary for the activation of the mastocytes responsible for chemical inflammation mediators. Application of ice and a means of compression affect the vascular state. Controlling the vascular state at this stage is necessary to limit both the haemorrhage and the inflammation. Ice also slows the cellular metabolism, thereby

protecting tissues from a secondary hypoxic injury. The earlier the ice is applied, the more beneficial the slowing of the metabolism will be.

### In practice
For optimum effectiveness, it is recommended that a maximum of 30 minutes be allowed between applications, for the first 4 hours following the trauma. For common cryotherapy, the treatment can be applied 20 to 30 minutes for deep structures and 10 to 15 minutes for superficial structures.[5, 6, 7]

## ACUTE PHASE (0 TO 4 WEEKS)

The purposes of treatment are the same as for the immediate post-traumatic phase. In addition, there is the need to effectively control pain and muscular spasms, ensure that the cleaning of the injured area to a certain extent, prevent trophic changes. After the first four hours following the injury, it is recommended that the patient continue to apply cold every hour or every second hour, for the first 24 to 48 hours. The application of cold during this acute period, such as following joint surgery, could cease the muscular inhibition caused by the effusion, and even facilitate contraction[8] of the inhibited muscle, and accelerate the return to functionality.[9, 10]

### In practice
During the acute phase, superficial thermotherapy, particularly heatwraps, is used a lot less than cryotherapy. It is, however, possible that certain forms of inexpensive superficial thermotherapy can be used to effectively treat pain, spasms and the sensation of stiffness[11, 12, ] even in the acute phase.

TENS can also be used effectively to reduce pain, and the use of analgesics, if the parameters are adequate[13]. The same applies to certain recent injuries, such as rib fractures. In these cases, TENS seems to be effective for controlling pain, even when compared to non-steroidal anti-inflammatories (NSAIDs)[14]. Moreover, in order to accelerate the return to functionality as long as the contraction does not exert any excessive pressure on the injured structures – the electrical stimulation of the muscles adjacent to the injured structure can be used as of the acute phase or following surgery, such as knee replacement.[15]

## SUB-ACUTE PHASE (4 TO 12 WEEKS)

During the sub-acute phase, the purpose of treatment is to control pain so that the patient can return to an active physiotherapy programme and his/her functional activities as soon as possible. The physical agents must also promote liquid and protein re-absorption, and act on persistent muscle spasms so as to limit muscle retractions, accelerate tissue healing, prevent atrophy and muscular imbalances, fight against painful inhibition, prevent the formation of adherences or retractions of soft tissues and, finally, prevent chronic pain.

### In practice
It is possible that the combined use of cryotherapy and exercises may be effective to attain these objectives at this phase.[5] Biofeedback could be useful at this stage to increase recruitment, or improve muscular coordination. Warming up the deep structures before stretching them, sometimes followed by cooling of the tissues in the extended position, will probably result in lasting gains in joint amplitude, as compared to simply stretching.[16, 17]

Certain physical agents are used for their ability to accelerate healing of the collagen tissue, particularly ultrasound, polarized currents such as high-voltage or micro-currents, laser, diathermy and pulsed electro-magnetic fields.

## TISSUE RE-MODELLING AND FUNCTIONAL GAIN PHASES

During these phases, the objective is to control pain related to persistent muscle tensions, tissue weakening, and the elimination of residual oedema that tend to produce a fibrosis of the connective tissue. Physiotherapists have to fight against tissue retractions and weakness, muscular asynchronisms, and focus on a return to normal functional activities. A muscle re-education programme should be implemented, increasing in intensity, and focusing on the isometric, concentric and excentric recruitment of the muscles if the patient's functional needs make this necessary. For this purpose, the techniques used during the sub-acute phase can continue to be used as long as they allow for an increase in intensity in the re-education programme or reduce the pain experienced during or after the physiotherapy programme.

## CHRONIC PHASE

When the injury is in the chronic phase, it is essential to identify and reduce, and even eliminate, if possible, the cause of the pain. Thus, the physical agents will fight tissue degeneration, the absence of complete healing, or the elimination of tissue calcification. At the same time, it is a good idea to use all means possible to fight chronic pain, to enable the patient to once again be autonomous in controlling his/her pain and, above all, act on the harmful effects of pain that can lead to the patient's inactivity. During this phase, physical agents can help physiotherapists attain their treatment objectives, as long as they are integrated in a plan to allow the patient to control his/her own pain and active treatments are preferred.

### In practice

Superficial heat provides a good cost-benefit ratio, and certain types of superficial heat seem to be effective on a short-term basis for the treatment of various conditions such as wrist pain.[18] TENS also provides a good cost-benefit ratio[19], and has been demonstrated to be effective for treating certain chronic conditions such as osteoarthritis of the knee[20] and back pain.[21]

Biofeedback has been used successfully for numerous types of chronic pain[22] helping to control muscle spasms and tension, while promoting active work of the muscle activation, or control deficits, or by acting on several biopsychosocial elements involved in chronic pain.

Although it is still controversial, depending on what a few well controlled studies have demonstrated, extra-corporal shock therapy can be useful in cases of chronic tendinopathies[23], and several types of devices have been approved in the United States by the Food and Drug Administration for the treatment of epicondylitis and plantar fasciitis.

Certain physical agents are used for their effect on the collagen tissue, particularly ultrasounds, polarized currents such as high-voltage or micro-currents, laser, diathermy and pulsed electromagnetic fields. Several of these techniques have positive effects on human beings for the treatment of delays in the consolidation of bones or chronic wounds. However, they have not yet been proved useful for degenerative or chronic lesions of ligament and tendon tissues in humans. Nevertheless, these techniques seem to be effective for reducing certain signs and symptoms of rheumatoid arthritis.[24, 25, 26, 27, 28] The laser can also play a positive role in the treatment of chronic joint pain if the dosage is adequate[29], or in the cases of capsulitis of the shoulder.[30] Positive effects have also been noted for a pulsed electromagnetic field in cases of osteoarthritis.[31, 32]

# 4. PHYSIOTHERAPY AND MEDICATION

The medications used for chronic pain are divided into three families:

- simple analgesics and non-steroidal anti-inflammatories;
- opioids;
- co-analgesics such as anti-depressants and anti-convulsants.

These medications and their effects are discussed in **Chapter 30**.

## PHYSIOTHERAPY TREATMENTS

The physiological and molecular effects[1, 2, 3] of physiotherapy treatments combine well with medication since they complement or can even replace it occasionally. However, inadvertently, through a lack of knowledge, or as a result of a poor physiotherapeutic diagnosis, a physiotherapy treatment may have effects that are contrary to those of the medication. In a medical context, it is essential for all of the information and therapeutic decisions to be transmitted from one professional to another and, as in any team, the objectives must be reviewed and shared on a regular basis.

When a patient is already taking medication, a physiotherapist must know which medications are being used, and which beneficial or other effects they have on the patient. For example, in the case of a patient receiving effective analgesic medication, I could focus my treatment on the objectives without hindering the analgesic prescribed. However, if the analgesic seems insufficient, I could add physical agents with analgesic impacts to complement the medication.

## SIMPLE ANALGESICS AND NON-STEROIDAL ANTI-INFLAMMATORIES

The means described in **Tables 2** and **3** have demonstrated analgesic and anti-inflammatory effects.[1, 2, 3, 4, 13, 14, 15] The analgesic effects are obtained to a large extent through stimulation of the neural system.

The anti-inflammatory effects are the result of a concrete effect on vascularization. The physical agents can be applied as a complement to or in place of certain medications.

TABLE 2: Physical agents with analgesic effects

| PHYSIOLOGICAL EFFECTS | PHYSICAL AGENTS |
| --- | --- |
| Increase or decrease in the activity of sensitive receptors and nerve depolarization of sensitive fibres by:<br>• Closing of the Melzack Wall gate<br>• Stimulation of Golgi tendon organs<br>• Inhibition of the neuromuscular spindle | Thermotherapy<br>Vibratory stimulations<br>Electric currents such as TENS and other related currents<br>Cryotherapy<br>Endermotherapy |
| Action on the motor unit recruitment:<br>• By nerve depolarization<br>• By reducing pain inhibition<br>• By direct stimulation of the muscle without the intermediary of the motor neuron<br>• Through awareness of the muscular contraction | Low or medium frequency neuromuscular stimulator (ex.: Russian current)<br>Cryotherapy, electro analgesia (ex.: TENS and related techniques)<br>Low frequency muscle stimulator with broad impulse duration<br>Biofeedback |

TABLE 3: Physical agents with anti-inflammatory effects

| PHYSIOLOGICAL EFFECTS | PHYSICAL AGENTS |
| --- | --- |
| Action on cellular metabolism<br>• Increase<br>• Decrease | Thermotherapy<br>Cryotherapy |
| Modification of vascularization by:<br>• Vasodilatation<br>• Vasoconstriction<br>• Increase in circulation back to the heart | Thermotherapy<br>TENS and related currents<br>Cryotherapy<br>Intermittent compression devices Endermotherapy<br>Rhythmic neuromuscular stimulation including slow frequency or pulsed with slow frequency TENS type devices |
| Cutaneous penetration of medication (ex.: dexamethasone, topical NSAID) | Iontophoresis: constant continuous current<br>Phonophoresis: ultrasound |

## OPIOIDS

The means described in **Table 4** have demonstrated opioid effects.[1, 2, 3] The opioid effects are obtained to a large extent by stimulation of the medullary system and the descending inhibition system. These two systems stimulate the production of endorphins and endogenous enkephalin.

When a patient is taking opioid medication that effectively treats his/her pain, the physiotherapist probably does not need to add physical agents of the same type, and in this case, could focus treatment on anti-inflammatory means, or co-analgesia through anti-convulsants. The analgesia obtained could be completed by focusing on another pain mechanism, since the physiotherapist already knows that the effect on the opioid receptors is beneficial. However, if the patient is not taking opioid medication, the physiotherapist could test a physical agent, and determine whether or not it is effective in the treatment of the pain.

TABLE 4: Physical agents with opioid effects

| PHYSIOLOGICAL EFFECTS | PHYSICAL AGENTS |
|---|---|
| Release of neurotransmitters such as endorphins and enkephalin | Cryotherapy and alternating hot and cold baths<br>TENS<br>Extracorporal and radial shocks |

## CO-ANALGESICS SUCH AS ANTI-CONVULSANTS AND ANTI-DEPRESSANTS

### Anti-convulsants .

The means described in **Table 5** have demonstrated anti-convulsant effects.[1, 2, 3] The anti-convulsant effects are obtained to a large extent through a reduction in neural conduction and the sensitivity threshold of pain receptors.

When a patient receives medication from the anti-convulsant family, the physiotherapist probably does not need to add physical agents of the same type. The treatment could be focused on anti-inflammatory or opioid means. The analgesia obtained could be complemented by focusing on another pain mechanism since the physiotherapist already knows that neuron conduction is being treated effectively. However, if the patient is not taking co-analgesic medication for that mechanism, the physiotherapist can test a physical agent, and determine whether or not it treats the pain effectively.

TABLE 5: Physical agents with anti-convulsant effects

| PHYSIOLOGICAL EFFECTS | PHYSICAL AGENTS |
|---|---|
| Decrease in activity of sensitive receptors and nerve depolarization of sensitive fibres by:<br>· Closing of Melzack Wall gate<br>· Stimulation of Golgi tendon organs<br>· Inhibition of neuromuscular spindle | Thermotherapy<br>Electric currents such as TENS and other related currents<br>Cryotherapy |
| Slowing of nerve conduction | Cryotherapy |
| Action on motor unit recruitment by:<br>· Nerve depolarization<br>· Reducing pain inhibition | Low or medium frequency neuromuscular stimulator (ex.: Russian current)<br>Cryotherapy, electroanalgesia<br>(ex. TENS and related techniques) |

## Anti-depressants

Anti-depressants are prescribed to treat pain. The action mechanisms are described in **Chapter 30**. As physiotherapists, we know that physical exercise has an impact on mood and the general perception of well-being. The stimulation of the descending inhibition system, and the release of endorphins and enkephalins are described by all those who take part in intense exercise on a regular basis as giving them a sensation of euphoria.

Patients suffering from chronic pain are, for the most part, generally out of condition. For this reason, the global approach in physiotherapy, like that used in pain clinics, includes a general physical conditioning programme. Following an evaluation of the patient's deficiencies and incapacities, the physiotherapist will start a programme as soon as possible, while respecting the patient's pain and capacities.

In the case of all types of pain, it is important to stimulate the neural system by various influxes from all parts of the body. Several means are available for cardiovascular re-education. By staying or getting back into shape, patients will feel that they still have physical capacities that can improve, and will observe that pain does not limit them in all spheres of their lives.

## 5. CONCLUSION

Patients frequently consult physiotherapists for nociceptive, neuropathic and chronic pain. The therapeutic tools we use to treat pain, in particular physical agents, have effects that are comparable to those of medication. However, as in the case of medication, there are no specific means for the treatment of a specific kind of pain. We must make choices based on scientific evidence, and conduct therapeutic tests. As a professional, I must make constant adjustments in order to obtain relief that is acceptable to the patient. In most cases, the purpose of this relief is to improve quality of life and also to lead to functional re-education that will enable patients to consolidate the physical components of an active and full life.

## REFERENCES

1.  BÉLANGER, AY. Evidence-Based. Guide to Therapeutic Physical Agents. Lippincott Williams & Wilkins, Baltimore, Philadelphie, 2002.
2.  BUSSIÈRES, P, et J. Brual. Les agents physiques en réadaptation : Théorie et pratique. Les Presses de l'Université Laval, Québec, 2001.
3.  KAHN, J. Principles and Practice of Electrotherapy, 4e edition. Elsevier - Health Sciences Division, 2000.
4.  MERRICK, MA. Secondary injury after musculoskeletal trauma: a review and update. J Athl Train, 2002 (37), 209-17.
5.  BLEAKLEY, C, and S. McDonough. The use of ice in the treatment of acute soft-tissue injury. A systematic review of randomized controlled trials. The American Journal of Sports medicine, 2004 (32), 251-61.
6.  MACAULEY, D. Ice therapy: How good is the evidence? Int J Sports Med, 2001 (22), 379-84.
7.  HO, SSW, RL Illgen, RW Meyer, PJ Torok, MD Cooper and B. Reider. Comparison of various icing times in decreasing bone metabolism and blood flow in the knee. Am J Sports Med, 1995 (23), 74-6.
8.  HOPKINS, JT, CD Ingersoll, J. Edwards and TE Klootwyk. Cryotherapy and Transcutaneous Electric Neuromuscular Stimulation Decrease Arthrogenic Muscle Inhibition of the Vastus Medialis after Knee Joint Effusion. J Athl Train, 2002 (37), 25–31.
9.  HUBBARD, TJ, SL Aronson and CR Denegar. Does cryotherapy hasten return to participation? A systematic review. J Athl Train 2004 (39), 88-94.
10. HUBBARD, TJ, CR Denegar. Does cryotherapy improve outcomes with soft tissue injury? J Athl Train, 2004 (39), 278-9.
11. NADLER, SF, DJ Steiner, SR Petty, GN Erasala, DA Hengehold and KW Weingand. Overnight use of continuous low-level heatwrap therapy for relief of low back pain. Arch Phys Med Rehabil 2003(84), 335-42.
12. NADLER, SF, DJ Steiner, G Erasala, DA Hengehold, S Abeln and KW Weingand. Continuous low-level heatwrap therapy for treating acute non-specific low back pain. Arch Phys Med Rehabil, 2003 (84), 329-34.
13. BJORDAL, JM, MI Johnson and AE Ljunggreen. Transcutaneous electrical nerve stimulation (TENS) can reduce postoperative analgesic consumption. A meta-analysis with assessment of optimal treatment parameters for postoperative pain. Eur J Pain, 2003 (7), 181-8.
14. ONCEL, M, S Sencan, H Yildiz, N Kurt. Transcutaneous electrical nerve stimulation for pain management in patients with uncomplicated minor rib fractures. Eur J Card Thor Surg, 2002 (22), 13-7.
15. AVRAMIDIS, K, PW Strike, PN Taylor, ID Swain. Effectiveness of electric stimulation of the vastus medialis muscle in the rehabilitation of patients after total knee arthroplasty. Arch Phys Med Rehabil, 2003 (84), 1850-3.
16. KNIGHT, CA, CR Rutledge, ME Cox, M Acosta and SJ Hall. Effect of superficial heat, deep heat, and active exercise warm-up on the extensibility of the plantar flexors. Phys Ther 2001 (81), 1206-14.
17. PERES, SE, DOP Draper, KL Knight and MD Ricard. Pulsed shortwave diathermy and prolonged long-duration stretching increase dorsiflexion range of motion more than identical stretching without diathermy. J Athl Train, 2002 (37), 43-50.
18. MICHLOVITZ, S, L Hun, GN Erasala, DA Hengehold and KW

Weingand. Continuous low-level heat wrap therapy is effective for treating wrist pain. Arch Phys Med Rehabil, 2004 (85), 1409-16.

19. CHABAL, C, DA Fishbain, M Weaver and LW Heine. Long-term transcutaneous electrical nerve stimulation (TENS) use: Impact on medication utilization and physical therapy costs. Clin J Pain, 1998 (14), 66-73.

20. OSIRI, M, V Welch, L Brosseau, B Shea, J McGowan, P Tugwell, et al. Transcutaneous electrical nerve stimulation for knee osteoarthritis (Review). The Cochrane Database of Systematic Reviews, 2000 (Issue 4).

21. WILSON, I, AS Lowe-Strong and DM Walsh. Evidence for transcutaneous electrical nerve stimulation in the management of low back pain? Phys Ther Rev, 2002 (7), 259-65.

22. PULLIAM, CB and RJ Gatchel. Biofeedback 2003. Its role in pain management. Critical Reviews in Physical and Rehabilitation Medicine, 2003 (15), 65-82.

23. ROMPE, JD, J Decking. Repetitive low-energy shock wave treatment for chronic lateral epicondylitis in tennis players. Am J Sports Med, 2004 (32), 734-43.

24. BROSSEAU, L, V Welch, G Wells, R DeBie, A Gam, K Harman, et al. Low level laser therapy (Classes I, II and III) for treating rheumatoid arthritis. The Cochrane Database of Systematic Reviews, 1998 (Issue 4).

25. CASIMIRO, L, L Brosseau, V Robinson, S Milne, M Judd, G Well, et al. Therapeutic ultrasound for the treatment of rheumatoid arthritis. Cochrane Database Syst Rev, 2002 (Issue 3).

26. Ottawa Panel Evidence-Based Clinical Practice Guidelines for Electrotherapy and Thermotherapy Interventions in the Management of Rheumatoid Arthritis in Adults. Phys Ther, 2004 (84), 1016-43.

27. PELLAND, L, L Brosseau, L Casimiro, V Robinson, P Tugwell and G Wells. Electrical stimulation for the treatment of rheumatoid arthritis (Review). The Cochrane Database of Systematic Reviews, 2002 (Issue 2).

28. BJORDAL, JM, C Couppé, RT Chow, J Tunér, EA Ljunggren. A systematic review of low level laser therapy with location-specific doses for pain from chronic joint disorders. Austr J Physioth, 2003 (49), 107-16.

29. GREEN, S, R Buchbinder, S Hetrick. Physiotherapy interventions for shoulder pain (Review). The Cochrane Database of Systematic Reviews, 2003 (Issue 2).

30. Agence d'évaluation des technologies et des modes d'interventions en santé (AÉTMIS). Thérapie du signal pulsé et traitement de l'ostéoarthrite. Rapport préparé par Alicia Framarin. (AÉTMIS 01-02 RF). Montréal, AÉTMIS 2001 : xiii-33 p.

31. HULME, J, V Robinson, R DeBie, G Wells, M Judd, P Tugwell. Electromagnetic fields for the treatment of osteoarthritis. The Cochrane Database of Systematic Reviews, 2002 (Issue 1).

32. MAJLESI, J, H Ünalan. High-power pain threshold ultrasound technique in the treatment of active myofascial triggers points: A randomized, double-blind, case-control study. Arch Phys Med Rehabil, 2004 (85), 833-6.

# MORRIS' STORY

**Morris K.,** Montreal, Quebec, Canada

(See other testimonials, pages 100, 246, 310, 372 and 382.)

*Morris survived a plane crash, and recuperated from a broken jaw and ankle, as well as fractures to the spine*

### We must do a lot to help ourselves.

During my recovery period, I continually asked questions of the doctors at the hospital clinic about new pains that I was feeling, but I rarely got answers. I started keeping notes as I found that once it was on paper I could focus my mind toward positive things, and not drown in the swamp of unanswered negativity.

I got on a merry-go-round for the next few years, going from doctor to doctor in search of answers. I saw neurologists, neurosurgeons, orthopaedists, surgeons, specialists in everything and anything. Most were reluctant to give a diagnosis. Some surgeons said that they could not promise to make it better, but it could become worse.

I had countless pages of unanswered questions. I learned to listen to my body and while all the actions I took were not necessarily recommended, they worked for me. I created strategies from my imagination, using logic or what was logical to me, and it got me through many years. It also took me through many years while I learned that the vast majority of medical doctors do not know what to do to help patients with chronic pain. Keeping a positive attitude does wonders.

One day in a casual conversation somewhere, 18 years after the plane crash, I heard about a pain clinic. **At my first appointment, I was astounded as I finally met a doctor who understood pain,** a doctor who I thought was nearly feeling my pain, a doctor who told me that pain is an illness. I did not know that doctors who understood pain like this doctor did even existed. Pain was **especially** not seen as an illness by doctors other than those who are pain specialists. What an eye-opener this was! I had just come through 18 years of banging my head against walls and doctors' doors, on the road to nowhere. That's 18 years in a very dark tunnel, losing hope of ever finding help to deal with these pains. Pain was just not an illness that doctors in general knew how to treat.

A plan of action was made, and explained to me by the doctor. We started with certain medications, and I gave feedback on their effectiveness. The doctor would decide on the next step. We only made one change at a time, giving me sufficient time to evaluate the latest change. Over time, we went from changes in medications to adding minimally invasive non-surgical treatments and procedures. We maintained the medications that were on record at that time, always evaluating for the desired benefits. Everything is a trial, but we keep on going. I have noted some pain relief, but we are trying for more.

My own strategy was to go day by day always keeping a positive attitude. I feel that it is most important to maintain this positive attitude. Any step forward was a positive achievement. I approach any new procedure in the same way. It will be successful. Other than that, I do not think about it consciously. That is my way of avoiding a negative disappointment. Rule number one is to listen to my body. Rule number two is never forget rule number one.

# OCCUPATIONAL THERAPY
## AND CHRONIC PAIN

Lucie Bouvrette-Leblanc, BSc OT, MAP (candidate), Montreal, Quebec, Canada

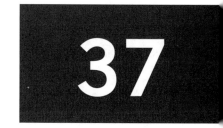

**37**

## ABSTRACT

Occupational therapists are health professionals. They may work in several health sectors with people of all ages. Chronic pain is one area in which occupational therapists work.

This chapter provides a brief explanation of occupational therapy, and describes some of the interventions occupational therapists undertake with respect to people with chronic pain.

**This chapter is intended to be informative. Anyone who wants to integrate these principles, in part or in full, should first be evaluated by an occupational therapist, or consult a physician, and follow their recommendations.**

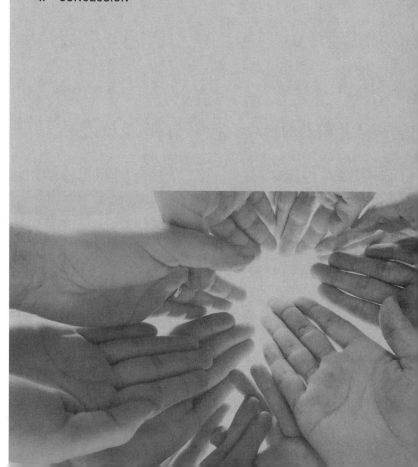

# 1. INTRODUCTION

Occupational therapists are health professionals. They have the opportunity to work with children, adults and the elderly in the field of physical and/or mental health. They work to promote health, prevent deficiencies, and promote the autonomy and social integration of individuals as they take part in their tasks, activities and significant occupations. Occupational therapy came into being particularly after the two world wars (Friedland & al 2000). Soldiers returning from the battlefield with physical injuries or mental health problems had to learn to live with their new condition. Occupational therapists helped these soldiers regain a certain amount of autonomy and quality of life.

# 2. CHRONIC PAIN AND OCCUPATIONAL THERAPY

In terms of chronic pain, the occupational therapist helps individuals suffering from chronic pain maintain or develop their functional capacity in terms of their daily activities and tasks, such as personal hygiene, leisure activities and productive activities (school, work, volunteer work, household chores, etc.), and improve their quality of life. The occupational therapist assesses and treats those suffering from chronic pain, regardless of where the pain occurs.

Several interventions in occupational therapy will focus on the principles of the self-management of chronic pain. These include, for example, the principles of energy conservation, body mechanics, good posture, good sleep habits, relaxation techniques, and many others. This is done while taking into account the individual's living environment. As needed, the occupational therapist will evaluate the possibility of modifying the individual's physical environment so as to facilitate a return to work or the performance of daily activities.

When the pain interferes with the individual's ability to perform certain daily activities, he/she is often referred to an occupational therapist. Nevertheless, the various administrative and government levels in the health care system are increasingly working on preventing the chronicity of pain. For example, referring the individual with a painful condition to occupational therapy or other disciplines before the pain becomes chronic, in order to reduce the rate of disability, as well as the loss of productivity and autonomy in the performance of daily activities.

The following points will cover certain principles concerning the self-management of chronic pain. It should be noted that, while the occupational therapist accompanies the individual who is suffering from chronic pain throughout the rehabilitation process, the occupational therapist is not the captain of the ship; the patient is. The occupational therapist can give the patient tools, but the individual is responsible for using them, and integrating them in his/her life. Moreover, the focus of chronic pain treatments is not on treating the pain, but on self-managing chronic pain and improving functional capacities and quality of life.

## EDUCATION ON THE CONDITION

In order to promote the activity participation of the individual, he/she must understand what chronic pain is in terms of his/her condition, and what the intervention plan will involve in terms of occupational therapy as part of a multidisciplinary team.

## THE PRINCIPLES OF ENERGY CONSERVATION

There are four principles of energy conservation: planning, prioritization, pacing and posture. One tool that is essential for the first three principles is the use of an agenda.

### Planning

Planning involves planning the activities of the day, the week and the month. This involves the notion of time. When an activity is planned, it is important to evaluate the various aspects of the plan: who, what, where, when, how and how much.

**Who** are you going to delegate the task to, are you going to do it with someone else, or on your own...
**What** do you need to complete the activity?
**Where** are you going to do this activity?
**When** are you going to do this activity?

**How** are you going to do this activity? Are there parts of this activity that can be eliminated? Can the activity be simplified? Can the sequence of the tasks to be completed, be re-arranged in order to simplify the activity?
**How much** time do you think it will take to complete the activity?

- Here are some examples of ways in which to save energy.
- You're doing the laundry. Do you really need to put all of the clothes for the family away, or can each member of the family put their own clothes away? e.g. The clothing can be placed on the bed of each family member.
- You are making a meal. Prepare all of the ingredients and dishes/utensils before starting.
- You can use frozen food to make the job easier.
- When you cook, you can make a larger quantity, and freeze the rest.

- You can place a basket on a piece of furniture at the top or bottom of the stairs, and place objects that have to be carried up or down in it. You or a family member going up or down the stairs can either carry the basket or a few objects. In this way you avoid having to go up and down the stairs repeatedly. If you can't carry certain objects up or down the stairs, don't hesitate to ask for help.
- Plan enough time to perform the task. Doing a task in a rush takes more energy.

It is also important to balance work and household chores, rest and leisure activities. Often leisure activities and time for yourself are the first aspects to be neglected. Balancing these three elements enables you to manage your level of energy better.

To ensure this balance, it is important that you plan an interesting activity every day and set aside time for unexpected events. One aspect to consider is to start by noting appointments and activities that absolutely must take on a give day at a specific time, before planning the rest of your schedule.

Moreover, clients suffering from chronic pain often report that they have days when they feel that they have more energy than they usually do. They get up one morning feeling full of energy. So they set out to complete their tasks one after another. Finally, the next day or the day after that, they feel drained of energy. They stay in bed or rest until they feel that they once again have the energy they need for their activities. Then, they experience another burst of energy and the situation is repeated all over again. In keeping with the principles for conserving energy, you have to be able to plan your activities day by day in order to avoid these large fluctuations in energy.

One way in which to evaluate how you use your energy throughout the day and the week is to use an agenda that includes the seven days of the week and the hours in each day. For each day, you write down the activities completed in the day. Then you can use three highlighters, one pink, one yellow and one green. You can use the pink to highlight the activities that require more energy, the yellow for those that require an average amount of energy and the green for the activities that require little energy. Then look at your week, and evaluate the distribution of the colours over the course of the week. If one day is mostly pink, and the following days are mostly green because you had no energy left, it might be beneficial to re-distribute some tasks from one day to another, so as to have each of the three colours for each day.

Moreover, if you feel like you're running for a good part of the day, but at the end of the day you feel as if you've accomplished almost nothing, you can write a list of the tasks you completed during the day, or a list of the things you have to do, and then cross them off as soon as they have been completed. This gives certain people a sense of accomplishment.

Several people wonder how they can plan their schedule when they don't know how they will feel on any given day. Don't forget that your plan must be flexible. If you had planned to do the grocery shopping one day, and then you don't feel as if you have the necessary energy, you can always do a task that requires less energy, such as a load of laundry, and postpone the grocery shopping to the next day. You must, however, do an activity, and not postpone all the activities. Otherwise you will feel overwhelmed by the list of things to do.

### Prioritization

Prioritization can also be done on a daily, weekly and monthly basis. This involves making a list of the tasks to be completed in order of importance (prioritize). It is also important to determine whether the tasks are obligatory, and if they can be reduced, eliminated or delegated to others. Moreover, if it is financially possible for you to hire people to provide certain services, such as housekeeping, snow removal and lawn care, etc., this will help you conserve energy for other activities.

### Pacing

In order to conserve your energy, it is preferable to take a break before you get tired. An activity can also be divided into several parts so that you can take breaks. For example:

- When you do the dishes, you can leave the pots soaking in soapy water. If you want to watch television, you can use the commercial breaks to wash the pots, and let them dry until the next commercial break, etc.;
- You can also clean one room in the house, condo or apartment and take a break before cleaning another room. It is important to take breaks before you start feeling tired;
- You can also use a timer to remind you to take breaks. For example, if you are working on the computer, you can set the timer to ensure you take a break when you need to, but you must take at least one break per hour, and do a few stretching exercises.

Moreover, taking a break does not necessarily mean stopping all activity and going to lie down, relax or even watch television. It also involves changing the type of activity in order to give your musculoskeletal system time to rest. For example, if you are doing a standing activity, you can, after a certain amount of time, continue that activity, or do another one while sitting. It is important to vary your activities so that you don't do the same activity, in the same manner, for a long period of time.

## Posture

Posture is another principle for conserving energy. First, performing a task while sitting instead of standing requires much less energy. Nevertheless, regardless of whether you are sitting or standing, postural alignment is important in order to conserve your energy. If, for example, an individual is seated with his/her back hunched over forward, and his/her head tilted forward, gravity will exert force on the person's head, and it will take more energy for the back muscles to maintain that position than if he/she were seated with a good postural alignment. When the head is aligned with the trunk, it takes less energy to maintain that position.

## POSTURAL HYGIENE

Postural hygiene is one of the essential principles for conserving energy. This refers to the standing, lying or sitting position in which the muscles and ligaments supporting the posture exert the least tension and effort.

Postural alignment serves to:
- Keep the bones and joints aligned so as to use the muscles as efficiently as possible;
- Prevent the abnormal wear of joint bones;
- Reduce stress on the ligaments;
- reduce back and joint stress;
- prevent fatigue/conserve energy;
- manage pain.

(Source: Cleveland Clinic)

Postural hygiene is based on individual needs. If, for example, an individual has a kyphotic posture and osteoarthritis of the spine, recommendations will be made in keeping with his/her condition to satisfy particular needs. Something that satisfies the needs of one individual may not satisfy the needs of another. For this reason, it is important for each individual to be assessed by an occupational therapist before making changes to his/her posture or workstation. **The following principles are general, and should not be applied before an occupational therapist has made an evaluation.**

Postural alignment requires:
- Flexibility;
- Muscular strength;
- Balance in the muscular strength of the agonist and antagonist muscles;
- Perception and awareness of current posture so that it can be improved;
- Knowledge of postural hygiene.

(Source: Cleveland Clinic)

A lack of flexibility, muscular strength or balance in the muscular strength of the agonist and antagonist muscles will influence posture.

### Posture when standing

- The ear lobes should be aligned with the centre of the shoulders.
- The spine should be straight or, in other words, it should not be tilted left, right, forward or backward, and the natural spinal curves, cervical, thoracic and lumbar, should be maintained.
- Imagine a thread attached to the top of your head, pulling your head toward the ceiling.
- Contract your abdominal muscles slightly so as to keep from tilting your pelvis too far forward or backward.
- Feet should be separated by a distance slightly less than the width of your shoulders.
- Knees should be slightly bent.
- Wear shoes with arch support, without high heels.
- It is important to balance the weight of your body evenly between your two legs or to shift your weight from one leg to the other (right–left) either from side to side or forward-backward while maintaining a certain amount of weight on both feet.

(Source: Cleveland Clinic)

### Posture in the kitchen

When standing in the kitchen, some clients will open a cupboard under the counter in order to place a foot on the edge of the cupboard, and then change feet. This shifts the load from one leg to the other and helps maintain body alignment. You must, however, take care not to bump into the open cupboard door.

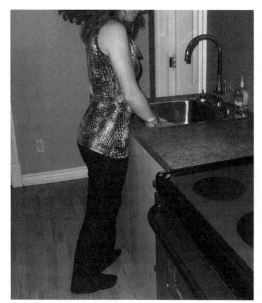

No postural alignment

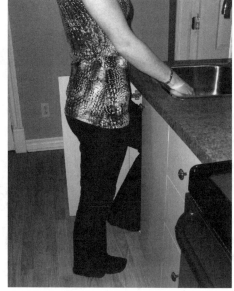

Postural alignment

You can place a reminder on your kitchen counter, such as a ribbon on the soap dish, to remind you to use a proper posture.

## Posture when sitting

The first part of the body to be positioned is the pelvis. If the pelvis is tilted too far forward or backward, this will influence the position of your trunk, and your head and can affect the movement of your shoulder joints.

Therefore, it is important to have support for your lower back so that you can maintain the lumbar curve, and promote better postural alignment. You can use a lumbar cushion, or roll up a towel, and use it as a lumbar support. Furthermore, if you are sitting in a chair without any armrests, for example in a waiting room, you can use your coat or purse to support your arms.

## Posture when sitting at the computer

The primary objective of ergonomics is to facilitate work and ensure the safety of the client's workstation. Although there are general principles of ergonomics, the workstation must be adapted to the physiological and psychological characteristics, anthropometric measurements, as well as the worker's capacities and needs.

Ergonomics is based on needs. Something that may satisfy the needs of one individual may not satisfy those of another. For this reason, it is important for each person to be assessed by an occupational therapist before making changes to his/her posture or workstation. **The following principles are general and should not be applied before an occupational therapist has made an evaluation.**

At work or at home, when you are seated at a computer, you should have an ergonomic chair:
· With 5 wheels;
· Adjustable height;
· With lumbar support in the back;
· The back must be adjustable in terms of height so that the height of the lumbar support can be adjusted;
· Armrests that can be adjusted in terms of height. If necessary, armrests that can be adjusted in terms of width so as to increase or reduce the space between the two arm rests so that they are not too close to or too far from your body.

## To adjust the chair
· Adjust the height of the back, so as to provide support for your lumbar curve.
· The space between the back of your knee and the seat should be equivalent to 2 or 3 finger width, so as to prevent creating pressure at the back of the knees, and to support the thighs.
· When you are seated, your hips should be at a 90-degree angle, with the possibility up to 110 degrees.
· The knees should be bent at an angle between 90 and 130 degrees.
· The height of the armrests should support your arms when your elbows are bent at a 90-degree angle.
· When you relax your arms at each side of your body, your armrests should be positioned under your forearms. Otherwise, you will have to adjust the distance between your armrests.
· Following this, position your chair in front of your computer, and adjust the height so that your hands are at the same level as your keyboard. If your feet do not touch the ground, you will have to use a footrest, while maintaining the angle of your hips.

## To adjust the height of your screen
· The top of the screen should be at the level of your eyes when you look straight ahead.
· When you relax your eyes, you will automatically be looking in the centre of the screen.
· However, if you wear bifocals, the screen should be somewhat lower.
· If you use a laptop computer, you can place your computer on a support specifically designed for that type of computer in order to raise the computer, and position the screen appropriately. You can also add an external keyboard and a wireless mouse. This will enable you to adopt a position that is more adequate.

This represents only few elements related to ergonomics. Computer ergonomics includes many other aspects.

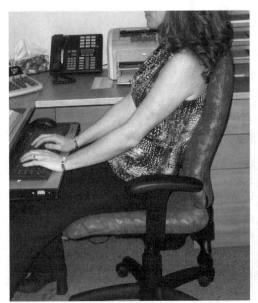

No postural alignment

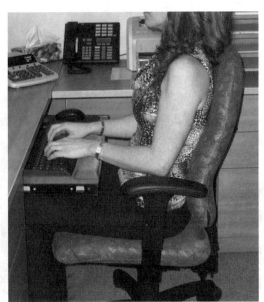

Postural alignment

## Posture when lying down

In order to facilitate sleep, it is important that you have an adequate posture. First, a cervical pillow will help maintain the alignment of your spine at your neck. Choosing a pillow is very personal. A latex pillow may please one person, while another may prefer a contour foam pillow.

Often, cervical pillows have a higher curve on one side of the pillow. This is intended to satisfy individual needs. If you are a small individual with a less pronounced cervical curve, you will probably use the side of the pillow with the smallest curve. If you are a large individual, and your cervical curve is more pronounced, you will probably use the side of the pillow with the highest curve, so as to obtain the necessary support. Moreover, if you sleep on your side, you will probably need to use the side of the pillow with the highest curve.

If you have lumbar spine problems, it is important to support it in order to decrease the muscular-skeletal tension. To do this, place a pillow under your knees when you are lying on your back. If you have pain in your shoulders, you can also place pillows under your arms when you are lying on your back. When lying on your side, you can use a body pillow to support your arm and your leg. This will prevent the rotation of your spinal column, and support your arm, as needed. Your arm that is not on the mattress will be supported by the body pillow and the arm that is in contact with the mattress should not be placed under your head. Nevertheless, you can place the pillow in front of your head.

It is preferable, if possible, to avoid sleeping on your stomach since this position causes a lot of tension in the spinal column (neck and back).

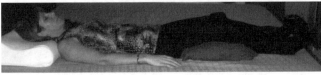

On your back

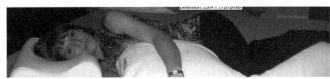

On your side

## SLEEP HYGIENE

Sleep is an essential need. It is not only a passive phase, but one in which tissues are repaired, learning is consolidated, emotions are cleaned up, stress is released, the immune system is activated, and many other important events take place.

Chronic pain interferes with sleep quality. When sleep does not restore you as much as it should, mood and cognitive functions such as attention and concentration can be affected. Certain means can help improve sleep. These means will be divided into two types: modifications of behaviours and modifications to the environment, so as to improve sleep.

**There are different means to modify behaviours in order to improve sleep, for example:**

· Develop a sleep routine. For example, complete your personal hygiene, take a bath, and/or use a relaxing technique;
· Go to bed every night at the same time, even on weekends;
· Don't drink coffee, use stimulants or drink alcohol in the evening;
· Do some low intensity aerobic exercises, but not during the evening;
· Manage stress and its hassles before you do your sleep routine;
· Use relaxation techniques when going to bed;
· Do not eat a large meal at night;
· Do not take naps lasting more than 20 to 30 minutes, unless you have to drive, and need more sleep.

**There are different means to modify the environment in order to improve sleep, for example:**

• Your bedroom should be a peaceful place, for intimacy, resting and sleeping;
• Never put your office in your bedroom. Your bedroom is the place where you relax;
• Do not have a television in the bedroom. The light produced by a television reduces the level of melatonin. Melatonin is a hormone produced by the pineal gland when it is dark and promotes sleep;
• Place a glass of water on your bedside table so you don't have to get up if you get thirsty;
• Put a pencil and paper on your night table. If you think of something that you're worried you might forget, write it down in order to relieve your fear that you won't remember it the next day;
• Keep the bedroom dark, neither too hot nor too cold;
• Light blankets – a goose down duvet is often appreciated;
• A mattress that is neither too firm nor too soft.

## RELAXATION TECHNIQUES

There are several relaxation techniques: Jacobson, visualization, Schultz… Nevertheless, don't forget the personal techniques that each individual uses to manage his/her own stress. For some people, this will involve listening to music, taking a walk in the woods, going to see a movie, talking on the telephone with a friend, or taking a candlelit bath. Most of the time, these means are set aside and attention is paid to the list of things to do. Don't forget that, in order to conserve your energy, work, leisure activities and rest must be in balance.

In order to relax, you can place a list of personal techniques on the refrigerator so that you will not forget to take time for yourself and to relax. Relaxation helps with the management of pain.

foot will stay on the ground while you will raise your left leg backward, and bend your hip and knee slightly to pick up an object from the floor, using your right hand. The individual can also sit on a chair, and bend from the hips while keeping his/her back straight. Finally there is also the skier technique: move your buttocks backward to maintain your lumbar curve, bend your knees slightly, and bend at the hip level in order to bend forward to pick up an object from the floor.

## BODY MECHANICS

Body mechanics refers to the movement of the body when performing daily activities. Here are some principles of body mechanics:

### Pushing instead of pulling
One of the principles of body mechanics involves pushing instead of pulling when moving an object so that it slides or rolls (ex.: pushing on a cart instead of pulling it).

### Picking up an object from a position below knee level
Another principle of body mechanics involves keeping the back straight and bending the knees when picking up an object from below knee level. Nevertheless, if the individual experiences knee pain, or is unable to perform these movements, the occupational therapist should consider other possibilities. If the object is light, and the individual has no problems with blood pressure or balance, the golfer technique is also another possibility. To perform the golfer technique, the individual should hold on to a stable piece of furniture with one hand. For example, if you hold on to the stable piece of furniture with your left hand, your right

### Avoid combining certain movement when completing daily activities
Several individuals use inadequate movements (flexion, rotation and extension) of the back when completing daily activities. A movement that combines bending with twisting may be harmful for the back. As a result, the individual must re-learn to move, using adequate body mechanics while performing his/her activities, so as to prevent further injury and manage pain. The individual must first develop an awareness of his/her body mechanics and posture in order to be able to correct them.

### Completing daily activities

The occupational therapist also works with individuals suffering from chronic pain who have lost part of their independence in completing daily activities. Therapists work with their patients to improve their level of autonomy and productivity while using the principles of body mechanics, good posture, sleep hygiene, means of compensation, technical aids if needed, and re-activation.

## REACTIVATION AND RETURNING TO WORK

Reactivation is an integral part of interventions in occupational therapy. Most of the time, those who suffer from chronic pain react by minimizing their activities. This leads to deconditioning. As a result of deconditioning, the individual tires more quickly. Deconditioning and fatigue affect the individual's productivity, and his/her psychological state. Everything increases the level of stress which in turn increases muscular tension, and consequently increases the level of pain and sleeping disorders. This vicious circle continues to spin until changes are made to the situation in order to break this vicious circle of pain.

Reactivation is an important element in breaking the vicious circle of pain, and managing the symptoms of chronic pain. Low intensity aerobic exercise helps to manage pain, and improves productivity, sleep quality, muscular strength, flexibility, cardiovascular capacity and well-being. Moreover, by facilitating deep sleep, it also encourages tissue repair.

Several people suffering from chronic pain take walks or swim as a low intensity aerobic activity. Nevertheless, any activity that is not contraindicated can be used. The important thing is that you enjoy doing the activity.

Reactivation, however, does not just involve exercise. Reactivation can be undertaken in order to return to work, or to improve an individual's capacities and endurance for performing daily activities. One of the means used in occupational therapy involves establishing periodic objectives. Working together with the person, this may entail preparing a daily schedule with daily and weekly objectives. For example, an individual may have to get up at 7:00 a.m. every day as if he/she were going to work, and take part in activities that simulate a portion of his/her work, or simpler tasks that require less energy. This will help him/her progress towards more demanding tasks, and tasks that require more time, in order to take part in simulations that are similar to the current tasks and activities in his/her work environment. It is important to engage in reactivation one step at a time in order for the body to gradually get used to the activities. Furthermore, the individual should complete activities on a daily basis in order to get back into condition.

## DISCHARGE AND FOLLOW-UP

Following discharge from occupational therapy services, the individual will have to continue incorporating the various tools learned throughout the services provided. As needed, the individual may contact the occupational therapist for follow-up if he/she has questions or needs to review certain exercise or other programmes, or if the clinician needs to see the individual in follow-up for a specific reason.

## 3. CASE HISTORY – MS. LEDUC

Ms. Leduc is 42 years old and has been diagnosed with fibromyalgia. She was diagnosed 9 months ago. She lives with her husband and two children, Gabrielle (12 years old) and Simon (16 years old). She has been off work for two months. She used to work four days a week as a speech therapist in a hospital. She adores her work and wants to return to it, but she is experiencing difficulty managing her symptoms. Her principle symptoms include: pain, fatigue and sleeping problems.

Ms. Leduc has received multidisciplinary rehabilitation services. These services focused on education, reactivation, and returning to work. With respect to education, she received information about what fibromyalgia is, stress management, sleep hygiene, energy conservation principles, postural hygiene, ergonomics at work, and the community resources she can use to continue to do low-intensity aerobic exercises in order to maintain the progress she made after being discharged. She also received information about and now practices various relaxation techniques. In addition to receiving information about sleep hygiene, the principles of energy conservation and postural hygiene, Ms. Leduc practised, took part in simulations, and integrated some of these principles into her daily activities.

In order to improve her sleep, Ms. Leduc changed her sleep routine. She now goes to bed at 10:00 p.m. every night. Forty-five minutes before going to bed, she completes her personnel care routine and uses a relaxation technique. She has reported that the quality of her sleep improves when she relaxes by taking a bath, or using a relaxation technique through visualization. Moreover, she now manages her concerns and schedule at the end of the day, and not when she goes to bed. She also reorganized her bedroom, so as to make it into an oasis of relaxation and intimacy, and has removed the television from it.

Moreover, in terms of posture hygiene, Ms. Leduc now uses a cervical pillow, and a body pillow to maintain her postural alignment when she goes to bed.

Doing low-intensity aerobic exercises for 45 minutes three times a week has also improved the quality of her sleep. She joined a group of people with fibromyalgia to do low-intensity aerobic exercises once per week, and walks outdoors or in a shopping mall once per week. She also swims once per week. She reports that she has more endurance since she has been doing exercise.

When she works in the kitchen, she now places one foot on the lower edge of the lower cupboard, so as to maintain her postural alignment. She also uses an anti-skid pad to keep the mixing bowls in place when she cooks. She has also integrated the principles of body mechanics into her daily activities.

Reactivation and preparation for a progressive return to work were also included in the treatments that Ms. Leduc received. Her workstation was also assessed in order to evaluate and recommend environmental recommendations, and equipment that will facilitate her return to work.

With respect to work, she also integrated ergonomic principles, and her work area has been modified to respond to her needs. Ms. Leduc was fearful about returning to work, but returned to her functions progressively. She now works four days per week, and has reported improvements in the quality of her personal, family and professional life.

# 4. CONCLUSION

Occupational therapists help people suffering from chronic pain improve their ability to manage their condition, as well as their level of autonomy and productivity. Occupational therapy also promotes the reintegration of people in society, their leisure activities and their occupations, so as to improve their quality of life, and enable them to become active members of society.

# REFERENCES

- Ask Dr. Weil, Polaris Health (Ed). Health Conditions – Insomnia Treatment, DrWeil.com. [Consulté le 03 janvier 2010]. http://www.drweil.com
- Canadien Association of Occupational Therapy [Consulté le 31 décembre 2009]. http://www.caot.ca/default.asp?ChangeID=279&pageID=286&francais=1
- Cleveland Clinic, [Consulté le 02 janvier 2010]. http://my.clevelandclinic.org/spine/posture.aspx
- Friedland, J.; I. Robinson & T. Cardwell (2001). L'histoire de l'ACE de 1926 à 1939, Actualités ergothérapiques, Vol. 3, No. 1. http://www.caot.ca/otnow/jan01-fr/jan01-history.cfm
- Montreuil, S. & A. Lajoie (2008). Ergonomie : travail de bureau avec écran de visualisation: guide de formation, 4e édition, 1-76.
- Passeport santé, [Consulté le 03 janvier 2010]. http://www.passeportsante.net/fr/Maux/Problemes/Fiche.aspx?doc=insomnie_pm
- Travail Sécuritaire Nouveau Brunswick. (2010). Guide d'ergonomie travail de bureau Guide pour la prévention des lésions musculo-squelettiques, Travail sécuritaire NB, 1-16.

# MORRIS' STORY

**Morris K.,** Montreal, Quebec, Canada

(See other testimonials, pages 100, 246, 300, 372 and 382.)

*Morris survived a plane crash, and recuperated from a broken jaw and ankle, as well as fractures to the spine.*

As I recovered, we noticed that we had lost some friends because they could not cope mentally with my tragedy. This is not what good friends are made of. Other supposed reasons may be that I had to adapt to a major change in my way of living; for example, no more movies as I can't sit on the soft cushy seats in the theatre. I still avoid crowds as being pushed or jostled could bring on trauma. Just the physical tension of walking through a crowd makes it not worth the price, no matter how big the star or show. I am always on guard as I approach someone or as someone comes over to say hello. A friendly hello slap on the back or shoulder usually brings on major trauma, and I found that I could not depend on people to remember. This new way of living may have helped shed some old friendships. On looking back, we see that none of our friends from before the accident are counted among our current friends.

**Doors closed and new doors opened**. Most important was getting on with life! That meant doing the things and going to the places that felt most comfortable for me.

Fortunately for me, my best friend — my wife — is always there for me. In my new life, we have made a whole new set of friends who accept me with my limitations as they are.

# ACUPUNCTURE AND
## CHRONIC PAIN

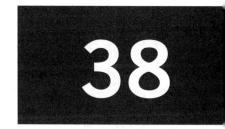

**38**

Sylvain Cardinal Ac, Rimouski, Quebec, Canada, for the Ordre des acuponcteurs du Québec

## ABSTRACT

Instinctively, we mistrust anything that stings. As a result, in nature, the attack of a wasp that has been interrupted in its work, or a brutal encounter with a thorny bush, can be more or less traumatizing moments for us.

From this point of view, acupuncture appears unsettling. How could it possibly relieve pain and even heal? **How is it even possible to think, if our minds push that line of thought a little further, that a beneficial effect can be obtained with simple needles that contain no medication?**

Yet, acupuncture derives its strength from this very characteristic. When inserted judiciously and at strategic places, these slender needles can have profound and lasting effects on the nervous system and the musculoskeletal framework, among other things.

Based on recent studies, neurophysiology attempts to explain the effects of this thousand-year-old therapy, by demonstrating that it could act by energizing the pain control paths, stimulate tissue repair, and re-establish a balance in the central nervous system.

The notions used in traditional acupuncture, which seemed unsettling or mysterious to our Western frame of mind, until recently, are now being explained progressively by contemporary physiology. Concepts such as the *QI*, the meridians, the *yin* and the *yang* reveal valuable notions that enable the acupuncturist to determine an optimal treatment.

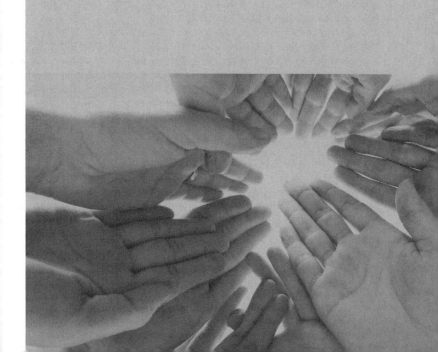

# 1. THE MEDICAL WORLD REDISCOVERS ACUPUNCTURE

With respect to the treatment of numerous painful syndromes that include a muscular component, the medical world first determined, through clinical experiments that were repeated many times, that myofascial pain[1] could be treated effectively by injecting local anaesthetics at the trigger points associated with that pain.

Then, several injectable solutions were tested in order to determine which pharmacological agent was the most effective. Following this, researchers were surprised to note that a simple saline solution – water and salt – was almost as effective as most of the pharmacological agents studied.[2]

The conclusion was obvious: the nature of the solution injected has no therapeutic effect; however, it is the pricking of the precise trigger point associated with this pain that determines the clinical result.

**In other words, medical research had just "rediscovered" the use of the needle in the treatment of myofascial pain, something acupuncture had been practising for a long time.**

According to traditional Chinese thinking, in fact, an obstruction of the circulation of the *QI* and the blood results in points that are painful upon palpation, namely the trigger points of modern medicine and that pricking these *ahshi* points is one means of treating musculoskeletal pain.

As a result, the medical world rediscovered, in its own manner, what clinical studies involving large groups of patients have demonstrated, namely that acupuncture is effective for relieving chronic musculoskeletal pain.[3]

# 2. THE MERIDIANS OF ACUPUNCTURE AND TREATING THE PAINFUL ZONE FROM A DISTANCE

Let us suppose that a patient suffering from headaches consults an acupuncturist for the first time. Not knowing quite what to expect, he/she will be quite surprised to note that the therapist starts the treatment by inserting a needle in the patient's foot! Has the therapist confused one patient with another? No, of course not. The acupuncturist is simply using a strategy that the medical world tries to explain by the paths for controlling pain, among other things. In other words, the new stimulation – caused by the needle – will somehow attract the attention of the central nervous system, and inhibit the painful signal from the mind. This analgesic effect involves various structures of the spinal cord and the brain that specialize in the processing of nociceptive signals[4]. The descending inhibition systems – that is what these nervous signals are called since they travel down the spinal cord – operate automatically, without our conscious involvement. These nervous fluxes will block the pain messages at the gate or, in other words, the entrance for the sensitive influxes of the spinal cord. In acupuncture, the energy currents or meridians remind the practitioner about the effective points for relieving pain, depending on its location. It is through these points that the descending inhibition systems can be triggered, or at least accentuated, even if the points chosen are located at a distance from the painful zone. **It should be noted that the effect occurs progressively from one treatment to another – we refer to this as a cumulative effect – which explains why several treatments are needed to produce an optimal effect[5].**

# 3. DE-ACTIVATING THE LIMBIC SYSTEM AND THE ARRIVAL OF THE *QI*

In the case of chronic pain for which the source cannot be eliminated, acupuncture helps reduce the suffering caused by the individual's injury. Occasionally, the pain experienced is not very intense, but it is no less uncomfortable, particularly if it lasts for a long time; this pain has an emotional component. In fact, if pain were not uncomfortable, we would not be determined to act to avoid it. Certain cerebral structures located in the limbic system come into play in the emotional component of pain; they are particularly active when an individual is suffering. Cerebral imaging has demonstrated that acupuncture treatments can deactivate the limbic system responsible for the uncomfortable aspect of pain.[6] Stimulating a certain type of nervous fibres – the A-delta fibres – can inhibit the limbic system and it has been observed that the acupuncture needles specifically stimulate these fibres. Where each needle is inserted, the patient will experience tingling, heaviness or numbness, all sensations which are characteristic of A-delta fibre stimulation, which is referred to as the arrival of the *QI* in acupuncture.

The practitioner can modulate pain by adjusting the needles meticulously in order to obtain these sensations. The arrival of the *QI* is often the sign that indicates an effective treatment.

# 4. ENERGY RE-EQUILIBRATION

One of the principal changes that the patient experiences after an acupuncture treatment is **a profound sensation of well-being**, which occurs as a result of the re-equilibration of the energy forces referred to as *yin* and *yang*. Some people compare this state of serenity to the sense of internal peace experienced during meditation. These observations highlight the regulating effect that acupuncture has on the psychological state, which is influenced by the state of the central nervous system. Laboratory studies tend to support these clinical observations. They suggest that acupuncture acts on the hypothalamus, which acts as an orchestra conductor for the regulatory activities of the central nervous system[7].

**Treat the patient and not the disease – this is the philosophy behind acupuncture. The practitioner examines the patient's symptoms as a whole, and not just the injury that originally caused the pain. The subsequent treatment is intended to re-create the energy balance the person needs for good health, an effect that translates into a sense of well-being associated with the treatment.**

The acupuncturist can use several treatment strategies to relieve the individual's suffering. For this reason, two patients with apparently identical problems may receive very different treatments.

# 6. THE EFFECTIVENESS OF ACUPUNCTURE TESTED BY THE GERMAN INSURANCE COMPANY STUDIES (GERAC)

At the beginning of this new millennium, several German insurance companies joined forces to sponsor clinical studies intended to verify the effectiveness and safety of acupuncture to treat various painful conditions. The effectiveness of acupuncture was even compared with the best traditional care available. These clinical studies, called GERAC, examined large numbers of patients, and focused on three painful syndromes: migraines[8], chronic back pain[9] and knee osteoarthritis[10].

Their conclusions can be summed up as follows:
- Acupuncture is equivalent to the best traditional medical treatments for preventing migraines;
- Acupuncture is superior to the best traditional medical treatments for chronic back pain and knee osteoarthritis.

# 7. A FEW PRACTICAL CONSIDERATIONS

The acupuncture needles are sterile, and used only once. They are generally inserted without causing any pain although the individual might feel a slight sting following by numbness, tingling or heaviness, sensations which the acupuncturist occasionally tries to cause, in order to ensure the effectiveness of the treatment.

Certain complementary techniques may also be used.
The most common include:
- Moxibustion, which involves burning wormwood (a herbaceous plant) over the needle or the acupuncture point so as to create a beneficial heat;
- The application of a suction cup over an acupuncture point or sliding one along a meridian.

Contemporary techniques include:
- Electrostimulation of the needles;
- The laser, which can even replace the needle.

# 8. *ORDRE DES ACUPONCTEURS DU QUÉBEC* (QUEBEC ORDER OF ACUPUNCTURISTS)

Every acupuncturist practising in Quebec must be a member of the *Ordre des acuponcteurs du Québec (OAQ)*. Like all other professional orders in Quebec, the *OAQ* has been given a mandate by the government to regulate the practice of acupuncture in Quebec in order to protect the public. For more information about the *OAQ* or in order to verify the official status of your acupuncturist, call **514-523-2282** or **1-800-474-5914**.

The Ordre des acuponcteurs du Québec (Quebec Association of Acupuncturists) (*OAQ*) is a non-profit private organization made up of acupuncturists from Quebec. The mission of the *OAQ* is to promote Chinese medicine in Quebec and defend the socio-economic interests of the profession. The *OAQ* can be reached at **514-982-6567** or at **1-800-363-6567** or by Internet at www.acupuncture.com (in French only).

Only one facility is authorized to teach acupuncture in Quebec; it is the *Collège de Rosemont*. For information about training to become an acupuncturist, contact the Department of acupuncture of the *Collège de Rosemont* at **514-376-1620**, ext. 353.

# REFERENCES

1.  Myofascial pain is muscular in origin and it is caused by relaxation points, namely hyper-irritable zones located within the affected muscle.

2.  T. M. CUMMING, et A. R. WHITE, 2001. «Needling therapies in the management of myofascial trigger point pain: a systematic review», Archives of Physical Medecine and Rehabilitation, 82 (7), p. 986-992.

3.  C. M. WITT, B. BRINKHAUS, T. REINHOLD et coll., 2006a. «Efficacy, effectiveness, safety and costs of acupuncture for chronic pain - results of a large research initiative», Acupuncture in medecine, 24 (Suppl): p. S33-S39.

4.  La nociception est l'enregistrement par le système nerveux d'un signal potentiellement dangereux pour l'intégrité corporelle. La nociception peut conduire ou non à une expérience de douleur.

5.  A. WHITE, M. CUMMINGS et J. FILSHIE, 2008. An Introduction to Western Medical Acupuncture, Churchill Livingstone, p. 43-47.

6.  K. K. HUI, J. LIU, N. MAKRIS et coll., 2000. «Acupuncturemodulates the limbic system and subcortical gray structures of the human brain: evidence from MRI studies in normal subjects», Human Brain Mapping, 9 (1): p.13-25.

7.  A. WHITE, M., CUMMINGS et J. FILSHIE, 2008. An Introduction to Western Medical Acupuncture, Churchill Livingstone, p. 54.

8.  H. C. DIENER, K. KRONFELD, G. BOEWING et coll., 2006. «Efficacy of acupuncture for the prophylaxis of migraine: a multicenter randomised controlled clinical trial», Lancet Neurology 5 (4): p. 310-316.

9.  C. M. WITT, S. JENA, D. SELIM et coll., 2006c. «Pragmatic randomised trial evaluating the clinical and economic effectiveness of acupuncture for chronic low back pain», American Journal of Epidemiology 164 (5): p. 487-496.

10. H. P. SCHARF, U. MANSMANN, K. STREITBERGER et coll., 2006. «Acupuncture and knee osteoarthritis – a three arm randomized trial», Annals of Internal Medicine 145 (1): p.15-20.

# ACUPUNCTURE, OSTEOPATHY AND YOGA: **THINKING DIFFERENTLY ABOUT CHRONIC PAIN**

Pierre Beauchamp Ac, DO, Lorraine, Quebec, Canada

## 39

## ABSTRACT

During the 20 years I have spent practising acupuncture and osteopathy, Tai Chi and yoga, 80% of the people who have come to me for treatment were dealing with an acute or chronic pain condition. My clinical experience, my reflections and my research have led me to consider osteopathy, acupuncture and yoga as perfect complements for anyone wanting to take charge of their body and soul when dealing with chronic pain. This chapter provides a discussion of acupuncture and osteopathy, with a particular focus on how to use these two therapeutic approaches to deal with chronic pain.

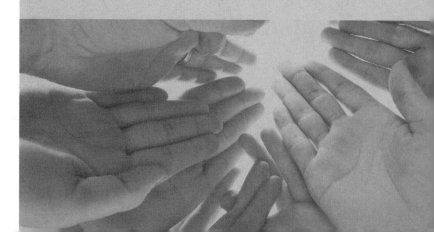

# 1. INTRODUCTION

**The body is more than the sum of its parts.** This is one of the first lessons I learned during my training in acupuncture. The strength of the therapeutic arts I practice is based on prevention and taking charge of the entire body and not just the region where the pain is located.

My role as a clinician is first to present my interpretation of pain to my patients and see that they understand: the macrocosm of their pain, namely the social and cultural influences, meteorological changes, the work and family climates, falls and accidents. The microcosm is the interpretation made by our brains and the manner in which our memories, experiences and emotions concerning pain are woven together.

# 2. WESTERN THOUGHT CURRENTS

In Latin, the word for "pain" is *pœna* and it means "chastisement, punishment".

In the Bible, the story of Job relates the life of a man affected not only by pain but also by the loss of his belongings, his family and his loved ones. Job found the psychological suffering much worse than the physical suffering, since well-meaning people came to comfort him during this troubled period. He believed that he had to have done something reprehensible for God to punish him so.

Job's story is not unique since, even today, people dealing with chronic pain believe to a certain extent that they are being punished somehow. This is part of their way of thinking and their belief system.

### TRANSPERSONAL PSYCHOLOGY AND JUNGIAN PSYCHOLOGY

Phineas Parkhurst Quimby lived in the United States at the beginning of the 19th century. He practiced magnetism and a form of hypnosis. He was the father of what we call «New Thought», which can easily be summed up as people developing an awareness of what they want in life (prosperity, health, harmony) and what they don't want (illness, poverty, disharmony). People achieve their objectives by working through God to create what they want. This is the thinking behind transpersonal and Jungian psychology.

### THE PATIENT'S MENTAL POWER

While treating one of his colleagues, Lucius Burkmar observed something that would change his clinical approach for the rest of his career. Burkmar had prescribed tea for one of his patients, a prescription that had produced few results. He then hypnotized the same patient. During the hypnosis session, Burkmar asked the patient to drink the same tea, telling him that the infusion would heal him. This time he obtained results. Quimby had remarked that the healing power was not in the tea, but in the **patient's mental power**. He concluded, "Your faith has healed you." (Mark 10:52)

### FAITH AND TREATMENT

Faith (combined with a healing method) that leads to healing is recognized as a placebo.

Dr. Andrew Weil, a physician and botanist from Harvard University, studied the placebo effect in several research studies. He concluded that it is the subconscious that controls the reaction to the placebo effect. Faith has no effect if it remains at the level of verbal or intellectual understanding. It must be more deeply buried in the strata of the brain and the field of consciousness in order to communicate directly with the nervous system.

### THE RELATIONSHIP BETWEEN BODY AND SOUL

One current of thought stipulates that all diseases are psychosomatic because they have physical and psychological components. We are no longer able to tell where the body starts, and where it ends. As a result, many doctors speak about the relationship between the body and the soul.

In his book, *Reinventing the body, resurrecting the soul*, Dr. Deepak Chopra discusses an experiment conducted on people who suffer from headaches when they use their cellular telephones. In a controlled environment, the participants were given cellular telephones. Some of them experienced pain as soon as the cellular telephone was placed close to their heads. An MRI demonstrated that, in the case of these patients, the part of the brain that controls the pain was more vascularized, indicating a certain irritation. All of the telephones given to the participants were fakes, but the pain was not imaginary.

# 3. THE NEUROLOGICAL MECHANISM OF PAIN

In order to understand the neurological mechanism of pain, we have to go 300 years back in time to La Haye, in Touraine (France), to the writings of mathematician, scientist and philosopher René Descartes. In his research into the union of the body and the soul, Descartes observed and documented the manner in which the nervous system functions through a diagram in which a little boy is seen sitting on a chair with one foot near a fire. Descartes traced a line (nervous stimulus) from the boy's foot along his leg and up to his back, continuing along the spinal column to the brain. Thus the boy moves his foot away from the fire when the heat becomes too intense.

In order to understand biology and the manner in which the body controls and interprets pain, let us return to 1973 and the research done by Ronald Melzack, psychologist, and Patrick Wall, biologist. Melzack and Wall developed the **gate theory**. This theory helps us understand how the body receives and controls pain.

After hitting his finger with a hammer, Martin experiences acute pain. At the time of contact, the pain receptors (rapid conduction receptor) in the region send a message to the spinal column, which in turn transmits it to the reticular activating system (RAS) of the medulla oblongata, which transmits it to the appropriate part of the brain (cortex prefrontal, thalamus), which interprets the signal and triggers the appropriate reaction. After a few choice words and an awkward dance, Martin's pain changes. It becomes less acute; the area remains sensitive, but not necessarily when moved or touched.

The signal from the pain receptors (rapid) is replaced by a slower signal from the sensory receptors. A different mechanism is used, namely a mechanism that helps moderate or control the pain. According to Melzack, these larger nerve fibres could inhibit the pain, or reduce its intensity. The brain then interprets the pain by using different memories and emotions that help the individual recognize the particular form of the pain. It is the part of the medulla oblongata that we refer to as the reticular activating system that filters the information, and forwards it in keeping with our past experiences and our thought patterns.

If you have never been burned or never seen fire, you will not have the reflex to avoid touching it. However, once you have had this experience, your brain will store the memory, and you will have the reflex to avoid any future contact with that form of stimulus. But the day when you burn yourself by accident, your brain will look through your memory to connect to the memory, and know how to react. In Martin's case, his brain does the same thing, determining the severity of the injury in order to react appropriately.

If I injure myself while playing hockey, my brain performs this exercise again to determine if focusing on my pain is more important that scoring a goal. The pain or the reaction could occur later. This is what I call a neurological association.

**Personal note:**
When my father passed away, it was a very difficult time for me. At the funeral home, as friends and relatives came by to give me their condolences, most of them combined their words with a small tap to my right shoulder. Several years later, at a party with friends, people shook my hand, or gave me a small tap on the right shoulder. For reasons I didn't understand at the time, I started thinking of my father. After reading *Personal Power* by Anthony Robbins , I understood how my brain had interpreted the stimulus of the tap on my shoulder. In his book, Robbins describes my experience as I lived through it. My brain had searched through all of my memories concerning my shoulder and the tap to it in order to cause my reaction... exactly as Melzack had described the relationship to pain.

The brain creates its own world. This is the point of view promoted by Melzack which, while being very philosophical, also takes into account what is represented by the world around us, our experiences, and the manner in which we integrate them, and use them in our lives. This is the part of the subconscious where every life experience is found. **One of the mysteries of chronic pain, and a good example, is phantom pain, namely the pain people who have had an amputation experience every day.**

The subconscious is responsible for 96% to 98% of our reactions to our external world. According to John Assaraf (*The Answer*), social ideologies are the source of the physical and emotional suffering of human beings.

## 4. STATISTICS

Dr. Angela Mailis-Gagnon, the manager of the pain clinic at Western Hospital in Toronto, explains that everyone suffers some form of pain, whether it is neuropathic in origin (damage to the nervous system, which is the most difficult to treat) or nociceptive (results from an injury or an illness affecting bones or muscles such as arthritis or a kidney stone). The way in which our experience of pain is made apparent depends on influences and genetic factors, our personality, our life experiences and our psychological state.

Many people suffer from chronic pain. Some experience pain on a daily basis, but it is not incapacitating; others experience pain every minute of the day, and it is incapacitating. According to Dr. Angela Mailis-Gagnon, one-third of the Canadian population suffers from chronic pain. This represents 9 million Canadians and of these 9 million people, 2 million suffer from neuropathic pain. Since the population is aging, this number could well increase in the coming decades.

A clinical study conducted by Dr. Mailis-Gagnon revealed that three patients out of four suffering from chronic neuropathic pain also suffered from anxiety or depression. Two-thirds of them were unemployed. Neuropathic pain affects 30% more men than women, and more people from 35 years to 49 years of age than other age groups.

Dr. Mailis-Gagnon concluded that there was no treatment to cure this type of pain. There are no treatments to control the intensity or duration of this pain. She recommended a combination of therapeutic arts such as exercise, acupuncture, massage, osteopathy, chiropractics, psychology, surgery and, if necessary, medication.

## 5. UNDERSTANDING THE SYMPTOMS OF CHRONIC PAIN

"Pain is in the brain!" – this is what Carl Jung and Sigmund Freud concluded in the 1920s. An individual in a state of chronic pain is not only constantly in pain, but also suffers from sleep disorders, depression and anxiety; he/she finds it hard to make simple decisions, and has mobility problems.

Professor Dante Chialvo, of the Northwestern University Feinberg School of Medicine, in Chicago, has been conducting research into chronic pain for several years. In February 2008, he worked with patients who suffered from chronic pain in their backs or elsewhere, and was able to use MRIs to open a path in the understanding of symptoms related to chronic pain.

Chialvo concentrated his efforts on the site in the brain where the neurological signal of patients suffering from chronic pain is altered. All of his patients had chronic back pain. His research indicated that, when the brain is healthy, all of the regions co-exist in a state of balance. This means that when one region is active, the others decrease their exchanges. In a brain dealing with chronic pain, the other regions continue their level of activity. The neurons continue their movements, while exhausting themselves, and modifying their links with the other neurons. This first observation of the state of the brain is directly related to the manner in which the brain reacts to pain.

Dr. A. Vania Apkarian, of the same university (Northwestern University Feinberg School of Medicine, in Chicago), speaks of shrinkage of the brain mass, of about 11%, corresponding to a loss equivalent to the effect of aging in a normal brain over a period of 10 to 20 years. After using MRIs to examine the brains of 26 patients, suffering or not from chronic pain, he observed a loss of 1.3 cubic centimetres of gray matter each year. Dr. Apkarian's research does not indicate whether these changes are permanent or not. This degeneration is not limited to the brain, but also affects the path taken by the signal from the region where the pain is located (the thumb, for example) to the nerves that transmit the signal to the spinal column and the frontal cortex. With years of overuse, the signal is altered by the transformation of the nerves it uses. Despite all these years of research, we still don't know how this happens, and even less how to remedy it.

## 6. A VISION OF THE ENTIRE BODY

Changing our vision of the body is a theory first advanced, according to the tradition of Greek mythology, by Asclepius, a hero of the Homeric period and god of medicine and healing. According to several historians, Asclepius was a human who was known for his knowledge and goodness who was later made divine. The asclepieia, or places where people could take refuge and regain their health, were based on the teachings attributed to Asclepius. Asclepius' art of medicine and healing was perpetuated by his descendants and followers, the most famous of whom was Hippocrates, the father of modern medicine.

In recent years, great steps have been taken to integrate a more holistic approach in the vision of the entire body, an approach which is endorsed by a large portion of the medical body. **Since the body is a whole, it must be seen and treated as such.** If your thumb hurts, that does not mean that your thumb is the source of your pain.

Well before, Asclepius, the Incas, the Taoists, Buddhists and Hindus had developed their own theories describing man and the universe as a whole. What exists between heaven and earth also exists in us: a movement of vital energy, the *QI*, perpetual and continuous, vibrates through us and everything that surrounds us. During one of the Apollo space missions (NASA, United States) in the 1970s, the astronauts deployed a net to capture the stellar particles that were floating in space. An analysis of the content of that net revealed that the particles found were the same elements that make up our planet, and are found in all beings living here.

In the past century, scientific discoveries that have been made have supported writings that were several thousand years old. At the end of the Newtonian era, science presented a very different picture from the one that had existed before. Neil Bohm, David Eisenberg and Max Planck announced the arrival of the period of quantum physics. $E=mc^2$ was a formula developed by mathematician Albert Einstein, who put forward the idea that everything is energy, and that all of the matter around us is made of particles of energy vibrating at a certain frequency that enables it to take form, such as a table, a flower, water, etc. According to these theories, we can change our approach and the way in which we perceive pain since it is merely a change in the frequency of the vibrations in our body at a given moment, whether the pain is acute or chronic.

**The body has an extraordinary capacity to heal itself. In my clinical approach, my goal is to reinforce the body in its vital energy so that it is better equipped to deal with any eventuality of a change in this vital energy, whether this change is internal in origin (emotional or subconscious) or external in origin (environmental, dietary, accidental or conscious).**

## 7. ACUPUNCTURE

On September 19, 1991, at 3,200 meters altitude, at the border between Italy and Austria, in theit Ötztal Alps, not far from the Italian dolomites, hikers made a very interesting discovery: a mummy. It was named Ötzi. According to Carbon-14 dating, the man had lived during the period between 3500 and 3100 BCE. Trapped in the ice, the body had been well preserved. On Ötzi's skin, 57 tattoos could be seen; they formed of small groups of lines that were either parallel or arranged in crosses, on the lumbar region, the knees and the ankles, at specific sites where several acupuncture sites are found. X-rays of these regions indicated that Ötzi was suffering from arthritis. Anthropologists had already noted that these types of marks were common in various ancient societies. It can be concluded that people during that period had access to someone in their tribe or their village who could help them with their health problems. These discoveries reveal the first form of acupuncture treatments.

A 3,000-year-old Chinese legend tells the story of a general who was renowned for his back pain. He had been struck by an arrow in his ankle, just below the lateral malleolus, an acupuncture point on the UB 62 bladder meridian, which is used to treat back pain today. Once his injury had healed, his back pain disappeared.

Chinese medicine is based on the duality of *yin* and *yang*. The *yin* is represented by rest, cold, the internal and the blood; the *yang* is represented by movement, heat, the external and the *QI*. When in balance, these two types of energy are synonymous of health. The *QI* is the movement of the *yang*; the blood is that of the *yin*. The *QI* and the blood circulate throughout the body by means of the meridians.

Each organ is represented by a group of meridians covering the body like an electrical circuit. They are connected to one another. The body is divided into *yin* (liver, heart, spleen, kidneys and lungs) and *yang* (gall bladder, small intestine, stomach, bladder and large intestine) organs. Each organ has very specific functions, and is linked to a single energy: the movement of the *QI* (*yang*) and the blood (*yin*) maintain fluid circulation of this energy in order to support the balance of the vital energy of the body. **On each meridian, there is a series of points at which the acupuncturists correct the movement of the energy by inserting needles. The points are selected in keeping with the Chinese energy diagnosis.**

### ACUPUNCTURE AND PAIN

In the case of acute or chronic pain, the painful region of the body is often strewn with sensitive points.

In acupuncture, we assess the balance and the movement through questions about the reasons for the consultation, of course, as well as the function of the organs:

- Breathing;
- Digestion;
- Sleep;
- Elimination (feces, urine, perspiration);
- Gynaecology;
- Pain;
- Senses (touch, smell , hearing, sight and taste);
- Emotional state;
- Observation;
- Posture;
- Movement and body shape;
- Face (colour, brightness, wrinkles, shape) where all the organs are represented;
- Tongue (shape, movement, tension, coating, marks, cracks and indents).

The Chinese energy pulse, taken at the wrist, indicates the state of energy movement in the body. Each organ is represented there. Disease results from an alteration in vital energy, with the symptoms and signs making up the face of the disease.

## Pain is an injury

Following a muscular injury, the body normally takes about eight weeks to recover (depending on the individual's age, gender, state of health and life hygiene). In the first days, pain is very present and intense, but over time it diminishes. After a few weeks, the pain occurs only periodically. After a month, there is no pain in daily movements, but there is still a certain weakness during sports activities when the limbs are solicited more intensely. Finally, the pain disappears completely.

## Friendly pain

This repair mechanism is very simple. Following a fall, our body has to drain away the debris caused by the damaged tissue, and once this has been done, it must repair the same tissues. Throughout this cycle, the nervous system communicates with the brain about the progress of the repairs. **In this case, pain becomes our best friend.** It tells us what we can do and what we can't do. It dictates how we are to limit our movements. When our movements are about to call on tissues that are still damaged or in the repair phase, the brain sends us a pain signal of the appropriate intensity. Throughout this cycle, the vital energy must work its way out of the blockage in order to return to its normal flow, namely a fluid flow without any obstruction.

## Chronic pain

"Humpty Dumpty sat on a wall.
Humpty Dumpty had a great fall.
All the king's horses and all the king's men
Couldn't put Humpty together again."
        - published in 1810

Here's a nursery rhyme that illustrates the definition of chronic pain well. Over time, the pain does not seem to diminish. It remains constant and regular in terms of nature, intensity and frequency. The body's energy is not sufficient to correct its movement.

In Chinese medicine, the liver is responsible for the flesh, namely the muscles and tendons. When pain moves from the acute phase to the chronic phase, the liver and its acolytes, the *QI* and the blood, are unable to correct the circulation. In addition to being responsible for the muscles and the tendons, the liver also governs the fluid and constant movement of energy through the meridians.

# 8. OSTEOPATHY

"There is one thing stronger than all the armies in the world, and that is an idea whose time has come."
Victor Hugo

Osteopathy is defined as a complete diagnostic and therapeutic system, based on the interconnectedness of anatomy and physiology for the study, prevention and treatment of illness. Osteopathy views the human organism as a whole, a machine that is in relation with its internal liquid environment, as well as its external environment. Osteopathy suggests that the organism, when fuelled in a healthy manner, functions to maintain itself, repair itself and heal itself, to the best extent possible, when its structure and physiology are in good order.

## HISTORY OF OSTEOPATHY

The origin of the practice of vertebral manipulations is very fuzzy. There are reasons to suppose that it dates back to the first people, since references to "bone-setters" putting bones and nerves back into place, can be found throughout the history of humanity. Therefore, it is not difficult to imagine that, during the course of such sessions, they would take part in vertebral manipulations.

The oldest writings to refer to such a practise are those of Hippocrates (in the chapter of the "Periarthron" on joints), those of a doctor in Antiquity, Galien, whose works were still considered to be authoritative up to the 18th century, those of the sophist Pausanias, who was originally from Syria and lived in Rome, as well as those of Ambroise Paré, a French surgeon during the Renaissance, who devoted the sixteenth chapter of his treatise to dislocations and one of the great English surgeons of the 19th century, Sir James Paget, who invited his colleagues to study the gestures and actions of the bone-setters.

Osteopathy is a therapeutic art developed by Andrew Taylor Still, an American physician who lived in Kirksville, Missouri (United States). In 1874, after 10 years of research and clinical work, Dr. Still started his new practice in osteopathy. The response to this practice on the part of his fellow physicians was lukewarm, but his patients and the citizens of Kirksville appreciated it. His reputation and his new form of medicine grew in popularity throughout the region. At the end of the 1880s, Dr. Still opened his osteopathy school.

## STRUCTURAL, VISCERAL AND CRANIAL OSTEOPATHY

Osteopathy focuses on three aspects: the structural, the visceral and the cranial.

### Structural osteopathy

Structural osteopathy involves the observation of the posture and body movements, an analysis of the muscles, ligaments, tendons and bones.

The osteopath uses mobilization techniques intended to re-establish the balance not only of the problem region, but also of the entire body. It is the circulation between the electrical signal that runs through the nerve, the blood movement, the lymph system and the primary respiratory movement that ensure health in the soft tissues of the body. This approach leads to long-term health.

### Visceral osteopathy

The human being is a whole: a set of bones, muscles and joints that enable it to move about. The viscera guarantee the functioning of this whole throughout one's life. The abdominal, pelvic, thoracic and cranial cavities contain sets of mobile viscera. When the body is affected by a pathology, the viscera become fixed. They lose their mobility in the cavity to which they belong and subject themselves to another structure. If the body is unable to adapt to this new situation, it will develop a functional problem that will, in turn lead to a structural problem if the adaptation is inadequate.

The role of the osteopath is to highlight the visceral fixation, since a loss of mobility results in a loss of motility. Each organ has its own mobility with respect to the axis of the movement, the space that is allocated to it for mobility. The purpose of osteopathy is to help the organ recover its continuous mobility so that it can once again function at a maximum.

### Cranial osteopathy (craniotherapy)

Craniotherapy was developed in 1932 by an osteopath named William Garner Sutherland. Based on the principles of osteopathy, cranial techniques involve mobilizing the bones of the skull, as well as those of the face. In ayurvedic medicine (yoga), we work with the *chakras*, in Chinese medicine with the *QI*, and in osteopathy with the primary respiratory mechanism (PRM). All of which are different terms used to designate the same energy movement.

The primary respiratory mechanism (PRM) is at its strongest in the skull, but can be perceived easily throughout the body. The brain, the cerebellum, the medulla oblongata, the spinal cord and all of the nerve ramifications that leave the spinal cord form a whole.

It is easiest to palpate and manipulate the PRM in the circulation of the cerebrospinal fluid and that is where the osteopath makes the correction. According to Dr. John E. Upledger, the cerebrospinal fluid acts as a pump or a hydraulic system. By mobilizing this system, the osteopath corrects the primary respiratory mechanisms as well as bodily problems.

When using cranial techniques, the osteopath places his/her hands on the bones of the calvaria or on the face, and occasionally even the mouth. The touch is light, with pressure of barely one to two ounces. This is probably one of the most relaxing and pleasant techniques. Many patients feel very relaxed and rested after a session.

# 10. YOGA

"Does there exist a British cancer, an Italian cancer and an Indian cancer? The human sufferings are the same ones, whether one is Indian or Western. The diseases are common to all the human beings, and yoga is given to us to cure these diseases."
B.S.K. Iyengar

Yoga is one of the six Indian Astika schools of philosophy. It is also a discipline that focuses on meditation, moral ascetics, and bodily exercises in order to achieve the unification of the human being in his/her physical, psychic and spiritual aspect.

Yoga does not exclude the metaphysical level from the physical and mental levels. It does not fundamentally separate matter from thought. Its method includes all knowledge, the structure of the apparent world, the formation of thoughts, the role of the energy that gives birth to one or the other and the beyond, the energy and creative force from which the world was born. Through the method of re-integration, it allows the individual to perceive the nature of mental representations and the conscious, and to arrive at a union with the subtle form of the being.

Yoga was already practised in the third millennium before our time, but it is relatively recent in the Western world, although it is well-established here. Almost immediately. it ensures mental and muscular relaxation. In the medium term, it develops flexibility and helps resolve various musculoskeletal problems. The regular practice of yoga can relieve serious health problems, and lead to better general health. Although yoga is basically a spiritual practice, it can be practised by anyone as a tool of health and healing.

## THERAPEUTIC APPLICATIONS

Yoga is probably the most complete form of exercise. It can result in major changes. A yoga session has three steps.

### Step 1: Prana and pranayama

The prana simply means respiration. The pranayama is respiration at a variable rhythm. Respiration is the first contact between the soul and the physical. Respiration on its own is a big step towards relaxation.

### Exercise

Close your eyes, take a deep breath through your nose, puffing up your belly. Now, breathe out through your nose and repeat.

### Step 2: The asanas

The asanas are the postures used in the practice of yoga. They are varied and often involve a certain amount of difficulty at the start. The purpose is to maintain the physical body and balance the energies on the seven levels of the being. By contracting and relaxing the muscular fibres, the body receives an internal massage. Originally, the asanas were static postures used to promote meditation. More than simple stretching exercises, the asanas open the energy channels (the *chakras*), and help centre the psychic energy. The asanas purify and reinforce the body, and the control the concentration of the conscious.

An asana must be performed in a stable, comfortable and firm manner that is also relaxed. Throughout a posture, respiration plays an important role in harmonizing the body, the soul and the conscious.

## Step 3: Meditation

**During meditation, you make changes in the perception of your pain.**

The term meditation (from the Latin *meditatio*) refers to a mental or spiritual practice. Meditation involves focussing our attention on a single thought or on ourselves.

Meditation is a practice that is intended to produce inner peace, mental emptiness, modified states of consciousness, or the progressive calming of the mental sphere, even simple relaxation, by becoming familiar with an external object (such as a real object or a symbol), or an internal object (such as the mind, a concept, or the absence of a concept). Meditation is letting go. This is where we control and chase away our compulsive, egocentric thoughts, and open new spiritual horizons. Our past is an old story, the future is a mystery, but the present is a gift.

# 11. CONCLUSION

Science has made a great deal of progress with respect to finding a solution for chronic pain. But, according to Dr. Weil, doctors have a success rate of 85% in the treatment of acute pain and 35% in the treatment of chronic pain. Often, the only resource they have is medication.

Acupuncture and osteopathy are tools that can help you get your muscles back into balance, improve your posture, and remove any blockage of the blood, nerve, lymphatic and energy movements. These treatments will also relax the soft tissues of your body significantly, and calm your mind. When combined with yoga (respiration, postures and meditation), they can help you change some of your limiting beliefs on your own.

> "If you change the way you look at things, the things you look at change!"
> **Dr. Wayne W. Dyer**

During your acupuncture and osteopathy assessment, you will receive the adjustments needed to bring your body back into balance, but this will not be enough. You will need to go a little further. The approach will require you to make an investment since, in reality, you **are the only one who can make a difference.**

From a clinical point of view, I prepare my treatments in four steps.

## Step 1: Acupuncture
Once the assessments have been completed, an energy diagnosis is prepared, a detailed treatment plan is developed and points are selected.

## Step 2: Prana (breathing)
Once the needles have been inserted they are left in place for 20 minutes. During this time, I ask the individual to practice a simple respiration exercise. This increases the relaxation, the letting go and the movement of the *Qi* in his/her body.

## Step 3: Osteopathy
The osteopathic techniques chosen are intended to correct and reinforce the weaknesses and lack of balance noted at the time of the assessment. During the cranial treatment, a small guided meditation is included.

## Step 4: "Homework"
I regularly assign "homework" or exercises to be done at home. This step accounts for 40 to 50% of the success of the treatments. It involves one or more exercises that will result in changes in the way you perceive your health and pain. Here is an example.

- Create a new mental and physical vision for your health (including pain).
- Create new statements that support the new vision.
- Create written or visual materials, physical exercises, subliminal messages or audios that will be filled with your new vision.
- Practice your training three times a day for 10-30 minutes per day for at least 30 days.
- Meditate.

**When you learn something new, whether it is physical or intellectual, it takes more or less 30 days for your body to adjust to it and accept it as a regular and constant activity.**

> "A journey of a thousand miles starts with a single step."
> Lao-Tseu (Tao Te Ching)

**Now it's up to you to take the first step.**

# TREATING CHRONIC NON-CANCER PAIN –
## TIME FOR A CHANGE?

Yoram Shir, MD, anaesthesiologist, Director, Alan Edwards Pain Management Unit,
McGill University Health Centre (MUHC), Montreal, Quebec, Canada.

## 1. INTRODUCTION

Chronic non-cancer pain (CNCP), defined as pain associated with a non-malignant condition or disease lasting for more than six months, has become a leading cause of human suffering, disability and health care utilization. Regardless of its etiology, the prevalence of CNCP has been rising continuously and is predicted to double over the next two decades. The mere statistics associated with chronic pain, its prevalence, cost to the individual patient and to society, and loss of working days is staggering. Still, these numbers do not reflect the amount of physical and emotional suffering endured by these patients and their families.

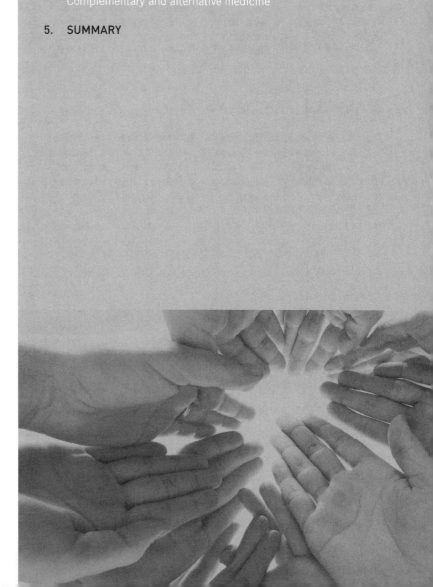

Take for example Mr. K, a 68-year-old patient of mine who has been suffering from intractable postherpetic neuralgias (chronic shingles) of the left chest for more than 5 years. His pain disease comprises ongoing burning, touch-evoked pain, and bouts of electric-shock-like pains in the affected area. Otherwise healthy, this unfortunate patient is almost completely incapacitated since even the simplest tasks aggravate his pain significantly.

A multitude of therapeutic approaches has been tried along the way by our multidisciplinary pain team, including oral non-opioid and opioid medications, invasive interventions like IV lidocaine infusions and nerve blocks, behavioural therapies and various complementary and alternative medicine (CAM) interventions. Unfortunately, none of these measures brought upon significant, long-lasting pain relief, a situation that is not expected to change in the future either. Mr. K. still visits our clinic regularly, at least finding some solace in the support and encouragement of the entire team.

Efforts to cure CNCP often fail due to a multitude of reasons, a discussion of which is beyond the scope of this article (for a comprehensive review please see: Brennan F, et al., Anesth Analg 2007; 105: 205-21).[1] Some authorities in the field now foresee that even with limitless medical resources at hand, we will not be able to cure many of the patients afflicted with CNCP. Since limitless resources are not available we are basically facing a cureless disease. Indeed, cure is seldom mentioned in conjunction with CNCP patients, where symptomatic relief is often the main goal. Even with the best available tools at hand the chances to cure CNCPs like post herpetic neuralgia, phantom limb pain, fibromyalgia, failed back surgery and complex regional pain syndromes, and even benign chronic low back pain are slim. For example, a recent Canadian survey following people with chronic neuropathic pain for two years shows that even when treated in multidisciplinary pain treatment centres, participants are not getting significantly better. This stands in sharp contrast to other more "respected" diseases like cancer, where the current cure rate could surpass 50%.

The picture is not necessarily brighter even if we accept the fact that curing patients with CNCP is not realistic, focusing instead on symptomatic pain relief and improved function. Take for example the efforts toward developing new pain-relieving medications. The multibillion dollar investments in new and promising products indeed have yielded novel medications with clear analgesic effects in a variety of CNCP conditions. For example, a study on the effect of pregabalin on pain in patients with fibromyalgia showed that approximately 50% of patients reported a statistically significant decrease in their pain (Arnold LM, et al., J Pain 9; 792: 2008).[2] This change, however, was in the magnitude of 2/10 on a 0–10 numerical pain scale, leaving patients with a significant amount of pain and suffering. Yet, the old, cheap and non-specific antidepressant amitriptylin is still regarded by some clinicians as the drug of choice in patients with fibromyalgia. One might ask, therefore, whether the substantial investment in medications whose effect amounts only to moderate palliation is justified. Could it be more beneficial to try to divert some of these funds into new therapeutic avenues? Since the outcome of our current therapy for CNCP is far from satisfactory, I believe we should change our approach to this disease and, consequently, allocate resources accordingly. Adhering to our traditional therapeutic habits will not, in my mind, lead to a significant improvement in the outcome of CNCP patients.

## 2. A CALL FOR A CHANGE

This chapter reviews my thoughts on a different approach to CNCP therapy. Before proceeding, I would like to make it clear that the dire need for other changes related to chronic pain (e.g. government and other official policies, federal and provincial budget allocation, and pain education, to mention just a few) are beyond the scope of this chapter, and will not be discussed.

The changes I suggest are in two main domains:
1. Focusing more on preventing CNCP from developing, rather than on traditional means of palliation;
2. Exploring novel palliative pain-relieving measures since the current conservative means that are used for treating CNCP frequently fail

# 3. PREVENTION OF CHRONIC NON-CANCER PAIN

Once developed, chronic pain is difficult to treat. Might it not be better, therefore, to invest more in preventing CNCP rather than focusing mainly on its palliation? This is not a trivial task since most human beings cannot predict when and in which circumstances they might develop CNCP. One might argue then that the only way to prevent CNCP could be by pre-emptive vaccination, an idea that until few years ago could be regarded as unrealistic. However, a research group from the U.S. has published in 2005 the results of a novel study on the role of vaccination in preventing acute herpes zoster and chronic postherpetic neuralgia.

This study, testing more than 40,000 elderly people, found that compared to non-vaccinated individuals, the prevalence of chronic shingles in the vaccinated group decreased by 66% (Oxman MN, et al., N Engl J Med 352; 2271: 2005).[3] To my knowledge, none of the existing palliative measures for shingles, or other CNCP diseases, was found to be as effective. However, vaccination has its limits. Although animal experiments show preliminary promising results of another vaccine, one that can limit nerve damage after trauma, it is unlikely that a vaccination could be found for other types of chronic pain.

A different way to approach CNCP prevention stems from one of its greatest mysteries, i.e. the fact that not every person undergoing the same trauma, injury or inflammatory process will develop CNCP. For example, out of 10 otherwise healthy males undergoing an elective surgery of inguinal hernia repair, one or two will develop chronic neuropathic postsurgical pain. This will happen even if the same surgeon performs all surgeries using the same surgical technique. **At present, we lack the tools to identify the individuals at risk for developing CNCP. If, however, we learn to recognize these individuals when still healthy, we could prepare them appropriately.**

For example, aggressive analgesic measures could be taken either before surgery to try to prevent the development of chronic postoperative pain, or immediately after trauma to prevent chronic post-traumatic pain.

---

**Identification of individuals at risk might be possible in two ways.**
**1. Finding genetic variances associated with the increased tendency to develop CNCP**
**2. Identification of individual characteristics associated with the tendency to develop CNCP (i.e. identifying individuals' phenotype)**

---

## 1. Finding genetic variances associated with the increased tendency to develop CNCP

Most of our current knowledge of genes vs. pain comes from experiments in rodents showing that 30 to 70% of the tendency for developing pain after injury is genetic. Although research on genetics vs. CNCP in humans is still in its infancy, there are data showing a strong association between the two. For example, people with parental history of chronic pain possess less internal capabilities to fight pain through their natural endogenous opioid system compared to people with healthy parents (Bruehl S, et al., Pain 124; 287: 2006).[4] Specific genetic variations are associated with increased response to opioid medications, and the tendency to develop chronic pain conditions like complex regional pain syndrome type I (Mailis A, et al., Clin J Pain 10; 210: 1994),[5] low back pain and temporomandibular joint pain. With the rapid advancement in the field, it is possible that genotyping will play a more central role in future pain therapies.

## 2. Identification of individual characteristics associated with the tendency to develop cncp (i.E. Identifying individuals' phenotype)

Preliminary data in healthy individuals show that it is possible to identify predictive behaviours associated with increased acute and chronic pain. In other words, we might have the ability to identify those of us possessing a "chronic pain proneness" phenotype. The evidence supporting this idea comes from the following observations.

*Early exposure to pain could permanently change our pain behaviour.*

Studies showed circumcision alters pain response to vaccination months later (Taddio A, et al., Lancet 349; 599: 1997),[6] neonatal pain, endured for example by newborns in the intensive care unit, could predict exaggerated pain behaviour later in life (Grunau RV, et al., Pain 56; 353: 1994)[7], and early injury can alter pain processing at adulthood (Fitzgerald M, Nat Neurosci Rev 6; 507: 2005).[8]

*The sensitivity of healthy individuals to benign experimental pain stimuli before elective surgery correlates significantly with their immediate and late postoperative pain levels.*

This has been shown for painful heat, cold and pressure stimuli (Strulov L, et al., J Pain 8; 273: 2007).[9] Although speculative at present, other stimuli, not necessarily painful, might also be found to differentiate between "normal" healthy individuals and the "chronic pain proneness" individuals (e.g. sensitivity to pungent smells, touch of various materials, etc.).

I argue that even with our current limited knowledge, we can start categorizing patients according to their risk of developing acute pain and CNCP. In fact, a first step toward creating such a pain risk score has already been taken in 2006 for acute postoperative pain (Pan PH, et al., Anesthesiology 104; 417: 2006).[10] The risk scale for CNCP could include scoring of cultural, ethnic and social backgrounds, previous chronic pain history, familial history of pain, psychological status, and the response to defined painful/unpleasant stimuli. Hopefully, future research will improve the scoring system by adding environmental risk factors (see below), specifying genetic profiling for "pain genes", and finding more sophisticated associations between the individual's phenotype and the increased pain tendency.

It is unlikely that CNCP could be eradicated just by taking preventive measures, efficient as they may be. Among the many tools that could be suggested to enrich the CNCP palliation armamentarium I would like to mention two: the environment and complementary and alternative medicine (CAM).

# 4. EXPLORING DIFFERENT PALLIATIVE TOOLS

## A. THE ENVIRONMENT

Environmental determinants of health are well recognized as having a pivotal role in the development of major ailments like coronary heart disease and cancer. There is no reason to ignore, therefore, the possible role of the environment in CNCP, which is confirmed by preliminary animal and human experiments. In rodents, factors such as the experimental site, identity of the cage-mates, levels of congestion in living facilities, weather conditions (e.g. ambient temperature and barometric pressure) and dietary constituents can all augment or decrease chronic pain behaviour. In humans, there are indications that compromised housing conditions, previous exposure to pain, dietary constituents, the weather and environmental toxins can aggravate pain. Of these, the weather and dietary constituents have been especially fascinating for me.

### Weather

Patients often comment on the effect of weather conditions on their CNCP. Just like old sailors that can smell a storm far in advance, many patients with CNCP can actually predict weather changes before they arrive by experiencing changes in their chronic pain levels. Other CNCP patients report that their pain is at least partially weather-dependent. I am sure that many among the readers will agree that humid weather tends to aggravate some types of CNCP. One would expect, therefore, that this universal variable will be the subject of vigorous pain research. The sad truth is that the medical community has almost totally ignored this topic: less than five studies have ever examined it. **These studies showed, however, a direct association between pain and weather conditions.** For example, a recent study done in the U.S. found that air pressure and temperature are independently associated with levels of chronic osteoarthritis knee pain (McAlindon T, et al., Am J Med 120; 429-34: 2007).[11]

### Diet

Multiple studies to date show that specific dietary constituents are beneficial in ailments like cancer, cardiovascular diseases, depression and rheumatic disease. Although less investigated for their effect on pain, there are preliminary data showing that certain types of dietary fats, carbohydrates and amino acids possess analgesic properties. For example, sweetened liquids decrease procedural pain in infants (Akman I, et al., J Pain 3;199:2002)[12], and omega-3 polyunsaturated fatty acids are associated with decreased inflammatory pain (Cleland LG, et al., Drugs 63: 845: 2003).[13] Yet, serious clinical research on the analgesic properties of diet is almost non-existing. To my knowledge, our research group is one of the few to explore this area, testing the analgesic properties of dietary constituents like soy protein in patients with CNCP.

Even if found to directly affect CNCP, not all environmental factors could be changed; most of us will have to cope with our local weather and housing conditions. However, we could control other harmful environmental conditions if proven to increase CNCP. What is missing is solid scientific proof implicating specific environmental parameters as pain modifiers or amplifiers. However, the paucity of current research makes it unlikely that environmental change could play a significant role in treating patients with CNCP in the near future.

## B. COMPLEMENTARY AND ALTERNATIVE MEDICINE

The lack of scientific evidence supporting the use of complementary and alternative medecine (CAM) by patients with CNCP is in stark contrast to its popularity and widespread use. The proportion of CAM users among the general population in North America has been growing steadily, probably passing the 50% mark. While chiropractors and massage therapists account for nearly one half of all visits to CAM professionals, multiple other disciplines gained popularity as well. Preliminary studies show that patients with CNCP utilize CAM more frequently than the general population (Boisset et al., J Rheumatol 21; 148-52: 1994).[14] Actually, pain-related disorders are the most commonly reported conditions for which patients use CAM, and CAM therapies are probably chosen more frequently than conventional therapies to treat CNCP. Surprisingly, all this is happening with minimal scientific proof justifying the use of CAM in CNCP. Even though high-quality scientific data is missing in most CAM domains, clinical observations of its efficiency cannot be ignored. For example, a recent German survey evaluated the effect of acupuncture in almost 500,000 patients with chronic headache, osteoarthritis and low back pain. Effectiveness of acupuncture was rated by the treating physicians and was found to be marked in 22% and moderate in 54% of the patients (Weidenhammer W, et al., Complement Ther Med 15; 238: 2007).[15]

The use of CAM in medicine in general, and in CNCP conditions in particular, remains controversial not only because of the lack of solid scientific data; physicians and patients often fail to inquire or report the use of CAM, and physician/patient disagreements on the validity and effectiveness of individual CAM therapies.

Safety concerns are as important in disciplines such as manipulation therapy, herbal supplements, megavitamins and folk remedies. **Some of these remedies could contain toxic ingredients or cause significant adverse reactions when taken in conjunction with prescribed medications.**

In light of the limitations of conventional medicine to supply appropriate pain palliation in many CNCP patients, CAM could be a valuable alternative. This could not happen, however, as long as we lack concrete scientific evidence of its efficiency, safety and limitations.

## 5. SUMMARY

There are few epidemiological studies looking at the long-term outcome of CNCP patients. Nevertheless, I doubt whether patients with CNCP fare significantly better at present compared to a decade or two ago, a frustrating situation for patients and healthcare providers alike. This stagnation happens regardless of the great efforts to improve the outcome of CNCP, for example by advanced basic research seeking targets for novel medications. Unfortunately, only few such targets have materialized into novel therapies due to a lack of clinical effect or intolerable side effects. I believe that the time has come, therefore, to divert some of our attention from traditional therapeutic areas to novel and sometimes less lucrative directions. I am not suggesting neglecting these traditional approaches; exploring new types of pharmacological interventions, for example targeting more specific pain mechanisms in more defined CNCP conditions could be found to be very effective. Rather, I suggest combining these efforts with different approaches and modes of therapy that might prevent the development or improve the outcome of CNCP.

## REFERENCES

1. Brennan, F, DB Carr & M. Cousins. Pain management: a fundamental human right. Anesth Analg, 2007; 105: 205-221.
2. Arnold, LM, IJ Russell, EW Diri, WR Duan, JP Young, U. Sharma,SA Martin, JA Barrett & G. Haig. A 14-week, randomized, double-blind, placebo-controlled monotherapy trial of pregabalin in patients with fibromyalgia. The Journal of Pain, 2008, 9(9): 792-805.
3. Oxman, MN et al. A vaccine to prevent herpes zoster and postherpetic neuralgia in older adults. New England Journal of Medicine, 2005, June 2; 352(22): 2271-2284.
4. Bruehl, S. et al. Parental history of chronic pain may be associated with impairments in endogenous opioid analgesic systems. Pain, 2006, Volume 124, Issue 3, 124; 287.
5. Mailis A. et al. Etiology, clinical manifestations, and diagnosis of complex regional syndrome in adults. Clinical Journal of Pain, 1994,10; 210.
6. Taddio A. et al. Effect of neonatal circumcision on pain response during subsequent routine vaccination. Lancet, 1997, 349; 599.
7. Grunau RV et al. Pain, plasticity, and premature birth: a prescription for permanent suffering? Pain, 1994, 56; 353.
8. Fitzgerald, M. The development of nociceptive circuits. Nature Reviews Neuroscience 6, 2005; 507-520.
9. Strulov L. et al. Pain Catastrophizing, Response to Experimental Heat Stimuli, and Post–Caesarean Section Pain. Journal of Pain, Volume 8, Issue 3, 2007; 273-279.
10. Pan, PH et al. Survey of the Outcome Measures Used in Postoperative Pain Research. Anesthesiology, Volume 104, 2006; 417-425.
11. MAClindon, T. et al. Changes in Barometric Pressure and Ambient Temperature Influence Osteoarthritis Pain. American Journal of Medicine, Volume 120, Issue 5, 2007; 429-434.
12. Akman I, et al. Sweet solutions and pacifiers for pain relief in newborn infants. Journal of Pain, Volume 3, Issue 3, 2002; 199-202.
13. Cleland, LG et al. The Role of Fish Oils in the Treatment of Rheumatoid Arthritis. Drugs, Volume 63, Issue 9, 2003; 845-853.
14. Boisset et al. Complementary and alternative medicine in rheumatology. Journal of Rheumatology, Volume 21, 1994; 148-152.
15. Weidenhammer W, et al. Acupuncture for chronic pain within the research program of 10 German Health Insurance Funds—Basic results from an observational study. Complementary Therapies in Medicine, Volume 15, Issue 4, 2007; 238-24.

# THE CROSSING

Louise O'Donnell-Jasmin, BEd, Laval, Quebec, Canada

(See other testimonials, pages 84 and 26. See Chapter 1, page 3.)

A small silhouette reached the top of the dunes, her long black coat floating around her in the beach grass sloped by wind. It was an old black coat, used by years of wandering, its tail floating in the wind like two black wings, slowly hovering over her. Long and black, the colour of her despair. Impassive sea birds ran toward the shore, pecking at food that was not there, ignoring the invisible presence on the dunes. The silhouette of a woman barely alive.

How many years did she stand on the dunes of pain, on the threshold of life?

The sea suddenly stood still, as much out of fear of the woman finally walking toward the waves as her falling before she got there.

As her final quest, she finally recognized the music haunting her suns and her moons: the rolling and rumbling sound of waves breaking near the beach, the sound of Life. The sound she had waited for and followed, the sound she had searched for was there, majestic, at last within her reach. She knew she could walk from one infinity to the next along the shores, refreshing her body and soul, letting Life inside her again.

She now had to choose: to go on and cross the threshold leading to the sea or let the desert of pain win the battle. She had to move beyond pain. She knew it was the answer.

Life stood still. In the ruins of her world, where desert meets sea, she walked toward the threshold, the very last door. She stood haunted by the darkness of pain and memories. The wind was wings to help her fly again. To live again. She would use it for the crossing. It was her only chance. She asked herself if the wind wasn't love pushing her on to cross the limits she had set for herself. Wasn't the wind love that pushed her along the way when she stopped trying to go on? Wasn't that what the wind was made of?

She finally followed the soft rumbling of the sea. There was hope, there was Life, with pain or without it. She chose to live and love. She would find a way out of pain.

And then she crossed the threshold.

# LIVING WITH PAIN: TOOLS TO HELP OURSELVES - A TESTIMONIAL

**Penny Cowan,** Rocklin, California, USA,
Executive director, American Chronic Pain Association (ACPA)

www.theacpa.org

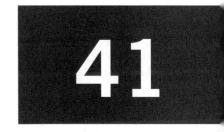

**41**

## ABSTRACT

A person with pain is like a car with four flat tires. When we find the right medicine, we can fill one of our tires; however, we still have three flat tires and are unable to move forward. For many, the expectation is that medication will solve their pain problem. Instead of looking at other areas of pain management, they continue to seek out medications to resolve their pain. This chapter will explore what a person with pain needs to know to make his/her journey from patient to person. We discuss the basics of pain management as we explore the American Chronic Pain Association (ACPA) *Ten Steps From Patient to Person*.

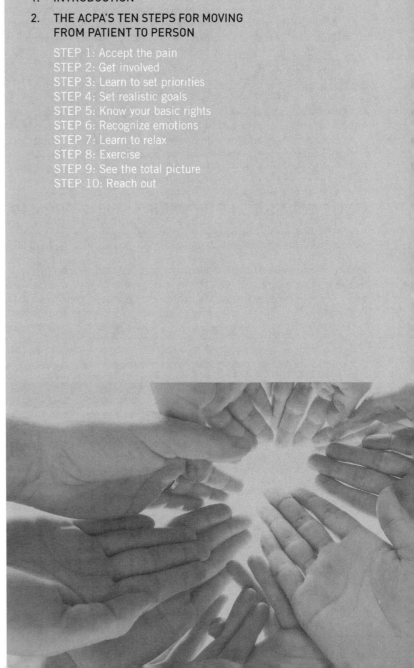

# 1. INTRODUCTION

Looking for a simple solution to managing pain usually turns into an endless journey of tests, treatments and hoping to find the magic bullet that will eliminate the pain. Our expectation is that if we can find the right medication or the right treatment, our pain will be gone, and we can get on with our life. What we don't realize is that there may be a medication out there that will provide us with as much relief as anything available, but there will still be some level of pain. Pain that we may have to live with... if we can.

This chapter presents the ten steps or coping skills provided by the American Chronic Pain Association (ACPA) to help people living with pain deal with their condition in a more positive and constructive manner. (See **Chapter 48**.)

**The problem for so many of us is that pain becomes our identity.** As much as I fought it, after a six-year journey to find a solution to my pain, I lost who I was, and defined myself by my pain, or rather by the ability that my pain allowed me. I became so consumed with my pain that all of my energies were focused on the pain and how to rid my body of unrelenting pain, so that I could go back to life the way it was *before* the pain. The problem was that, like so may others, I looked for the quick fix, the magic that would instantly make my pain vanish. It made no sense to me that with all of medicine's there was now way to relieve my pain. What I didn't realize was how complex chronic pain is, and how many areas of my life — and those of my family — that the pain had invaded.

In the six-year journey to find relief, I did not realize just how much of myself I relinquish to my pain. The fix could not be simple; it could not be as easy as taking a pill or discovering the "miracle" cure. No, the solution would take an approach that was completely foreign to me, as it would be for anyone who travelled on the same road. Perhaps the best way to describe how I finally made my journey from the disabled patient to that of a functional person, is to use a simple analogy.

A person with pain is like a car with four flat tires. When we find the right medicine we can fill one of our tires, however we still have three flat tires, and are unable to move forward. The solution requires far more than we anticipated. It requires us asking what else do we need to fill our other three tires so that we can resume our life's journey. Unlike traditional medicine where the "patient" is a passive participant, living a full life with pain requires that we take an active role in the recovery process. We need to work with our healthcare providers to find what we need to fill up our other three tires. For each of us it will be different depending on our medical and personal needs. Biofeedback, physical therapy, counselling, pacing, nutritional counselling, and a host of medical modalities are but a few of the choices.

The American Chronic Pain Association has developed *Ten Steps from Patient to Person*, a road map of sorts to help a person with pain along their journey. These steps are not meant to be followed in any particular order, but rather according to personal needs. Below is an overview of each of those steps. However, much more is needed to continue the journey. Working with your healthcare provider will help direct you on a path and guide you as you continue your journey.

# 2. THE ACPA'S TEN STEPS FOR MOVING FROM PATIENT TO PERSON

## STEP 1: ACCEPT THE PAIN

Learn all you can about your physical condition. Understand that there may be no current cure and accept that you will need to deal with the fact of pain in your life. That does not mean that you have to relinquish your life to your pain, but rather do not allow it to become your identity — simply just a part of what makes you who you are. Your pain does not define you!

## STEP 2: GET INVOLVED

Take an active role in your own recovery. Follow your doctor's advice and ask what you can do to move from a passive role into one of partnership in your own healthcare. In the traditional role of a patient, you look to the healthcare community to take care of you. Living with chronic pain changes the playing field. You are an important member of the team. Ask your healthcare provider what you can do to take an active role in moving from patient to person.

## STEP 3: LEARN TO SET PRIORITIES

Look beyond your pain to the things that are important in your life. As pain slowly took over your life, many of your activities fell by the wayside. Looking back, you are overwhelmed by how many things that have piled up. It is time to sort through all those things, and ask yourself what is the most important thing in your life at this time. One way to identify your priorities is to make a list of everything you can think of that has any significance for you. It helps to put each item on a separate card to allow for easier sorting later. Once you think you have completed your list, take each card, and lay it face up on a table so that you can see all the issues you have been carrying around. Now, ask yourself what is the most important item you have identified, and pick up that card. You have now identified your first priority, and defined a starting point.

## STEP 4: SET REALISTIC GOALS

We all walk before we run. Yet, like so many people with pain, we have good days and bad days. Unfortunately, on a good day we try to accomplish as much as possible to make up for all the days when we cannot perform. We quickly learn that being too active increases our pain, so we eliminate any activities that we think might increase our pain. The problem is that we have become so deconditioned since our pain began that no matter what we do, we will probably experience more pain. The key is to be realistic; don't set yourself up for failure. If you have a good day, why not take it slow and pace your activities so that you enjoy the day, not suffer because of it.

The problem for people with pain is they cannot see their progress from day to day. It is like watching their hair grow. We fail to see that in spite of the fact that we may still have some level of pain, we are actually more active and enjoying life more, and our abilities may have increased. Setting goals and tracking your progress will allow you to see improvements over time. The American Chronic Pain Association has charts, such as its *Pain Log*, to help a person with pain set goals and track progress from week to week.

## STEP 5: KNOW YOUR BASIC RIGHTS

We all have basic rights. Among these are the right to be treated with respect, say no without guilt, do less than humanly possible, make mistakes, and not need to justify our decisions, with words or pain. Having pain doesn't change the fact that we still have rights. Yet, we tend to push ourselves trying to regain some sense of "normal" life whenever possible. What we need is to assert ourselves and realize that we do not have to be perfect. Below are the basic rights that the American Chronic Pain Association uses to help people on their journey from patient to person. We suggest that people use them whenever possible.

**YOUR BASIC RIGHTS (American Chronic Pain Association)**
1. The right to act in a way that promotes your dignity and self-respect.
2. The right to be treated with respect.
3. The right to make mistakes.
4. The right to do less than you are humanly capable of doing.
5. The right to change your mind.
6. The right to ask for what you want.
7. The right to take time to slow down and think before you respond.
8. The right to feel that you don't have to explain everything you do and think.
9. The right to say "no" and not feel guilty.
10. The right to ask for information.
11. The right to feel good about yourself.
12. The right to ask for help or assistance.
13. The right to disagree.
14. The right to ask "why?"
15. The right to be listened to and taken seriously when expressing your feelings.

## STEP 6: RECOGNIZE EMOTIONS

Our body and mind are one. It is impossible to separate them. What we experience emotionally will have a physical effect on us and vice-versa. There is a great book called *The Angry Book* by Theodore Rubin that discusses all different forms of anger. The key message in his book, however, is what we do with our anger. Instead of recognizing feelings as they occur, many of us tend to bury them for fear of being viewed as "angry" or negative. The problem is those feelings don't go away. They build up inside of us until we reach a point where they are just too powerful to hold on to. When that happens, we tend to explode, releasing all of our emotions at an inappropriate time usually on the wrong person. If we would just recognize and deal with feelings as they occur, it would make our life a bit more manageable. It takes a tremendous amount of energy to keep those feelings buried. Keep in mind that there are no wrong feelings, only inappropriate reactions. Expressing your feelings is okay! Emotions directly affect physical well being. By acknowledging and dealing with your feelings, you can reduce stress and decrease the pain you feel.

## STEP 7: LEARN TO RELAX

Pain increases in times of stress. Relaxation exercises are one way of reclaiming control of your body. Think about this: count from 1 to 25 and at the same instant say the alphabet to yourself. Try hard. You cannot do it can you? Why? Because we really do have a one-track mind. We cannot think about two things at exactly the same time. So, if you can redirect your thought toward things other than your pain, you might find that you are reducing your sense of suffering. Deep breathing, visualization and other relaxation techniques can help you to better manage the pain with which you live. However, keep in mind these are learned skills, and must be practised on a regular basis.

## STEP 8: EXERCISE

Most people with chronic pain fear exercise. Unused muscles feel more pain than toned flexible ones. With your doctor, identify a modest exercise program that you can do safely. The problem for so many of us is that we want to feel better yesterday. If we believe that exercise will help, and are encouraged by our healthcare provider to start a program, we might mistakenly jump in with both feet, so to speak. We have to keep in mind the concept of pacing. Remember, we do not want to set ourselves up for failure. Perhaps we need to start out at a snail's pace, and slowly and gradually add increased repetitions and exercises over time. As you build strength, your pain can decrease. You will feel better about yourself, too.

## STEP 9: SEE THE TOTAL PICTURE

As you learn to set priorities, reach goals, assert your basic rights, deal with your feelings, relax, and regain control of your body, you will see that pain does not need to be the centre of your life. You can choose to focus on your abilities, not your disabilities. You will grow stronger in your belief that you can live a normal life in spite of chronic pain. You also need to realize that your pain has not just affected you, but all those around you, especially your family. They actually experience the same life changes as you do. The only real difference between you and your family members when it comes to chronic pain is that they do not feel the physical pain. Keep that in mind as you begin your journey; share with your family what you are learning to help them cope with the changes in their life since your pain began.

## STEP 10: REACH OUT

It is estimated that one person in three suffers with some form of chronic pain. In the United States, both direct and indirect costs related to chronic pain amount to an estimated $250 billion a year in. It is an epidemic and one that cannot be ignored. There are millions of people like you who need to know that they are not alone. They need to know that their pain is real, that someone understands what it is like to live in a body that looks "normal" yet is completely controlled by pain. It is up to each of us to reach out to others, to invite them to come along on the journey from patient to person. We do not have all the answers, we cannot take away their pain, but hopefully we can help them to help themselves to reduce their sense of suffering and improve the quality of their life. Living with chronic pain is an ongoing learning experience. We all support and learn from each other.

# LIVING WITH COMPLEX REGIONAL PAIN SYNDROME (CRPS): A TESTIMONIAL

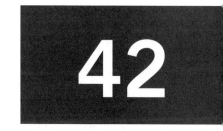

## 42

**Helen Small** BA, BEd, St. Catharines, Ontario, Canada
Executive director, PARC: Promoting Awareness of RSD/CRPS in CANADA

www.rsdcanada.org

*"Self healing is the privilege of every human being."*
Yogi Bhajan

## ABSTRACT

Having complex regional pain syndrome (CRPS) can be frightening, confusing and just plain difficult. This chapter is a guide to finding your way once you are diagnosed. Little is known about how to successfully treat this mysterious disease. As a 20-year veteran of the CRPS wars, valuable insight is offered to CRPS patients and their family who struggle to comprehend the puzzling changes in their loved ones. Various alternative therapies, exercise, pain issues and coping strategies are offered along with my personal journey from pain patient to Executive Director of Promoting Awareness of RSD and CRPS in Canada (PARC: www.rsdcanada.org). My deepest hope is that this chapter be beneficial to CRPS patients and all readers who live with pain, and whose sheer determination has shown me the potential and power of the human spirit.

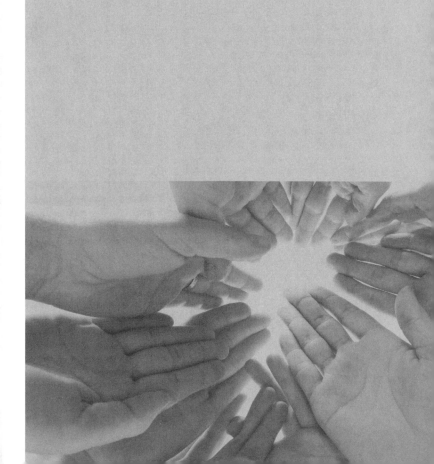

# 1. INTRODUCTION TO COMPLEX REGIONAL PAIN SYNDROME

Conventional medicine does not have all the answers for complex regional pain syndrome (CRPS). It is still slowly unravelling its mysteries. We don't know why some people develop CRPS and some don't. Why do some cases spontaneously resolve? Why do some people have very severe cases in spite of the best treatment? Why do some treatments work for one person, and not for the other? Why do some people get CRPS after an injury, and some don't? (See **Chapter 4**.)

Progress is being made in many areas: diagnostic criteria, treatments, and developing new tests. However, we still have many mysteries to solve. In the meantime, how do we as patients cope and manage the illness each day?

This chapter presents suggestions in finding medical help, choosing therapies best suited for you, focusing on you, and finding coping strategies. Many pain issues will also be discussed.

Life is not just about existing, but living, and you can still have a life even with CRPS. There is a major upheaval in your life when you get such an illness. Many things change medically, socially and emotionally. Financial and legal issues surface, work and home situations change. It is not easy; often you stumble and fall. Change happens quickly, or not quickly enough. There is so much to absorb when you are first diagnosed, and so many people to meet.

# 2. FINDING MEDICAL HELP

The first place to start is to find a general practitioner who will listen to you and be open to receiving CRPS information. Doctors with a good heart will help even if they do not know about CRPS. Others may take the time to learn. Unfortunately, not all doctors have the time or inclination to learn. If you feel uncomfortable, or your questions are ignored, switch doctors. Find one you are comfortable with and who is willing to work with you. The doctors are the quarterbacks. They call the plays. It is essential to develop a good relationship with them. Approach the relationship as an important collaboration between you and the doctor. Work together.

Quite often patients will copy a huge amount of information for the doctor who really does not have the time to read it. Start with a summary page about CRPS. Each subsequent visit you can bring another page relevant to your situation. Ask yourself what you want out of your patient appointment. Planning ahead for each appointment will help you get the most of your visit.

## PLANNING A MEDICAL APPOINTMENT

- Start a pain diary.
- Supply a list of medications and treatments. Indicate results of each.
- Supply test results ahead of time or bring with you.
- Answer questions about pain. (OPQRST)

OPQRST refers to pain questions about:
**O**nset: when did the pain start?
**P**rovokes: what makes it better or worse?
**Q**uality: what does it feel like? Describe the pain.
**R**adiates: does the pain travel?
**S**ite: where do you feel the pain?
**T**iming: when do you get pain (morning, afternoon, evening) and how long does it last?

- Respect the time given by the doctor. Edit your story: mention symptoms and include relevant information.
- Write questions ahead of time. Allow time for the doctor to answer. If someone is accompanying you to the appointment, have him/her record the doctor's answers.

Source: Dillard, J. M.D. The Chronic Pain Solution, Bantam, 2002.

Next, a tougher job, is finding a good pain management doctor or one with an interest in CRPS. Check with your local medical school, Canadian Pain Society, local teaching hospital or pain clinic, or call PARC for this information. Verify qualifications of doctors with medical associations or through official medical Web sites. Quite often the local support group can also supply some names of doctors. It is helpful if the pain specialist is open to integrative medicine, which is combining conventional medicine and alternative treatment.

Pain education in Canada is fragmented. The Canadian Pain Society survey found that doctors receive an average of 19 hours of pain training in medical school whereas veterinarians receive 98 hours. Nevertheless, specialities like anaesthesia, rehabilitation (physiatry), neurology and psychiatry deal with pain. Make sure the doctor is board certified, and that they treat pain specifically.

Rarely does anyone know a great deal about CRPS when they are first diagnosed, so consider it your job to learn. Replace fear of the unknown about CRPS with concrete knowledge about what CRPS is, and how it behaves and affects you personally. CRPS affects everyone differently and effectively communicating with your family about what you have learned immediately includes them in the loop. Often spouses do not understand the illness simply because it was never explained to them. Getting family support and advocacy comes from good communication and understanding of the illness. Family may avoid the illness, marriages are tested by it, and relationships can deteriorate. Initial support is the key to the newly diagnosed patient making any progress. Support is the foundation on which the patient builds their self-management program.

# 3. THERAPIES

Pain is often too complicated to treat with one therapy. Use a combination of therapies that can work together. Assemble your own medical support team. Pain affects you physically, mentally and emotionally, so a variety of therapies can address each aspect of pain. Some therapies work in conjunction with each other to have a synergistic effect.

The following therapies have been found to be helpful. Everyone is different and therapies will work for some people and not for others. Do what works for you.

- Acupuncture
- Aqua therapy or physical therapy, mirror therapy
- Autogenic training: biofeedback
- Chiropractic
- Chronic pain diet
- Cognitive behaviour therapy (CBT)
- Craniosacral Therapy
- Exercise program (graded)
- Homeopathy
- Massage
- Music
- Myofascial release or trigger point therapy
- Naturopathic medicine
- Nutrition
- Photon therapy (laser)
- Psychological support
- Qi Gong
- Relaxation techniques: e.g. progressive muscle relaxation, guided imagery, meditation
- Sleep hygiene
- Stretching program
- Support group or network
- Yoga, pilates

Discuss with your doctor which therapies you'd like to try. Be open to anything reasonable, safe and non-invasive.

You can start with an easy therapy, determine its effectiveness and gradually add another therapy. Use small steps. Look for slow improvements, and do not expect instant cures. You can try a combination of therapies. Various therapies in different intensities and frequencies can be very helpful. Adapt, improvise, or adjust therapies if needed.

## KEEPING A THERAPY AND ACTIVITY JOURNAL

The next step is to keep a therapy and activity journal. In a notebook, make four vertical columns on each page: date/time, pain level, recent activities, action taken/ results. This journal is a good tool to fight pain.

Keeping a journal helps you to think and discover patterns. It will help you identify triggers, what eases pain, and what aggravates it. It helps you identify when you feel best and why, when you feel worst and why, what you can do about it, what action you have taken and what was the result.

---

**Make a chart of seven vertical columns on a sheet of paper. Print a title for each one.**

- Therapy
- Goal of therapy
- Dosage taken or frequency used
- Length of trial
- Results
- Side effects
- Is it worthwhile to continue this therapy?

Source: Dillard, James MD, The Chronic Pain Solution, Bantam 2002, p. 76

---

## EXERCISE

If someone with chronic pain does not exercise, the consequences are not as serious as if it was a CRPS patient. For the CRPS patient, exercise is particularly difficult not only due to pain but to a lack of oxygen in the skeletal muscle, as found in studies, making exercise difficult for some. There are also serious movement issues (dystonia) unique to CRPS that may result if exercise is not done. (See **Chapters 23, 24, 25, 28, 35, 36,** and **37.**)

**Most long term patients find exercise to be one of the most important parts of their success.**

# 4. FOCUSING ON YOU

**"You are the CEO of your own life".**
E. Covington, Cleveland Clinic

You are the CEO of your own life and, even though doctors are medical experts, you have the power to make decisions for yourself given the medical input that you need. Your doctor is your partner in your medical care. Make informed choices in your medical care by educating yourself on the options. To self-manage an illness you need to take charge, be proactive, and make informed choices. CRPS is a tough, uphill mental battle.

Once you have been diagnosed and you have read up on CRPS, you may fall into the trap of believing everything you read: that CRPS is progressive, everyone will be totally disabled and very ill. The truth is that there are mild, moderate and severe cases of CRPS, and everyone is different. For some, the disease does not progress, and for some it does. If this worry is present in your daily life, every day it will cause more stress, and elevate your pain. Why add more stress?

Changing your way of thinking is critical to success. Positive thinking is desperately needed early on in your journey toward recovery. Focusing on your goals and dreams is more uplifting than focusing on your pain. Pain is still there but it will be on the sidelines if you set your sights on your goals. Negative thinking is prevalent in chronic pain. If you can, recognize what your negative thinking pattern is and learn to re-frame your thoughts. If others see this negative thought process happening or you know that you can't help yourself, there are psychologists who will guide you. It is called cognitive behaviour therapy and is very successful for chronic pain or CRPS.

**"What you think can disable you."**
E. Covington, Cleveland Clinic

# 5. PAIN ISSUES

People who live with CRPS have to deal with many pain issues and often feel that no one understands the challenges they face. But many people with CRPS have shared their experiences about the issues addressed in this section.

### Finding a balance
While you live with pain, you are in survival mode, and you do what you need to do to get through each day. You are forced to focus on your diagnosis, treatments, management and doctor's visits. Survival mode is often interpreted as selfishness, not thinking about others in the family. It is hard to find a balance between looking after yourself and taking care of others. Make a conscious effort to consider others as well as yourself.

### Understanding pain
Some people will never understand what it is like to experience pain. Some will eventually understand if you have the time and patience to educate them. Some will never take the time to listen and have no frame of reference. Most comments are made out of ignorance and fear.

### Relationships
Having complex regional pain syndrome affects all relationships. For some, the primary relationship with the spouse or partner strengthens if the relationship is already on a solid footing. For others, an already rocky relationship can deteriorate and crumble. A counsellor can help both parties understand what it is like to deal with pain and disability.

Most of us have a few good friends we can count on for help and support, who really understand us and believe us when we say we have pain. Having someone to help is essential to managing the illness since the illness requires more time to manage than anything else.

### Social disbelief
People sometimes don't believe that pain is real. Pain is invisible. Many people won't believe you are in as much pain as you say you are. If your family does not believe your pain is real, then it must be dealt with.

### Entitlement
Nobody would have to suffer in a perfect world, but life isn't fair. People do suffer and at some point in our life we feel pain. Certainly we all deserve better but probably that will not happen.

### Self-blame
You may think you should be able to control your pain much better. If you are taking your pain medications as directed and participating in treatments, there is no need to blame yourself.

### From blaming to healing
Blaming others for your illness allows you to continue to focus on illness, disability and pain. Blaming allows you to shift the responsibility of taking care of your illness to another person or situation. You may be angry at what happened. However, prolonged anger places undue stress on the body, and you do not move forward. Blaming is an obstacle to healing. If you are blaming, you are not healing.

## Measuring progress against others' progress

Measuring yourself against others' progress is counterproductive and frustrating. As long as you are improving slowly and setting realistic goals in small steps, you are moving forward.

## Overactivity

People often conclude that their activity level is related to the severity of the pain. They push until they feel pain and have to stop. Then, due to the pain, they do nothing. This is the overactivity/inactivity cycle is a trap into which we can all fall. Too many of us use the "all or nothing" theory where we do it all and suffer or do nothing. Pacing and activity are part of the solution.

## Inactivity

Not moving or protecting the painful part of your body is a short-term solution to avoiding pain. However, long-term immobility causes problems. Doing what feels good now can cause more difficulty in the long term. Lack of movement will eventually contribute to weakness, muscle atrophy, more pain and less mobility. Consistent lack of movement can lead to no movement or lack of function of the entire limb. At a certain point the function cannot be restored.

## Personality and pain

Each personality deals with pain differently, based on their type and the traits they possess. If you know what your strengths are, you can use them to cope more effectively. Once identified, weaknesses can become your challenges. Counselling can help you deal with your pain more effectively.

## The magic bullet

There is no magic pill or treatment to cure pain. Spending time searching for the magic bullet is energy you could be using to recover. Solutions for pain are found on a trial and error basis.

## Re-injury

For CRPS patients, re-injury is a real possibility. Avoiding certain activities because you're afraid of re-injury can lead to disability. If you believe that the activity will cause injury, it can worsen pain. When pain increases, you continue to avoid activity and become physically deconditioned, and possibly disabled. What you think can disable you physically and emotionally. Worrying, being anxious about re-injury and negative thinking all contribute to pain. Not only are these thought patterns negative, they can interfere with your coping skills in daily life and dealing with real life situations.

# 6. COPING STRATEGIES

Some coping strategies presented here deal with your pain condition and everyday activities. You can develop your own strategies once you begin to look for solutions.

## Accept the situation

Acceptance is a central issue. Are you a CRPS patient or a patient with CRPS? What is the difference? A CRPS patient is a person whose illness is their life. A patient with CRPS is a person whose life includes illness, but living their life to the best of their ability is the focus, not the illness.

Adjusting to CRPS is a process. Having CRPS is a lot like the stages of grief.

    Denial: denying you have an illness.
    Blame: finding someone to blame
    Anger: at the world, people or the disease itself
    Bargaining: making a deal with yourself or God
    Acceptance: final acceptance of what you have

## Identify pain triggers

Keeping a daily journal will help you identify all triggers. Some triggers are very subtle and hard to discover unless a pattern emerges from writing and reading your journal.

If a pain suddenly increases, stop what you are doing, evaluate the situation and rest. It is not wise to push through the pain at this point since your body is giving you a warning signal. Pushing to complete what you are doing will only result in more pain. If you can find the source of the pain, perhaps it is a trigger that can be eliminated.

## Control your pain

It is easier to keep pain under control than it is to get it under control.

Pain is better controlled by taking pain medicine as directed. It is the best way of knowing if this medicine is working properly for you. Getting pain under control when it is an 8 or 9 out of 10 on the pain scale is much harder than taking pain medicine on a regular basis.

## Cope with flare-ups

Inevitably, people have flare-ups of CRPS. Have a plan in place for a flare-up. Pacing is often the key to avoiding flare-ups. Advance planning and pacing can improve matters, and help you minimize the effect of known triggers.

## Outwit pain with thoughts

Distract yourself from pain, for example, by listening to music or meditating.

## Save your energy

Often we waste our time on things that are not important. People with CRPS do not have much energy to spare so it is important to focus on what is truly essential, and what can wait. Break up the tasks you must do into several moments of the day or several days. Find ways to rest during the day such as after lunch or before dinner. Even if you do not sleep, the body is remaining calm and resting.

### Know your limits

By keeping a pain journal, you will discover your limits, and staying within them will avoid flare-ups. Listen to your body and you may receive warning signals before a pain flare-up.

### Plan ahead and pace yourself

When taking part in a special activity, decide if the activity is worthwhile. If so, plan ahead for a flare-up by having extra medications or breakthrough medicines on hand. Plan ahead. Pace yourself as much as possible by using the "activity/rest/activity/rest" cycle. Try to anticipate and head off any possible problems by breaking the activity into smaller steps. Set a goal and work toward it gradually. Remember to be flexible. If your pain is more severe on a given day, do more resting and less activity. Vary the activity/rest cycle according to how you feel that day. The important thing to remember is to actively move each day.

### Join a support group

Support can come from a support group through online chat or groups, or even a local group meeting. Participants learn from each other and talk about treatments and therapies. They take comfort in the feeling that someone really understands them. Staying positive and working toward better treatment outcomes is the focus of the group. Humour is also appreciated.

It is essential to share with others what works for you. In return, others will gain knowledge from you and also share with you. There is a reciprocity that happens here, which forms a bond of friendship. There is comfort in knowing that there is someone who understands what it is like to be in pain. These bonds are strong and cannot be broken.

### Make anger work for you

It's okay to be angry when you have pain. Rather than take it out on your family or friends, use it to your advantage, in a constructive way. For example, channel anger into an activity or exercise program, or calm it with relaxation techniques.

### Learn from mistakes

We all make mistakes in our life, and we can learn form the mistakes of others: they are warnings to the rest of us. You will meet others with pain and see how they approach their pain management, what works for them, how you learn from their errors, and what can you learn from your own errors.

### Pick your battles

Fighting every battle that comes along drains the energy of a CRPS patient. Pick the battles that are important to you and that you need to fight and concentrate your energy on those situations.

### Stay positive

When pain is all that you experience, it is hard to stay positive all the time.

Here are some ideas to keep you going:
- **Be grateful for five things each day;**
- **Find the gift that comes with pain.** It may be that you are more compassionate with others or a better listener, learning to be patient, meeting new people who are supportive and caring, or making new friendships;
- **Use positive self-talk;**
- **Help others.** You have the power to help others in pain;
- **Volunteer your time in your community or with a charity;**
- **Find a positive support network;**
- **Stay focused.** Your goal is wellness and better quality of life.

### Don't give up!

This is probably the most important concept about coping with pain. Rest, recharge the batteries and start fresh tomorrow. Support from family and friends is essential when you feel yourself giving up.

### Ask for help

Most people have difficulty coping with the pain, limitations and changes in their lives, and often refuse to ask for help. Asking for help helps keep a positive focus.

### Share your story

Your story has power. It can hold the attention of the audience and be used to affect change. Your story can be the catalyst for change. Personal experience with pain is always an eye-opener for those who have not experienced it first hand.

## 7. CONCLUSION

Living with CRPS is a challenge. We learn by trial and error. We must expect that we will not always have success. Failure need not deter us from our goal. We change our approach, modify our thinking and find another goal. We have to get up again and start over and build on small successes. Remember that there is hope. Hope lives!

# MY STORY

**Helen Small** BA, BEd, St. Catharines, Ontario, Canada
Executive director, PARC: Promoting Awareness of RSD/CRPS in CANADA
www.rsdcanada.org

See other testimonial, page 386. See chapter 46, page 353)

In the summer of 1989, I was on summer holiday at my trailer, and opened an overhead cupboard door. Suddenly, a coffee jar fell on my left foot, and I forgot about it until I woke up a week later and couldn't walk. It was only a coffee jar! You can't have that much pain, can you?

The pain was out of proportion to my injury, the foot was swelling, the skin changed temperature and colour, and I was sweating profusely. I was now sensitive to noise and light and could not bear weight. My family doctor had no idea what I had, and sent me to the orthopedic doctor. He could not find anything wrong, and sent me to the rheumatologist who diagnosed me with Reflex Sympathetic Dystrophy (RSD), now known as complex regional pain syndrome (CRPS).

I received a series of painful injections between the toes and in the bone of the foot and I still couldn't walk. It made it worse. I didn't know that it was the wrong treatment, and valuable had time passed. I had a gut feeling that things were not right since there was no improvement. I convinced my doctor to refer me to a major university hospital clinic where they confirmed the diagnosis. I was referred to a physiatrist who specialized in CRPS. Finally, I received treatment quickly, but it was too late for complete recovery because too much time had passed.

I had to stop teaching, a job I loved but couldn't do anymore because I couldn't walk, was on crutches, and had constant pain and disability. I now had time to find out what this disease was, and which drugs and treatments were available to me. I found out that you have to be diagnosed early in the first three months with proper treatment for complete recovery.

I applied for a pension and spent many hours calling, faxing and sending letters for nearly a year with no result. I had no job and no money. One day I decided that enough was enough and drove 75 miles (120 km) in anger and considerable pain to the pension office with all my papers and told them I would be there until it was resolved. They stalled for three hours until I finally threatened with the "L" word: lawyer. The money appeared a week later.

I checked the Internet, and to my surprise, there is no organization in Canada that dealt with CRPS. Why not? In 1995, I started attending conferences to learn more about this mysterious disease. The word got around and people called me for advice. I eventually talked to over 500 people with CRPS, and found out that many were not believed, and treated as psychiatric patients. This was outrageous!

The phrase "my doctor doesn't know about it" was heard in every phone call I received. Why was that? I heard many stories about disbelief, pain, anger, disability and mistreatment. I was angry and decide to do something about it.

I learned more by attending conferences in Tampa, San Diego, Chicago, Orlando, Phoenix, Holland and Canada—14 conferences in 20 years — where I developed a network with leaders of CRPS groups, prominent doctors and researchers.

In 2002, along with an RSD friend, Barbara, I started a non-profit charitable organization called Promoting Awareness of RSD/CRPS in Canada (PARC). The charity developed a web site (www.rsdcanada. org) a PARC newsletter and a CRPS self-management program. I know what works for one does not work for everyone, but the list of ideas and advice is practical and based on a 20-year experience.

A survey confirmed what those 500 phone calls said was true: two out of three patients see three or more doctors before diagnosis and only 40% are diagnosed early. There is so much work to do!

# PATIENT ASSOCIATIONS IN CANADA, QUEBEC AND THE UNITED STATES

# CANADIAN PAIN COALITION (CPC)

**Lynn Cooper** BES, Oshawa, Ontario, Canada
President, Canadian Pain Coalition

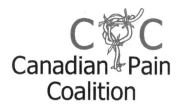

## 1. HISTORY

The Canadian Pain Coalition (CPC) is a partnership of people with pain groups, health professionals caring for people in pain and scientists studying more effective ways of managing pain. The CPC began in 2002 and was incorporated as a non-profit organization in 2004. It is a volunteer run organization.

## 2. CPC MISSION

The Canadian Pain Coalition is the national voice of people with pain, representing them at national government levels, partnering with professional and people in pain groups, and providing education about pain and pain management.

## 3. CPC VISION

The vision of the Canadian Pain Coalition is:
· To help people with pain have a better quality of life by providing information to them so they can make informed decisions, therefore better managing their pain and their self care;
· To have pain recognized nationally so that it is understood by decision makers as a key health issue that can be managed;
· To have people with pain involved in establishing research and health education priorities and to have the Canadian Pain Coalition at decision tables.

The CPC provides education about pain and pain management through sponsoring or hosting public events about pain, distributing print materials and, via the Pain Resource Centre, www.prc.canadianpain-coalition.ca. The Pain Resource Centre is a joint project of the CPC and the Canadian Pain Society that provides one central place on the web where Canadians can access resources and reliable information about pain and pain management.

## 4. PROMOTING PAIN AWARENESS

Since its inception, the CPC has promoted awareness of the pain issues in Canada. In 2003, the CPC created the "Charter of Person with Pain Rights and Responsibilities" which is an important document for awareness building. In 2004, the CPC secured, the Senate Declaration of National Pain Awareness Week as the first full week in November and has run yearly awareness activities surrounding this week. In 2007, the CPC partnered with the Canadian Pain Society and the Canadian Pain Foundation to create Painexplained.ca, a national pain awareness campaign.

## 5. SUPPORTING ITS MEMBERS

The CPC supports its member organizations though educational grants and provides information and updates to its membership via the e-newsletter and e-bulletins.

The CPC supports Canadians who live with pain by providing the person with pain perspective wherever decisions and policy are being made about pain care.

## 6. ACTIVE CPC VOLUNTEERS

The volunteers of the CPC, many of whom live with pain themselves, are dedicated to the sustained improvement in the diagnosis, treatment and management of all types of pain in Canada. For more information about the Canadian Pain Coalition visit www.canadianpaincoalition.ca or email: office@canadianpaincoalition.ca

## 7. COORDINATES

1143 Wentworth St. W.
Suite 202
Oshawa, ON, L1J 8P7
Office: T: 905-404-9545
Office: F: 905-404-3727

# ASSOCIATION QUÉBÉCOISE
## DE LA DOULEUR CHRONIQUE (AQDC)
### QUEBEC CHRONIC PAIN ASSOCIATION

**Jacques Laliberté**, St. Bruno, Quebec, Canada
Founding Director and volunteer president of the Association québécoise de la douleur chronique
**Line Brochu**, Quebec City, Quebec, Canada
Founding director and volunteer secretary of the Association québécoise de la douleur chronique

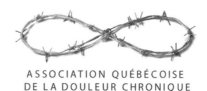

ASSOCIATION QUÉBÉCOISE
DE LA DOULEUR CHRONIQUE

## 1. *ASSOCIATION QUÉBÉCOISE DE LA DOULEUR CHRONIQUE* QUEBEC CHRONIC PAIN ASSOCIATION

### HISTORY

The *AQDC* held its first meeting in January 2004, thanks to the vision and dedication of Dr. Aline Boulanger. She was the driving force behind the first meeting of those who would become the founding directors of the *AQDC*. Nine of the founding members of the association, of the 12 directors on the board of directors, were individuals who suffered from chronic pain. These directors represented, as patients, the major pain clinics in Quebec. All of the founding members were volunteers who wanted to make a difference for people suffering from chronic pain.

Since 2005, the *AQDC* has represented Quebecers who suffer from chronic pain at the Canadian Pain Coalition (CPC), of which it is a member. It also serves on the advisory committee of that coalition.

The Association incorporated on September 23, 2005 and has been recognized as a charitable organization since the first quarter of 2005. (N/E 860295633RR0001)

After four years of public life, in 2010, the *AQDC* had over 4,000 members. More than 1.5 million pages on its Internet site (www.douleurchronique.org) are now consulted each year.

## 2. THE *AQDC*'S MISSION

To improve the condition and reduce the isolation of people suffering from chronic pain in Quebec.

## 3. THE *AQDC*'S OBJECTIVES

- To gather people suffering from chronic pain from all the regions of Quebec together within a single energetic and influential association;
- To make the public aware of chronic pain and inform them about the extremely harmful consequences that chronic pain may have on the patient, his/her loved ones and society;
- To make health professionals and the public aware that chronic pain is an illness;

- To ensure that pain is targeted as a priority in our health care system, and increase the funding provided substantially;
- To create different information tools to communicate with our members, and facilitate the dissemination of new knowledge in the field of pain;
- To communicate with the political authorities in order to improve the services provided to people suffering from chronic pain.

### THE *AQDC*'S LONG-TERM OBJECTIVES

- To increase the content dedicated to the evaluation, management and treatment of pain in educational institutions so that these notions are systematically taught to health care professionals working in the field (ex.: doctors, nurses, psychologists, physiotherapists, etc.);
- To improve first-line health care with regards to chronic pain, particularly with general practitioners;
- To substantially increase the number of centres and specialized clinics in the evaluation and multidisciplinary treatment of chronic pain;
- To substantially increase the financing granted for research in the field of pain in order to identify new strategies to not only treat chronic pain better, but also to prevent it;

- To organize fund-raising campaigns to support the association's activities, and bring financial support to chronic pain research.

### FUTURE VISION

- The *AQDC* is recognized by all stakeholders as the association that represents all Quebecers suffering from chronic pain. Its leadership is undisputed and it even serves as a model for other associations. If the past guarantees the future, its other projects will be brought to fruition in the near future. Thus, the *AQDC* will offer seminars on chronic pain and will train support groups in the regions of Quebec in 2010.

## 4. THE *AQDC*'S PUBLIC ACTIVITIES

The *AQDC* has fulfilled its objectives in recent years through its public activities, among other things, and in particular through its involvement with the *Réseau Universitaire en Santé (RUIS)* and the *Programme ACCORD*, its Internet site, and by granting clinical research bursaries.

### PARTICIPATION IN THE *RÉSEAU UNIVERSITAIRE INTÉGRÉ POUR LA SANTÉ (RUIS)*

Since 2008, the *AQDC* board members, representing the users, have attended meetings organized by the various groups that belong to the *Réseau universitaire intégré pour la santé (RUIS)* in order to take part in writing the first application for the certification of its chronic pain expertise centres; this includes the McGill University *RUIS*, the *RUIS Université de Montréal*, the *RUIS Université de Sherbrooke* and the *RUIS Université Laval*.

In 2010, the Quebec Minister of Health and Social Services signed designation letters for the four facilities that will form chronic pain expertise centres associated with the *RUIS* for the *Université de Montréal*, the *Université Laval*, the *Université de Sherbrooke* and *McGill University*.

### PARTICIPATION IN THE *PROGRAMME ACCORD*

Throughout 2008, the *AQDC* took part in developing the *Programme ACCORD*, chaired by Dr. Manon Choinière, PhD., who is a member of the *AQDC* Board of Directors. The *Programme ACCORD* is a research programme focused on the transfer of knowledge. The objective is to improve the condition of people suffering from chronic pain in Quebec. The Programme ACCORD brings together the efforts of more than 50 Quebec researchers who will ensure an improved and joint management

of chronic pain in Quebec. The *AQDC* represents people suffering from chronic pain in each segment of this vast research field.

### *AQDC* WEB SITE

The *AQDC* Web site and a pamphlet were created during the course of 2005 and 2006. Since 2010, the *AQDC* Web site has become the portal for several other chronic pain sites in Quebec. Among other things, it provides a pain resource centre and a large number of video-conferences.

News about developments in the field of pain is posted on the site regularly.

### CLINICAL RESEARCH BURSARIES

In order to fulfil its mission, the *AQDC* promotes, among other things, clinical training for health professionals through an annual clinical training bursary programme. This programme offers study bursaries so that health professionals (physicians, nurses, physiotherapists, occupational therapists, psychologists, pharmacists or others) can perfect their knowledge in the field of pain.

## 5. THE ADVANTAGES OF BECOMING AN *AQDC* MEMBER

One of the main advantages in becoming a member of the *AQDC* is avoiding isolation and knowing that there is an association that works for you and with you. The more members we have, the more they contribute collectively to the association's influence with all stakeholders and those who make decisions concerning chronic pain in Quebec and elsewhere.

**Membership is free.**

Members of the *AQDC* are:
- people suffering from chronic pain, no matter what its origin may be, and interested in promoting our objectives;
- family members or loved ones of people suffering from chronic pain;
- members of the medical or paramedic community and all others interested in chronic pain;
- all groups, collectives, incorporated or registered associations, all moral persons wishing to promote our objectives, having similar objectives to ours and wishing to be recognized as an *AQDC* supporter.

## 6. CONCLUSION

People suffering from chronic pain must not be passive when it comes to their pain. Self-management of pain is possible. The days when people could go to the doctor's office and say, "Doctor, I'm in pain. Do something!" are over. If necessary, we must make up our own treatment team, unless we have access to one in a multidisciplinary pain treatment centre.

As patients, we must take part in our healing and the way in which we react to pain is very important. The more we fear pain, the more pain we will feel since we will stop moving and our bodies will become less alert, lose their strength and isolation and depression will become omnipresent in our lives.

Therefore, it is very important to continue doing exercise and to take part in activities that are very beneficial for us: walking, even for short periods of time, increasing the duration through small, attainable objectives, reading, yoga, visualization, volunteer work for people who need us, regardless of our condition, etc. Pain must not be a focus of attention, because that causes our health problems and our psychological distress to increase.

As a result of the aging of the population, the incidence of pain or chronic discomfort will increase 70% over next 20 years. In 2010, more than 1,500,000 people suffered from chronic pain in Quebec.

The *AQDC* is not qualified to provide medical advice, but we do tell people who are suffering from chronic pain to take charge of their pain, to refuse to accept that they are not believed, to refuse to let people say no to them, to accept the aid that is offered to them, and to never give up until they are satisfied with the treatments they are offered. People who suffer chronic pain should not wait to be evaluated and treated.

# ThE PRESENT MOMENT

Lucie Moisan, St-Eustache, Quebec, Canada

(See other testimonials, pages 136 and 174.)

> «The present moment is a frail bridge. If you weigh it down with yesterday's regrets and tomorrow's concerns, the bridge will give way, and you will fall.»
>
> Sister Odette Prévost, sister of Charles de Foucault, assassinated in Algeria on November 10, 1995 Translated from: http://blogdelapaix.over-blog.com (In French only)

As time passes, I understand more and I grow more. I wanted to fight for a past that was no longer and a future that didn't exist. I was looking back; I was looking ahead. However, I had forgotten the most important thing: The present moment. People say that today is a gift, and that's why we call it the present moment. Saying goodbye to the past is never easy, but sometimes it's an essential part of fulfilment.

Life led me along a very particular path for a certain time. That period of my existence opened my eyes, helped me to progress and to reinforce my beliefs in my priorities. It caused me to discover how peaceful it is to live in the present moment. It also made me realize that being there for someone is priceless, intangible, made up of pure sentiments, a gift of one's self. There can be a lot of joy in making others happy despite our own situation. The grief that we share reduces and divides the pain while shared happiness can only multiply. If we only counted the things that cannot be bought, we would feel immensely richer. We feel so happy when we create a little warmth and comfort around us, when we can relieve someone's suffering or pain. A person's beauty is not what they reflect outward, but what their heart beholds.

Time is a priceless gift and I have learned that we must live and appreciate the present moment. No one can predict the future; changes arrive unannounced. So, let's savour all the seconds that life gives us and remember to live them fully.

# CHRONIC PAIN ASSOCIATION
## OF CANADA (CPAC)

**Barry D. Ulmer**, Executive Director, Chronic Pain Association of Canada, Edmonton, Alberta, Canada

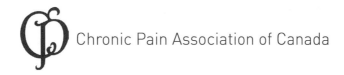 Chronic Pain Association of Canada

## 1. CHRONIC PAIN: A CANADIAN REALITY

Adequate treatment of pain is essential to alleviate suffering, yet studies show that patients with chronic pain often receive inadequate pain relief. The large number of conditions, which include pain as part of the illness, and the number of personal experiences of chronic pain sufferers, indicate that the problem of chronic pain in our society is far greater than we realize. Studies have shown the incidence of chronic pain in our society ranges from 16 to 44% of our population and causes untold suffering, as well as a huge financial expense to our health care system.

Although universally acknowledged, pain is experienced in ways that vary with ethnicity, gender, age, social class, and condition. The implications to health care are obvious. If culture is a lens through which the world is perceived and understood, each refraction will depend on the particular prism employed. People bring their culturally determined values, behaviours and biases to all consequential experiences, especially interpersonal encounters. The meaning pain holds for sufferers

and those attending them determines the intensity with which it is perceived and the response it generates. Substantial differences among patients, families, and caregivers in their perceptions of and reactions to pain affect the ways pain is expressed, the ways in which relief is requested, and how it is administered.

The importance of decision-making is nowhere more striking than in the health care setting. Issues of control and choice, influenced by cultural background, current illness, perceived obligations, and education are brought into sharp focus as people from different vantage points grapple with complex and emotion-laden dilemmas. Ultimately, the pain experience must be accepted as what the patient says it is, and compassion must speak in the most forceful and universal tongue to relieve pain.

## 2. PAIN FACTS

Millions of Canadians suffer from chronic pain. Surveys indicate over 18% of Canadians suffer from severe chronic pain. At any given moment, half of all Canadians will have experienced some kind of pain. A majority of Canadians experience head pain at least monthly. People suffering from chronic pain do not receive adequate treatment. While over 70% of cancer patients experience moderate to severe pain during their illness, fewer than half receive adequate pain relief. A study at one large medical centre found that the majority of patients who were in moderate to severe pain were not even asked by their doctors or nurses if they were having pain.

Pain is devastating to individuals and families. When pain persists at these levels, a persons entire life becomes impacted. It becomes difficult to concentrate, to remember things, to perform routine tasks, to think about anything except the pain. Lost wages and medical costs are often financially devastating to many people. One of the most common reasons that people buy books on suicide and physician assisted suicide, is the fear of living in severe intractable pain.

Pain is costly to society. The annual cost of chronic pain, including medical expenses, lost income, and lost productivity, but not the social costs, is estimated to exceed $10 billion.

Most pain is treatable. According to many experts, 90% of cancer pain can be relieved through relatively simple means. The truth is that fewer than half of cancer patients get adequate treatment for pain. A recent survey in the Medical Post indicated that 55% of physicians in Canada felt their peers were not doing enough to treat cancer pain.

Most pain is under treated. One recent study of chronic pain patients involved in litigation concluded that the overall rate of inaccurate or incomplete diagnosis at time of referral was 40 to 67%. In a large survey of oncologists, 86% of respondents felt that the majority of patients with pain were under treated. Another study indicated that only 30% of practising neurologists felt adequately trained to treat the entire spectrum of pain disorders. In general, the lack of medical training in pain management and the uneasiness of both healthcare providers and patients to deals with pain leads to widespread under treatment of both acute and chronic pain.

Most pain sufferers are under medicated. Although 91% of respondents in a recent survey believe prescription medication is effective in relieving pain, 2 out of 3 said that when they are in "fairly serious" pain they avoid taking pain medication until they really can not bear the pain. Research clearly indicates this only serves to worsen the pain.

Pain is stigmatized by society. Patients and healthcare professionals are embarrassed about pain, reluctant to acknowledge and talk about it candidly, thus they are often judgemental and ineffectual in dealing, or in managing pain. Society has taught us that we should "learn to live with it" or "it will make you a better person". No one should ever have to suffer unbearable pain for even short periods of time.

## 3. THE CHRONIC PAIN ASSOCIATION OF CANADA (CPAC)

The Chronic Pain Association of Canada (CPAC) is a not-for-profit charitable consumer association with the primary goals of advancing the treatment and management of chronic pain and encouraging the development of research projects to promote the discovery of a cure for this disease. The education of pain patients, health professionals and the general public are the primary means of accomplishing these goals.

## 4. CPAC HISTORY

### Position statement

CPAC grew out of a need for change and support for people suffering from chronic pain. In the mid 1980's, a small group of individuals met in a physician's office, and after discovering that they were all there for the same reason, decided to meet together and support each other in their struggle to survive the nightmare of constant pain. As the meetings progressed, it was decided that change must happen in the acceptance and the treatment of the very real pain that people had. Efforts were put forward on an ad hoc basis over the next few years. Because most of the people in the group suffered from pain, it was very hard to maintain a persistent and productive level of work.

It was decided in 1993, that the Association should incorporate as a not for profit society and register as an official charity. This was accomplished with the assistance of close family members. Efforts then increased in contacting various medical professionals, government departments and others who could help us reach our goals. The work carried out by the Chronic Pain Association of Canada has been done primarily by volunteers, most of who suffer with pain, with the help of one full-time executive director. Some of our initiatives and successes are listed below.

- We have successfully convinced the Faculty of Medicine and Oral Health at the University of Alberta to include the diagnosis and treatment of chronic pain in the new curriculum starting in 1999.
- We have, through the support of the Edmonton Community Foundation, written a comprehensive *Support Group Manual* that is used by support groups formed under our association.
- We have successfully held over 40 Chronic Pain Awareness and Education Forums in the Edmonton and surrounding areas, and over 3,500 people have attended these forums.
- We have successfully networked with other groups to help inform their members of all the methods available to help manage pain.
- We have developed relationships with medical research groups, clinicians, and practitioners around the world, to increase our knowledge about chronic pain.
- We have initiated contacts with Health Canada to develop a means of influencing all teaching facilities in Canada, to adopt the new curriculum which the University of Alberta has begun.
- We have initiated contacts with Alberta Health to work with our association to improve the area of pain education.
- We have contacted the regulatory bodies to begin a partnership to create awareness about the need to properly treat people in chronic pain.
- We are working within the regions to establish complete multidisciplinary pain management centres.
- We have developed a speaker's bureau and speak regularly to service clubs and other groups who request information concerning chronic pain.
- We worked with the Department of Continuing Medical Education to develop continuing education seminars to help those physicians seeking to improve their knowledge about chronic pain management.
- Lately, we have worked with the Canadian Pain Society, who have developed and published an excellent Position Statement on Pain Relief. We have forwarded this paper to all the Medical Boards and Associations in Canada. We encouraged them to take it to their members and discuss adopting the principles in this statement.

### CPAC's position statement on pain relief

- Almost all acute and cancer pain can be relieved, and many patients with chronic non-malignant pain can be helped. Patients have the right to the best pain relief possible.
- Unrelieved acute pain complicates recovery. Unrelieved pain after surgery or injury results in more complications, longer hospital stays, greater disability and potential long-term pain.
- Routine assessment is essential for effective management. Pain is a subjective and highly variable experience. Therefore patient's self-report of pain should be used whenever possible. For patients unable to report pain, a nonverbal assessment method must be used. Health professionals have a responsibility to assess pain routinely, to believe patients' reports, and to document pain reports, and to intervene in order to prevent pain.
- The best pain management involves patients, families, and health professionals. Patients and families must be informed that they have a right to the best pain relief possible and encouraged to communicate the severity of their pain. Patients, families and health professionals need to understand pain management strategies, including non-pharmacological techniques and the appropriate use of opioids.

While we are very proud of these initiatives and accomplishments, we know that there is still much work to be done. There is still the trend of dealing with chronic pain and its subsequent disability by denying its reality. We will continue to work towards meeting our goals and ensuring that the condition of chronic pain does not remain in the dark, does not continue to destroy lives and that sufferers of chronic pain can find the help they need. Short changing people when they are the most vulnerable should not be the way pain is handled.

## 5. MISSION STATEMENT

**CPAC is a non-profit consumer association with two primary goals:**

1. The advancement of the treatment and management of chronic intractable pain;
2. The development of research projects to promote the discovery of a cure for this disease.

Education of both the health care community and the public will be the primary means of accomplishing our mission.

We do not recommend any one treatment. We do promote the education of all the options concerning pain management so you and your doctor can make the best choice for you.

### CPAC GOALS

- To advance the treatment and management of chronic pain.
- To increase the understanding of how pain affects the lives of those who suffer and use this understanding to improve their quality of life.
- To educate all who are involved in the field of pain management; patient, caregivers, families, friends, employers, and co-workers.
- To develop partnerships between patients and caregivers.
- To ensure patients realize their responsibilities within the partnership of pain management.

### CPAC'S MAJOR ACTIVITIES

- To provide a meeting place for the consideration and discussion of questions concerning pain that affects the interests of the community.
- To provide information to the general public concerning the treatment of chronic pain.
- To work towards establishing multidisciplinary pain centres that use all the methods of treating and managing pain.
- To improve the way the medical profession is educated about the treatment and management of pain.

### PATIENT SUPPORT GROUPS

### Support group statement of purpose

The Chronic Pain Association of Canada support groups will offer those suffering from chronic pain the opportunity to improve their quality of life and knowledge of all the treatments that are available to help manage their pain. The support groups will end the isolation of sufferers by showing that they may rely on others like themselves for understanding and help. Through their personal knowledge and experience, the gathering of information, and the advocacy of education and research, members will improve their quality of life and ultimately change how all sufferers are treated. These support groups are a key to promote self-management treatment therapies for people in pain and help insure they are part of their own pain management team. CPAC develops and supports patient support groups across Canada. (See **Chapter 50**.)

## 6. CPAC PROFILE

CPAC is a grass roots organization that has grown because of a desperate need for relief of chronic pain. Thousands of humans are crying in agony with unrelenting pain that has no end. With the proper education and the most up to date treatment, there is no need to suffer so much.

**After all, patients have the right to:**
- Have their pain treated;
- Be believed;
- Be treated with respect;
- Have access to all the best possible technology in pain management;
- Know about all the pain management options so they can make best decisions for their own pain;
- Live with the least amount of pain possible.

## 7. COORDINATES

**The Chronic Pain Association of Canada (CPAC)**
Suite 7 – 10329, 61 Avenue
Edmonton, Alberta
Canada T6H 1K9

**Postal address**
PO Box 66017 Heritage Postal Station, #130
2323-111 Street Edmonton
AB, T6J 6T4
Canada

**If you have any questions:**
Please contact our office between 9:00 am and 4:00 pm Monday to Friday.
Tel: (780) 482-6727
Fax: (780) 433-3128
Email: cpac@chronicpaincanada.com
Website: www.chronicpaincanada.com
Executive Director: Barry D. Ulmer

# PARC: PROMOTING AWARENESS
# OF RSD AND CRPS IN CANADA

**Helen Small** BA, BEd, St. Catharines, Ontario, Canada
Executive director, PARC: Promoting Awareness of RSD/CRPS in Canada

www.rsdcanada.org

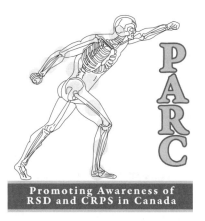

**Promoting Awareness of
RSD and CRPS in Canada**

## 1. MISSION

The mission of PARC (Promoting Awareness of RSD and CRPS in Canada) is to support, educate and inform persons with Reflex Sympathetic Dystrophy (RSD) (otherwise known as Complex Regional Pain Syndrome - CRPS), the community and the medical professionals treating RSD/CRPS about the utmost importance of early diagnosis and treatment. The suffering of those afflicted must also be recognized.

## 2. WHAT WE DO

· Offer support, information and encouragement to CRPS patients, their family and friends.
· Promote awareness of CRPS through education and disseminate information at educational events.
· Assist patients in finding doctors and healthcare practitioners who have treated and managed CRPS.
· Support research into the causes, controls and cures for CRPS.

## 3. CRPS PATIENTS: VICTIMS OF IGNORANCE

PARC began forming in late 1990's in the minds of two Canadian CRPS patients: Barbara Barry and myself. We both had long-term CRPS, and were acutely aware of unjust treatment of CRPS patients. Too many times we were told, "It's all in your head." We were aware of the negative atti-tudes surrounding psychological issues, lack of awareness, and a pervasive belief in the medical community that CRPS did not exist. Many patients had difficulty convincing their doctor that it was a real disease, intense pain was involved, disability could follow, early treatment was needed and early diagnosis would ensure a good prognosis for patients. However, this rarely happened due to lack of knowledge about the disease. Those afflicted with CRPS were the victims of ignorance.

In addition, Workplace Safety and Insurance Board (WSIB, Ontario, Canada) and insurance claims for CRPS went unrecognized. Often patients with an early diagnosis were left untreated or treatment was delayed, and came too late to be effective.

Early diagnosis is occurring more often in recent years, but still not often enough. Most doctors do not know that early treatment is essential for success. A PARC survey found that 66% of patients saw 3 or more doctors before diagnosis. The survey also found that 3 out of 5 patients were diagnosed in first year, and that only 30% were diagnosed in the first 3 months, when the success rate for treatment is the highest. The overall success (self-rating) was rated as 50%, or less by 2 out of 3 patients. When asked to rate their current status, 63% said their CRPS was worse.

## 4. AWARENESS

Awareness of CRPS was the first goal of PARC, and remains just as important to this day. Distributing information continues to be one of PARC's main ways to promote awareness.

To promote awareness of CRPS, PARC offers:
- **An information package** to each patient and professional who requests it;
- **A help line** where we answer countless calls for information, advice and support. We assist patients in finding doctors and healthcare practitioners that treat and manage CRPS. We give non-medical advice on how to cope each day;
- **The Pocket Card**, a wallet card for patients featuring warning signs and symptoms that encourage early diagnosis, which is instrumental in educating about CRPS;
- **A DVD** featuring Drs. Pollett, Rhydderch and Shulman, three excellent pain-management doctors who treat CRPS in their daily practice. The DVD eliminates the confusion surrounding CRPS diagnosis and treatment, and provides a clear path of understanding for doctors and other healthcare professionals;
- **A self-management program for CRPS** when members join PARC. It treats many aspects of the condition and life with CRPS, including examples of combinations of traditional and alternative medicine treatments that have proven effective. Based on 20 years' experience and 14 CRPS conferences, the program provides a firm basis from which each person can develop their own strategies to cope with CRPS;
- **The PARC Web site**, which was launched in 1999. It has grown into an extensive site full of information on the latest news about CRPS, conferences, survival tips, research and current CRPS information from all corners of the world. In 2002, when PARC officially became a non-profit organization, more people visited and gleaned information from its pages. The site continues to be updated and new information is added as it happens. Through the site, PARC has been able to reach thousands of people diagnosed with CRPS, giving them the assistance they need. PARC is a CRPS portal;
- **Seminars** offered since 2005. PARC began holding events in the Niagara and Toronto areas to educate the public and professionals. PARC has also spoken in front of Rotary and Lions clubs and local groups;
- **Participation in conferences.** PARC takes part in national chronic pain conferences and events to raise awareness of chronic pain and CRPS. Since 1995, PARC has also attended 14 CRPS conferences, and shares new developments with everyone;
- **Financial contributions to research on CRPS.** PARC has donated funds to researchers at McGill University (Montreal, Quebec) who are studying CRPS. PARC continues to raise funds every year;
- **The RIDE TO CONQUER CRPS 2008**, organized by PARC, where Dr. David L. Shulman, a chronic pain specialist and triathlete, took time from his busy practice to travel the 3,767 km from Ontario to St. John's, Newfoundland (Canada), by bike in 21 days. Along the way, he promoted awareness of CRPS and spoke at a CRPS seminar at Montreal General Hospital (Quebec) along with researchers from McGill University. Funds from this ride were also donated to McGill research;
- **To offer training for health professionals, our next goal.**

The PARC survey revealed that 66% of patients saw 3 or more doctors prior to diagnosis and a mere 19% of patients saw only 1 doctor before diagnosis. After one year, 1 in 4 still had not been diagnosed. Moreover, the average time between onset and diagnosis of CRPS is 30 months. These facts are inexcusable, and point toward lack of education about CRPS in the medical community. There is confusion about how to diagnose, treat and manage CRPS. Many clinicians still refuse to believe it exists. That is why PARC's aim is to educate every doctor in Canada on this disease and make it as recognizable as diabetes or heart disease. It is our hope that more patients will be diagnosed early, thereby avoiding the suffering from CRPS and ensuing lifetime of pain.

**PARC is the "small charity with big dreams.**

# ASSOCIATION QUÉBÉCOISE
# **DE LA FIBROMYALGIE (AQF)**
## QUEBEC FIBROMYALGIA ASSOCIATION

Élisabeth Marion, AQF, Quebec, Canada

## 1. HISTORY

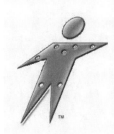

The *Association québécoise de la Fibromyalgie* (*AQF* - Quebec Fibromyalgia Association) was founded in 1989. The first directors were: Ms. Marguerite-Rose Pesant-Bédard, patient; Mr. Paul-André Pelletier, Rhumatologist; Ms. Bernadette Picard, patient.

## 2. MISSION

Since it was founded, the primary mission of the *AQF* has been to make the general public aware of this disease by defending the collective rights of patients from various regions of Quebec. Each of the regions accredited by the provincial association has a mission to support people with this disease by organizing activities, providing written and visual information, holding conferences, as well as through any other activity that could satisfy the expectations of patients.

In the future, the *AQF* wants to create a sense of belonging to the cause of fibromyalgia using all means possible and uniting the efforts of all associations around the organization's mission.

## 3. ROLE

The role of the association is to support people suffering from fibromyalgia, provide information about this disease and prepare activities for patients.

## 4. SPECIFIC CODE

The *Association québécoise de la Fibromyalgie* is an organization that works to defend the collective rights of people suffering from this syndrome. It has been in operation since April 1989, when it was incorporated, and the organization now covers five regions.

Other groups representing people with fibromyalgia are located throughout the province. These associations are autonomous by choice, but they also provide assistance to people with fibromyalgia. As you may note, fibromyalgia affects all regions in the province of Quebec. It also affects all levels of society and particularly women, since out of ten people diagnosed with this disease, nine are women.

This syndrome has serious consequences for the person suffering from it, ranging from loss of employment, unrecognized disability, impoverishment, depression, isolation, etc.

The *Association québécoise de la Fibromyalgie* has taken steps with the *Ministère de la santé et des Services sociaux* (Quebec) to implement a SPECIFIC CODE for the syndrome of fibromyalgia that would complement the existing International Classification of Diseases (CM10).

## 5. COORDINATES

**Association québécoise de la Fibromyalgie**
208-333 Lacombe Boulevard
Le Gardeur, Quebec J5Z 1N2 (Canada)
Telephone: 450 582-3075 or 1-866-582-3075
Fax: 450 582-0674
Email: aqf@aqf.ca
Web site: www.aqf.ca (in French only)

# 6. USEFUL LINKS

**Association québécoise de la fibromyalgie**
333, boul. Lacombe, suite 208
Le Gardeur (Québec) J5Z 1N2
Telephone : 450 582-3075 Toll-free : 1-866-582-3075
Fax : 450 582-0674
Email : aqf@aqf.ca
Web site : www.aqf.ca

**Association de la fibromyalgie de l'Estrie**
1013, rue Galt Ouest
Sherbrooke (Québec) J1H 1Z9
Telephone : 819 566-1067
Fax : 819 566-0111
Email : fmestrie@aide-internet.org
Web site : www.fibromyalgie.ca

**Association de la fibromyalgie Manicouagan/
Haute-Côte-Nord**
1250, rue Lestrat, bureau R-134
Baie Comeau (Québec) G5C 1T8
Telephone : 418 589-2229
Fax : 418 589-2229
Email : fibromyalgie.manicouagan@globetrotter.net

**Association de la fibromyalgie Mauricie/Centre-du-Québec**
109, rue Brunelle
Trois-Rivières (Québec) G8T 6A3
Telephone : 819 371-1458
Fax : 819 371-1736
Email : afmcq@videotron.ca
Web site : www.info-fibro.com

**Association de la fibromyalgie de la Montérégie**
1278, rue Papineau
Longueuil (Québec) J4L 3L1
Telephone : 450 928-1261
Toll-free : 1-888-928-1261
Fax : 450 670-7667
Email : fibromyalgiemonteregie@bellnet.ca

**Association fibromyalgie Saint-Eustache et Basses-Laurentides**
184, rue Saint-Eustache
Saint-Eustache (Québec) J7R 2L7
Telephone : 450 623-3574
Fax : 819 797-8874
Email : lfortiers@videotron.ca

**Association de la fibromyalgie de l'Abitibi-Témiscamingue**
380, avenue Richard, bureau 208
Rouyn-Noranda (Québec) J9X 4L3
Telephone : 819 797-0874
Fax : 819 797-8874
Email : afat@cablevision.qc.ca

**Association de la fibromyalgie du Bas-Richelieu**
71, De Ramesay, bureau 209
Sorel-Tracy (Québec) J3P 3Z1
Telephone : 450 730-0251

**Association de la Fibromyalgie du Bas-Saint-Laurent**
P.O. Box 252
Rimouski (Québec) G5L 7C1
Telephone : 418 724-5613
Email : fibro_bsl@hotmail.com
Web site : www.pages.globetrotter.net/fibro.bsl

**Association de la fibromyalgie des Bois-Francs**
P.O. Box 282
Victoriaville (Québec) G6P 6S9
Telephone : 819 752-4616

**Association de la fibromyalgie Chaudière/Appalaches**
81, rue Saint-Antoine, bureau 127
Sainte-Marie-de-Beauce (Québec) G6E 4B4
Telephone : 418 387-7379
Toll-free : 1-877-387-7379
Fax : 418 387-7379
Email : afrca-@hotmail.com
Site web : www.afrca.ca

**Association de la fibromyalgie de Duplessis**
690, boul. Laure, bureau 222-E
Sept-Îles (Québec) G4R 4N8
Telephone : 418 968-1999
Toll-free : 1-866-968-1999
Fax : 418 968-1999
Email : ass.fib.dup@globetrotter.net

**Association de la fibromyalgie Île-de-Montréal**
1140, rue Jean-Talon Est, bureau 300
Montréal (Québec) H2R 1V9
Telephone : 514 259-7306
Fax : 514 259-2526
Email : afim_mtl@yahoo.ca
Web site : www.afim.qc.ca

**Association de la fibromyalgie de Lanaudière**
144, rue Saint-Joseph, bureau 310
Joliette (Québec) J6E 5C4
Telephone : 450 755-1184
Toll-free : 1-888-223-0227
Fax : 450 755-1084
Email : arfl@citenet.net
Web site : www.fibromyalgielanaudiere.com

## 6. USEFUL LINKS (CONT'D)

**Association de la fibromyalgie des Laurentides**
723, rue Labelle
Saint-Jérôme (Québec) J7Z 5M2
Telephone : 450 569-7766
Fax : 450 569-7769
Email : afl@videotron.ca
Web site : www.fibromyalgie-des-laurentides.ca

**Association de la fibromyalgie de Laval**
1435, boulevard Saint-Martin ouest, bureau 301
Laval (Québec) H7S 2C6
Telephone : 450 933-1123
Fax : 450 933-1123
Email : info@fibromyalgielaval.org

**Association de la fibromyalgie de Québec**
840, Saint-Vallier Ouest, bureau 203
Québec (Québec) G1N 1C9
Telephone : 418 667-2224
Email : fibro.qc@oricom.ca
Web site : www.fibromyalgiequebec.info

**Association de la fibromyalgie Saguenay Lac-Saint-Jean**
605, rue Saint-Paul, bureau 309
Chicoutimi (Québec) G7J 3Z4
Telephone : 418 543-4959
Email : fibrosaglac@hotmail.com

**Association de la fibromyalgie Vaudreuil-Soulanges**
418, avenue Saint-Charles, bureau 305
Vaudreuil-Dorion (Québec) J7V 2N1
Telephone : 450 424-7722
Fax : 450 424-4810
Email : info@afsfc-vs.org
Web site : www.afsfc.vs-org

**Fédération québécoise de la fibromyalgie**
314, Chemin de la Côte-Sainte-Catherine
Outremont (Québec) H2V 2B4
Telephone : 514 259-7306
Fax : 514 259-2526
Email : fqf_@globetrotter.net
Web site : www.pages.globetrotter.net/fibro.bsl/fqf.htm

**Association québécoise de l'encéphalomyélite myalgique (AQEM)**
(Syndrome de fatigue chronique)
7400, boul. Les Galeries d'Anjou, bureau 410
Anjou (Québec) H1M 3M2
Telephone : 514 369-0386
Email : aqem@spg.qc.ca
Web site : www.aqem.org

**Association québécoise de la douleur chronique (AQDC)**
P.O. Box 61, Maison de la poste
Montréal (Québec) H3B 3J5
Telephone : 514 355-4198
Email : aqdc@douleurchronique.org
Web site : www.douleurchronique.org

## On grieving

Janice Sumpton, RPh, BSc Phm, London, Ontario, Canada

(See other testimonials, pages 194 and 222. See chapter 31, page 247.)

Accepting the "new me" takes time.
Grieving the loss of the "old me" is necessary.
I must remember that the soul of who I am has not changed.

# AMERICAN CHRONIC
# PAIN ASSOCIATION (ACPA)

**Penny Cowan,** Rocklin, California, USA,
Executive director, American Chronic Pain Association (ACPA)

*American Chronic Pain Association*

## 1. HISTORY

The American Chronic Pain Association (ACPA) was founded in 1980 by Penney Cowan, a person with chronic pain, in Pittsburgh (Pennsylvania, USA), and is now based in California (USA) with an international reach.

## 2. MISSION

- To facilitate peer support and education for individuals with chronic pain and their families so that these individuals may live more fully in spite of their pain; and

- To raise awareness among the health care community, policy makers, and the public at large about issues of living with chronic pain.

## 3. DISTINGUISHING CHARACTERISTICS

- The ACPA is the «voice» of real people with chronic pain; the only organization with direct contact with consumers;
- The ACPA offers a broad array of how-to materials that teach pain management life skills; created by a person with pain for people with pain;

- The ACPA is focused on enhancing quality of life and decreasing the sense of suffering through education and empowerment of the individual.

## 4. SERVICES OFFERED BY THE ACPA

- Peer support groups: Nearly 300 groups across the US and in several other countries; Writing Connection for those unable to attend groups; Growing Pains for young people with pain;
- Pain management tools: Pain management skills workbooks; family manual; relaxation tapes; videos; journals; coping calendar; more;
- Quarterly newsletter, *The Chronicle*;
- Web Site: www.theacpa.org provides basic pain management information, news, and links to other resources; about 700,000 hits/month (all-time high was 2,100,000).

## 5. RECENT SPECIAL PAIN AWARENESS PROJECTS

- Partners for Understanding Pain: more than 80 organizations working together to move pain to the top of the national health care agenda;
- Annual conferences;
- Distribution of Nurses' and Pharmacists' Pain Awareness Kits, posters and buttons;
- Support of the *Pain Care Act*;
- *Making Sense of Pain Relief*, an informational campaign to help people understand and make sound decisions about pain medications (September 2005);
- *Managing Your Risk*, an informational campaign helping people evaluate their risk factors for ulcers and better manage them (September 2005);
- *It Takes Nerve*, a neuropathic pain awareness campaign (2006);
- *Pain and the Emergency Department*, partnering with American College of Emergency Physicians (2007);
- *Growing Well with Pain*, working with farmers and ranchers to understand and manage persistent pain. (2008).

## 6. COORDINATES

**The American Chronic Pain Association (ACPA)**
PO Box 850
Rocklin, CA 95677
USA

Tel: 1-800-533-3231
Fax: (916) 632-3208
Email: ACPA@pacbell.net
Web site: www.theacpa.org/contact.asp

# CARE-RING VOICE
# **NETWORK**

**Samuelle Fillion,** Care-ring Voice Network, Montreal, Quebec, Canada

www.caringvoice.com

# *RÉSEAU ENTRE-AIDANTS*

NO CAREGIVER LEFT BEHIND

## 1. WHO ARE CAREGIVERS?

Caregivers are family members or friends who provide both short-term and ongoing care and assistance, without pay, to those in need of support due to physical, cognitive or mental health conditions. They are our parents, siblings, children of all ages, grandchildren, grandparents, friends and neighbours.

While caregiving includes immeasurable personal rewards, it may also involve physical, psychological, social and financial risks for the families and friends who assume this role.

**The Care-Ring Voice Network believes that taking care of caregivers is essential to the health of our communities.**

## 2. WHAT IS THE CARE-RING VOICE NETWORK?

The Care-ring Voice Network is managed by the Caregiver Support Centre of CSSS Cavendish (Montreal, Quebec). This free and confidential programme helps caregivers by giving them access to information and support through interactive tele-learning sessions. Caregivers connect by telephone, from home, at work or on the go, and benefit from workshops on caregiver-specific topics. Sessions are guided by professionals, generally last one hour, and include a period for questions and discussion.

**Founded in 2004, Care-ring Voice and has helped more than 12, 000 families and hosted over 225 tele-learning sessions. It is the largest tele-learning network in Canada supporting caregivers.**

## 3. WHY DO CAREGIVERS NEED THE CARE-RING VOICE NETWORK?

Of the 3 million caregivers in Canada, hundreds of thousands are overwhelmed by the daily tasks associated with caregiving. Caregivers frequently experience exhaustion, psychological and emotional distress, physical illness, isolation, loss of employment, and financial difficulties due to the strain of caregiving.

Through the programme, caregivers are able to obtain practical help and resources in a supportive environment by simply using the telephone. Care-ring Voice provides caregivers with the opportunity to seek help, break out of their isolation, and connect with others in similar situations. The flexibility, adaptability and facilitated access to the programme make it a wonderful alternative for caregivers who are unable to access information and support due to time, geographic, physical or psychological constraints.

## 4. THE NETWORK

Care-ring Voice has established a Canada-wide partnership network in order to enable other community and non-profit organizations to expand their services to include tele-learning. Care-ring Voice has brought together nearly two dozen network partners. These partners develop the educational content and host Care-ring Voice tele-learning sessions. Through the Care-ring Voice tele-learning model, these agencies are better able to meet the needs of their communities by providing simpler and more readily accessible assistance to families.

The current focus is on growing the Care-ring Voice Network in the province of Quebec. At the same time, a national partner recruitment initiative is underway.

## 5. CAREGIVERS PARTICIPATING IN TELE-LEARNING

The Care-ring Voice Network provides a telephone information line where caregivers can call to register for the tele-learning sessions as well as receive referrals to other services. Caregivers can also go online to the Care-ring Voice website at www.careringvoice.com to access the programme.

## 6. COORDINATES

Website: www.careringvoice.com
Care-ring Voice Info-line:
**1-866-396-2433**

# SUPPORT GROUPS FOR PEOPLE
# **WITH CHRONIC PAIN**

**Marie-Eve Richard,** Longueuil, Quebec, Canada, Member of the Montreal Chronic Pain Support Group (MCPSG),
Chronic Pain Association of Canada (CPAC), Montreal, Quebec, Canada
**Gary Blank**, Dollard-des-Ormeaux, Quebec, Canada
Group leader, Montreal Chronic Pain Support Group (MCPSG), Chronic Pain Association of Canada (CPAC),
Montreal, Quebec, Canada

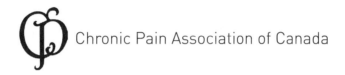

Chronic Pain Association of Canada

## 1. INTRODUCTION

Support groups for people dealing with a health issue first appeared at the end of the 20th century. This is a new form of mutual assistance that developed above all in the health field. This assistance is provided by peers, free of charge. At present, millions of people are members in various types of support groups throughout North America.

People who suffer from chronic pain are often poorly understood, alone and isolated, which is what makes support groups so important. Pain is a very solitary experience. Many myths, misunderstandings and false ideas are associated with pain. No one can feel or judge the suffering of another. Pain is a unique, emotional and physical experience that affects all aspects of the lives of those suffering from it.

## 2. NEEDS OF PEOPLE SUFFERING FROM CHRONIC PAIN

A support group responds to the numerous needs of people suffering from chronic pain: the need to know that they are not alone and that others are suffering like them, the need to share their helplessness, the need to be helped and supported, the need to know how others live their daily lives, the need to know their strategies for managing pain, the need to belong, and the need to know they can count on others who suffer like they do.

This relationship between people with a particular health issue who support one another is provided outside the health institutions. For the most part, these institutions do not yet offer support services for people dealing with chronic pain despite the fact that the need is so pressing and the outcomes so potentially positive for the patients. Moreover, few psychologists are trained to treat people suffering from chronic pain, most of them are not affiliated with a pain clinic, and their private services are often costly. This is why the existence of support groups for people suffering from chronic pain is so important; they need to know that they are not alone, and that help is available. The acceptance and the sharing of an experience that is common to all members of the group make interactions within the group much different than those that may exist with the family, friends and loved ones, for whom the daily repetition of the painful state may be tiresome and annoying.

## 3. MONTREAL CHRONIC PAIN SUPPORT GROUP

The Montreal chronic pain support group is a non-profit group administered by volunteers, affiliated with the Canadian Pain Association of Canada (CPAC, www.chronicpaincanada.com).

### THE PURPOSES OF THE SUPPORT GROUP

· To break isolation and provide moral support through discussion and through sharing experiences and information.
· To learn that it is possible to live with chronic pain on a daily basis.

### MEMBERS

The organizers and facilitators are volunteers who also suffer from chronic pain. The group is open to adults, both men and women, who have a common experience: chronic pain. The members range in age from 20 to 80. Most of them are Anglophones, but many are bilingual, and Francophones are most welcome. The majority can no longer work as a result of chronic pain. Some receive regular medical treatment at a pain clinic. Others have been placed on a waiting list for such a clinic. Still others have been discharged from the pain clinic, and are continuing their treatment with their family physician. Unfortunately, some don't receive medical treatment as a result of a shortage of resources in the Quebec health system.

### ACTIVITIES

The activities of the support group include a free two-hour monthly meeting and a few social activities organized throughout the year. Once a year, in November, as part of National Chronic Pain Awareness Week, the group organizes an event focused on the social changes that are needed in our society to deal with the epidemic of chronic pain, and its impact on the people suffering from it and on their loved ones and friends.

### GROUP MEETING PROCEDURE

At the beginning of each meeting, the group welcomes participants with compassion. The new participants introduce themselves and, if they feel comfortable doing so, talk about their condition. The members listen and respond to the questions and needs of the new participants. The participants talk to one another. Various topics may be discussed: frustration, irritability, depression, family problems, and problems with insurance or government claims. The facilitators provide new participants with information, resources and brochures, including one about My Tool Box Link: http://mytoolbox.mcgill.ca Announcements are made, followed by a break, and then the topic of the day is discussed. For example: How do you manage irritability and fatigue? Are you concerned about the upcoming holidays? What did you enjoy the most during the summer? What made you smile during the past month?

## 4. CONCLUSION

In the group, each individual is accepted and understood. Isolation is broken. Everyone is helped. Everyone supports one another in order to face their fears and regain their self-confidence. We share our experiences freely; we discuss strategies, exchange tips and suggestions to help manage our pain better on a daily basis. We learn to live with pain and take charge of it. There are changes that can be made in terms of our bodies, our thoughts, and our environment that can make chronic pain bearable. Finally, for several members, the group meeting is their only outing in the month other than medical appointments. Friendships are formed and several participants maintain contact outside the monthly meetings.

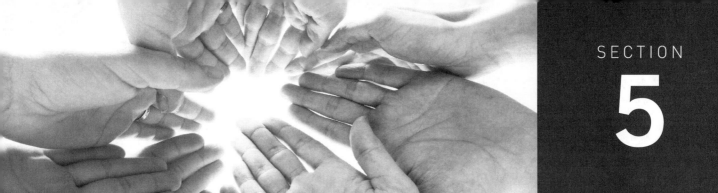

# PROFESSIONNAL ASSOCIATION
# FOR PAIN SPECIALISTS

# INTERNATIONAL ASSOCIATION
## FOR THE STUDY OF PAIN® (IASP®)

IASP®, Seattle, Washington, USA

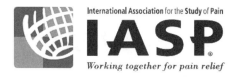

## 1. INTRODUCTION

The International Association for the Study of Pain® (IASP®) brings together scientists, clinicians, health care providers, and policymakers to stimulate and support the study of pain, and to translate that knowledge into improved pain relief worldwide. The IASP vision statement is:

Working together for pain relief throughout the world.

IASP currently has more than 6,500 members from over 120 countries, and more than 80 chapters around the world. Every two years, the association hosts the world's largest pain-related gathering: the World Congress on Pain®. The next such meeting — the 13th World Congress on Pain — took place in Montreal, Canada, from August 29 to September 2, 2010.

The following summary provides a brief overview of IASP. More details are available on the association's website: www.iasp-pain.org

## 2. HISTORY

IASP began in May 1973 with an interdisciplinary meeting that brought together scientists and clinicians from 13 countries. University of Washington anesthesiology professor Dr. John J. Bonica invited 350 participants to the gathering in Issaquah, Washington (near Seattle), in the United States. Recognizing the need for increased sharing of information on pain, the participants decided to form a multidisciplinary, professional organization dedicated to pain research and management, and they became founding members of IASP. They also agreed to launch a new journal, called PAIN®, to be edited by Dr. Patrick D. Wall. Initially a quarterly journal, PAIN published its first issue in March 1975. To this day, it remains the world's most widely read journal on the subject of pain.

At that first meeting, Dr. Bonica identified IASP's original mission: to provide an egalitarian, interdisciplinary, international forum to improve knowledge about pain, enhance the education of health care providers, and improve the care of patients. He drafted the association's bylaws, and IASP was officially incorporated one year later on May 9, 1974.

While other pain-related organizations have emerged in the 35 years since IASP was founded, it has kept its status as the world's largest and most respected pain-study organization.

## 3. MISSION

IASP is known for its global presence, the collaboration it fosters between researchers and health care professionals, and its shared mission. Its mission is to bring together scientists, clinicians, health care providers and policy makers to stimulate and support the study of pain, and to translate that knowledge into improved pain relief worldwide.

## 4. MEMBERSHIP

With members from many more than 120 countries and 80 chapters around the world — and growing — IASP is the leading professional forum for science, practice, and education in the field of pain. Membership in the association is open to all professionals involved in research, diagnosis, or treatment of pain. IASP currently has more than 6,500 members and 14 Special Interest Groups (SIGs) focusing on specific areas of pain research and treatment. Members may run for elected positions on the IASP Council (Board of Directors), and many also serve on its various Committees, Task Forces, and Working Groups.

## 5. SPECIAL INTEREST GROUPS

The dramatic growth in IASP's worldwide membership over the years reflects the rapid developments in pain research and treatment methods. As the knowledge base expands in the field of pain, it becomes increasingly important for researchers and health care professionals with specific interests in the pain field to have a forum to discuss certain pain topics in depth. IASP's Special Interest Groups (SIGs) offer participating members an opportunity to carry on intensive, in-depth discussions in key areas of pain, including acute pain, pain in childhood, pain in older persons, pain and movement, orofacial pain, pain in non-human species, and other topics. Membership in SIGs is open exclusively to members of IASP.

## 6. ORGANIZATIONAL STRUCTURE

IASP is a nonprofit organization governed by its elected Council, which is made up of a five-member Executive Committee (President, President-Elect, Immediate-Past President, Secretary, and Treasurer) and 12 Councilors. The current president is Dr G. F. Gebhart (USA), and the President-Elect is Dr. Eija Kalso (Finland).

## 7. PROGRAMS AND INITIATIVES

### GLOBAL YEAR AGAINST PAIN

Pain — particularly chronic pain — is a serious problem that affects people's quality of life. For this reason, IASP sponsors and promotes the **Global Year Against Pain**, a yearlong initiative designed to raise awareness of different aspects of pain worldwide.

As the average lifespan increases, the issues surrounding pain continue to grow. In developing countries in particular, while there are many serious diseases that can cause severe pain, there is often little or no pain relief available for those afflicted with such diseases. The control of pain has been a relatively neglected area of governmental concern in the past, despite the fact that cost-effective methods of pain control are available. Although few people die of pain, millions die in pain, and even more live in pain. Therefore, IASP's leaders and members believe it is essential to raise the profile of pain worldwide and promote the recognition of chronic pain as an important global health concern.

On the third Monday of each October, IASP launches a new Global Year Against Pain campaign theme focusing on a different aspect or type of pain, including the following:

- Pain Relief is a Human Right (2004–2005)
- Global Year Against Pain in Children (2005–2006)
- Global Year Against Pain in Older Persons (2006–2007)
- Global Year Against Pain in Women (2007–2008)
- Global Year Against Cancer Pain (2008–2009)
- Global Year Against Musculoskeletal Pain (2009–2010)
- Global Year Against Postoperative Pain (2010–2011)

For each of these 12-month campaigns, IASP makes resources and tools available to heighten awareness among health professionals, decision-makers, and the general population worldwide. These resources include a series of fact sheets that IASP translates into multiple languages and posts on its website. In addition, IASP's local chapters around the world organize meetings, symposia, media events, pain camps, and screening events for the public, and countless other activities designed to focus more attention on the specific area of pain highlighted by the **Global Year** campaign for that year.

More information about the **Global Year** initiative is available at: www.iasp-pain.org/GlobalYear

## GRANTS, AWARDS, AND FELLOWSHIPS

IASP offers its members an extensive selection of grants, awards, and fellowships to support investigators working in basic or clinical research, and to support pain education in developing countries. For example, its Collaborative Research Grants support collaborative, interdisciplinary research between two or more research groups located in different countries.

The association also offers the John J. Bonica Trainee Fellowship, which was named for its founder and supports training for pain pro-

fessionals in the early stages of their careers. In addition, the IASP Developing Countries Project funds educational support grants that address the need for improved education about pain, and its treatment in low-income countries. More details about IASP's various grants, awards, and fellowships — and the important work that they support — are available at: www.iasp-pain.org/Grants

# 8. EVENTS

## WORLD CONGRESS ON PAIN®

Every two years, IASP hosts the World Congress on Pain® in a different city around the world. The Congress is the world's largest pain-related gathering, attracting pain researchers and health care professionals from more than 100 countries. Like the IASP membership, Congress attendance is diverse and multidisciplinary, bringing basic and research scientists, physicians, nurses, dentists, surgeons, physical and occupational therapists, veterinarians, social scientists, and professionals from many other fields under one roof to share the latest pain research and treatment methods. While their backgrounds and areas of specialty vary, Congress delegates are all united in their desire to better understand and relieve pain.

Plenary sessions, workshops, poster sessions, and refresher courses comprise the Congress agenda, and attendees can receive continuing medical education credits for the sessions they attend. More information about the Congress, including previous and future Congresses, is available at: www.iasp-pain.org/WorldCongress

## IASP RESEARCH SYMPOSIA

IASP provides grants to fund symposia on specific pain-related topics of interest to both basic scientists and clinical researchers. The association sponsors one symposium every other year, alternating with the World Congress on Pain. Symposium topics have included:

- Opioid Sensitivity of Chronic Noncancer Pain (1998)
- Complex Regional Pain Syndrome: Current Research on Mechanisms and Diagnosis (2000)
- Spinal Cord Injury Pain: The Clinical Problem and Experimental Studies (2001)
- Hyperalgesias: Molecular Mechanisms and Clinical Implications (2003)
- Poststroke Pain: Retrospective and Prospective (2006)
- ICECAP Systematic Reviews and Meta-analyses in Pain: Lessons from the Past Leading to Pathways for the Future (2006)
- Fundamentals of Musculoskeletal Pain (2007)
- A Global Problem: Cancer Pain from the Laboratory to the Bedside (2009)

# 9. PUBLICATIONS AND RESOURCES

## JOURNAL PAIN®

*PAIN®* is the official journal of IASP, featuring 18 issues per year of original research on the nature, mechanisms, and treatment of pain. This peer-reviewed journal—consistently ranked as the premier and most-cited journal on the subject of pain—provides a forum for the dissemination of research in the basic and clinical sciences of multidisciplinary interest and is cited in Current Contents and Index Medicus. The current Editor-in-Chief of *PAIN* (2010) is Allan Basbaum.

## BOOKS FROM IASP PRESS®

IASP Press®, the publishing division of IASP, produces high-quality, reasonably priced books on pain. These publications, written and edited by leading experts in the field of pain, explore such topics as chronic pain, musculoskeletal pain, CRPS, neuropathic pain, psychological aspects of pain, spinal-cord injury pain, and many others.

While most books from IASP Press are intended primarily for pain researchers and clinicians, one of the publisher's most popular titles is a patient book, *Pain Management for Older Adults: A Self-Help Guide*. This book was designed specifically for mature adults seeking practical solutions for managing their chronic pain. Developed by husband-wife researchers Dr. Thomas Hadjistavropoulos and Dr. Heather D. Hadjistavropoulos of the University of Regina (Saskatchewan, Canada), and their contributors, this softcover, 200-page resource offers self-assessment checklists, progress charts, photos and illustrations, and simple instructions for managing persistent pain. The book — which was a 2009 Recipient of the *American Medical Writers Association Medical Book Awards, Honorable Mention* — has proved to be an essential "how to" resource not only for adults with chronic pain, but also for health care providers, physical therapists, fitness consultants, caregivers, and even family members of those in pain. More information is available at: www.iasp-pain.org/OlderAdults

## CLINICAL NEWSLETTER

IASP's clinical newsletter, *Pain: Clinical Updates*, aims to present information that is timely, relevant, and useful to clinicians seeking to practice rational and effective pain management. In 2008, for example, readers received seven timely issues (several related to that year's IASP Global Year against Pain in Women) on a range of topics, including:

· Gender, Pain, and the Brain;
· Screening for Opioid Abuse Potential;
· Gender Differences in Responses to Medication and Side Effects of Medication;
· Update on Fibromyalgia Syndrome.

## 10. CONTACT INFORMATION

Mailing/Postal Address:

International Association for the Study of Pain (IASP)
111 Queen Anne Avenue North, Suite 501
Seattle, WA 98109-4955
USA

Tel: +1 206-283-0311
Fax: +1 206-283-9403
Email: iaspdesk@iasp-pain.org
Website: www.iasp-pain.org

CANADIAN
# PAIN SOCIETY (CPS)

CPS: **Barry Sessle** MDS, PhD, Dsc(hc), FRSC, **Ellen Maracle-Benton**, Canada

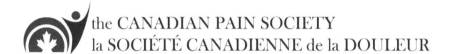

the CANADIAN PAIN SOCIETY
la SOCIÉTÉ CANADIENNE de la DOULEUR

## 1. PRESENTATION

The Canadian Pain Society (CPS) is a chapter of the International Association for the Study of Pain (IASP), and currently has approximately 850 members across Canada. The CPS includes as members a variety of people interested in pain:
- Physicians, dentists, nurses, physiotherapists, psychologists, and other clinicians involved with management of pain;
- Scientists involved in the design of improved methods of pain management and the identification of basic mechanisms of pain and analgesia;
- Professionals involved in education, training, and publication of new information in the field of pain;
- Lay persons with an interest in the field of pain.

## 2. MISSION

The aims of the Canadian Pain Society are:
- To foster and encourage research on pain mechanisms and pain syndromes and to help improve the management of patients with acute and chronic pain by bringing together the basic scientists and health professionals of various disciplines and backgrounds who have an interest in pain research and management;
- To promote education and training in the field of pain;
- To promote and facilitate the dissemination of new information in the field of pain;
- To promote and sponsor regional scientific and educational meetings;
- To encourage the adoption of a uniform classification, nomenclature, and definition regarding pain and pain syndromes;
- To encourage the development of local, regional, and possibly even national and international data banks, and to encourage the development of a uniform records system, with respect to information relating to pain mechanisms, syndromes, and management;
- To inform the general public of the results and implications of current research in the area of pain;
- To advise national, regional, and local agencies and institutions on standards relating to the use of drugs, appliances, and other procedures in the therapy of pain;
- To engage in such other activities as may be incidental to or in furtherance of the aforementioned purposes.
- The Canadian Pain Society became an incorporated entity in 2009 and is currently expanding its mandate to further promote pain awareness, treatments and solutions for pain-related issues across Canada.

## 3. COORDINATES

Canadian Pain Society Office
1143 Wentworth Street West
Suite 202
Oshawa, ON L1J 8P7
CANADA
Tel: 905-404-9545
Fax: 905-404-3727
Website: www.canadianpainsociety.ca

# MORRIS' STORY

**Morris K.**, Montreal, Quebec, Canada

(See other testimonials, pages 100, 246, 300, 310 and 382.)

I will be forever grateful to the doctors and staff that helped me at the pain clinic.
**Pain doctors, thank you for your dedication!**
**You do make a difference!**

# SOCIÉTÉ QUÉBÉCOISE DE LA
## DOULEUR (SQD)
### QUEBEC PAIN SOCIETY

**Roderick Finlayson** MD, FRCPC, anaesthesiologist, Montreal, Quebec, Canada
President, Société québécoise de la douleur

# 53

When this chapter was written, the author was president of the SQD. Christian Cloutier, BSc, MD, FRSC was the SQD president when this book was published.

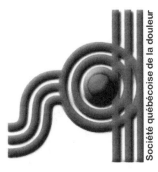

## 1. HISTORY OF THE SOCIÉTÉ QUÉBÉCOISE DE LA DOULEUR (SQD)

In 1990, Mr. Doucet, of the Astra company, asked Dr. Yves Veillette, an anaesthesiologist at the Hôpital Maisonneuve Rosemont, if he was interested in re-creating the «Pain Club» that had existed in Montreal in the 1980s. It had a budget of approximately $3,000 per year.

Instead, Dr. Veillette proposed that they create a Quebec pain society since he knew doctors specializing in pain in both Quebec City and Montreal. In fact, Dr. Veillette had a degree in medicine from Université Laval and had done part of his specialization in Quebec City. He knew Dr. Truchon, Dr. Beauvais, Dr. St-Pierre, Dr. Dolbec, Dr. Montreuil, Dr. Parent, and Dr. Buissières of Quebec City, as well as Dr. Laperrière of Trois-Rivières since he was now working in Montreal. Moreover, he also knew Dr. Catchlove, Dr. Germain, Dr. Blaise and Dr. Fugère.

At the time, they wanted a name that was not going to define a specific group but rather the specific work involved in the treatment of pain. As a result, they chose the name the *Association des algologistes du Québec* (Quebec association of algologists). According to the charter, the association's goals were to bring together the various stakeholders working in the field of pain in Quebec, to promote multidisciplinarity, to educate, by means of an annual conference, to train new experts and, finally, to gain recognition for multidisciplinary centres.

**ALGO:** pain (Greek)
**LOGY:** study (Greek)

Founded in 1993, the association started recruiting anaesthesiologists, psychologists and physical therapists interested in pain. A quarterly letter appeared three years later under the direction of Dr. Pierre Dolbec. The name never really caught on and was quickly connected to the world of anaesthesiologists. It was replaced by the *Société québécoise de la douleur (SQD)* in April 2000, which better reflects the multidisciplinary nature of the therapeutic approach.

The *SQD* has maintained its mission to promote the treatment of chronic pain in Quebec and, in recent years, the members of its executive have been the principal stakeholders behind the Quebec advisory committee on chronic pain and the resulting expert centre projects. The annual conference also remains an important event in the continuous training activities conducted in Quebec.

## 2. CONTACT INFORMATION

Société québécoise de la douleur
7400, Les Galeries d'Anjou boul., suite 410
Anjou, Quebec (Canada) H1M 3M2
Telephone: 514 355-8001
Fax: 514 355-4159
Email: sqd@spg.qc.ca
Website: www.sqd.ca

## THERE IS A BRIGHT SPOT SOMEWHERE

**Terry Bremner,** Stillwater Lake, Nova Scotia, Canada
National Support Group Coordinator, Chronic Pain Association of Canada (CPAC),
President, Action Atlantic, Pain support group leader, Chronic Pain Association of Canada (CPAC)

(See other testimonial, page 110.)

There is always a bright spot somewhere. You just have to find it.

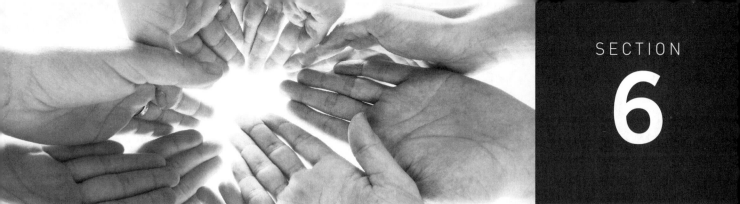

# PAIN CLINICS AND PHYSICAL
# REHABILITATION AND ADAPTATION CENTRES

# THE SERVICES OF THE STE. ANNE'S HOSPITAL
# PAIN MANAGEMENT CLINIC, VETERANS' AFFAIRS CANADA (VAC)

## 54

**Monique Allard** RN, BSc Nursing, Nurse coordinator, Ste. Anne's Hospital Pain Management Clinic,
Ste-Anne-de-Bellevue, Quebec, Canada
Read by Simon Laliberté, PhD, psychologist, Ste. Anne's Hospital Pain Management Clinic,
Ste-Anne-de-Bellevue, Quebec, Canada

Since 2005, Ste. Anne's Hospital has offered specialized pain management services to veterans of all ages. Following an analysis of the needs of our clientele, several initiatives were implemented. Over the years, the services offered have evolved and are now offered under the banner of the Pain Management Clinic (PMC), as we know it today.

## 1. INTRODUCTION

Pain is part of the human experience and, more specifically, the experience of illness. The causes of pain are numerous, its manifestations are varied and the effects of pain are often devastating for the individual, both physically and psychologically. According to the International Association for the Study of Pain (IASP 1979), pain is defined as "an unpleasant sensory and emotional experience associated with actual or potential tissue damage, or described in terms of such damage." Chronic pain is defined in terms of its persistence beyond the usual amount of time required for an injury to heal (3-6 months).

Up to 20% of Canadian men and 24% of Canadian women live with chronic pain. Chronic pain is the principal reason for medical consultations and more than 50 million people in the United States suffer from it. More than $100 billion in health care services annually is spent on chronic pain each year[1]. For certain more vulnerable groups these figures are even higher. Elderly people and people suffering from operational stress injuries (OSI) are often more vulnerable to pain.

### THE ELDERLY PERSON AND PAIN

Since painful medical conditions become more concentrated as a result of aging, a very large number of elderly people have to deal with the difficulties of chronic pain. The under-treatment of this pain remains a constant concern, particularly with respect to this more vulnerable population. According to certain statistics, more than 50 % of this population does not benefit from an optimum quality of life as a result of pain[1]. According to Gloth (2004), 50% to 80% of residents living in a long-term care setting apparently experience pain, compared to 25% to 40% of the elderly people living in the community. (See **Chapter 13**.)

### PAIN AND MENTAL HEALTH

Several studies have demonstrated that in certain people there is a link, called a comorbidity, between presence of chronic pain and mental health issues. The presence of unrelieved chronic pain has a major impact on the quality of life of these people and contributes to their distress and their suffering in a significant manner.

### VETERANS COPING WITH PAIN

According to Poundja et al (2006), 86.9% of the 130 veterans treated at the National Centre for Operational Stress Injuries (NCOSI) of Ste. Anne's Hospital (Sainte-Anne-de-Bellevue, Quebec, Canada) indicated that they suffer significant pain. The mutual maintenance of a post-traumatic stress syndrome (PTSS) and chronic pain is a phenomenon that has not been studied extensively to date, particularly in a population of veterans.

## 2. SERVICES PROVIDED AT STE. ANNE'S HOSPITAL

At Ste. Anne's Hospital, our mission is to offer veterans and our other clients a range of programmes and a continuum of high quality care and services while respecting their dignity and their autonomy. These leading-edge programmes meet both their needs and those of their families. The hospital takes veterans in for long-term or respite care. The **Day centre** offers support services to those still living in the community. **The National Centre for Operational Stress Injuries** offers mental health and short-term hospitalization services for veterans and other clients.

Ste. Anne's Hospital offers services to a varied clientele requiring chronic pain care. As we wish to improve our services on an ongoing basis and offer quality care to our particular clientele, several initiatives have been implanted for managing pain. Since October 2000, we have implemented a policy and a specific procedure for the relief of pain. Moreover, we have created tools to evaluate pain, we have set up an advisory committee on pain relief and we use the concept of pain as a fifth vital sign.

Despite these initiatives, a study of the needs of the clientele of the **Ste. Anne's Operational Stress Injury Clinic** and those of our long-term patients, has indicated that they require better support in the management and relief of pain. Considering the complexity of their health problems, the links with certain comorbidities such as anxiety, depression and post-traumatic stress syndrome (PTSS), the Ste. Anne's Hospital established the **Pain Management Clinic** (PMC) in 2005, in order to take all of these factors into consideration, and attempt to treat them together.

## 3. THE PAIN MANAGEMENT CLINIC

### OUR MISSION

The mission of the **Pain Management Clinic** (PMC) is to maximize the relief of the chronic pain and suffering of its clients. **The Clinic's mission is based on the hospital's organizational conviction that pain relief is a legitimate therapeutic objective, essential for the quality of life of veterans.**

### OUR APPROACH

The interdisciplinary team of the **Pain Management Clinic** prefers a biopsychosocial approach in which the client manages his pain and the client is supported by the team in this process. We believe that respect for the individual's choices, his involvement in the process, the support he receives from the interdisciplinary team and his/her loved ones are important aspects of the treatment process.

The team also believes that pain relief requires a **personalized treatment plan** (PTP) integrating all aspects of pain:
- physical;
- psychological;
- social and spiritual.

This overall vision of the individual and his/her health serves, in our opinion, to optimize the relief of pain and lead to an improvement in the quality of life of these individuals dealing with persistent pain.

### OUR OBJECTIVES

Our objectives are as follows:
- to reduce the intensity of pain and suffering;
- to improve the client's quality of life;
- to involve the client and his/her loved ones in the development and application of the treatment plan.

### OUR SPECIFIC OBJECTIVES

Our specific objectives are as follows:
- to optimize the client's functional capacities;
- to reduce the emotional distress and the social isolation related to the pain;
- to provide education to the client and his/her loved ones concerning pain management;
- to increase the client's ability to handle the management of his/her pain after leaving the clinic.

# 4. CLIENTELE SERVED BY STE. ANNE'S HOSPITAL PAIN MANAGEMENT CLINIC

## INTERNAL CLIENTELE AND REFERRAL PROCESS

The **Pain Management Clinic** offers services to the residents of the Ste. Anne's Hospital, the clients of the **Liaison Centre**, the **veterans in the network of operational stress injury clinics**, the eligible clients of the **VAC district offices** and the active service people in the process of being discharged who experience chronic pain (lasting more than three months) which is not relieved by usual treatments.

The referral process for the PMC varies according to the type of client. The internal resource person is still the attending physician in the care unit. For people outside the Ste. Anne's Hospital, such as clients of the **district offices**, the sector case advisor/manager is the resource person. Members of the **Canadian Forces** (CF) must go through their case manager or other resource people.

developed. It is implemented in cooperation with our partners. There are various treatments that may be offered either in the PMC or in the client's community, such as:

- Psychiatry treatment;
- Physiotherapy treatment (physical activation, manual traction);
- Osteopathy;
- Information about his/her diagnosis, good living habits, medication management, etc.;
- Brief therapy with the psychologist (management of pain, pacing,

## EXTERNAL CLIENTELE AND REFERRAL PROCESS

For external clients, we ask:
- For a request from the physician or other specialist treating the client;
- That the request be handled first by the district office or by the CF case manager;
- For a registration form to be completed;
- For the pertinent medical file;
- Compliance with the eligibility criteria.

Once an individual is admitted to the PMC, an appointment is made for an evaluation day. The individual is on hand for the day to meet with the various professionals. The schedule for the day is as follows:

After the client is evaluated, the personalized treatment plan is

relaxation, mental imaging);
- Other.

Once the condition is stabilized, and the patient is familiar with the pain management tools and has the resources needed in his/her community to ensure follow-up, if necessary, the patient can be discharged from the PMC.

# 5. CONCLUSION

As we can observe, chronic pain is widespread in the general public. It can have a major impact on several spheres of the life of the individual who suffers from chronic pain, on society and the health system. Its duration and complexity as well as the factors that affect it or maintain it must, therefore, be taken into consideration during the treatment. It should be noted that chronic pain cannot usually be "cured". At this point in time, we speak more of managing pain through a multidimensional approach, through the involvement of the various health professionals and by treating the comorbidity at the same time as the chronic pain.

Veterans live with several comorbidities that must be treated at the same time, which makes the treatment more complex. Very often, these veterans, who have operational stress disorders, suffer intense physical pains, experience significant emotional distress and have to cope with

a greater level of interference and disability in daily life. Since the incidence of PTSS in the case of the people who are referred for pain treatment varies between 20% and 34%, which is significantly higher than in the general population (where it is 9% during the course of a life), particular attention must be paid to this population and professionals must intervene as quickly as possible.

Finally, more than 80% of the veterans questioned live with chronic pain that varies in intensity. Therefore, the PMC meets the needs of this specific clientele and makes an active contribution to the high quality of care. The Ste. Anne's Hospital Pain Management Clinic represents an innovation in the field of chronic pain and mental health and is constantly evolving.

# REFERENCES

1. Gloth M. Pain, Pain, Everywhere… Almost, In: Handbook of pain relief in older adults: an evidence-based approach. Édité par F. Michael Gloth III MD FACP. Publié par Humana Press, Totowa, NJ, É.-U., 2004, 264 pp.

2. Poundja J., D. Fikretoglu, A. Brunet. Co-occurrence of PTSD symptoms and pain : is depression a mediator? Journal of Traumatic Stress, 2006; 19 (5): 747-751.

3. Sharp Timothy. The prevalence of post traumatic stress disorder in chronic pain patients. Current Pain and Headache Reports, 2004; 8: 111-115.

4. Asmondsun G., S. Coons Taylor, J. Katz, PTSD and the experience of pain : research and clinical implications of shared vulnerability and mutual maintenance models. Can J Psychiatry, Dec. 2002; 47(10): 930-937.

5. Otis J. D., T. M. Keane, R. D. Kerns. An examination of the relationship between chronic pain and Post-traumatic Stress Disorder. Journal of Rehabilitation Research & Development, 2003; 40(5): 397-405.

6. Guay, S. et A. Marchand, Les troubles liés aux évènements traumatiques — Dépistage, évaluation et traitements, Montréal, PUM, 2006, p. 42.

# TESTIMONIAL

André Léonelli, for Ste. Anne's Hospital Pain Management Clinic, Ste-Anne-de-Bellevue, Quebec, Canada

My name is André Léonelli. I began my military career with the Canadian Armed Forces in September 1975 as a combat soldier with the 3rd battalion of the Royal 22nd Regiment at Valcartier (Quebec, Canada). I then joined the 1st commando of the Canadian Airborne Regiment in 1976 in Edmonton (Alberta, Canada), after which I returned to Valcartier in 1978, still as part of the 3rd battalion of the Royal 22nd Regiment.

I was deployed to Cyprus (Europe) in 1979, as part of the UN peace-keeping force. In 1980, I had to transfer to a trade in the aviation sector as a result of the deterioration of my physical condition. I was already suffering from chronic pain at the time. Later, in 1989, I was deployed to Sinai as part of Squadron 420 ETAH (Valcartier) for the Multinational Force and Observers, as a security system technician. Then, in 1992, I was deployed to Nairobi (Africa) with troops from the Canadian Forces base at Trenton (Ontario, Canada) to provide humanitarian aid. I left the regular Canadian Forces in 1994, to join the Reserve Forces in 1995, at the Saint-Hubert base (Quebec, Canada), where I remained until June 2005.

I am being treated for a chronic pain condition at Ste. Anne's Hospital Pain Management Clinic. The clinic has helped me not only learn to live with my pain, but also to control it while maintaining the objective to improve my quality of life significantly. The personalized approach that prevails there enables us to have a better relationship with the care providers and to make the most of effective follow-up. As a result of the cooperation, willingness to listen and humanity of the Clinic personnel, we feel like real people and not just simple numbers. The clinic's health care team and the atmosphere that prevails there enhance and accelerate the recovery of the people treated there. I was privileged to benefit from the quality service provided by the St. Anne Hospital. Thanks to the entire health care team!

**St. Anne Hospital**
305 des Anciens-Combattants boul.
Sainte-Anne-de-Bellevue (Quebec) H9X 1Y9 (Canada)
Tel.: (514) 457-3440
Toll-free: 1 800 361-9287
Email: steanne@vac-acc.gc.ca

# CHRONIC PAIN
# AND REHABILITATION
## (CONSTANCE-LETHBRIDGE REHABILITATION CENTER)

## 55

**Geneviève Côté-Leblanc** OT, Program manager
**Geneviève Lefebvre**, Director of rehabilitation programs
**Martine Leroux** OT
Constance Lethbridge Rehabilitation Centre (CLRC), Montreal, Quebec, Canada

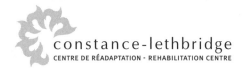

constance-lethbridge
CENTRE DE RÉADAPTATION - REHABILITATION CENTRE

Chronic pain leads to both physical and psychosocial disabilities. As a result, the individual's life habits and social roles, at home, at school, in the community and at work, are affected considerably.

The **Constance-Lethbridge Rehabilitation Centre (CLRC)** offers specialized and ultra-specialized rehabilitation services that help clients achieve greater autonomy and participate in community life to the fullest extent possible

The CLRC chronic pain management program is intended for clients who experience chronic pain of various origins such as neurological, arthritic and musculoskeletal affections. This programme is composed of two occupational therapists, one physiotherapist, two psychologists, one social worker, a special care counsellor and a physical educator.

**The interventions of the chronic pain management program are intended to allow the return to all life habits while focusing on interventions that specifically target chronicity risk factors. Specifically, the objectives are as follows:**

- Reduction in fear of movement;
- Self-management of pain;
- Reduction of pain behaviours and modification of cognitions;
- Management of stress, emotions, mood and sleep;
- Strategies for energy conservation, healthy posture and bodily mechanics;
- Improvement of physical and functional capacities;
- Reduction of deconditioning syndrome;
- Improvement in eating habits;
- Education about chronic pain, the importance of good physical and psychological condition, in addition to a progressive reactivation process and using the pain management strategy appropriately;
- Integration of knowledge acquired in the clinical setting as well as in the community;
- Planning and supervision of a gradual return to work.

Our specialized or ultra-specialized services are offered individually or in groups. The specialized services are offered to clients who have experienced disruption of several life habits as a result of their chronic pain syndrome. The ultra-specialized services are offered to clients who, in addition to their pain syndrome, have also experienced conditions associated with drug abuse, mental health issues (depression, anxiety, post-traumatic stress syndrome, etc.) or associated medical conditions that can affect their prognosis. The interventions are also more intense and involve the contributions of all of the program's therapists .

The duration of the interventions is adjusted in keeping with the client's needs individually (for example, two intensive weeks if he/she lives in a distant region, two days/week if the client is working, etc.). For group interventions, the maximum duration is 14 weeks (alternating activities at the centre and activities in the community and/or at work). This structure has the advantage of ensuring the transfer of knowledge and generalization of the progress made. Moreover, we offer re-assessment sessions, as well as meetings with family members and significant others.

The CLRC has been designated by the *Quebec Ministère de la Santé et des Services sociaux* (Canada) to offer services to Anglophones as well as the cultural communities. Thus, our services are offered in French and English and we call on interpreters as needed. The CLRC is a member of the McGill RUIS (*Réseau universitaire intégré de santé*) and is currently taking part in the development of a continuum of services for chronic pain. This continuum is intended to promote the continuity of services and ensure that the rehabilitation services are offered at the opportune time.

The Health and Social Services Ministry (*MSSS*) has recently designated (2010) the MUHC (McGill University Health Center) and the CLRC as centres of expertise in chronic pain.

# MORRIS' STORY

**Morris K.,** Montreal, Quebec, Canada

(See other testimonials, pages 100, 246, 300, 310 and 372.)

*Morris survived a plane crash, and recuperated from a broken jaw and ankle, as well as fractures to the spine.*

At a rehabilitation centre in Montreal, Quebec, Canada, I was seen by a doctor, psychologist and physiotherapist, each who interviewed me separately to assess my needs. Some weeks later, I was on their waiting list and finally I was accepted into their program.

I went through a series of seminars showing aids and ways to help bodies that work only partially. I was taught all sorts of things such as energy conservation strategies, pain and nutrition, joint protection, washing and drying my clothes, using the broom, dusting, cleaning and how to lift things, just to name a few of the ordinary everyday things that we encounter or must do. I realized how many of these techniques I had already developed on my own years ago. It is amazing what we can devise on our own when it's a matter of survival.

Soon I was introduced to their warm water therapy pool and to my water physiotherapist. The pool is kept at 94°F to 96°F. It was incredible, and felt so good that I never wanted to leave the water. The physiotherapist showed me a group of exercises, and was always there to answer questions. It was a group session. Everyone had a different problem. She kept an eye on everyone, and added new exercises for individuals according to how each individual was progressing. My body felt so good while I was in the water. It was actually traumatic for me when I was discharged.

My plan was to get back to walking 30 minutes on the treadmill. My hips slowed me down from my routine speed of 3.6 mph two years ago. I have built back up to 30 minutes walking on the treadmill, but at 3.0 mph. I will add to the speed when my body tells me to. I also do 30 minutes on the bicycle and 55 minutes in an aqua fitness group. The instructor shows us what she wants us to do and I adapt all exercises to suit what I think I can safely do, without annoying my body. It is very tricky as there are so many switches from one exercise to another. I do not have the luxury of time to sit and think about it. There are times that I come away in pain, but that is the price that was known in advance. At these times, I put my thinking cap on, and try to figure out which movement was causing the pain. I then alter the culprit, and try again. **The only alternative is to be dormant and that is not acceptable.**

# THE CHRONIC PAIN ADAPTATION CLINIC
## OF THE LUCIE-BRUNEAU
## READAPTATION CENTRE (CRLB)

## 56

**Jean-Marc Miller** MPs, psychologist, Lucie Bruneau Rehabilitation Centre (LBRC), Montreal, Quebec, Canada

www.luciebruneau.qc.ca (in French only)

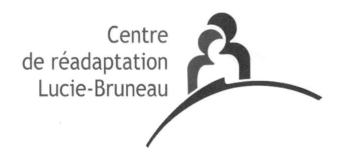

## HISTORY OF THE CENTRE DE RÉADAPTATION LUCIE-BRUNEAU

The history of the *Lucie-Bruneau Rehabilitation Centre (LBRC)* is based on the vision and determination of Lucie Bruneau, a woman who was ahead of her time. When she founded the *Association catholique de l'aide aux infirmes* in 1926, Ms. Bruneau demanded the right to live a full and complete life for people with physical limitations, in terms of work, leisure activities and housing. Throughout her life, Ms. Bruneau did everything in her power to improve the quality of life of these people, going so far as to petition the government for a vacant piece of land where she could build a large residence for people with physical problems.

Today, the *LBRC* offers personalized, specialized, and super-specialized services in adaptation/rehabilitation, social and professional integration to people with motor or neurological problems, integration support, assistance and coaching services for families and significant others, along with alternative housing resources all in order to enable them to take part in society and maximize their quality of life.

## CHRONIC PAIN ADAPTATION CLINIC

Despite progress made in terms of research, medicine does not always manage to completely eradicate pain following an accident or an illness. This ongoing pain can have a major impact on the social, education or professional integration of the individual while also affecting his/her ability to take part in activities. In order to respond to this problem, the *LBRC* developed expertise over the years in providing interdisciplinary support for people who suffer chronic pain.

The *LBRC* chronic pain adaptation clinic is part of a consortium of facilities affiliated with the *Université de Montréal* (Quebec, Canada). The professionals at this clinic teach users, whose pain is not associated with cancer but is persistent, how to integrate strategies to improve their quality of life.

## THE VICIOUS CIRCLE OF PAIN

It is known that intractable and persistent pain is often accompanied by other problems, such as depression, concerns about the future, insomnia, inadequate use of medication, fear of moving or exacerbating one's condition, and interpersonal difficulties resulting from increased irritability. Since they are all interrelated, all of the problems associated with chronic pain are commonly referred to as the **vicious circle of pain.** (See next page.)

Through individual and group interventions, the clinicians at the *LBRC* chronic pain adaptation clinic help individuals identify the best strategies for dealing with the harmful aspects of their pain. Since the various problems that make up the vicious circle of pain are interrelated, working on one aspect could well result in benefits on other levels. An individual who takes part in this programme must, as a result, learn how to change certain habits and occasionally learn to look at life differently in order to improve his/her quality of life. This task is not always easy, but with a team of physicians, psychologists, physiotherapists, kinesiologists, occupational therapists and social workers, who work closely and involve the participant in all decisions that concern him/her, the person who suffers chronic pain can learn, with good tools, not to allow the pain to become overwhelming.

Anyone who wants to be admitted to the *LBRC* Chronic Pain Adaptation Clinic must provide a medical referral confirming that he/she has been suffering from on-going pain for at least six months, that an in-depth medical investigation has been made, and that medical treatment is no longer able to provide relief.

Before starting the programme, the individual will also be evaluated in order to make sure that he/she is sufficiently motivated to change certain aspects of his/her way of functioning, and integrate appropriate strategies for self-managing his/her condition.

# THE VICIOUS CIRCLE OF PAIN

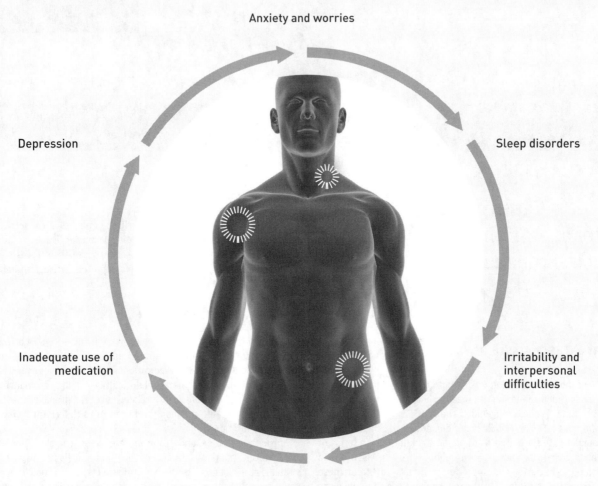

Anxiety and worries

Sleep disorders

Depression

Irritability and
interpersonal
difficulties

Inadequate use of
medication

Inactivity and fear
of movement

# PHYSICAL REHABILITATION AND CHRONIC PAIN
## INSTITUT DE RÉADAPTATION EN DÉFICIENCE PHYSIQUE DE QUÉBEC (IRDPQ)

**Marie-Josée Gobeil** OT, Quebec City, Quebec, Canada
Institut de réadaptation en déficience physique de Québec, Quebec, Canada

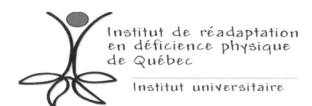

## 57

The *Institut de réadaptation en déficience physique de Québec (IRDPQ)* is a public facility classified as a physical disability rehabilitation centre in keeping with the *Act respecting health* services and social services. It offers adaptation, rehabilitation and social integration services to people of all ages who experience handicaps as a result of their hearing, motor, visual, speech and language disabilities, as well as coaching and support for significant others. The institution serves the people in the region of Quebec (03) and provides highly specialized, national or back-up services for other regions under agreements with regional rehabilitation facilities.

The *Institut de réadaptation en déficience physique* is affiliated with *Université Laval* (Quebec city, Quebec, Canada). Since 1995, it has been designated as a university institution – the only one operating in the field of physical disability rehabilitation in Quebec – in keeping with the *Act respecting health services and social services*. It is renowned for its leading edge experts, its clinical organization through programmes and its evaluation, teaching, training and research activities.

Since 1989, the institution has provided a rehabilitation programme specifically dedicated to clients suffering with chronic pain. Originally intended for workers dealing with chronic back pain, the programming and services have gradually grown to include a larger clientele dealing with the functional impacts of persistent pain.

For more details about the services available and to find out how to contact us, please visit the institution's web site: www.irdpq.qc.ca (in French only).

## FOCUSING ON YOU

Helen Small, BA, BEd, St. Catharines, Ontario, Canada

(See testimonial, page 340. See Chapter 41, page 333 and Chapter 46, page 353.)

You are the CEO of your own life and, even though doctors are medical experts, you have the power to make decisions for yourself given the medical input that you need. Your doctor is your partner in your medical care. Make informed choices in your medical care by educating yourself on the options. To self-manage an illness you need to take charge, be proactive and make informed choices.

# CHRONIC PAIN SERVICES AT THE JEWISH REHABILITATION **HOSPITAL (JRH)**

Patricia Piché OT, PÉDIP* Coordinator, Jewish Rehabilitation Hospital (JRH), Laval, Quebec, Canada

*\*PÉDIP: Programme d'évaluation, de développement et d'intégration professionnelle (Evaluation, development and professional integration programme)*

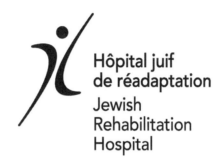

Hôpital juif
de réadaptation
Jewish
Rehabilitation
Hospital

## 1. THE JEWISH REHABILITATION HOSPITAL (JRH)

The Jewish Rehabilitation Hospital (JRH) is a specialized hospital dedicated to rehabilitation. It is also the regional centre for adult and paediatric clients with physical disabilities in Laval. It offers clients with incapacities resulting from physical health problems and/or physical disabilities, specialized intensive functional rehabilitation, socio-professional, socio-residential and community services, as well as housing in non-institutional residences and technical aid services. These services focus on the recovery of optimal independence, as well as the social reintegration of clients into their communities.

When faced with an injury to their physical integrity, clients regularly have to deal with pain that can interfere with the rehabilitation process. This pain must be taken into consideration quickly so as to limit the impacts. As a result, interdisciplinary teams have developed expertise in addressing these problems in their interventions. The actions taken can be preventive or curative depending upon the clientele served in the facility's various programmes.

However, when pain becomes the primary cause limiting a client's return to previous activities, a programme of adapted and specific interventions must be implemented. In order to respond to the needs of individuals living with such a situation, the JRH recently developed services under the banner of the Activation programme. The JRH also offers services to people suffering from fibromyalgia through group follow-up as part of the ambulatory services programme.

## 2. ACTIVATION PROGRAMME

The clinicians assess the barriers that prevent a return to previous activities, including work, taking into account not only the main injury but the person as a whole and his/her environment. The team prefers an interdisciplinary approach that focuses on the individual.

**Our intervention goals are to:**

· improve physical condition;
· restore basic routines (sleep, diet, etc.);
· optimize pain and energy management;
· increase participation in various activities (including work);
· reduce kinesiophobia;
· reduce catastrophic thoughts;
· improve the feeling of self-efficacy;
· reduce the perception of physical incapacity;
· promote self-awareness and more optimal regulation of thoughts, emotions and behaviours so as to facilitate the management of pain and energy.

The team prefers an active pain management approach in which the client plays the central role. Methods of symptoms management and problem solving techniques are taught and tested in order to enable the client to regain control over his/her pain problem. The various professionals guide the individual in a search for solutions that will have an impact on his/her involvement in various daily activities (preparing meals, sleep, and housekeeping). The support offered throughout the process enables the individuals to address their fears and beliefs with respect to persistent pain and a return to regular activitiess, including work. Cognitive and behavioural approaches are given priority in order to help the individual learn to plan and manage his/her activities so as to ensure maximum control and satisfaction despite the pain. The means and duration of the interventions vary according to programme and clientele.

## FIBROMYALGIA PROGRAMME

The purpose of this programme is to provide education to clients, promote the integration of healthy living habits and help clients develop strategies for managing their disease.

The interdisciplinary team offers programme activities to groups of ten, over a period of ten weeks.

For more information about our services and the means for accessing them, please visit the JRH web site at www.hjr-jrh.qc.ca